D0214625

Canola and Rapeseed

Production, Processing, Food Quality, and Nutrition

AOCS Mission Statement

To be a global forum to promote the exchange of ideas, information, and experience, to enhance personal excellence, and to provide high standards of quality among those with a professional interest in the science and technology of fats, oils, surfactants, and related materials.

Canola and Rapeseed

Production, Processing, Food Quality, and Nutrition

Edited by **Usha Thiyam-Holländer**
N. A. Michael Eskin • Bertrand Matthäus

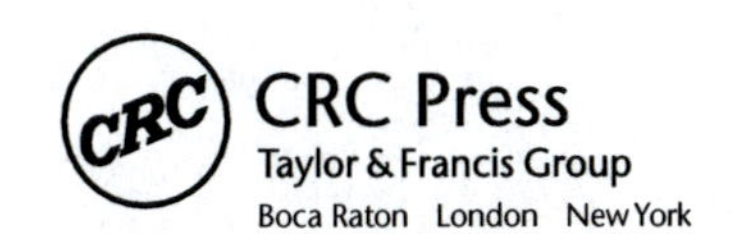

CRC Press is an imprint of the
Taylor & Francis Group, an **informa** business

CRC Press
Taylor & Francis Group
6000 Broken Sound Parkway NW, Suite 300
Boca Raton, FL 33487-2742

Printed in the United States of America on acid-free paper
Version Date: 20121011

International Standard Book Number: 978-1-4665-1386-0 (Hardback)

Visit the Taylor & Francis Web site at
http://www.taylorandfrancis.com

and the CRC Press Web site at
http://www.crcpress.com

Contents

Preface....vii
Editors....ix
Contributors....xi

Chapter 1 Canola Research: Historical and Recent Aspects....1
N.A. Michael Eskin

Chapter 2 An Update on Characterization and Bioactivities of Sinapic Acid Derivatives....21
Ayyappan Appukuttan Aachary and Usha Thiyam-Holländer

Chapter 3 Valuable Vinylphenols from Rapeseed and Canola: Decarboxylative Pathways....39
Usha Thiyam-Holländer, Narsireddy Meda, K. Misra and Ahindra Nag

Chapter 4 Processing of Canola Proteins: A Review....59
L. Xu and Levente L. Diosady

Chapter 5 Future of Omega-9 Oils....79
Asim Syed

Chapter 6 Modification of Seed Oil Formation in *Brassica* Oilseed Species....101
Crystal L. Snyder and Randall J. Weselake

Chapter 7 Measurement of Oil Content by Rapid Analytical Techniques....125
Véronique J. Barthet

Chapter 8 The Potential for Ultrasound and Supercritical Fluid Extraction for Value-Added Processing of Canola....145
Curtis B. Rempel and M.G. Scanlon

Chapter 9 Processing of Virgin Canola Oils....171
Bertrand Matthäus

Chapter 10 Rapeseed Proteins: Recent Results on Extraction and Application 187

Frank Pudel

Chapter 11 Frying Stability of High-Oleic, Low-Linolenic Canola Oils 203

Bertrand Matthäus

Chapter 12 Biodiesel from Mustard Oil........ 217

Titipong Issariyakul and Ajay K. Dalai

Chapter 13 Canola Oil and Heart Health: A Historical Perspective 245

Bruce E. McDonald

Chapter 14 Canola Oil: Evolving Research in Obesity and Insulin Resistance 251

Danielle Hanke, Karin Love, Amy Noto, Peter Zahradka and Carla Taylor

Chapter 15 Rapeseed and Canola Phenolics: Antioxidant Attributes and Efficacy........ 277

Usha Thiyam-Holländer and Karin Schwarz

Chapter 16 Nutritional Impact of Fatty Acid Composition of Canola Oil and Its Effect on the Oxidative Deterioration 299

Kazuo Miyashita

Chapter 17 Effect of Canolol on Oxidation of Edible Oils........ 317

Bertrand Matthäus

Chapter 18 Canola Oil, Canolol and Cancer: Evolving Research 329

Pablo Steinberg

Chapter 19 Canolol as a Promising Nutraceutical: Status and Scope 337

Dayanidhi Huidrom and Usha Thiyam-Holländer

Index........ 349

Preface

This book is based on a canola workshop originally held at the Richardson Centre for Functional Foods and Nutraceuticals, University of Manitoba, Winnipeg, Manitoba, Canada in May 2010. The title was expanded to include rapeseed, as this term is still used in Europe where it refers to the low erucic acid and glucosinolate varieties. This book presents the most recent state-of-the-art information on the chemistry of the minor constituents of canola and rapeseed and their relevance to health not covered by existing reference books. It also includes the most recent technological and scientific advances on the bioactives present in canola and rapeseed by-products and oil. This book covers the pharmacological properties of the minor components and bioactives and identifies new areas of research and opportunities for the industrial application of functional foods and nutraceuticals from canola and rapeseed. This book's chapters are authored by experienced researchers in this field and have been expanded considerably to include a number of areas not included in the original workshop in order to provide a more comprehensive coverage of this very important crop.

Chapter 1 covers the historical development of canola and the extensive research conducted on the properties and performance that led to the worldwide success of the oil. Chapter 2 discusses the characteristics and bioactivities of sinapic acid derivatives, followed by Chapter 3, which updates the importance of sinapic acid derivatives and the decarboxylation pathways leading to their formation. Chapter 4 provides a good up-to-date review of the processing of canola proteins. Chapter 5 covers the development of high omega-9 canola oils and their future applications. A detailed discussion of the modification of *Brassica* oilseeds can be found in Chapter 6. Chapter 7 discusses a number of rapid analytical methods for measuring the oil content while Chapter 8 presents the potential of ultrasound and supercritical fluid extraction for producing value-added by-products from canola meal. The importance of processing virgin rapeseed oils in Europe is the subject of Chapter 9 followed by a review of the extraction and application of canola protein in Chapter 10. The frying stability of high-oleic low-linolenic acid canola oils is an important topic discussed in Chapter 11. The potential of mustard oil, an oil related to the Brassica family, for biodiesel is described in Chapter 12. The remaining chapters focus on health and include a discussion of the beneficial effects of canola oil on cardiovascular disease in Chapter 13 followed by the possible role of canola oil in obesity and insulin resistance in Chapter 14. The importance of canola phenolics as antioxidants is covered in Chapter 15 while Chapter 16 examines the nutritional impact of canola oil and its effect on oxidative deterioration. This is followed by a discussion of the antioxidant properties of canolol in Chapter 17. Chapter 18 describes the antimutagenic and anticancer properties of canola oil and canolol with the final chapter, Chapter 19, covering the potential nutraceutical status of canolol.

The editors have tried to bring together a diverse group of chapters that represents a broad view of the latest and future development in canola and rapeseed for the world market. We are extremely grateful to the AOCS Press and editors of CRC Press, Taylor & Francis for their encouragement and assistance in getting this book completed. We hope this book will be useful to researchers in both university and industry who wish to better understand canola and rapeseed as important sources of oil and protein.

Usha Thiyam-Holländer
N.A. Michael Eskin
Bertrand Matthäus

Editors

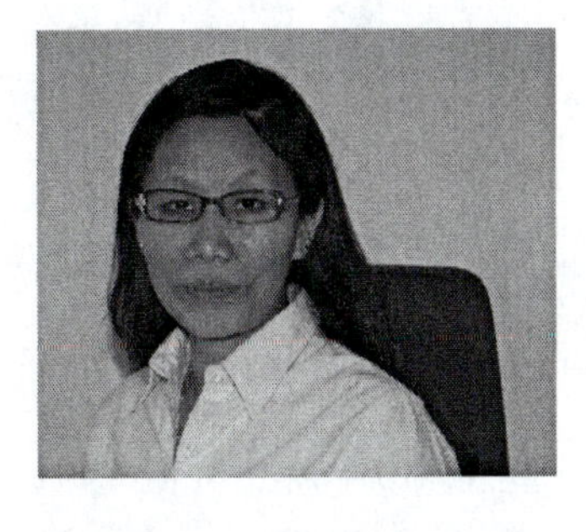

Usha Thiyam-Holländer holds a PhD from the University of Kiel, Germany. Immediately after receiving her doctoral degree, she worked at the prestigious Fraunhofer Institute of Process Engineering and Packaging, Freising, as a post-doc (2005–2006), where she concentrated on rapeseed phenolics and proteins. Since 2007, she has been an assistant professor at the Department of Human Nutritional Sciences, based at the Richardson Centre for Functional Foods and Nutraceuticals, University of Manitoba, Canada, where she researches the impact of various novel aspects of processing on canola oil and minor components. She recently completed more than 10 years in this area of research. Her work also focuses on plant-based functional foods and nutraceutical ingredients and the impact of innovative technology, isolation and optimization. Her interests include biorefining and environmentally friendly processes for deriving functional ingredients. Thiyam-Holländer teaches 'Food Quality Evaluation' and 'Lipid Chemistry' at the University of Manitoba. She holds patents in the field of lipid oxidation, processing and minor components of canola and other oilseeds. She has also published extensively in these areas. In 2008, 2010 and 2011, she organized and chaired workshops on 'Sensory aspects of canola oil', 'Value-addition to canola' and 'Current controversies in polyphenols' at the University of Manitoba. She has served as the vice-chair for the AOCS Lipid Oxidation and Quality (LOQ) Division since 2010; as its secretary/treasurer 2009–2011, and helped organize and support the LOQ networking session. In 2008–2009, she was the representative for the LOQ technical program committee. In 2007, she was co-vice-representative for the LOQ Division; and has been a member-at-large since 2007. Dr. Thiyam-Holländer is also involved in student mentoring sessions at AOCS.

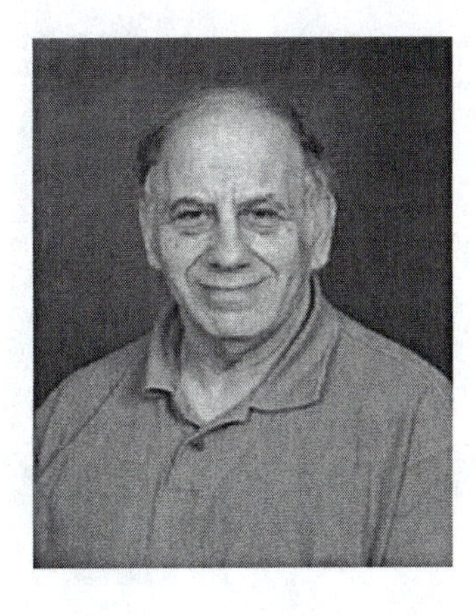

N.A. Michael Eskin is a professor and associate dean in the Department of Human Nutritional Sciences, Faculty of Human Ecology, University of Manitoba, Canada. He has done extensive research on edible oils and was involved in the early development of canola oil. Dr. Eskin has published 120 research papers and 11 books including *Canola: Chemistry, Production, Processing and Utilization* with Jim Daun and Dave Hickling released in May 2011 by AOCS Press. He has garnered a number of awards including the AOCS Timothy Mount's Award for excellence in the science and technology of edible oils and the Canadian Institute of Food

Science and Technology W.J. Eva Award for outstanding contribution to Canadian Science and Technology. He is also the 2012 recipient of the prestigious Institute of Food Technology (IFT) Stephen S. Chang Award for significant contributions to lipid or flavour science. Dr. Eskin is a fellow of the American Oil Chemists' Society, the Canadian Institute of Food Science and Technology and the Institute of Food Science and Technology in the United Kingdom. He sits on the editorial boards of six international journals and was recently selected as co-editor of *Lipid Technology*.

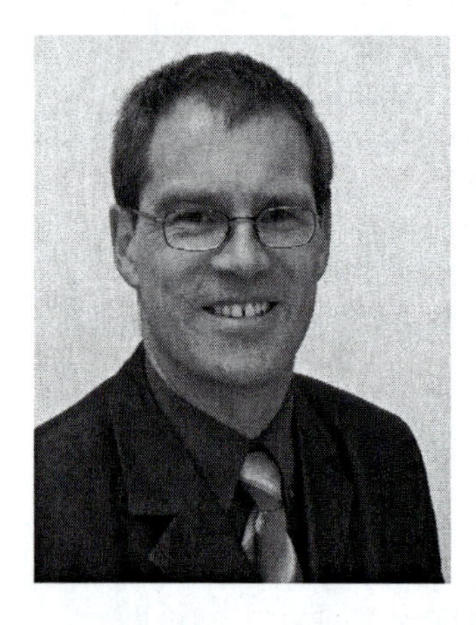

Bertrand Matthäus received his PhD in food chemistry in 1993. Since then, he has headed a laboratory at the Max Rubner-Institute, Federal Research Institute for Nutrition and Food, in the Department of Lipid Research of the German Federal Ministry for Nutrition, Agriculture and Consumer Protection. In this position, he is responsible for research dealing with the improvement of the quality of fats and oils, especially canola oil. His work focuses on the investigation of frying processes, with contaminants such as 3-MCPD esters, acrylamide, phthalates or 4-hydroxy-2-*trans*-nonenal and the investigation of the oxidation of edible fats and oils. He has published more than 180 articles, scientific papers and book chapters. He has worked with industry to evaluate and improve the quality of frying oils and cold-pressed canola oil. He has organized and coorganized several symposia and workshops on fats and oils for those in industry. He is also a member of a panel for the sensory evaluation of virgin edible oils.

Contributors

Ayyappan Appukuttan Aachary
Department of Human Nutritional Sciences
University of Manitoba
Winnipeg, Manitoba, Canada

Véronique J. Barthet
Canadian Grain Commission
Grain Research Laboratory
Winnipeg, Manitoba, Canada

Ajay K. Dalai
Department of Chemical Engineering
University of Saskatchewan
Saskatoon, Saskatchewan, Canada

Levente L. Diosady
Department of Chemical Engineering and Applied Chemistry
University of Toronto
Toronto, Ontario, Canada

N.A. Michael Eskin
Department of Human Nutritional Sciences
University of Manitoba
Winnipeg, Manitoba, Canada

Danielle Hanke
Department of Human Nutritional Sciences
University of Manitoba
Winnipeg, Manitoba, Canada

Dayanidhi Huidrom
Department of Human Nutritional Sciences
University of Manitoba
Winnipeg, Manitoba, Canada

Titipong Issariyakul
Department of Chemical Engineering
University of Saskatchewan
Saskatoon, Saskatchewan, Canada

Karin Love
Department of Human Nutritional Sciences
University of Manitoba
Winnipeg, Manitoba, Canada

Bertrand Matthäus
Department for Lipid Research
Max Rubner-Institut
Detmold, Germany

Bruce E. McDonald (Deceased)
Department of Human Nutritional Sciences
University of Manitoba
Winnipeg, Manitoba, Canada

Narsireddy Meda
Department of Human Nutritional Sciences
University of Manitoba
Winnipeg, Manitoba, Canada

K. Misra
Department of Chemistry
Indian Institute of Technology Kharagpur
West Bengal, India

Kazuo Miyashita
Bio-Functional Material Chemistry
Faculty of Fisheries Sciences
Hokkaido University
Hakodate, Japan

Ahindra Nag
Department of Chemistry
Indian Institute of Technology
Kharagpur
West Bengal, India

Amy Noto
Department of Human Nutritional
Sciences
University of Manitoba
Winnipeg, Manitoba, Canada

Frank Pudel
Pilot Pflanzenöltechnologie
Magdeburg e.V.
Magdeburg, Germany

Curtis B. Rempel
Department of Food Science
University of Manitoba
Winnipeg, Manitoba, Canada

M.G. Scanlon
Department of Food Science
University of Manitoba
Winnipeg, Manitoba, Canada

Karin Schwarz
Institute of Human Nutrition and
Food Science
University of Kiel
Kiel, Germany

Crystal L. Snyder
Department of Agricultural, Food
and Nutritional Science
University of Alberta
Edmonton, Alberta, Canada

Pablo Steinberg
Institute for Food Toxicology and
Analytical Chemistry
University of Veterinary Medicine
Hannover, Germany

Asim Syed
Healthy Oils Applications
DowAgro Sciences
Indianapolis, Indiana

Carla Taylor
Department of Human Nutritional
Sciences and Physiology
University of Manitoba
and
Canadian Centre for Agri-Food
Research in Health and Medicine
St. Boniface Hospital Research Centre
Winnipeg, Manitoba, Canada

Usha Thiyam-Holländer
Department of Human Nutritional
Sciences
University of Manitoba
Winnipeg, Manitoba, Canada

Randall J. Weselake
Department of Agricultural, Food
and Nutritional Science
University of Alberta
Edmonton, Alberta, Canada

L. Xu
Department of Chemical Engineering
and Applied Chemistry
University of Toronto
Toronto, Ontario, Canada

Peter Zahradka
Departments of Human Nutritional
Sciences and Physiology
University of Manitoba
and
Canadian Centre for Agri-Food
Research in Health and Medicine
St. Boniface Hospital Research Centre
Winnipeg, Manitoba, Canada

1 Canola Research
Historical and Recent Aspects

N.A. Michael Eskin

CONTENTS

1.1 Introduction 2
1.2 Development of Canola 3
1.3 Canola Oil 4
1.4 Room Odour 6
1.5 Stability of New Low Linolenic Acid Canola Oil 8
1.6 Sedimentation Phenomenon 9
1.7 Minor Components 12
1.8 Rapid Method for Assessing Shelf-Life Stability 16
References 16
Further Reading 19

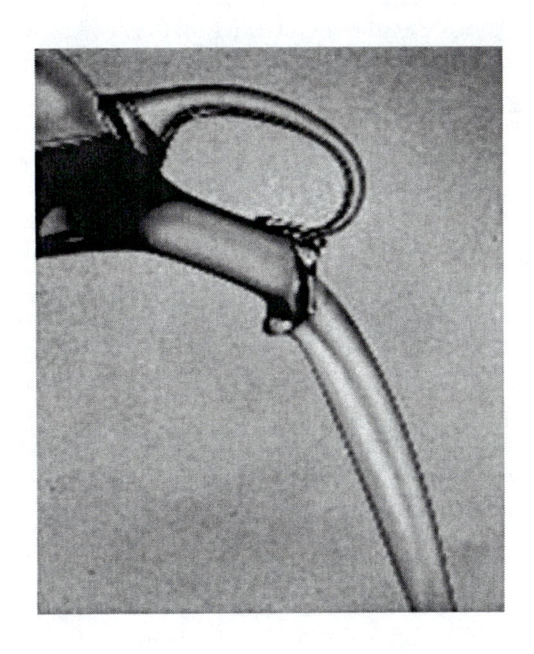

1.1 INTRODUCTION

Canola, previously known as rapeseed, is Canada's Cinderella crop that is now ranked among the top three oilseeds worldwide. The first recorded Canadian production of rapeseed was in Saskatchewan in the 1930s when an immigrant farmer from Poland, Mr Fred Solvoniuk, planted seeds sent to him by a Polish friend. The seeds adapted well to the soil conditions, and were later shown to be from *Brassica campestris*, now referred to as *B. rapa* L. species. The outbreak of the Second World War and the subsequent blockade of European and Asian sources of rapeseed oil made the commercial production of rapeseed a high priority by the Canadian government. The reason for this was because rapeseed oil was an excellent lubricating oil for marine engines. Under extreme heat and steam, rapeseed oil adhered to metal surfaces better than any other source of oil. In 1942, the Head of the Forage Crop Division of Canada Department of Agriculture was given the mandate for production in Canada. To relieve the desperate shortage of rapeseed oil, the total 1942 crop of 2600 lb or 42 bushels of *B. napus* was needed for planting in 1943. A further 41,000 lb of Argentine type seeds, *B. napus*, was purchased from US seed companies. The earlier Polish type (*B. campestris* now *B. rapa*) and the Argentine type (*B. napus*) both adapted extremely well to the Canadian prairies and grew fast with excellent yields. With a reduced demand for marine lubricants and the move to diesel engines, however, the Canadian rapeseed acreage dropped precipitously from 80,000 acres in 1948 to barely 400 acres in 1950. After the Second World War, alternative markets were sought for rapeseed including food. However, because of its green colour, sharp taste and high acid content, rapeseed had limited use as a food oil. It was not until the late 1950s that Baldur Stefannson at the University of Manitoba and Keith Downey in Saskatoon carried out their ground-breaking breeding research on rapeseed. As a young researcher, who had barely heard of rapeseed, I arrived in Winnipeg in 1968 to take up a position as an assistant professor in the Department of Foods and Nutrition at the University of Manitoba. This was followed shortly afterwards by the arrival of Bruce McDonald. We were both brought to the University of Manitoba by the late Lewis Lloyd, the first dean of the Faculty of Human Ecology, who certainly changed the course of my professional life. Being part of the development of canola and seeing it blossom into a major world crop was a unique opportunity not fully appreciated until many years later.

While I also conducted research on mucilage, phytate, phytase and sinapine in canola (Ismail and Eskin, 1979; Eskin et al., 1979; Atwal et al., 1980; Ismail et al., 1980; Latta and Eskin, 1980; Eskin and Wiebe, 1983; Kim and Eskin, 1987; Lu et al., 1987; Eskin, 1992; Khattab et al., 2010), this chapter will focus primarily on my work with canola oil. Before proceeding further, however, I would like to acknowledge a wonderful mentor and friend, the late Professor Marion Vaisey-Genser, with whom I had the privilege to work with for almost 30 years. As a leading sensory specialist, our expertise not only blended well but working with her was a delight and an inspiration. I would like to dedicate this chapter to her blessed memory.

1.2 DEVELOPMENT OF CANOLA

The journey that took an obscure, inedible oilseed, such as rapeseed, to become one of the healthiest edible oils on the world market today is a testament to the perseverance and ingenuity of both Baldur Stefansson and Keith Downey. They were two plant breeders who toiled using traditional plant breeding techniques that changed the face of Canadian agriculture. Today this multi-billion dollar crop has generated processing plants and hundreds of thousands of jobs in Canada and around the world. Not bad for a couple of Prairie boys in the outbacks of Canada. These breeders earned the title of the '*fathers of canola*' and are in the Canadian Agricultural Hall of Fame. Keith Downey took over the responsibility for the rapeseed breeding program at the Canada Agriculture Research Station in Saskatoon in 1957 while Baldur Stefansson was a professor in the Department of Plant Science at the University of Manitoba. A crucial aspect to the success for both these breeders was the development of gas–liquid chromatography (GLC). Using GLC for the precise analysis of erucic acid was key to the success of both breeders' research.

An important discovery by Keith Downey and his graduate student Bryan Harvey was that erucic acid was controlled by the genotype of the developing embryo in the seed rather than the maternal plant. In other words, seeds from the same plant could in fact differ in erucic acid content. They developed the 'half-seed method' in which the oil could be analysed by GLC for erucic acid which accelerated the development of low erucic acid varieties of rapeseed. Using this tool they were able to screen the world's rapeseed germplasm. In 1960, a major breakthrough for Stefansson was identification of Liho, the European forage rapeseed, with 10% erucic acid. I should point out here that the late Dr. Frithjof Hougen, a professor in the Department of Plant Science, did the analytical work that significantly contributed to Stefansson's success. His role is often overlooked and I would like to emphasize the importance of his work as a key research partner in this work. Stefansson provided some of the Liho seed to Downey who successfully transferred the low erucic acid characteristic to a *B. napus* variety. This resulted in the development of the first LEAR variety, ORO. While ORO was a significant scientific achievement it proved to be an agronomic failure as it was quite inferior to the high erucic varieties. In addition, the availability of cheap sunflower oil in the USSR essentially eliminated the demand for the higher priced LEAR (ORO) oil.

Downey then passed on the low erucic acid characteristic to *B. campestris*, which accounted for the majority of rapeseed grown in the Prairies. After examination of countless seeds, he finally identified a Polish sample with very low erucic acid with one seed containing zero erucic acid. Using a half seed technique to grow a new plant, five invaluable seeds led to the successful *B. campestris* breeding program with the release of the first low erucic acid *B. campestris* variety in 1971.

Besides erucic acid, Downey and Stefansson also turned their attention to glucosinolates in the meal. A rapid GLC developed by Young and Wetter in 1967 at Prairie Regional Laboratory (PRL) in Saskatoon allowed for the rapid and accurate measurement of glucosinolate levels in the meal. A line of low-glucosinolate summer *B. napus* detected by Dr. Jan Krzymanski and brought into Canada in

1967 facilitated the development of a *B. napus* variety low in both erucic acid and glucosinolates by these breeders in 1973. A healthy competition ensued between Stefansson and Downey with Stefansson developing an agronomically superior Tower variety which Agriculture Canada registered in 1974 as the world's first zero-erucic acid, low-glucosinolate *B. napus*. Not to be beaten, Downey, together with the plant breeder Sid Pawlowski, developed the first zero-erucic acid, low-glucosinolate *B. campestris* variety, Candle which was better suited to Northern growing conditions where Tower's later maturity was a problem.

1.3 CANOLA OIL

The development of the double low rapeseed placed Canada at the forefront of rapeseed breeding in the world. To distinguish the superior edible products derived from double-low varieties of *B. napus* and *B. campestris*, the Western Canadian Oilseed Crushers' Association trademarked the term 'canola' in 1978. The word canola stands for Canadian oil, low acid. This trademark was subsequently transferred to the Canola Council of Canada (the name also changing from the Rapeseed Association of Canada) in 1980. The success of canola can be seen from the approximate 7 million tonnes of canola seed produced in Canada each year, of which half is exported with the remainder crushed domestically. In Canada, approximately 90% of canola oil is used for salad and cooking oils while 50% of shortening and margarine oils are produced from canola.

The change to canola had a dramatic effect on the composition of the oil as the erucic acid content was reduced to <1% while the oleic acid content increased substantially (to approx. 60%). This was accompanied by smaller increases in linoleic (to approx. 20%) and linolenic acid (to approx. 10%). My initial interest was primarily on the oxidative stability of the new oil, particularly in light of its high linolenic acid content. This commenced following my sabbatical year at the Faculty of Agriculture of the Hebrew University in Rehovoth, Israel in 1974–1975. It was during that year that I worked with another visiting professor from Rutgers University, Chaim Frenkel. He was studying the ageing of plants, in particular tomatoes, and invited me to join him. At that time, I was interested in lipoxygenase and noticed he used a reagent, titanium tetrachloride, to measure inorganic peroxides. This was based on the fact that peroxides were traditionally used in geology to detect titanium in rocks. I wondered whether it would measure organic peroxides and set up a lipoxygenase assay and found that it did. I immediately realized that I had a new method for measuring rancidity, as during those days, there were only a relatively few reliable methods available. On my return to the University of Manitoba, I ordered titanium tetrachloride and set about developing the method. Preliminary work showed that the reagent did not react with organic peroxides but only with organic hydroperoxides as it required the presence of the labile hydrogen. It was not too long before a method for measuring rancidity based on the formation of hydroperoxides was developed and subsequently published in the *Journal of the American Oil Chemists' Society* (Eskin and Frenkel, 1976). I was amused to read the comments from one of the reviewers who stated 'Why on earth do this on rapeseed oil, after all it isn't even edible?' The method proved to be easy and rapid, and unlike the Peroxide Value, did not depend on identifying the elusive titration end point. It simply required dissolving 0.5 g of the oil in 10 mL acetone in a Pyrex centrifuge tube followed by the addition of 0.5 mL of titanium reagent (20% $TiCl_4$ in conc. HCl). After mixing the solution thoroughly, the titanium–hydoperoxide complex formed which was then precipitated by the addition of 2 mL conc. NH_4OH. After centrifuging for 5 min, the supernatant was discarded and the precipitate redissolved in 4 N nitric acid, with the final volume adjusted to 10 mL. The titanium–hydroperoxide complex formed a peak with a maximum absorbance at 415 nm which increased during Schaal Oven storage over 16 days compared to an equivalent blank (Figure 1.1). The method proved to be a very simple and rapid procedure for monitoring rancidity as hydroperoxide value (HV) and correlated with the other chemical tests (TBA and PV methods) as well as Odour Intensity Value (OIV) (Table 1.1). The main drawback was it required the use of strong acids, which, by today's standards, was definitely not environmentally friendly. Nevertheless, it proved to be a very useful method and many visitors to our laboratory were impressed by its simplicity and reliability. This study introduced me to oil chemistry and a long and successful collaboration with the late Professor Marion Vaisey-Genser. Using this and other methods, combined with sensory evaluation, we soon published a number papers that clearly established the suitability of canola oil as a salad and frying oil (Eskin and Frenkel, 1977; Stevenson et al., 1983, 1984a,b). We also showed that the presence of too much dockage had a detrimental effect on canola oil quality (Ismail et al., 1980).

Professor Vaisey-Genser and I were commissioned by the Canola Council of Canada to write a booklet on canola oil suitable for dietitians and related health professions as part of their global strategy to introduce the oil to the world market. The first booklet covering all aspects of canola oil came out in 1978 and was followed

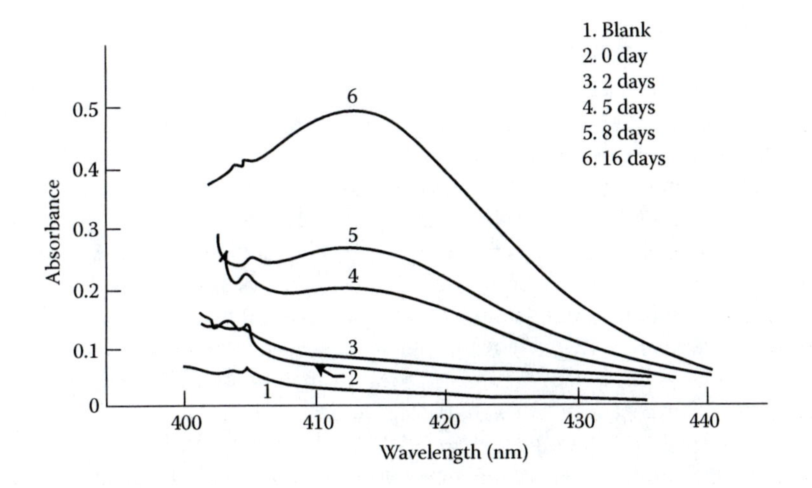

FIGURE 1.1 Change in absorption spectra for titanium–hydroperoxide formation in rapeseed oil samples over 16 days at 65°C. (From Eskin, N.A.M. and Frenkel, C. 1976. *J. Am. Oil Chem. Soc.* 53: 746–747. With permission.)

TABLE 1.1
Regression Equations and Coefficients of Determination (r^2) for Methods Used for Assessing Rancidity of Rapeseed Oil

Methods[a] Compared	Linear Regression ($y = a_1x + a_0$)	Coefficient of Determination (r^2)
PV and HV	HV = 0.003 PV + 0.03	0.98
PV and TBA	TBA = 0.004 PV + 0.14	0.93
PV and OIV	OIV = 0.04 PV + 1.14	0.87
HV and TBA	TBA = 1.20 HV + 0.10	0.98
HV and OIV	OIV = 12.16 HV + 0.70	0.93
TBA and OIV	OIV = 10.27 TBA − 0.38	0.98

Source: From Eskin, N.A.M. and Frenkel, C. 1976. *J. Am. Oil Chem. Soc.* 53: 746–747. With permission.

[a] TBA = thiobarbituric acid, PV = peroxide value, HV = hydroperoxide value, OIV = odour intensity value.

by a number of editions, some of which were translated into French, German and Spanish (Vaisey-Genser and Eskin, 1978, 1979a,b, 1980, 1982, 1983, 1987). The final 1987 edition of the booklet was used in a lipid graduate course taught at the University of California at Davis.

In addition to my association with Professor Vaisey-Genser, I had the privilege to work on many challenging problems with a number of outstanding scientists including Dr. Roman Przybylski, Dr. Linda Malcolmson, Dr. Rachel Scarth, Dr. Costas Biliaderis and more recently Dr. Michel Aliani with excellent technical support by Donna Ryland. The following chapter covers many aspects of this work.

1.4 ROOM ODOUR

One of the first problems associated with high linolenic acid edible oils, such as canola and soyabean, was the development of room odour during frying. A study published with Professor Vaisey-Genser and Dr. Przybylski in 1989 (Eskin et al., 1989) tried to address this problem. We examined three oils, a laboratory refined low and high C18:3 canola oil and a high C18:3 commercially refined canola oil containing 1.9%, 9.0% and 8.5% C18:3, respectively. Both high C18:3 oils had slightly lower C18:1 and C18:2 fatty acid levels compared to the low C18:3 variety. The oils were heated at 185°C for 10 min under air or nitrogen with odour intensity assessed by an 8-membered trained panel at 50°C using a 15 cm semi-structured line scale. The results summarized in Table 1.2 showed significant differences between the low and high C18:3 oil samples but no differences between the lab refined or commercially refined high C18:3 oils. In addition, less oxidative changes were evident when heated under nitrogen compared to air. While there was a marked reduction in room odour between the oil containing 8–9% and 1.9% C18:3, room odour was still too strong and unacceptable to 56% of the panelists. Since using a nitrogen blanket was not feasible, touch hydrogenation was considered a suitable technique-obviously unacceptable by today's standards.

TABLE 1.2
Effects of Heating on the Chemical and Sensory Indices of Oxidation of Low and High Linolenic Acid Canola Oils (Average of Duplicate Values in Two Replications)

	Low C18:3, Laboratory Refined			High C18:3, Laboratory Refined			High C18:3, Commercially Refined			Least Significant
Index[a]	Unheated	Heated N_2	Heated Air	Unheated	Heated N_2	Heated Air	Unheated	Heated N_2	Heated Air	Difference
PV	0.30	1.00	2.30	0.50	1.80	4.00	0.00	2.10	3.50	1.67
TBA	0.01	0.31	0.84	0.03	1.90	2.57	0.03	2.09	3.14	0.83
FFA	0.03	0.05	0.15	0.05	0.08	2.16	0.15	0.06	0.27	0.09
DIEN.	0.01	0.16	0.58	0.03	0.44	1.54	0.02	0.91	1.64	0.51
CARB.	0.62	3.15	7.45	1.50	4.44	13.04	0.72	8.54	17.40	8.20
OIV	0.40	4.60	7.20	2.00	6.80	11.10	1.00	9.30	12.20	2.66
ACCP. (%)	100	94	44	100	62	19	100	31	0	—

Source: From Eskin, N.A.M. et al. 1989. *J. Amer. Oil Chem. Soc.* 66: 1081–1085. With permission.

[a] PV = Peroxide value (Meq/kg); TBA = thiobarbituric acid value; FFA = free fatty acids (%); DIEN. = dienals (unsaturated carbonyls); CARB. = carbonyls; OIV = odour intensity value (max. 15); ACCP. = acceptability (%).

1.5 STABILITY OF NEW LOW LINOLENIC ACID CANOLA OIL

In the early 1990s, we were asked to test a new experimental low C18:3 Stellar canola seed developed by Rachel Scarth and Baldur Stefannson. The Stellar variety oil had 3.1% C18:3 compared to 11.3% for Westar. It was slightly higher in C18:1 but much higher in C18:2 compared to Westar. Using the Schaal Oven Test at 60°C for 12 days, a trained panel assessed odour intensity and pleasantness while the chemical tests for rancidity include TBA, PV, hydroperoxide value (HV), as well as carbonyl values and dienals (a new method developed by Dr. Roman Przybylski). This study found that the chemical indices for rancidity were markedly lower for Stellar (Figure 1.2)

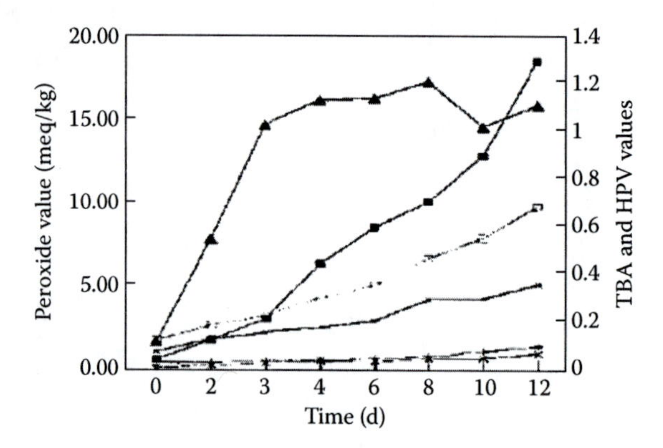

FIGURE 1.2 Effect of storage at 60°C on the development of PV, TBA and HVin Westar and LLCO oils. Westar: (■) PV, (▲) TBA, (*) HV: LLCO: (□)PV; (×) TBA; (×) HV. (From Przybylski, R., Biliaderis, C.G. and Eskin, N.A.M. 1993a. *J. Amer. Oil. Chem. Soc.* 70: 1009–1015. With permission.)

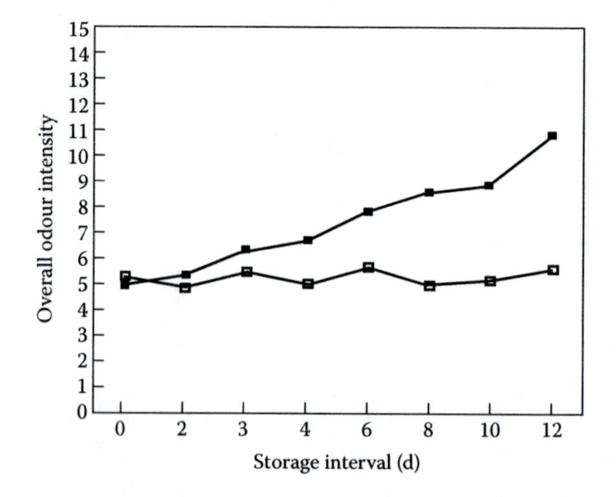

FIGURE 1.3 Effect of storage at 60°C on the overall odour intensity of Westar (■) and LLCO (□). (From Przybylski, R., Biliaderis, C.G. and Eskin, N.A.M. 1993a. *J. Am. Oil Chem. Soc.* 70: 1009–1015. With permission.)

(Przybylski et al., 1993). In addition, Westar exhibited an overall increase in odour intensity over the 12 days of storage while Stellar showed little change (Figure 1.3). High correlations were observed between sensory and chemical and instrumental methods with poor correlations for Stellar. These results indicated a marked improvement in stability for Stellar over Westar which resulted in Stellar being selected by McCain's for use in their healthy fries.

1.6 SEDIMENTATION PHENOMENON

Canola oil, with a very low level of saturated fatty acids, could be used in salads without winterization (Biliaderis and Eskin, 1991; Eskin and McDonald, 1991; Eskin et al., 1996). However, subsequent reports by processors indicated that canola oil occasionally developed cloudiness on storage even though it may have passed the cold test. The latter test is generally used as an index of winterizing by measuring the resistance of an oil to crystallization at 0°C. The exact reason for this phenomenon in canola oil was unknown although sunflower oil, which has always had a haze or sedimentation problem, has been associated with the presence of waxes. The reason we got involved with this problem followed a meeting with Dr. Jim Daun, then head of the Oilseed Section in the Grain Research Laboratory (GRL) in Winnipeg. He had carried out initial work on canola oil sediment in which he reported that the clouding material consisted mainly of wax esters and some high-melting triacylglycerols (Daun and Jeffery, 1991). Since this area was not within the mandate of GRL, he asked us to consider continuing this research, which we did with great enthusiasm. I spearheaded a successful application for an NSERC Strategic Grant with Drs. Przybylski, Biliaderis and Scarth which allowed us to hire a postdoc to look into this cause of this problem. We visited a Canola Oilseed Processing Plant in Morden, Manitoba and were surprised to find they winterized the oil. This plant previously processed sunflower oil which required winterization and even though they changed over to canola oil they still winterized the oil. We were particularly delighted as we were able to take substantial amounts of the sediment back to our lab and compare it with the sediment we isolated from our own canola oil.

The major components in canola oil sediment were found to be wax esters (78.1%) (Table 1.3). Other minor components included free fatty alcohols (2%), di- and triglycerides (3%) and a small amount of free fatty acids (0.2%). Thus, the major clouding material in canola oil was composed of waxes as in the case for sunflower oil haze (Hu et al., 1993). However, our work showed a large amount of other material in canola oil sediment not found in sunflower oil sediment, possibly complex carbohydrates or very long-chain wax esters (Liu et al., 1993, 1994, 1995a,b,c, 1996a,b; Przybylski et al., 1993). The composition of fatty acids and alcohol in canola oil sediment isolated from isolated winterized filter cake is shown in Table 1.4 (Liu et al., 1993). The major fatty acids in canola oil haze were C20:0 and C22:0 while the predominant fatty alcohols were C24:0, C26:0 and C28:0. Comparing canola and sunflower oil sediments illustrated significant differences between the corresponding haze-causing material. Sunflower oil sediment was composed mainly of wax esters (99%) while canola oil sediment contained 75–80% waxes. In addition,

TABLE 1.3
Composition of Canola Oil Sediment Isolated from an Industrial Filter Cake Collected after Winterization

Component	Content (%) ± s.d.
Wax esters	78.1 ± 1.0
Triacylglycerols	Trace
Free fatty acids	0.2 ± 0.1
Free fatty alcohols	2.0 ± 0.1
Diacylglycerols	2.7 ± 0.2
Others	17.7 ± 9.6

Source: From Liu, H. et al. 1993. *J. Amer. Oil Chem. Soc.* 70: 441–448. With permission.

Note: s.d. = standard deviation.

TABLE 1.4
Composition of Canola Oil Sediment Isolated from an Industrial Filter Cake

Fatty Acid (%)		Fatty Alcohol (%)	
16:0	3.0	16:0	0.5
18:0	1.8	17:0	0.3
20:0	35.4	18:0	0.4
21:0	0.8	19:0	3.9
22:0	20.4	20:0	0.4
23:0	0.7	21:0	6.7
24:0	8.0	22:0	1.4
25:0	0.6	23:0	4.9
26:0	7.1	24:0	14.3
27:0	0.5	25:0	5.0
28:0	8.9	26:0	23.6
29:0	0.4	27:0	5.7
30:0	3.2	28:0	12.2
31:0	0.1	29:0	1.7
32:0	0.4	30:0	6.7
		31:0	0.2
		32:0	6.2

Source: From Liu, H. et al. 1993. *J. Am. Oil Chem. Soc.* 70: 441–448. With permission.

the presence of longer chain length fatty acids and alcohols combined with the low sediment content appeared to contribute to the unique sediment formation in canola oil. A hexane-insoluble fraction from Canadian canola hull lipids had fatty acid and alcohol profiles as well as an x-ray diffraction pattern similar to the corresponding oil sediment.

Further studies showed that sedimentation in canola oil was a physicochemical process involving phase transitions. The high-melting lipid constituents are initially soluble in the oil but crystallize from the bulk oil forming the haze. Consequently, the melting and crystallization properties of the sediment were studied using differential scanning calorimetry (DSC). Figure 1.4 shows the narrow temperature range over which the canola oil sediment melted with a peak temperature at around 75°C. This melting temperature was higher than that for the sunflower sediment as the longer chain fatty acids and alcohols in canola sediment would melt at a higher temperature. The heterogeneity of the canola sediment was evident in the crystallization curve. A peak plus shoulder occurring throughout the crystallization process corresponded to the solidification of the various components in the sediment. X-ray diffraction studies showed the crystalline structure of the canola sediment was similar

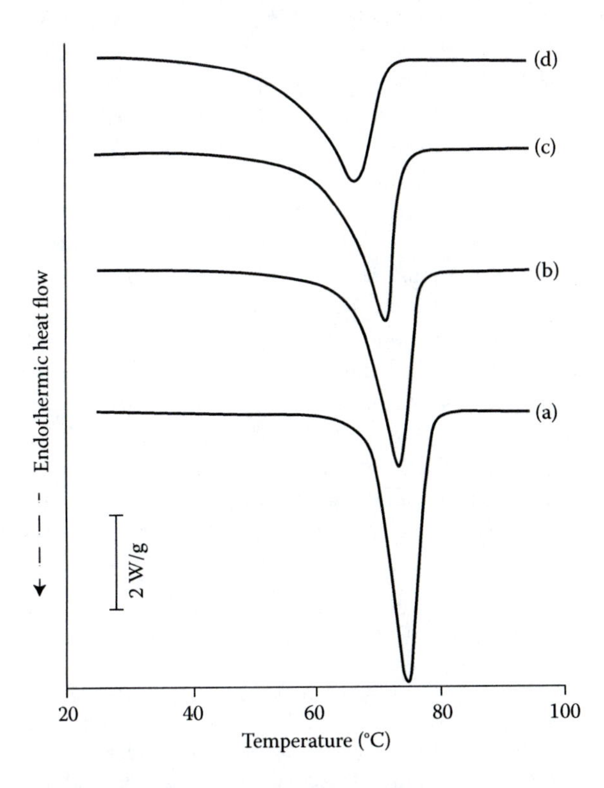

FIGURE 1.4 DSC thermal curves of canola sediment oil mixture. Sediment concentration: (a) 100%, (b) 80.3%, (c) 50.2% and (d) 19.6%, respectively. (From Liu, H. et al. 1993. *J. Am. Oil Chem. Soc.* 70: 441–448. With permission.)

TABLE 1.5
Clouding Time (Days) of Canola Oil at Various Sediment Concentrations at Different Storage Temperatures

Temp.	Sediment Levels (ppm)							
(°C)	25	50	75	100	150	200	250	300
0	6	4	3	3	2	1	<1	<1
5	3	2	1	1	1	<1	<1	<1
10	5	2	1	1	1	<1	<1	<1
25	>30	2	1	—	1	1	<1	<1
32	nd	—	—	>30	23	23	<1	<1

Source: From Liu, H., Przybylski, R. and Eskin, N.A.M. 1996b. *J. Am. Oil Chem. Soc.* 73: 1137–1141. With permission.
Note: nd = not determined.

to that of other waxes. The morphology of the sediment crystals showed the canola oil sediment exhibited needle-like crystals in the oil. At a very low cooling rate and a low sediment content, however, large leaf-like crystal structures were observed.

Examination of storage temperature and sediment concentration on haze formation in canola oil showed if the sediment concentration was <50 ppm more than 24 h was required to observe a sediment irrespective of the temperature (0–32°C). At 25°C, canola oil samples containing 50 ppm required 2 days before it became cloudy. Oil samples containing 25 ppm sediment, however, remained clear for a month. The optimum temperature for sediment formation appeared to be 5°C (Table 1.5).

In an effort to determine as well as predict the formation of a sediment in canola oil, a method was developed based on solvent precipitation. Our studies indicated that the addition of 30–40% acetone addition to canola accelerated crystallization of the sediment (Liu et al., 1996c). The relationship between turbidity and sediment formation in canola oil was shown to be non-linear. As can be seen in Figure 1.5, the presence of phospholipids also influenced turbidity as the addition of 2% lecithin increased turbidity by 23%. A review of this work can be found by Liu et al. (1998).

1.7 MINOR COMPONENTS

While a number of studies reported improvements in frying stability for modified vegetable oils compared to regular oils, other studies reported no significant improvement in frying stability (Liu and White, 1992; Warner and Mounts, 1993; Mounts et al., 1994). This suggested to us that fatty acids alone could not adequately explain or accurately predict the stability of frying oils. It was apparent that the primary focus of breeding was based on the premise that altering the fatty acids would improve frying stability while totally ignoring the minor components present

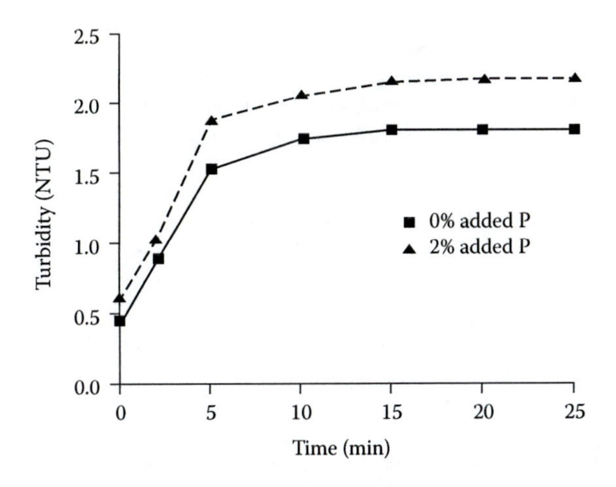

FIGURE 1.5 Turbidity of canola oil containing 50 ppm of sediment as a function of cooling time at 0°C. The turbidity for corresponding oils with 2% lecithin was also shown in broken line. (From Liu, H., Przybylski, R. and Eskin, N.A.M. 1996b. *J. Am. Oil Chem. Soc.* 73: 1137–1141. With permission.)

in the oil. It was our opinion that minor components played a significant role in oil stability particularly if their levels changed substantially during modification. A study by Xu et al. (1999) showed that the level of linolenic acid was crucial to the deep-frying performance of three high oleic acid canola oils. However, they did not examine the minor components in these oils. We examined the frying stability of three modified canola oils (high oleic acid canola oil (HOCO), low linolenic acid canola oil (LLCO) and a high oleic and low linolenic acid canola oil (HOLLCO) compared to a regular canola (RCO) by monitoring the formation of oil degradation products as well as tocopherols.

The initial quality of the oils all had PV <1.1 meq/kg and free fatty acids <0.11%. The modified oils were substantially lower in linolenic acid (3.0–6.7%) compared to 10.2% for regular canola oil. In addition, the modified canola oils were all higher in oleic acid (62.7–74.4%) compared to 57.4% for regular canola. With the exception of low linolenic acid canola oil, the other modified oils were also lower in linoleic acid. While the total polyunsaturated fatty acids (PUFAs) for HOCO and HOLLCO were approximately 50% of that in regular canola oil, LLCO was similar with 27.7%. Two replications of 72-h deep-frying trials were conducted using the four oils per trial in 2-L capacity domestic deep fryers. The oils were heated to 175 ± 2°C and kept at this temperature for 6 days. To accelerate the deterioration process, French fries were fried for 6 min each morning and evening. A 1:6 ratio of food to oil was used as this ratio was recommended by Morton and Chidley (1988). Samples were taken at predetermined times throughout frying, flushed with nitrogen and frozen until analysed.

A comparison of the formation of total polar compounds (TPC) showed no significant differences in the rates of TPC formation between LLCO and HOCO

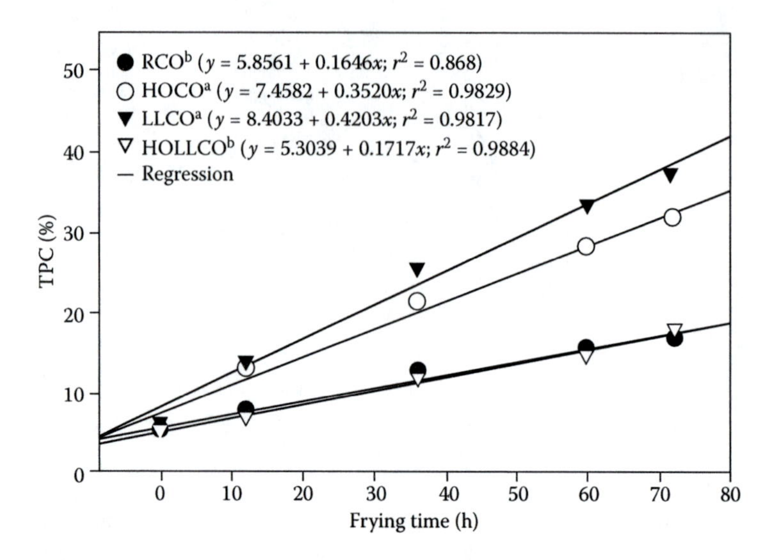

FIGURE 1.6 Total polar compounds (TPC) over frying time for canola oils. Oils with the same letter as subscript displayed no significant differences in rates of TPC formation at $p < 0.05$. (From Normand, L., Eskin, N.A.M. and Przybylski, R. 2001. *J. Amer. Oil Chem. Soc.* 78: 369–373. With permission.)

during frying (Figure 1.6). However, they both exhibited significantly ($p < 0.05$) faster rates of TPC formation compared to RCO and HOLLCO. Since TPC represent the products of oil degradation, LLCO and HOCO were significantly less stable during frying compared the other two canola oils. The superior frying stability of RCO over LLCO and HOCO was unexpected as both modified oils were lower in PUFA and, by all accounts, should have been less susceptible to oxidative breakdown. Warner et al. (1994) reported that HOCO was stabler than RCO based on the level of formation of TPC during frying. However, they only conducted the frying over 18 h and looked at the levels of TPC not the rate of formation. However, an earlier study by Warner and Mounts (1993) found no significant differences in TPC between regular canola and a low linolenic acid canola oil over 40 h of frying. In our study no significant differences in TPC formation were found between RCO and HOLLCO. This was also unexpected as HOLLCO had only half the levels of PUFAs compared to RCO.

Tocopherols, important minor components in these oils, showed HOLLCO had the highest level of 893 mg/kg compared to 468–601 mg/kg for the other three canola oils. This study was the first to examine the rate of tocopherol degradation during frying and showed the rates varied greatly between the four oils studied (Figure 1.7). In the case of LLCO and HOCO, the total tocopherols were reduced by 50% in the first 3–6 h of frying. In comparison, a 50% reduction in tocopherols occurred between 40 and 60 h of frying for HOLLCO and had still not been reached by ROCO after 72 h of frying. The following table (Table 1.6) shows the time required to reduce the original tocopherol levels by 50%. The data clearly shows RCO was the stablest

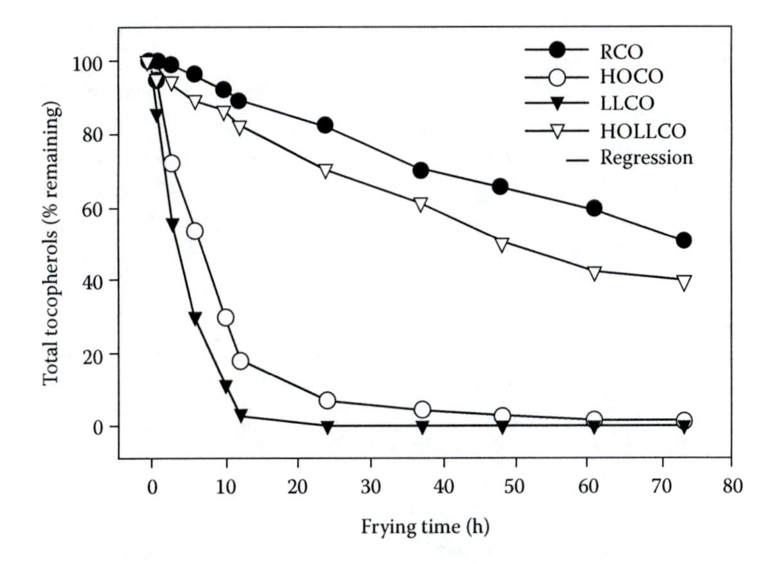

FIGURE 1.7 Total tocopherols remaining over frying time for canola oils (% original amount). (From Normand, L., Eskin, N.A.M. and Przybylski, R. 2001. *J. Am. Oil Chem. Soc.* 78: 369–373. With permission.)

oil during frying followed by HOLLCO while the least stable oils were HOCO and LLCO. Oils with faster rates of tocopherol degradation also had faster rates of TPC formation. Elimination of the possible role of trace metals was confirmed as negligible levels for Fe, Ni and Cu were found in all of the four canola oils studied. This study pointed to the danger of focusing solely on the fatty acid composition when

TABLE 1.6
Total and Individual Tocopherol Degradation Rates[a]

	Time (h) Required to Reduce Original Levels by 50% (Rate of Degradation ppm/h)		
Oil	**Total Tocopherols**	**Tocopherol α**	**Tocopherol γ**
RCO	>72 (3.3)	>72 (1.4)	60–72 (2.6)
HOCO	3–6 (50.1)	3–6 (15.0)	3–6 (35.1)
HOLLCO	48–60 (7.4)	>72 (8.0)	36–48 (6.3)
LLCO	3–6 (33.0)	3–6 (12.5)	3–6 (26.5)

Source: From Normand, L., Eskin, N.A.M. and Przybylski, R. 2001. *J. Am. Oil Chem. Soc.* 78: 369–373. With permission.

Note: RCO = Regular canola oil; HOCO = high oleic canola oil; HOLLCO = High oleic, low linolenic canola oil; LLCO = Low linolenic canola oil.

[a] All values are average of duplicate analysis.

studying the frying stability of oils and must also take into account such minor components as tocopherols.

Subsequent work by Zambiazi and Przybylski (1998) also showed that fatty acid composition could only explain half of the oxidative stability of vegetable oils including canola oil. The other half was attributed to the amount and composition of endogenous minor components which can shorten or extend the shelf-life of an oil. Such endogenous components were later discussed by Przybylski and Eskin (2006) and included tocopherols, mono- and diacylglycerols, free fatty acids, phospholipids, chlorophylls and derivatives, carotenoids, phytosterols, phenolic compounds and trace metals. In addition, the position that the fatty acid occupies in the triacylglycerol can also affect stability. For example, the location of linolenic and linoleic acids on the *sn*-2 position has been reported to cause faster oxidation and lower stability compared to the same fatty acids on *sn*1- and *sn*-3 positions. In contrast oleic acid at the *sn*-2 position proved stabler compared to its location on *sn*-1 and *sn*-3 positions (Neff et al., 1994, 1997).

1.8 RAPID METHOD FOR ASSESSING SHELF-LIFE STABILITY

This work led to further funding by a consortium of oil processors to develop a rapid method for determining the stability of their oils using breeder size samples. Our choice of instrument was the Iatroscan, which is relatively cheap and very user friendly. In fact, we used the Iatroscan quite often including adapting it as an effective and reliable method for separating and quantifying phospholipids in solvent extracted, expeller and degummed canola oil in the submicrogram range (Przybylski and Eskin, 1991). We also used the Iatroscan to develop a simplified method for analysing cereal lipids (Przybylski and Eskin, 1994). In addition to using small samples, the universality and sensitivity of the flame ionization detector made it a very effective tool. On a personal note when assessing rancidity, I like a method that gives me a defined end product. I do not like methods that give me an arbitrary number based on the transition of 1 or 2 electrons. This method is based on the formation of polar components as a measure of oxidation and uses the Iatroscan, TLC-FID instrument (Wu et al., 2006). Without giving too much detail about the method, which will be published shortly, suffice it to say that it can be used to measure the stability of breeder-size oil samples from seeds. The proposed method can be applied for stability comparison to help select the best line for further development.

I believe my research on canola oil has come full cycle starting with developing the titanium method for measuring the hydroperoxides in 1976, which required 0.5 mL (<0.5 g) of canola oil, and ending with the Iatroscan which used merely 20–30 μg of oil. The latter method required 1/10,000th of the oil needed for the titanium method and is a much more environmentally friendly.

REFERENCES

Atwal, A.S., Eskin, N.A.M., McDonald, B.E. and Vaisey-Genser, M. 1980. The effect of phytate on nitrogen utilization and zinc metabolism in young rats. *Nutr. Rep. Inter.* 21: 257–267.

Biliaderis, C.G. and Eskin, N.A.M. 1991. Canola oil, in *Encyclopedia of Food Science and Technology* (Y. Hui, ed.-in-chief), Vol. 2, John Wiley & Sons, New York, pp. 264–277.

Daun, J.K. and Jeffery, L.e. 1991. Sedimentation. In Canola, 9th Report, Canola Council of Canada, Winnipeg, pp. 436–440.

Eskin, N.A.M. 1992. Effect of variety and geographical location on the incidence of mucilage in canola seeds. *Can. J. Plant Sci.* 72: 1223–1225.

Eskin, N.A.M. and Frenkel, C. 1976. A simple and rapid method for assessing rancidity based on the formation of hydroperoxides. *J. Am. Oil Chem. Soc.* 53: 746–747.

Eskin, N.A.M. and Frenkel, C. 1977. A study of the deterioration of soybean and rapeseed oils by measurement of hydroperoxides. *Proceedings of the 13th World Congress of the International Society of Fat Research.* Section 1. Autooxidation and Thermooxidative Alteration. Marseille, France, pp. 1–9.

Eskin, N.A.M., Mag, T., Przybylski, R., McDonald, B.E., Malcolmson, L.J., Scarth, R., Adolph, D. and Ward, K. 1996. Canola oil, Chapter 1, in *Bailey's Industrial Oil and Fat Products*, 5th edition (Y. Hui, ed-in-chief), Vol. 2, Wiley Interscience, John Wiley & Sons Inc., New York, pp. 1–95.

Eskin, N.A.M. and McDonald, B.E. 1991. Canola oil. *Br. Nutr. Bull.* 1: 138–147.

Eskin, N.A.M., McDonald, B.E. and Vaisey-Genser, M. 1979. A study of the nutritional functional significance of phytate for removal or reduction from protein sources. *Final Report DDS Contract 025U. 01531-7-0448*, Agriculture Canada, pp. 97.

Eskin, N.A.M., Vaisey-Genser, M., Durance-Tod, S. and Przybylski, R. 1989. Stability of low linolenic acid canola oil to frying temperatures. *J. Am. Oil Chem. Soc.* 66: 1081–1085.

Eskin, N.A.M. and Wiebe, S. 1983. Changes in phytase activity and phytate during germination of two fababean cultivars. *J. Food Sci.* 48: 270–271.

Hu, X., Daun, J.K. and Scarth, R. 1993. Characterization of sediments in refined canola oils. *J. Am. Oil Chem. Soc.* 70: 535–537.

Ismail, F. and Eskin, N.A.M. 1979. A new quantitative procedure for sinapine. *J. Agric. Food Chem.* 27: 917–918.

Ismail, F., Eskin, N.A.M., and Vaisey-Genser, M. 1980. The effect of dockage on the stability of rapeseed oil. *6th Progress Report on Canola Seed, Oil, Meal and Meal Fractions.* Canola Council of Canada Publication. No. 5, 234–239.

Khattab, R., Eskin, N.A.M., Aliani, M. and Thiyam, U. 2010. Determination of sinapic acid derivatives in canola extracts using high-performance liquid chromatography. *J. Am. Oil Chem. Soc.* 87: 147–155.

Kim, S. and Eskin, N.A.M. 1987. Isolation and characterization of phytase from canola var. Candle. *J. Food Sci.* 52: 1353–1354.

Latta, M. and Eskin, N.A.M. 1980. A simple and rapid colorimetric method for phytate determination. *J. Agric. Food Chem.* 28: 1313–1315.

Liu, H. and White, P.J. 1992. Temperature stability of soybean oils with altered fatty acid composition. *J. Am. Oil Chem. Soc.* 69: 533–537.

Liu, H., Biliaderis, C.G., Przybylski, R. and Eskin, N.A.M. 1993. Phase transition of canola oil sediment. *J. Am. Oil Chem. Soc.* 70: 441–448.

Liu, H., Biliaderis, C.G., Przybylski, R. and Eskin, N.A.M. 1994. Effects of crystallization conditions on sedimentation in canola oil. *J. Am. Oil Chem. Soc.* 71: 409–415.

Liu, H., Biliaderis, C.G., Przybylski, R. and Eskin, N.A.M. 1995a. Solvent effects on phase transition behaviour of canola oil sediment. *J. Am. Oil Chem. Soc.* 72: 603–608.

Liu, H., Biliaderis, C.G., Przybylski, R. and Eskin, N.A.M. 1995b. Physical behaviour and composition of low and high-melting fractions of canola oil sediment. *Food Chem.* 53: 35–41.

Liu, H., Eskin, N.A.M. and Przybylski, R. 1998. Composition, physicochemical properties, and phase behaviour of canola oil sediment. *Recent Res. Dev. Oil Chem.* 2, Part II, 105–115.

Liu, H., Przybylski, D.K., Eskin, N.A.M. and Biliaderis, C.G. 1996a. Comparison of the composition and properties of canola and sunflower oil sediment with canola seed hull lipids. *J. Am. Oil Chem. Soc.* 73: 493–498.

Liu, H., Przybylski, R. and Eskin, N.A.M. 1996b. Influence of solvent content on phase-transition temperatures of oil sediment and solution viscosity in acetone/canola oil systems. *J. Am. Oil Chem. Soc.* 73: 1137–1141.

Liu, H., Przybylski, R. and Eskin, N.A.M. 1996c. Turbidimetric measurement of haze in canola oil by acetone. *J. Am. Oil Chem. Soc.* 73: 1557–1560.

Liu, H., Przybylski, R., Eskin, N.A.M. and Biliaderis, C.G. 1995c. Molecular origin, phase transitions, and formation mechanism of sediment in refined canola oil. *Proc. 9th Intern. Rapeseed Congress, Cambridge, England.* Vol. 3, 894–896.

Lu, S.-Y., Kim, S., Eskin, N.A.M., Johnson, S. and Latta, M. 1987. Changes in phytase activity and phytate during the germination of six canola cultivars. *J. Food Sci.* 52: 173–175.

Morton, I.D. and Chidley, J.E. 1988. Methods and equipment in frying. In *Frying of Food: Principles, Changes, New Approaches*, eds G. Varela, A.E. Bender, and I.D. Morton, Ellis Harwood Ltd., (Chichester). pp. 37–51.

Mounts, T.L., Warner, K. and List, G.R. 1994. Performance evaluation of hexane-extracted oils from genetically modified soybeans. *J. Am. Oil Chem. Soc.* 71: 157–161.

Neff, W.E., Mounts, T.L. and Rinsch, W.M. 1997. Oxidative stability as affected by triacylglycerol composition and structure of purified canola oil triacylglcerols from genetically modified, normal and high stearic and lauric acid canola varieties. *Lebensm. Wiss. U. Technol.* 30: 793–799.

Neff, W.E., Mounts, T.L., Rinsch, W.M., Konishi, H. and El-Agaimy, M.A. 1994. Oxidative stability of purified canola triacylglycerols with altered fatty acid compositions as affected by triacylglycerol composition and structure. *J. Am. Oil Chem. Soc.* 71: 1101–1109.

Normand, L., Eskin, N.A.M. and Przybylski, R. 2001. Effect of tocopherols on the frying stability of regular and modified canola oils. *J. Am. Oil Chem. Soc.* 78: 369–373.

Przybylski, R., Biliaderis, C.G. and Eskin, N.A.M. 1993. Formation and partial characterization of canola oil sediment. *J. Am. Oil Chem. Soc.* 70: 1009–1015.

Przybylski, R. and Eskin, N.A.M. 1991. Phospholipid composition of canola oils during the early stages of processing as measured by TLC with flame ionization detector. *J. Am. Oil Chem. Soc.* 68: 241–245.

Przybylski, R. and Eskin, N.A.M. 1994. Two simplified approaches to the analysis of cereal lipids. *Food Chem.* 51: 231–235.

Przybylski, R. and Eskin, N.A.M. 2006. Minor components and the stability of vegetable oils. *INFORM.* 17(3): 187–189.

Przybylski, R., Malcolmson, L.J., Eskin, N.A.M., Durance-Tod, S., Mickle, J. and Carr, R. 1993b. Stability of low-linolenic acid canola oil to accelerated storage at 60°C. *Lebensmittel u-wiss Technologie.* 26: 205–209.

Stevenson, S.G., Eskin, N.A.M., Hougen, F.W., Jefferey, L. and Vaisey-Genser, M. 1983. Quality evaluation of canola frying fat. *Proc. Intern. Rapeseed Congress., France.* Vol. II, pp. 1678–1683.

Stevenson, S.G., Jefferey, L., Vaisey-Genser, M., Fyfe, B., Hougen, F.W. and Eskin, N.A.M. 1984a. Performance of canola and soybean fats in extended frying. *Can. Inst. Food Sci. Techno. J.* 17: 187–194.

Stevenson, S.G., Vaisey-Genser, M. and Eskin, N.A.M. 1984b. Quality control in the use of deep frying oils. *J. Am. Oil Chem. Soc.* 61: 1102–1108.

Vaisey-Genser, M. and Eskin, N.A.M. 1978. *Canadian Rapeseed Oil: Properties, Processes and Food Quality.* Publication No. 54, Rapeseed Association of Canada, Winnipeg, pp. 40.

Vaisey-Genser, M. and Eskin, N.A.M. 1979a. *L'huille de Canola: Properties Traitment et Qualites Alimentaires.* Bulletin No. 55, Rapeseed Association of Canada, Winnipeg, pp. 40.

Vaisey-Genser, M. and Eskin, N.A.M. 1979b. *Canola oil: Processes and Food Quality.* Publication No. 55, Rapeseed Association of Canada, Winnipeg, pp. 40.

Vaisey-Genser, M. and Eskin, N.A.M. 1980. *Canola-Ol. Bescgaffenheiten, herstellungsverfahren und lebensmittel-qualitat.* Publication No. 55. Canola Council of Canada. pp. 40.

Vaisey-Genser, M. and Eskin, N.A.M. 1982. *Canola Oil: Properties and Performance.* Publication No. 60, Canola Council of Canada, Winnipeg, pp. 50.

Vaisey-Genser, M. and Eskin, N.A.M. 1983. *Aceite Canola. Propiedades y Funcions.* Publication N. 60. Canola Council of Canada, pp. 40.

Vaisey-Genser, M. and Eskin, N.A.M. 1987. *Canola Oil: Properties and Performance.* Revised edition. Publication No. 60. Canola Council of Canada, pp. 50.

Warner, K. and Mounts, T.L. 1993. Frying stability of soybean and canola oil with modified fatty acid compositions. *J. Am. Oil Chem. Soc.* 70: 983–988.

Warner, K., Orr, L., Parrott, L. and Glynn, M. 1994. Effects of frying oil composition on potato chip stability. *J. Am. Oil Chem. Soc.* 71: 1117–1121.

Wu, J., Przybylski, R. and Eskin, N.A.M. 2006. Rapid method for assessing the quality of breeder size oilseed samples. Abstract. *96th Annual Conference of the American Oil Chemists' Society*, Cincinnati, USA.

Xu, X-Q., Tan, V.H., Palmer, M., White, K. and Salisbury, P. 1999. Chemical and physical analyses and sensory evaluation of six deep-frying oils. *J. Am. Oil Chem. Soc.* 76: 1091–1099.

Zambiazi, R.C. and Przybylski, R. 1998. Effect of endogenous minor components on the oxidative stability of vegetable oils. *Lipid. Technol.* 10: 58–62.

FURTHER READING

Daun, J., Hickling and Eskin, N.A.M, D. 2011. *Canola: Chemistry, Production, Processing and Utilization.* American Oil Chemists' (AOCS) Press, Urbana, IL, pp. 370.

Eskin, N.A.M. and McDonald, B.E. 2000. Canola oil. In *Encyclopedia of Food Science and Technology*, 2nd edition (M. Francis, ed.). John Wiley & Sons, New York, pp. 248–262.

Eskin, N.A.M. and Przybylski, R. 2003. *Rapeseed/Canola Oil. Encyclopedia of Food Science and Nutrition*, Academic Press, New York, pp. 4911–4916.

Przybylski, R., Mag, T., Eskin, N.A.M. and McDonald, B.E. 2005. *Canola oil.* Chapter 2 in *Bailey Industrial Oil and Fat Products*, 7th edition (F. Shahidi, editor-in-chief), Vol. 6, John Wiley & Sons, Inc., New York, pp. 135–195.

2 An Update on Characterization and Bioactivities of Sinapic Acid Derivatives

Ayyappan Appukuttan Aachary
and Usha Thiyam-Holländer

CONTENTS

2.1 Introduction ... 21
2.2 Distribution of Sinapine and Related Compounds in Brassica ... 23
2.3 Formation of Canolol ... 24
2.4 Quantification and Characterization of Sinapine ... 25
2.5 Synthesis and Estimation of Canolol ... 25
2.6 Antioxidant Activity of Sinapine ... 27
2.7 Antioxidant Activity of Canolol ... 28
2.8 Bioactivities of Sinapine, Sinapic Acid ... 29
2.8.1 Effects on Cell Permeability ... 29
2.8.2 Neuroprotective Effects ... 29
2.8.3 Effects on Nutrient Digestibility and Growth ... 30
2.8.4 Anxiolytic Effects ... 31
2.9 Bioactivities of Canolol ... 32
2.9.1 Antimutagenic Activities ... 32
2.9.2 Anticancerous Effects ... 32
2.9.3 Protective Effects on Damages due to Oxidative Stress ... 33
2.10 Conclusion and Future Perspectives ... 34
Acknowledgements ... 34
References ... 35

2.1 INTRODUCTION

Phenolic compounds are an inherent part of our dietary consumption through the large ingestion of fruits, vegetables and plants. Phenolic compounds are also part of several plant-based pharmaceuticals, functional foods, nutraceuticals and other natural products. Special attention has been paid to phenolic compounds which exhibit protection against coronary heart disease and carcinogenesis due to the ever-increasing incidences of these conditions. *Brassica napus* L., spp. *oleifera* commonly known as rapeseed is one among the 100 species in the *Brassica* genus and is an excellent source of phenolic antioxidants. However, the use of *B. napus* for human or animal consumption is limited by the presence of erucic acid and glucosinolates considered toxic for many years until now. In the 1970s, very intensive breeding programs produced high-quality varieties that were significantly lower in erucic and glucosinolates. Rapeseed '00' denominates the reduction in erucic and glucosinolate levels. The term 'canola' refers to those varieties of *B. napus* that meet low levels of erucic acid (2%) and glucosinolates (<30 μg/g). A historical perspective and in-depth information on 'double zero' rapeseed and the term 'canola' is presented in Chapters 1 and 6.

An impressive and growing number of bioactive compounds have been identified that have potentially important health benefits. These compounds can act as antioxidants, enzyme inhibitors and inducers, inhibitors of receptor activities, and inducers and inhibitors of gene expression, among other actions. Antioxidants are emerging as prophylactic and therapeutic agents. Antioxidants are substances which counteract oxidative stress, which is defined as an imbalance between oxidants and antioxidants in favour of the oxidants, potentially leading to damage (Sies, 1997). The oxidative stress is caused by highly reactive molecules or chemical species containing unpaired electrons known as free radicals. These can greatly reduce the adverse damage due to oxidants by crumbling them before they react with biologic targets, preventing chain reactions or preventing the activation of oxygen to highly reactive products (Azzi et al., 2004). Dietary antioxidants are 'substances which can (sacrificially) scavenge reactive oxygen/nitrogen to stop radical chain reactions, or can inhibit the reactive oxidants from being formed in the first place' (Huang et al., 2005, p. 1842). Fruit and vegetable juices are predominately rich sources of polyphenols and carotenoids, and these constituents act as antioxidants. Brassica plants and oilseeds canola, mustard and sunflower are potential rich sources of naturally occurring phenolic compounds such as sinapic acid derivatives and chlorogenic acid derivatives. Rapeseed contains more phenolic compounds than most of the other oilseeds (Naczk et al., 1998).

Sinapine, sinapic acid and recently canolol are potent antioxidants as demonstrated by various *in vitro* assays relevant to food products. Chapter 17 outlines the role of canolol for use in frying. Research conducted in our laboratory in the past 9 years indicates that phenolics are retained in the meal in significant amounts when the oil is pressed from the seeds. Thus, we have aimed for and further investigated extractability and tested the extracts rich in phenolics in food relevant model systems. In addition to the meal, some of these phenolics are also found in crude rapeseed oil (Koski et al., 2003) and canola oil. The most significant of these phenolic compounds in rapeseed and canola is sinapine, the choline ester of sinapic acid (Kozlowska et al., 1990) in the seed and meal. Sinapic acid in rapeseed and canola also exists as the glucosidic ester, glucopyranosyl sinapate (Amarowicz and Shahidi, 1994). Studies indicate that the main phenolic compounds in rapeseed meal are sinapine while the sinapic acid was also found with one-tenth that of sinapine (Naczk et al., 1998). Typically the amount of sinapic acid derivatives in rapeseed meal varies between 6390 and 18370 μg/g depending on the variety of oilseed plant and the oil-processing method (Kozlowska et al., 1990). This chapter summarized the knowledge related to the bioactivities of these phenolics.

2.2 DISTRIBUTION OF SINAPINE AND RELATED COMPOUNDS IN BRASSICA

Sinapic acid, an important hydroxycinnamic acid is the most significant phenolic compound in rapeseed and forms 70.2–85.4% of free phenolic acids in defatted canola meals. Esterified forms of these phenolic acids constitute about 99% of total phenolics in rapeseed flour of which the sinapine, the choline ester of sinapic acid, is the main ester. A phenolic glucoside namely glucopyranosyl sinapate is also reported in canola (Amarowicz and Shahidi, 1994). Figure 2.1 shows the structures of sinapic acid, sinapine and glucopyranosyl sinapate.

The Shikimate/phenylpropanoid pathway in Brassica plants is responsible for the synthesis of sinapate which is later converted into a broad spectrum of *O*-ester conjugates (Milkowski and Strack, 2010). It is reported that 1-*O*-sinapoylglucose is the first major compound produced in this pathway by an enzyme known as UDP-glucose:sinapate glucosyltransferase during seed development and is later transformed to sinapine by sinapoylglucose:choline (Milkowski and Strack, 2010). The physiological significance of sinapine is that it functions as a storage molecule for the immediate supply of choline for biosynthesis of phosphatidylcholine in young seedlings. Due to limited variation in seed sinapine content within the assortment of *B. napus* cultivars, low sinapine lines cannot be generated by conventional breeding giving rise to genetic engineering of sinapate ester metabolism as a promising means. The recent trends in the identification of genes involved in sinapate ester metabolism and characterization of the encoded enzymes have been reviewed by

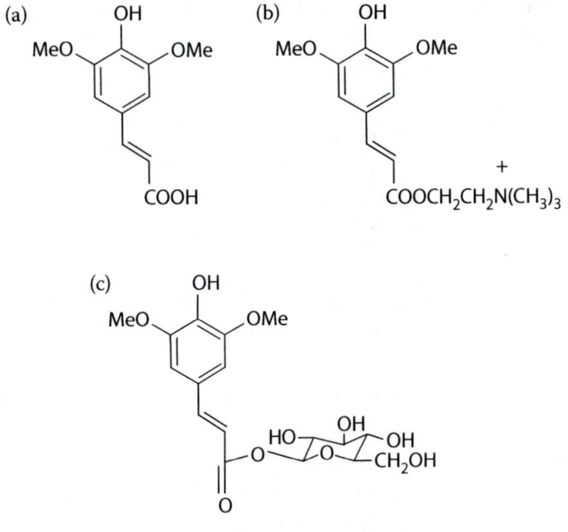

FIGURE 2.1 Structures of (a) sinapic acid, (b) sinapine and (c) sinapoyl glucose identified from rapeseed.

Milkowski and Strack (2010). The evolution of sinapate ester metabolism and strategies of targeted metabolic engineering, designed to generate low-sinapate ester lines of *B. napus,* have been discussed.

Brassica is not the only source of sinapine and related compounds. Bouchereau et al. (1991) investigated the total contents of sinapine in seeds of cruciferous species belonging to *Arabis, Brassica, Cakile, Diplotaxs, Eruca, Hesperis, Matthiola, Raphanobrassica, Raphanus* and *Sïnapis* and detected sinapine in many of these groups of plants. The distribution patterns of sinapine in these plants are genus-characteristic and the capacity of plants to accumulate and store sinapine in seeds is highly variable within the genus *Brassica*. Similarly, the distribution of sinapine in Semen Sinapis Albae, Semen Brassicae Junceae, Semen Raphani and Semen Lepidii was also reported (Liu et al., 2006). It is suggested that the environmental conditions influence the aromatic choline ester content in Brassica. On a similar line, Aires et al. (2011) analysed the biological role of six different Brassica vegetables (*Brassica oleracea* L. and *Brassica rapa* L.) as a natural source of antioxidants.

2.3 FORMATION OF CANOLOL

Canolol or 4-vinylsyringol is not reported to be a naturally occurring phenol in rapeseed, canola and other Brassica plants. Canolol was isolated from crude canola oil and Wakamatsu et al. (2005) designated it canolol. The chemical structure of canolol was determined to be 4-vinyl-2,6-dimethoxyphenol (Figure 2.2). Among various compounds identified from canola oil, 4-vinylsyringol is a highly active antioxidant and potent lipidperoxyl radical scavenger (Koski et al., 2003; Wakamatsu et al., 2005) traced to be formed due to heat treatment while pressing and extracting canola. This highly potent antioxidant molecule exhibits antimutagenic properties (Koski et al., 2003; Kuwahara et al., 2004; Vuorela et al., 2004, 2005a,b; Wakamatsu et al., 2005) and interestingly, the antimutagenic potency of canolol is higher than that of α-tocopherol and flavonoids (Kuwahara et al., 2004). The amount of canolol in crude canola oil was approximately 200 ppm (Wakamatsu, 2001; Tsunehiro et al., 2002).

Canolol is formed by the elevated temperatures arising during the pressing of rapeseed (Koski et al., 2003) or during roasting of seeds (Wakamatsu et al., 2005). Zacchi and Eggers (2008) reported the effect of temperatures on the concentration of minor compounds (polyphenols) during thermal conditioning of pre-treated seed, and its influence on the oil and the oxidative stability. Thus, the food value of the rapeseed and rapeseed oil may be enhanced by elevating the canolol content through press processing or the roasting of rapeseed before pressing (Spielmeyer et al., 2009). The samples of unfiltered rapeseed oil of the first and second press were analysed

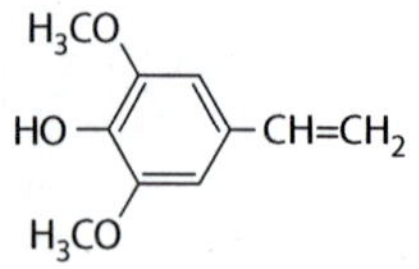

H_3CO

HO — [benzene ring] — $CH{=}CH_2$

H_3CO

FIGURE 2.2 Molecular structure of canolol or 4-vinylsyringol.

and the latter was characterized by higher temperatures and pressure. The result indicated a significant difference between the first and second press process with respect to canolol content in the oil and suggested the potential effects of the conditions of the press process on the canolol content of the oil.

Because of its potent bioactive potential, the increase of canolol content in rapeseed oil would theoretically produce oil with enhanced food value and as well as longer shelf life (Spielmeyer et al., 2009). Canolol is thermally unstable, even though it is being produced from sinapic acid at higher temperatures. An exponential decrease in the canolol content from 81.4 to 11.0 μg/g in oil was observed when it is exposed to a heat treatment up to a temperature of 180°C for 20 min.

Recently, Harbaum-Piayda et al. (2010) demonstrated the possibility of new compounds such as *cis*- and *trans*-diastereomers of 4-vinylsyringol dimer [*cis*-4,6-dimethoxy-5-hydroxy-1-methyl-3-(30,50-dimethoxy-40-hydroxyphenyl) indane and *trans*-4,6-dimethoxy-5-hydroxy-1-methyl-3-(30,50-dimethoxy-40-hydroxyphenyl) indane] and the vinylsyringol trimer in commercial rapeseed oils, as well as in a commercial by-product of oil refining, the deodistillate. The newly identified canolol dimer was present in the deodistillate of processed rapeseed oil in significant amounts (~3.50 g/kg). Trace amounts of phenylindane was also detected in commercial rapeseed oils. According to Harbaum-Piayda et al. (2010), this newly identified phenylindane compound had a high antioxidative potential and stressed its potential as an important phenolic compound to add value to the commercial deodistillate and rapeseed oils.

2.4 QUANTIFICATION AND CHARACTERIZATION OF SINAPINE

Different methods (Table 2.1) have been reported for the quantification and characterization of sinapine and related compounds (Ismail and Eskin, 1979; Fenwick, 1981; Ismail et al., 1981; Thies, 1991; Lacki and Duvnjak, 1996; Wang et al., 1998; Amarowicz and Kolodziejczyk, 2001; Li and El Rassi, 2002; Zhou et al., 2005; Liu et al., 2006; Khattab et al., 2010; Huang et al., 2011). With respect to its electrochemical properties, the sinapine gives an electrochemical response at a pyrolytic graphite electrode (Zhou et al., 2005). The peak current in the cyclic voltammogram is linear in the concentration range from 1.9×10^{-6} to 2.5×10^{-4} mol/L and the limit of detection is 9.9×10^{-7} mol/L. This highly selective, sensitive and stable electrochemical method can be applied to accurately detect the sinapine content of medicinal plants and oil seeds.

2.5 SYNTHESIS AND ESTIMATION OF CANOLOL

4-Vinylsyringol content of rapeseed can be increased through the decarboxylation of sinapic acid via roasting treatments (Spielmeyer et al., 2009). Among the various roasting conditions evaluated, 160°C was found to be optimum for the canolol formation and showed an increase in canolol content by a factor of 120 in relation to the unroasted sample. Previously, it has been reported that 4-vinylguaiacol and 4-vinylphenol are formed from ferulic and *p*-coumaric acids during the heating of soyabean flour (Olsen and Adler-Nissen, 1979).

TABLE 2.1
Various Analytical Methods for Sinapine and Related Compounds

No.	Method	Remarks	Reference
1.	Chromatography	Reversed-phase high-performance liquid chromatography (RP-HPLC) to detect sinapine from selected cruciferous plants	Liu et al. (2006)
2.	Combined chemical/ enzymatic method	Alkali treatment of sinapine to choline and sinapic acid followed by enzymatic hydrolysis of choline to betaine by choline oxidase	Li and El Rassi (2002)
3.	Chromatography	Ion-exchange column purification procedure using CM-Sephadex C25 to estimate sinapine content in the seed or meal	Wang et al. (1998)
4.	Capillary electrophoresis	Used for separating 1-*O*-glycopyranosyl sinapate from rapeseed	Amarowicz and Kolodziejczyk (2001)
5.	Spectrometry	Liquid-assisted surface desorption atmospheric pressure chemical ionization mass spectrometry (DAPCI-MS) to detect sinapine in radish taproot tissue	Huang et al. (2011)
6.	Calorimetric method	Sinapine formed a coloured complex with titanium tetrachloride	Ismail and Eskin (1979)
7.	Calorimetric method	Based on the yellow colour of sinapine in alkaline media and the weakening of the intensity of the red coloured Fe-sulphosalicylic acid complex in the presence of phytic acid.	Thies (1991)
8.	Enzymatic method	Enzymatic reduction of sinapic acid ester content in canola meal using polyphenol oxidase from the fungus *T. versicolor*	Lacki and Duvnjak (1996)

4-Vinylphenols, useful compounds for industrial applications, were obtained by decarboxylation of 4-hydroxycinnamic acids under microwave irradiation in the presence of 1,8-diazabicyclo[5.4.0]undec-7-ene (DBU) as base and basic aluminium oxide as solid support (Bernini et al., 2007). This methodology can be applied for the synthesis of canolol. Terpinc et al. (2011) prepared 4-vinylphenol, 4-vinylguaiacol, 4-vinylsyringol and 4-vinylcatechol by thermal decarboxylation of the corresponding hydroxycinnamic acids *p*-coumaric, ferulic, sinapic and caffeic acid, respectively, of these 4-vinylsyringol/canolol is more important. LC–MS followed by NMR analysis was used for confirmation of canolol.

Generally, the canolol is analysed by normal-phase HPLC/UV and the structure is confirmed by NMR and MS techniques. The component which showed the best radical scavenging activity in the polar fraction was obtained in the study conducted by Koski et al. (2003). The authors performed NMR spectrometry and mass spectrometry and identified as vinylsyringol (4-hydroxy-3,5-dimethoxystyrene, or 2,6-dimethoxy-4-vinylphenol). This compound exhibited a UV spectrum characteristic of benzoic acids, with an absorption maximum occurring at 275 nm. The compound also exhibited a strong fluorescence, with an excitation maximum occurring at 273 nm and an emission maximum at 328 nm.

Wakamatsu et al. (2005) were successful in determining the chemical structure of canolol. They confirmed the absence of neither nitrogen nor sulphur in the molecular structure of canolol using elemental analysis. The molecular mass of canolol is estimated to be 180 using a high-resolution MS of atmospheric pressure chemical ionization (APCI) plus LC/MS method. Based on these results, Wakamatsu et al. (2005) proposed the structure of canolol as $C_{10}H_{12}O_3$ and with the help of ^{1}H-NMR data, the authors concluded that this active component is 4-vinyl-2,6-dimethoxyphenol. Canolol had absorption peaks at 218 and 269 nm. The molecular extinction coefficient in water was 29,000 at 218 nm and 13,000 at 269 nm. Canolol exhibited a fluorescence emission maximum at 325 nm which was used for quantifying upon HPLC (Wakamatsu et al., 2005).

2.6 ANTIOXIDANT ACTIVITY OF SINAPINE

In biological systems, an antioxidant can be defined as any substance that, in low concentration compared with the oxidizable substrate, significantly delays or prevents oxidation of that substrate. The substrate, that is, the oxidizable compound, is usually a lipid, but can also be a protein, DNA, or carbohydrate. In the case of lipid oxidation, the main mechanism of antioxidants is to act as radical chain-breakers. Another mechanism is to act as preventive antioxidant oxygen scavenging or blocking the pro-oxidant effects by binding proteins that contain catalytic metal sites (Frankel and Meyer, 2000).

Several studies have shown that phenolic compounds have antioxidant properties. According to Wanasundara and Shahidi (1994), most powerful antioxidative component of rapeseed meal is glucosyl sinapate, the glucose ester of sinapic acid. Sinapic acid itself is an effective scavenger of the peroxyl radical (Natella et al., 1999) and inhibits oxidation in various model systems, including bulk methyl linoleate (MeLo) (Cuvelier et al., 1992), emulsified MeLo (Pekkarinen et al., 1999), methyl esters of lard and sunflower oil (Marinova and Yanishlieva, 1994) and low-density lipoprotein *in vitro* (Natella et al., 1999). Wanasundara et al. (1996) indicated that rapeseed phenolic extracts with sinapine as the main phenolic compound could act as excellent antioxidants for the oxidation of liposomes and low density lipid particles. This indicates that sinapine is the major contributor to the antioxidant activity. Their results implied that in addition to the total phenolic content, other compounds contribute to overall antioxidant activity of rapeseeds.

Amarowicz et al. (2000) and Matthäus (2002) investigated the effect of rapeseed phenolics on radical scavenging. The antioxidant activity of ethanolic (95%) extract of rapeseed meal towards the oxidation of rapeseed oil was better than that of some widely used synthetic antioxidants (Wanasundara and Shahidi, 1994). Phenolic compounds present in crude rapeseed oil have also shown antioxidant properties (Koski et al., 2003) in bulk and emulsified methyl linoleate and lecithin–liposome systems. Amarowics et al. (2003) investigated the antioxidant activity of phenolic fractions of rapeseed (total three fractions) using a β-carotene–linoleate model system and enhanced chemiluminescence and photochemiluminescence methods. A measure of 176 mg/g of total phenolics was present in fraction III; however, UV spectra indicated that derivatives of phenolic acids were dominant in all fractions.

Rapeseed phenolics isolated by Vuorela et al. (2004) were tested for radical scavenging and for liposome and low-density lipoprotein (LDL) model systems. The inhibition of hexanal and conjugated diene hydroperoxides formation was reported (>90% and >80%, respectively). All isolates also exhibited inhibition of LDL particles oxidation by >90%. The antioxidant activity of methanol and acetone extracts of canola hulls in a β-carotene-linoleate model system was comparable to that displayed by butylated hydroxyanisole (Naczk et al., 2005). These extracts showed more than 95% scavenging effects (at 40 μ/assay on DPPH radical). Vuorela et al. (2005a,b) indicated that rapeseed phenolics were excellent antioxidants towards oxidation of phosphatidylcholine membrane (liposomes) and rapeseed oil (crude) phenolics were effective radical scavengers (DPPH test). The authors suggested that these phenolic isolates from rapeseed are safe and bioactive for possible food applications including functional foods intended for health benefit.

Investigations on the free-radical-scavenging activity of sinapic acid and sinapine indicate that sinapine had a significant but lower activity as compared to sinapic acid (Thiyam et al., 2006). The experiments indicate that in contrast to tocopherol mixtures addition of sinapic acid causes increasing inhibition of hydroperoxides formation when enhancing the concentration from 50 to 500 μmol/kg oil. Sinapine was not able to inhibit the formation of hydroperoxides, compared to sinapic acid. This indicates that sinapic acid-rich extracts, as compared to sinapine-rich fractions, could better inhibit the lipid oxidation in bulk lipid systems. Rapeseed press cake and proteins contain significant amounts of sinapic acid, in the free and esterified form (Thiyam et al., 2009). Both syringeldehyde and canolol were not found in the investigated protein isolate.

2.7 ANTIOXIDANT ACTIVITY OF CANOLOL

Literature on the antioxidant activity of their 4-vinyl derivatives, especially 4-vinylsyringol or canolol, is scarce as compared to the volumes of parent hydroxycinnamic acids originating from plant and oilseeds. Most of the work done on 4-vinyl derivatives or volatile phenols are in the context of their significance to flavour and at a mild level linked to indirect antioxidant and high shelf life. The presence of volatile phenolic compounds is appreciated in certain beer styles. Values up to 1.45 ppm *p*-coumaric acid, 13.10 ppm ferulic acid, 4.65 ppm sinapic acid, 2.696 ppm 4-vinylphenol and 4.373 ppm vinylguaiacol have been encountered in beer. However, there is no report on the presence of canolol in beer (Wackerbauer and Kramer, 1982). Canolol, as a scavenger of the DPPH radical, is highly effective (Koski et al., 2003; Vuorela et al., 2004, 2005a,b) and inhibits protein and lipid oxidation (Vuorela et al., 2005a,b). Kuwahara et al. (2004) showed its scavenging capacity against the endogenous mutagen peroxynitrite. Similarly, Wakamatsu et al. (2005) exhibited its peroxyl radical-scavenging activity. Reports on systematic evaluation of the antioxidant properties of canolol under different conditions are lacking.

Koski et al. (2003) showed that canolol is attributed to the better stability of the crude rapeseed oils and the polar fraction containing vinylsyringol showed lipid antioxidative activity comparable to that of gamma-tocopherol. Furthermore, vinylsyringol appears to account for most of the detected total phenol content.

Canolol was prepared by thermal decarboxylation of the sinapic acid (Terpinc et al., 2011) and evaluated its antioxidant potential, in scavenging the alkylperoxyl radical generated in an emulsion system. Canolol revealed weaker antioxidant activity in a homogeneous polar medium than the sinapic acid. In the emulsion system, the activity for canolol was higher than was the activity of their corresponding phenolic acid. Terpinc et al. (2011) also showed that the canolol responds successfully to different radical or oxidant sources. The authors also assessed whether decarboxylation of hydroxycinnamic acid has any effect on its antioxidant potential. The phenolic acids and their decarboxylation products showed different antioxidant activity, which is attributed to their different structural characteristics, substitutions on the aromatic ring, partitioning properties between lipid and aqueous phase and intermolecular hydrogen bond interactions. Recently, Azadmard-Damirchi et al. (2010) suggested the use of microwave to treat rapeseeds before extraction by press, and the authors reported a relatively good recovery of oil with a high stability and high amount of nutraceuticals. The results also indicated that the new process promotes formation of canolol.

A very recent study by Galano et al. (2011) gives insights into the antioxidant activity mechanism of canolol, in aqueous and lipid solutions. Interestingly, canolol is predicted to react about 3.6 times faster in lipid media than in aqueous solution. The OOH radical scavenger activity of canolol is predicted and it is similar to that of carotenes but higher than that of allicin and melatonin. The predicted overall rate coefficients in aqueous and lipid media are 2.5×10^6 and 6.8×10^5/Ms, respectively. This is the first time that the branching ratios for the different channels of reaction are reported. The main channel of reaction was identified to be the hydrogen atom transfer from the phenolic moiety in canolol and it contributes to the overall reactivity of canolol towards •OOH by more than 99%, regardless of the polarity of the environment.

2.8 BIOACTIVITIES OF SINAPINE, SINAPIC ACID

2.8.1 Effects on Cell Permeability

There is only a single reference on the effects of rapeseed/canola phenolics on cell permeability. Satu et al. (2005) indicated that the crude rapeseed oil phenolic extract had no significant effect on the permeability of the model drugs. However, rapeseed meal phenolics enhanced the permeability of verapamil and ketoprofen indicating that they may have an impact on drugs and other components being actively transported across the cell membrane.

2.8.2 Neuroprotective Effects

The neuroprotective effects of sinapic acid and sinapine have been reported (Zou et al., 2002; Yang and He, 2008; Kim et al., 2010). Zou et al. (2002) reported that sinapic acid has a peroxy nitrite scavenging effect, and suggested that sinapic acid might play a crucial role in the neuronal protection against the peroxy nitrite-associated diseases. Yun et al. (2008) observed that sinapic acid had an anti-inflammatory effect in RAW264.7 macrophages, due to its suppressions of cyclooxygenase-2, tumor necrosis factor-a and inter leukin-1b expression. Furthermore, sinapic acid exerts an anxiolytic effect via the GABAergic neurotransmitter system in mice (Yoon et al., 2007). Additionally, sinapic acid markedly potentiated GABA currents and reactive IGABA increased to 1.8 times at 1 mM of sinapic acid, suggesting that sinapic acid is potential $GABA_A$ receptor agonist (Yoon et al., 2007). The neurotoxicity induced by glutamate receptor agonist or amyloid b peptide can be blocked by $GABA_A$ receptors activation (Louzada et al., 2004; Paula-Lima et al., 2005). Sinapic acid has a $GABA_A$ receptor agonistic property and free radical scavenging activity.

Kim et al. (2010) investigated the neuroprotective effects of sinapic acid on kainic acid (KA)-induced hippocampal brain damage in mice. Oral administration of sinapic acid (10 mg/kg) showed an anticonvulsant effect on KA-induced seizure-like behaviour and attenuated KA-induced neuronal cell death in the CA1 and CA3 hippocampal regions when administered as late as 6 h after KA. In addition, the effect of sinapic acid administered immediately after KA has been blocked by flumazenil, a $GABA_A$ antagonist, but not the effect of sinapic acid administered 6 h after KA. Reduced levels of reactive gliosis, inducible nitric oxide synthase expression, and nitro tyrosine formation in the hippocampus were followed by this. In the passive avoidance task, KA-induced memory impairments were ameliorated by sinapic acid. Kim et al. (2010) concluded that the potential therapeutic effect of sinapic acid is due to its attenuation of KA-induced neuronal damage in the brain via its anti-convulsive activity through $GABA_A$ receptor activation and radical scavenging activity.

Previous studies have clearly demonstrated that sinapine is a potent free radical scavenger and a nature anti-radiation chemical. The work by Yang and He (2008) is primary research for the neuroprotective effect of sinapine. They established the neuroprotective effects of sinapine against $Na_2S_2O_4$-induced toxicity of PC12 cells. The results showed that pretreatment with sinapine significantly reduced the cell death of PC12 cells. The sinapine reduced the apoptotic rate, LDH release, the lipid peroxidation and mitochondrial membrane potential depolarization. These findings provide insights into the role of sinapine as a protective molecule against the neurotoxicity in PC12 cells. Sinapine inhibited the loss of mitochondrial membrane potential and reduced the apoptosis rate (Yang and He, 2008). Additional experimental and clinical studies will be required to assess the potential for clinical application of sinapine or its derivatives.

2.8.3 Effects on Nutrient Digestibility and Growth

Two experiments were conducted to delineate the effect of dietary sinapic acid on broiler chickens, in terms of performance, toxicity and nutrient digestibility (Qiao et al., 2008). In the first experiment on 80 male broiler chicks with feeding of sinapic acid, performance from 0 to 18 days of age and the relative size of all the internal organs and intestines were not affected by dietary treatment. The result also implied that there was no damage to skeletal muscle, heart muscle, liver, kidneys, or brain as assumed from the no change of on the serum activity of creatine kinase and lactate dehydrogenase.

Qiao et al. (2008) in their second experiment investigated the effect of sinapic acid on nutrient retention and the retention of sinapic acid in the digestive tract of male broiler chicks. Dietary sinapic acid at the 0.025% level increased feed intake, and resulted in weight gain. However, dietary sinapic acid did not affect the relative weights of bursa of Fabricius, liver, kidney, or digestive tract, nitrogen-corrected AME and protein digestibility. The apparent ideal digestibility of Met, Thr, Ser, Pro, Gly, Ala and Phe followed a negative linear relationship with dietary sinapic acid level and it implied that sinapic acid may have a negative effect on amino acid digestibility at higher levels.

Previously, Vermorel et al. (1987) studied the effects of sinapine and other phenolic compounds on food intake and nutrient utilization in growing rats. The intake of sinapine and other phenolic compounds significantly reduced the dry matter intake and live weight gain of the rats during the first 8 days of feeding study. However, after this adaptation period, their performances were similar to those of the control group. Later, Qiao and Classen (2003) investigated the impact of dietary rapeseed meal and sinapine on broiler chickens. Sinapine bisulphate and sinapine ethanol extract did not affect feed intake and performance of broiler chickens. Sinapine bisulphate increased diet apparent metabolizable energy (AME) while sinapine ethanol extracts increased diet AME and faecal protein digestibility in comparison with the control diet.

Qiao and Classen (2003) also reported minor effects caused by dietary treatment of sinapine on tissue measurements. The authors proposed that the hind gut might be an important metabolic site for sinapine because all the diets containing sinapine reduced the empty weight of caeca. The ileal digestibility of SNP was 35–42%, 27–38% and 30–46% for sinapine bisulphate, sinapine ethanol extract and rapeseed meal sinapine, respectively, while faecal digestibility values were 68–72%, 65–75% and 54–63% for the same treatment groups. A major metabolic pathway of sinapine via hydrolysis into sinapic acid and choline in the digestive tract was identified.

In an earlier study, Josefesson and Uppström (1976) evaluated the influence of sinapine on the nutritional value of rapeseed meal and white mustard meal. However, the effect of sinapine was not highly significant. In another *in vivo* study, Pearson et al. (1980) found that sinapine did not reduce the ability of chicks or laying hens to oxidize trimethylamine. Since the amount included in the diet was similar to that which would be provided by a diet containing 10% rapeseed meal, it was concluded that sinapine is not involved in the depression of TMA oxidation that occurs when the meal is fed and acts solely as a source of TMA in the consequent production of egg taint.

2.8.4 Anxiolytic Effects

Sinapic acid is a phenylpropanoid and with the exception of its antioxidant activities, the pharmacological properties of sinapic acid have been rarely reported. Yoon et al. (2007) characterized the putative anxiolytic-like properties of sinapic acid using an elevated plus-maze (EPM) and hole-board test. Interestingly, sinapic acid (4 mg/kg, p.o.) significantly increased the percentages of time spent in the open arms of the elevated plus-maze test. The number of head-dips at 4 mg/kg was also significantly increased in the hole-board test by sinapic acid. It is also observed that the anxiolytic-like properties of sinapic acid examined in the elevated plus-maze test were blocked by flumazenil or bicuculline, which are $GABA_A$ antagonists. The GABA current in single cortical neurons has been significantly potentiated by the sinapic acid in a dose-dependant manner. These results suggested that anxiolytic-like effects of sinapic acid are mediated via $GABA_A$ receptors and potentiating Cl^- currents (Yoon et al., 2007).

2.9 BIOACTIVITIES OF CANOLOL

Koski et al. (2003) were the first to report the antioxidant activity of canolol and reported that its lipid protective activity is similar to that of γ-tocopherol. Shortly after, Kuwahara et al. (2004) found that canolol reduces intracellular oxidative stress-induced cellular apoptosis to a significant extent, in a dose-dependent manner. These authors also found that canolol prevents DNA strand breakage induced by ONOO•. Wakamatsu et al. (2005) proposed that canolol is more efficient as an alkyl peroxyl radical scavenger than α-tocopherol, vitamin C, β-carotene, rutin and quercetin. Taking into account that the reactivity of peroxyl radicals is significantly lower than that of other reactive oxygen species (ROS), canolol seems to be a promising chemical agent to prevent and fight oxidative stress. This is a very desirable property because oxidative stress has been associated with the development of a large number of health disorders, such as cancer, cardiovascular disorders, atherosclerosis and Alzheimer's disease.

2.9.1 Antimutagenic Activities

In their study, Kuwahara et al. (2004) reported that canolol inhibited mutation of *S. typhimurium* strain TA102 of 18% at a concentration of 8 μM. The anti-peroxyl radical activity and protection against apoptotic cell death induced by treatment with *Tert*-butyl hydroperoxide (*t*-BuOOH) were evaluated with human colon cancer SW480 cells (Fang et al., 2002, 2003). Canolol at concentrations of 5.6–56 μM suppressed pegylated zinc protoporphyrin (PEGZnPP) (25 μM)-induced oxidative stress to a significant degree. Even though *t*-BuOOH at 50 μM caused about 33% cell death; interestingly about 50% of this apoptosis was suppressed by 56 μM canolol (Kuwahara et al., 2004). However, at higher concentration (560 μM), the canolol was toxic.

The DNA strand breakage induced by the endogenous oxidant $ONOO^-$ has been prevented by canolol and it followed in a dose-dependent manner. Antioxidative effect or terminations of oxy radical-induced strand breaks are responsible to this. The capacity of canolol to suppress ONOO-induced cell damage, killing of bacteria and mammalian cells and bacterial mutation as well as plasmid DNA strand breakage have been established with this study (Kuwahara et al., 2004). Canolol prevented oxidative stress-induced cellular apoptosis to a significant extent in SW480 cells.

2.9.2 Anticancerous Effects

Oxidative stress is linked to gastric carcinogenesis because of its ability to damage DNA. Cao et al. (2008) examined antioxidative and anti-inflammatory effects of canolol on *Helicobacter pylori*-induced gastritis and gastric carcinogenesis using a Mongolian gerbil model. The results indicated the beneficial effects of canolol. Expression of interleukin-1b (IL-1b), tumour necrosis factor-a (TNF-a), scores for cyclooxygenase-2 (COX-2) and inducible nitric oxide synthase (iNOS) mRNA in the gastric mucosa, and serum 8-hydroxy-20-deoxyguanosine (8-OHdG), anti-*H. pylori* IgG and gastrin levels were also significantly lower in canolol-treated groups. In addition to this, the incidence of gastric adenocarcinoma was markedly reduced in canolol-treated group compared to the control group. These data imply without doubt that canolol to be effective for suppressing inflammation, gastric epithelial cell proliferation and gastric carcinogenesis in *H. pylori*-infected Mongolian gerbils. Importantly, canolol appears to suppress induction of mRNAs for inflammatory cytokines. In conclusion, oral administration of canolol significantly reduced anti-*H. pylori* IgG antibody titres and gastrin levels in serum, without apparently suppressing *H. pylori* colonization (Cao et al., 2008). A lack of any type of direct correlation between anti-*H. pylori* IgG antibody titres and number of colonies was previously reported by Murakami et al. (2005).

Canola oil is conventional cooking oil in many countries. The canolol content of crude canola oil (220–1200 ppm) could provide doses similar to that used in a study by Cao et al. (2008). It should be noted, however, that the concentration in refined canola oil is significantly lower (Wakamatsu et al., 2005) so that alternative strategies have to be proposed. Supplementation of canola oil with extracted or synthesized canolol will be an effective method to enrich and add value to the oils.

An anti-inflammatory agent or cancer-preventive agent comprising canolol has been developed (Maeda et al., 2009, US Patent). According to the inventor's claim, this anti-inflammatory agent is suitable for treatment of one or more diseases selected from the group consisting of gastro-duodenitis, gastro-duodenal ulcer, gastritis, bronchitis, rheumatism, hepatitis, colitis, conjunctivitis, pneumonitis, pancreatitis, stomatitis, pharyngitis and burn. They also claimed that this compound can suppress inflammation by suppression of 8-oxodeoxyguanosine formation, inhibition of COX-2 activity, inhibition of iNOS activity, or suppression of NO production inhibition of cytokine induction.

2.9.3 Protective Effects on Damages due to Oxidative Stress

In the pathogenesis of age-related macular degeneration, the role of oxidative stress damage to retinal pigment epithelial (RPE) cells is highly significant. The protective effect of canolol against oxidative stress-induced cell death in ARPE-19 cells and its underlying mechanism has been reported (Xin et al., 2011). Canolol showed relatively high safety for ARPE-19 cells and recovered the cell death caused by *t*-BuOOH dose dependently at a concentration of 50–200 μM. The *t*-BuOOH-induced intracellular ROS generation has been reduced by the canolol and thus protected ARPE-19 cells from cell apoptosis. After treatment with different concentrations of canolol for 24 h, various markers such as *HO-1*, catalase, *GST-pi* and *Nrf-2* were elevated in ARPE-19 cells. Moreover, the extracellular signal-regulated kinase (ERK) phosphorylation in ARPE-19 cells under the condition has been stimulated by canolol, with or without *t*-BuOOH. The protection of ARPE-19 cells from *t*-BuOOH-induced oxidative damage by canolol and the associated mechanism may be related with the upregulation (activation) of antioxidative enzymes, probably through an ERK-mediated pathway (Xin et al., 2011).

The anti-alkylperoxyl radical activity of canolol is better than that of the well-known antioxidants like vitamin E, vitamin C and quercetin. Eid (2010) investigated antioxidative effects of canolol under oxidative stress *in vivo* using broiler chickens. The result indicated that the body weight gain was significantly decreased by stress (corticosterone treatment), but canolol retained body weight gain under the stress. The breast muscle weight also followed a similar trend. The feed efficiency was decreased significantly under stress, and this effect was minimized by canolol treatment. However, both stress and canolol had no effect on feed consumption. Canolol markedly reduced the markers of lipid peroxidation and oxidative stress and maintained a fairly high level of α-tocopherol concentrations in liver and muscles. Even though, Eid (2010) pointed out the efficacy of canolol to enhance the broiler performance under oxidative stress, further studies are needed to clarify the most effective dose and the possible methods of application.

2.10 CONCLUSION AND FUTURE PERSPECTIVES

Identifying bioactive compounds and establishing their health effects are active areas of global research. The endogenous bioactive principles of canola such as sinapic acid, sinapine and canolol have great potential as therapeutic agents to maintain and improve health and well-being. These minor components with potent antioxidant activity can be incorporated into many food and non-food products. There are, however, several questions that still need to be answered. Data are supportive that sinapine and sinapic acid have been long a part of the human diet through Brassicaceae vegetables. There are reports on the antioxidant and other bioactive attributes of sinapine and sinapic acid in several *in vitro/in vivo* systems. Available experimental evidences support the hypothesis that canolol can offer an opportunity to prevent or mitigate cancer.

Even though encouraging results have been obtained for other plant phenolics in preliminary clinical trials, the data on canolol are limited. More investigations are required to further elucidate the mechanisms involved in the anti-cancerous effects of canolol. Similarly, the neuroprotective effects of sinapine have to be evaluated in new animal models. The observations made in this review and published information on quantification, characterization, evaluation of antioxidant properties and other biological effects of sinapine and canolol give a distinct direction to future research. Furthermore, the challenge of the future exploitation of these benefits into authentic nutrition and health issues remains a challenge. Moreover, the discovery of novel health effects of canola minor components will provide the scientific basis for future efforts to use biotechnology to modify/fortify foods and food components as a means to improve public health.

ACKNOWLEDGEMENTS

The authors thank Canola Council of Canada, Natural Sciences and Engineering Research Council of Canada (NSERC) and Syngenta Crop Protection Inc, Canada, for the financial support. The authors also thank Dr. Michael Eskin, University of Manitoba for the prior review of the manuscript. Gayatri Thiyam is gratefully acknowledged for her skillful literature search and further review for the presentation at the 2010 Canola Workshop that shaped this review.

REFERENCES

Aires A, Fernandes C, Carvalho R, Bennett RN, Saavedra MJ, Rosa EA. 2011. Seasonal effects on bioactive compounds and antioxidant capacity of six economically important Brassica vegetables. *Molecules*, 16(8):6816–6832.

Amarowics R, Raab B, Shahidi F. 2003. Antioxidant activity of phenolic fractions of rapeseed. *Journal of Food Lipids*, 10(1):51–62.

Amarowicz R, Shahidi F. 1994. Chromatographic separation of glucopyranosyl sinapate from canola meal. *Journal of American Oil Chemists Society*, 71:551–552.

Amarowicz R, Kolodziejczyk PP. 2001. Application of capillary electrophoresis for separating 1-*O*-glycopyranosyl sinapate from rapeseed. *Food/Nahrung*, 45:62–63.

Amarowicz R, Naczk M, Shahidi F. 2000. Antioxidant activity of various fractions of nontannin phenolics of canola hulls. *Journal of Agriculture and Food Chemistry*, 48:2755–2759.

Azadmard-Damirchi S, Habibi-Nodeh F, Hesari J, Nemati M, Fathi B. 2010. Effect of pretreatment with microwaves on oxidative stability and nutraceuticals content of oil from rapeseed. *Food Chemistry*, 12:1211–1215.

Azzi A, Davies KJA, Kelly F. 2004. Free radical biology—Terminology and critical thinking. *FEBS Letters*, 558:3–6.

Bernini R, Mincione E, Barontini M, Provenzano G, Setti L. 2007. Obtaining 4-vinylphenols by decarboxylation of natural 4-hydroxycinnamic acids under microwave irradiation. *Tetrahedron*, 63:9663–9667.

Bouchereau A, Hamelin J, Lamour I, Renard M, Larher F. 1991. Distribution of sinapine and related compounds in seeds of Brassica and alliedgenera. *Phytochemistry*, 30(6):1873–1881.

Cao X, Tsukamoto T, Seki T, Tanaka H, Morimura S, Cao L. 2008. 4-Vinyl-2,6-dimethoxyphenol (canolol) suppresses oxidative stress and gastric carcinogenesis in *Helicobacter pylori* infected carcinogen-treated *Mongolian gerbils. International Journal of Cancer*, 122:1445–1454.

Cuvelier ME, Richard H, Berset C. 1992. Comparison of the antioxidative activity of some acid-phenols: Structure—Activity relationship. *Bioscience Biotechnology Biochemistry*, 56:324–325.

Eid YZ. 2010. Novel antioxidant canolol reduces glucocorticoid induced oxidative stress in broiler chickens. *Egyptian Poultry Science*, 30(IV):917–926.

Fang J, Sawa T, Akaike T, Akuta T, Sahoo KS, Greish K, Hamada A, Maeda H. 2003. *In vivo* antitumor activity of pegylated zinc protoporphyrin: Targeted inhibition of heme oxygenase in solid tumor. *Cancer Research*, 63:3567–3574.

Fang J, Sawa T, Akaike T, Maeda H. 2002. Tumor-targeted delivery of polyethylene glycol-conjugated D-amino acid oxidase for antitumor therapy via enzymatic generation of hydrogen peroxide. *Cancer Research*, 62:3138–3143.

Fenwick GR. 1981. The quantitative determination of sinapine using titanium tetrachloride. Comments relating to the specificity of the method. *Food/Nahrung*, 25(8):795–798.

Frankel EN, Meyer AS. 2000. The problems of using one-dimensional methods to evaluate multifunctional food and biological antioxidants. *Journal of Science of Food and Agriculture*, 80:1925–1941.

Galano A, Francisco-Márquez M, Alvarez-Idaboy JR. 2011. Canolol: A promising chemical agent against oxidative stress. *Journal of Physical Chemistry B*, 115(26):8590–8596.

Harbaum-Piayda B, Oehlke K, Sönnichsen FD, Zacchi P, Eggers R, Schwarz K. 2010. New polyphenolic compounds in commercial deodistillate and rapeseed oils. *Food Chemistry*, 123(3):607–615.

Huang D, Luo L, Jiang C, Han J, Wang J, Zhang T, Jiang J, Zhou Z, Chen H. 2011. Sinapine detection in radish tap root using surface desorption atmospheric pressure chemical ionization mass spectrometry. *Journal of Agricultural Food Chemistry*, 59(6):2148–2156.

Huang D, Ou B, Prior RL. 2005. The chemistry behind antioxidant capacity assays. *Journal of Agricultural and Food Chemistry*, 53(6):1841–1856.

Ismail F, Eskin NAM. 1979. A new quantitative procedure for determination of sinapine. *Journal of Agricultural and Food Chemistry*, 27(4):917–918.

Ismail F, Vaisey-Genser M, Fyfe B. 1981. Bitterness and astringency of sinapine and its components. *Journal of Food Science*, 46(4):1241–1244.

Josefsson E, Uppström B. 1976. Influence of sinapine and *p*-hydroxybenzyl glucosinolate on the nutritional value of rape seed and white mustard meals. *Journal of the Science of Food and Agriculture*, 27(5):438–442.

Khattab R, Eskin M, Aliani M, Thiyam U. 2010. Determination of sinapic acid derivatives in canola extracts using high-performance liquid chromatography. *Journal of American Oil Chemists Society*, 87(2):147–155.

Kim DH, Yoon BH, Jung WY, Kim JM, Park SJ, Park DH, Huh Y et al. 2010. Sinapic acid attenuates kainic acid-induced hippocampal neuronal damage in mice. *Neuropharmacology*, 59:20–23

Koski A, Pekkarinen S, Hopia A, Wähälä K, Heinonen M. 2003. Processing of rapeseed oil: Effects on sinapic acid derivative content and oxidative stability. *European Food Research and Technology*, 217:110–114.

Kozlowska H, Naczk M, Shahidi F, Zadernowski R 1990. Phenolic acids and tannins in rapeseed and canola. In: *Canola and Rapeseed. Production, Chemistry, Nutrition and Processing Technology*. Shahidi F (Ed.). Van Nostrand Reinhold, United States of America, pp. 193–210.

Kuwahara H, Kanazawa A, Wakamatsu D, Morimura S, Kida K, Akaike T. 2004. Antioxidative and antimutagenic activities of 4-vinyl-2,6-dimethoxyphenol (canolol) isolated from canola oil. *Journal of Agricultural and Food Chemistry*, 52:4380–4387.

Lacki K, Duvnjak Z. 1996. Comparison of 3 methods for the determination of sinapic acid ester content in enzymatically treated canola meals. *Applied Microbiology and Biotechnology*, 45(4):530–537.

Li J, ElRassi Z. 2002. High performance liquid chromatography of phenolic choline ester fragments derived by chemical and enzymatic fragmentation processes: Analysis of sinapine in rape seed. *Journal of Agricultural and Food Chemistry*, 50(6):1368–1373.

Liu L, Wang Y, Li H, Ji Y, Se Pu. 2006. Study of distribution of sinapine in commonly used crude drugs from cruciferous plants. *Chinese Journal of Chromatography*, 24(1):49–51.

Louzada PR, Lima AC, Mendonca-Silva DL, Noël F, DeMello FG, Ferreira ST. 2004. Taurine prevents the neurotoxicity of b-amyloid and glutamate receptor agonists: Activation of GABA receptors and possible implications for Alzheimer's disease and other neurological disorders. *The FASEB Journal*, 18:511–518.

Maeda H, Tsukamoto T, Tatematsu M. 2009. Anti-inflammatory agent and cancer-preventive agent comprising canolol or prodrug thereof and pharmaceutical, cosmetic and food comprising the same, 2009, United States Patent Application 20090163600, Application Number:12/294972.

Marinova EM, Yanishlieva NV. 1994. Effect of lipid unsaturation on the oxidative activity of some phenolic acids. *Journal of American Oil Chemists Society*, 71:427–434.

Matthäus B. 2000. Isolation, fractionation and HPLC analysis of neutral phenolic compounds in rapeseeds. *Nahrung* 42:75–80.

Milkowski C, Strack D. 2010. Sinapate esters in brassicaceous plants: Biochemistry, molecular biology, evolution and metabolic engineering. *Planta*, 232(1):19–35.

Murakami M, Ota H, Sugiyama A, Ishizone S, Maruta F, Akita N, Okimura Y, Kumagai T, Jo M, Tokuyama T. 2005. Suppressive effect of rice extract on *Helicobacter pylori* infection in a *Mongolian gerbil* model. *Journal of Gastroenterology*, 40:459–466.

Naczk M, Amarowicz R, Sullivan A, Shahidi F. 1998. Current research developments on polyphenolics of rapeseed/canola: A review. *Food Chemistry*, 62(4):489–502.

Naczk M, Amarowicz R, Zadernowski R, Shahidi F. 2005. Antioxidant capacity of phenolics from canola hulls as affected by different solvents. Phenolic compounds in foods and natural health products, Chapter 6, 2005, pp. 57–66, ACS Symposium Series, Volume 909.

Natella F, Nardini M, di Felice M, Scaccini C. 1999. Benzoic and cinnamic acid derivatives as antioxidants: Structure—activity relation. *Journal of Agricultural and Food Chemistry*, 47:1453–1459.

Olsen HS, Adler-Nissen J. 1979. Industrial production and application of soluble enzymatic hydrolysate of soy protein. *Process Biochemistry*, 14:7–10.

Paula-Lima AC, De Felice FG, Brito-Moreira J, Ferreira ST. 2005. Activation of ABAA receptors by taurine and muscimol blocks the neurotoxicity of b-amyloid in rat hippocampal and cortical neurons. *Neuropharmacology*, 49:1140–1148.

Pearson AW, Butler EJ, Fenwick GR. 1980. Rape seed meal and egg taint: The role of sinapine. *Journal of the Science of Food and Agriculture*, 31(9):898–904.

Pekkarinen SS, Stockmann H, Schwarz K, Heinonen IM, Hopia AI. 1999. Antioxidant activity and partitioning of phenolic acids in bulk and emulsified methyl linoleate. *Journal of Agricultural and Food Chemistry*, 47:3036–3043.

Qiao H, Classen HL. 2003. Nutritional and physiological effects of rapeseed meal sinapine in broiler chickens and its metabolism in the digestive tract. *Journal of the Science of Food and Agriculture*, 83(14):1430–1438.

Qiao HY, Dahiya JP, Classen HL. 2008. Nutritional and physiological effects of dietary sinapic acid (4-hydroxy-3,5-dimethoxy-cinnamic acid) in broiler chickens and its metabolism in the digestive tract. *PoultryScience*, 87(4):719–726.

Satu V, Kreander K, Karonen M, Nieminen R, Hämäläinen M, Galkin A et al. 2005. Preclinical evaluation of rapeseed, raspberry and pine bark phenolics for health related effects. *Journal of Agricultural and Food Chemistry*, 53(5):5922–5931.

Sies H. 1997. Oxidative stress: Oxidants and antioxidants. *Experimental Physiology*, 82:291–295.

Spielmeyer A, Wagner A, Jahreis G. 2009. Influence of thermal treatment of rapeseed on the canolol content. *Food Chemistry*, 112:944–948.

Terpinc P, Polak T, Šegatin N, Hanzlowsky A, Ulrih NP, Abramovic H. 2011. Antioxidant properties of 4-vinyl derivatives of hydroxycinnamic acids. *Food Chemistry*, 128:62–69.

Thies W. 1991. Determination of the phytic acid and sinapic acid esters in seeds of rapeseed and selection of genotypes with reduced concentrations of these compounds. *Lipid/Fett*, 93(2):49–52.

Thiyam S, Stöckmann H, Felde TZ, Schwarz K. 2006. Antioxidative effect of the main sinapic acid derivatives from rapeseed and mustard oil by-products. *European Journal of Lipid Science and Technology*, 108(3):239–248.

Thiyam U, Claudia P, Jan U, Alfred B. 2009. De-oiled rapeseed and a protein isolate: Characterization of sinapic acid derivatives by HPLC–DAD and LC–MS. *European Food Research and Technology*, 229:825–831.

Tsunehiro J, Yasuda F, Wakamatsu D, Nakai C. 2002. Isolation and characterization of lipid-radical scavenging component in crude canola oil. In *Third International Conference and Exhibition on Nutraceuticals and Functional Foods: From Laboratory to the Real World and the Marketplace*, Nov. 17–20, 2002; San Diego, CA; American Oil Chemists' Society: Champaign, IL, 2002.

Vermorel M, Hocquemiller R, Evrard J. 1987. Valorization of rapeseed meal. 5. Effects of sinapine and other phenolic compounds on food intake and nutrient utilization in growing rats. *Reproduction Nutrition Development*, 27(4):781–790.

Vuorela S, Kreander K, Karonen M, Nieminen R, Hämäläinen M, Galkin A, Laitinen L et al. 2005a. Preclinical evaluation of rapeseed, raspberry, and pine bark phenolics for health related effects. *Journal of Agricultural and Food Chemistry*, 53:5922–5931.

Vuorela S, Meyer AS, Heinonen M. 2004. Impact of isolation method on the antioxidant activity of rapeseed meal phenolics. *Journal of Agricultural and Food Chemistry*, 52:8202–8207.

Vuorela S, Salminen H, Makela M, Kivikari R, Karonen M, Heinonen M. 2005b. Effect of plant phenolics on protein and lipid oxidation in cooked pork meat patties. *Journal of Agricultural and Food Chemistry*, 53:8492–8497.

Wackerbauer K, Kramer P. 1982. Bayerische Weizenbierseine Alternative. *Brauwelt*. 18:758–762.

Wakamatsu D, Morimura S, Sawa T, Kida K, Nakai C, Maeda H. 2005. Isolation, identification, and structure of a potent alkyl-peroxyl radical scavenger in crude canola oil, canolol. *Bioscience Biotechnology Biochemistry*, 69(8):1568–1574.

Wakamatsu D. 2001. Isolation and identification of radical scavenging compound, canolol in canola oil. MS Thesis, Graduate School of Natural Science, Kumamoto University, 2001; pp. 1–48.

Wanasundara UN, Amarowicz R, Shahidi F. 1996. Partial characterization of natural antioxidants in canola meal. *Food Research International*, 28:525–530.

Wanasundara UN, Shahidi F. 1994. Canola extracts as an alternative natural antioxidant for canola oil. *Journal of American Oil Chemists Society*, 71:817–822.

Wang SX, Oomah DB, McGregor DI. 1998. Application and evaluation of ion-exchange UV spectrophotometric method for determination of sinapine in Brassica seeds and meals. *Journal of Agricultural and Food Chemistry*, 46(2):575–579.

Xin D, Li Z, Wang W, Zhang W, Liu S, Zhang X. 2011. Protective effect of canolol from oxidative stress-induced cell damage in ARPE-19 cells via an ERK mediated antioxidative pathway. *Molecular Vision*, 17:2040–2048.

Yang CY, He L. 2008. Neuroprotective effects of sinapine on PC12 cells apoptosis induced by sodium dithionite. *Chinese Journal of Natural Medicines*, 6(3):205–209.

Yoon BH, Jung JW, Lee JJ, Cho YW, Jang CG, Jin C, Oh TH, Ryu JH. 2007. Anxiolytic-like effects of sinapic acid in mice. *Life Sciences*, 81(3):234–240.

Yun KJ, Koh DJ, Kim SH, Park SJ, Ryu JH, Kim DG, Lee JY, Lee KT. 2008. Anti-inflammatory effects of sinapic acid through the suppression of inducible nitric oxide synthase, cyclooxygase-2, and pro inflammatory cytokines expressions via nuclear factor-kB inactivation. *Journal of Agricultural and Food Chemistry*, 56:10265–10272.

Zacchi P, Eggers R. 2008. High temperature pre-conditioning of rapeseed: A polyphenol-enriched oil and the effect of refining. *European Journal of Lipid Science and Technology*, 110(2):111–119.

Zhou H, Huang Y, Hoshi T, Kashiwagi Y, Anzai J, Li G. 2005. Electrochemistry of sinapine and its detection in medicinal plants. *Analytical and Bioanalytical Chemistry*, 382(4):1196–1201.

Zou Y, Kim AR, Kim JE, Choi JS, Chung HY. 2002. Peroxynitrite scavenging activity of sinapic acid (3,5-dimethoxy-4-hydroxycinnamicacid) isolated from *Brassica juncea*. *Journal of Agricultural and Food Chemistry*, 50:5884–5890.

3 Valuable Vinylphenols from Rapeseed and Canola

Decarboxylative Pathways

Usha Thiyam-Holländer, Narsireddy Meda, K. Misra and Ahindra Nag

CONTENTS

3.1 Introduction 39
3.2 Decarboxylation of β-Ketocarboxylic Acids by Base 40
3.3 Transition Metal-Catalysed Decarboxylation 41
  3.3.1 Copper-Catalysed Decarboxylation 41
  3.3.2 Copper-Catalysed Decarboxylation in Presence of Quinoline or Pyridine 41
  3.3.3 Mercury-Catalysed Decarboxylation (Pesci Reaction) 43
  3.3.4 Silver-Catalysed Decarboxylation of Ortho-Substituted Benzoic Acids 43
  3.3.5 Pd-Catalysed Decarboxylation 44
  3.3.6 Barton Decarboxylation 46
  3.3.7 Greener Protocol for Transformation of Substituted Cinnamic Acid 47
3.4 Decarboxylation for Generation of Vinylphenols from Food Sources 49
  3.4.1 Temperature-Sensitive Production of Vinylphenols 50
  3.4.2 Decarboxylation for Generation of Substituted Vinylphenols (Canolol) from Substituted Cinnamic Acid 50
  3.4.3 Decarboxylation Involving Enzymes 51
3.5 Decarboxylation and Production of Canolol by Thermal Treatment 54
References 56

3.1 INTRODUCTION

Carboxylic acids (RCO_2H) are distributed widely in nature in fruits and vegetables as well as commercially available. Decarboxylation of carboxylic acids is documented as one of the most important functional group transformations in organic synthesis (Yoshimi et al., 2010). It is a chemical reaction that releases carbon dioxide.

$$RCOOH \longrightarrow RH + CO_2$$

SCHEME 3.1

In chemistry, decarboxylation refers to a reaction of carboxylic acids, in which a carbon atom is removed from the carbon chain as carbon dioxide (Scheme 3.1).

Metals, especially copper compounds (Wiley and Smith, 1963), are usually required and such reactions proceed via the intermediates composed of metal carboxylate complexes. Alkylcarboxylic acids and their salts, however, do not always undergo decarboxylation readily (March, 1985).

The background and detailed mechanisms of decarboxylation are very extensive, and therefore this chapter will discuss some specific pathways of decarboxylation. In addition, we have highlighted recent cases of decarboxylation relevant to hydroxycinnamic acids in wine, beer and camelina and attempted to reason if such strategies can be transferred for value addition to processing of rapeseed and canola. An update on the recent thermal decarboxylation to form canolol, a phenol of interest in rapeseed and canola processing, is discussed in the last part of this chapter.

3.2 DECARBOXYLATION OF β-KETOCARBOXYLIC ACIDS BY BASES

Decarboxylation under mild conditions is a general property of both cyclic and acyclic (open chain) β-ketocarboxylic acids (Scheme 3.2). The mechanism of decarboxylation involves a concerted process during which bond breaking and bond formation take place simultaneously without any intermediates being involved. Hence, activation energies are low and reaction takes place under mild conditions. This mechanism also proceeds through the formation of a stable six-membered transition state (Scheme 3.3).

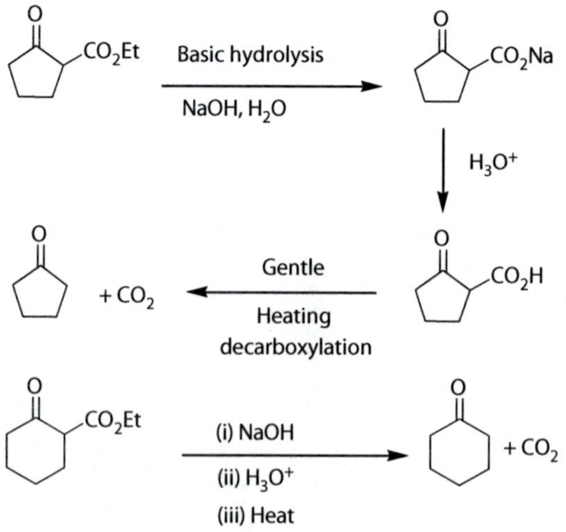

O
CO_2Et Basic hydrolysis
NaOH, H_2O
O
CO_2Na
H_3O^+
O
$+ CO_2$
Gentle
Heating
decarboxylation
O
CO_2H
O
CO_2Et
(i) NaOH
(ii) H_3O^+
(iii) Heat
O
$+ CO_2$

SCHEME 3.2

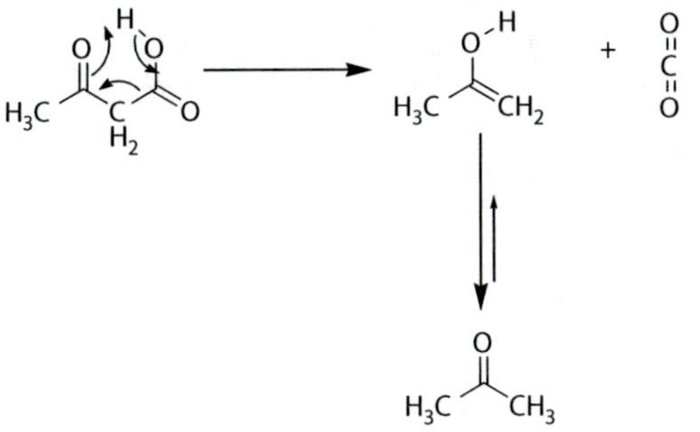

SCHEME 3.3

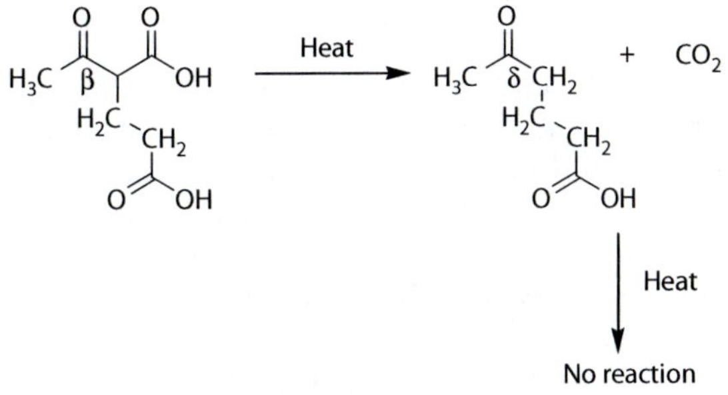

Heat
Heat
No reaction

SCHEME 3.4

The evidence for the mechanism is shown in Scheme 3.4.

Decarboxylation of ketocarboxylic acids leads initially to the formation of an enol and CO_2. The enol then tautomerizes to corresponding ketone. However, in cases where enol formation is unfavourable, the relevant ketocarboxylic acid will be resistant to decarboxylation.

3.3 TRANSITION METAL-CATALYSED DECARBOXYLATION

3.3.1 Copper-Catalysed Decarboxylation

Decarboxylation of 3-halofuroic acid occurred simply by heating the substances at temperatures between 210°C and 300°C. 3-Chlorofuroic acid and 5-chlorofuroic acid proved to be stabler and could not be decarboxylated in this way. Copper prepared by reducing the oxide at 300–400°C effectively catalysed the decarboxylation (Scheme 3.5).

3.3.2 Copper-Catalysed Decarboxylation in Presence of Quinoline or Pyridine

Heat-triggered decarboxylation of aromatic carboxylic acids in quinoline solution in the presence of copper metal or copper salts (the copper–quinoline decarboxylation)

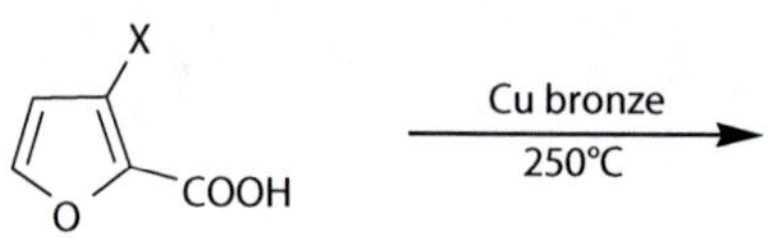

X, COOH → (Cu bronze, 250°C) → X

SCHEME 3.5

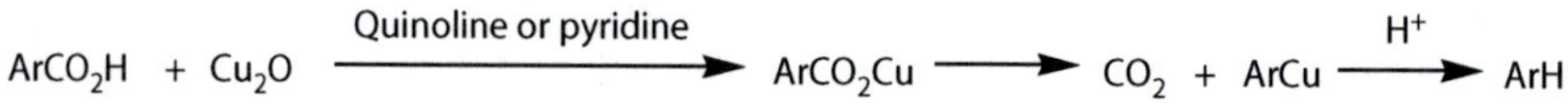

$ArCO_2H + Cu_2O \xrightarrow{\text{Quinoline or pyridine}} ArCO_2Cu \longrightarrow CO_2 + ArCu \xrightarrow{H^+} ArH$

SCHEME 3.6

is widely practised since its discovery by Shepard et al. (1930). The same work indicates that cuprous and cupric salts decarboxylate at approximately the same rate. Cohen et al. (1978) performed the reaction easily by heating the acid in quinoline under an inert atmosphere in the presence of cuprous oxide (Scheme 3.6).

Jones and Chapman, (1993) developed a method for the decarboxylation of indole-2 carboxylic acids derivatives by microwave-assisted thermolysis using copper (5–25 mol%) in the presence of quinoline (Scheme 3.7).

Goossen et al. (2007) developed a method for the decarboxylation of deactivated benzoic acid derivatives using 10 mol% of copper catalyst in the presence of quinoline (Scheme 3.8).

Recently, an effective protocol was developed that allows the smooth protodecarboxylation of diversely functionalized aromatic carboxylic acids within 5–15 min. In the presence of at most 5 mol% of an inexpensive catalyst generated *in situ* from copper(I) oxide and 1,10-phenanthroline, even non-activated benzoates were converted in high yields and with great preparative ease (Scheme 3.9) (Goossen et al., 2009a).

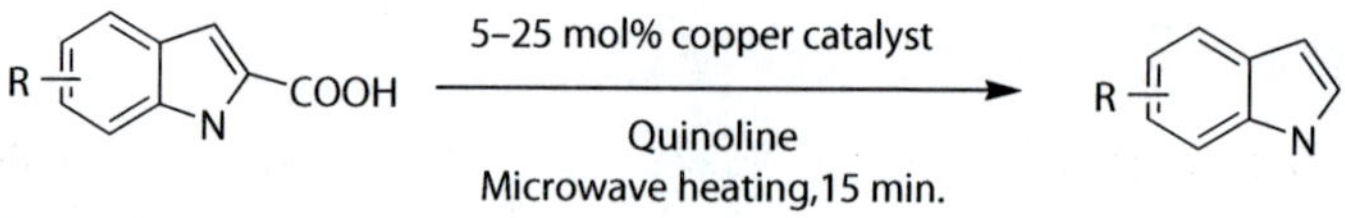

R, N, COOH → (5–25 mol% copper catalyst; Quinoline; Microwave heating,15 min.) → R, N

SCHEME 3.7

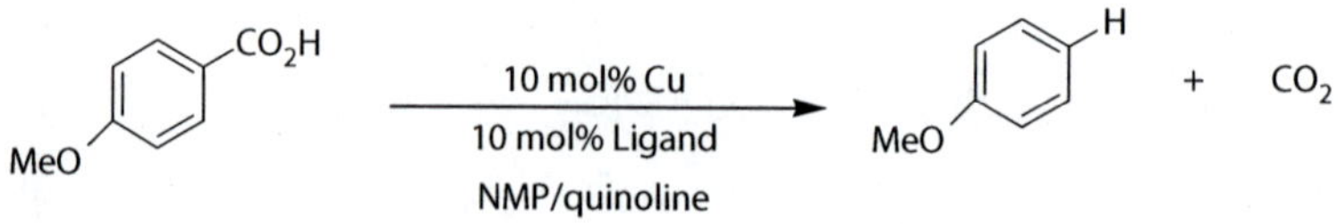

MeO, CO_2H → (10 mol% Cu; 10 mol% Ligand; NMP/quinoline) → MeO, H + CO_2

SCHEME 3.8

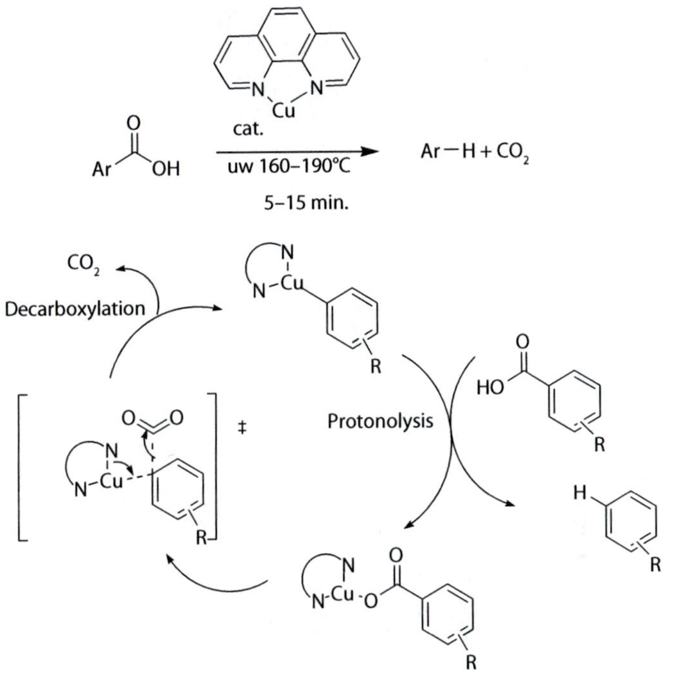

SCHEME 3.9

3.3.3 Mercury-Catalysed Decarboxylation (Pesci Reaction)

In the early studies, naphthoate series was hydrolyzed to its dicarboxylate anion and treated *in situ* with HgO in acetic acid and water (effectively $Hg(OAc)_2$). The Hg species possibly adds initially between the carboxyl groups, and then into the arene ring displacing one or other of the carboxylate groups, which is then released as CO_2, giving the anhydro organo-mercury isomers (2a,b) in typically quantitative yield in all cases. These are very stable compounds that can be isolated and oven dried. They are thought to exist in polymeric chains, which probably account for their low solubility in organic solvents. Acidic hydrolysis (or hydride reduction) releases Hg as its salt to yield the arene mono-acids (3a,b) (Moseley and Gilday, 2006) (Scheme 3.10).

3.3.4 Silver-Catalysed Decarboxylation of Ortho-Substituted Benzoic Acids

The metal-mediated protodecarboxylation of benzoic acids had limited scope, involved harsh conditions (200°C) and the use of stoichiometric amounts of Cu(I) or Hg(II) salts. Recently, a catalytic version of this reaction using a Cu_2O/phenanthroline/quinoline system with a broad scope was reported, but still required high temperatures (160–190°C). To overcome these problems, a silver-based catalyst system was discovered that effectively promotes the protodecarboxylation of various

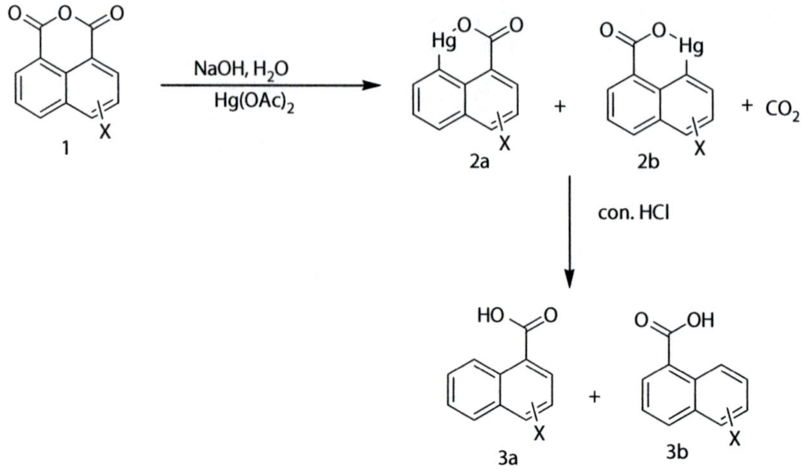

SCHEME 3.10

ArCOOH —(10 mol% AgOAc, 15 mol% K_2CO_3; NMP, 120°C)→ ArH + CO_2

SCHEME 3.11

aromatic carboxylic acids at temperatures of 80–120°C more than 50°C below those of the best-known copper catalysts (Goossen et al., 2009b) (Scheme 3.11).

Then this method was then extended to ortho-substituted benzoic acids (Cornella et al., 2009). In this method, they screened various silver catalysts such as AgOAc, Ag_2CO_3, Ag_2O and $AgOCOCF_3$ and solvents such as dimethyl sulfoxide (DMSO), dimethylformamide (DMF), toluene, dioxane and AcOH, and found that the combination Ag_2CO_3/DMSO gave the best results in the decarboxylation of ortho-substituted benzoic acids (Scheme 3.12).

This method is also further extended to decarboxylation of heteroaromatic carboxylic acids (Scheme 3.13) (Lu et al., 2009).

3.3.5 Pd-Catalysed Decarboxylation

The decarboxylation of free carboxylic acids is often difficult except for some activated acids such as aryl carboxylic acid. Conversion of the free carboxylic acids into proper derivatives such as acid anhydrides or esters makes the transition metal-catalysed decarboxylation reaction easy and these have also been applied to various coupling reactions. Water in a supercritical stage (374°C, 22 MPa) was used for decarboxylation of free carboxylic acids using 10 wt% Pd on active carbon in a closed pot (Matsubara et al., 2004) (Scheme 3.14).

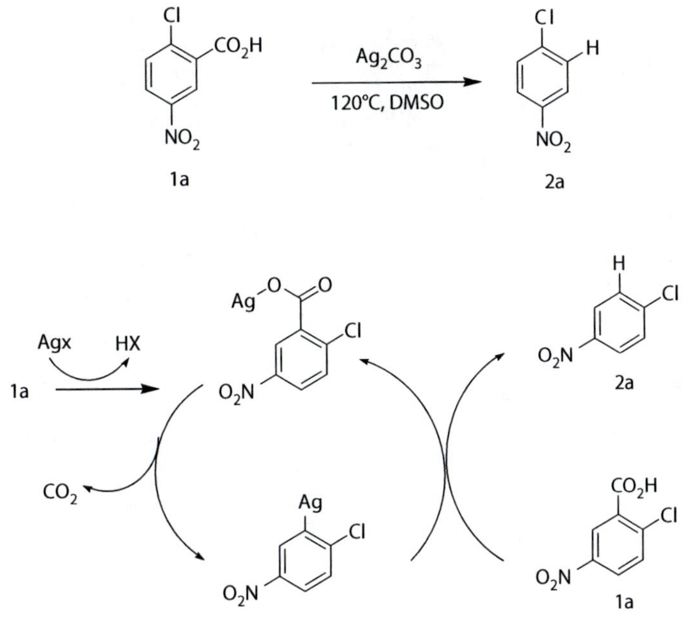

Cl CO2H Ag2CO3 120°C, DMSO Cl H NO2 1a NO2 2a

Agx HX 1a Ag O O Cl O2N H Cl O2N 2a CO2 Ag Cl O2N CO2H Cl O2N 1a

SCHEME 3.12

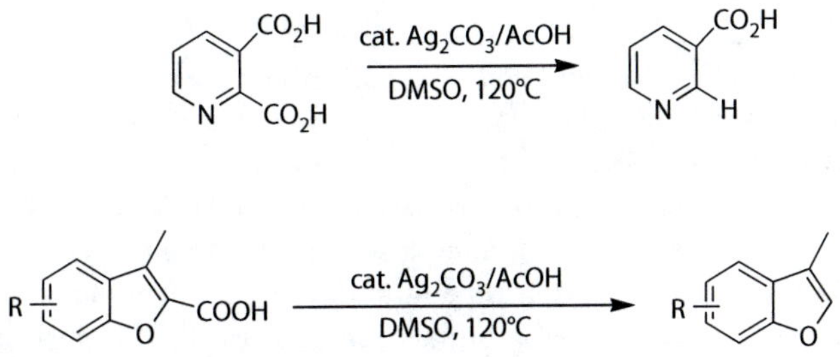

CO2H N CO2H cat. Ag2CO3/AcOH DMSO, 120°C CO2H N H

R O COOH cat. Ag2CO3/AcOH DMSO, 120°C R O

SCHEME 3.13

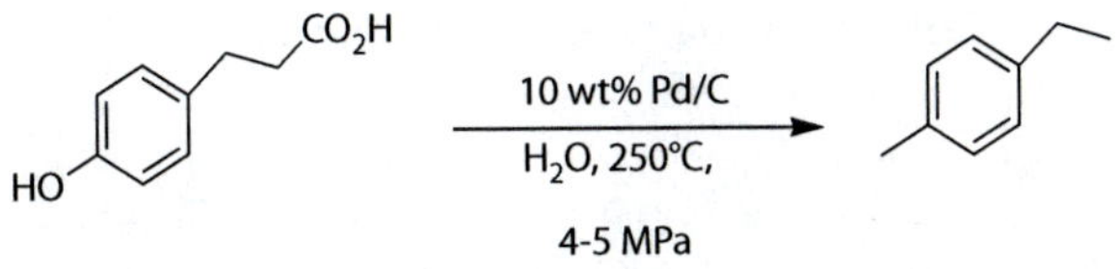

CO2H HO 10 wt% Pd/C H2O, 250°C, 4-5 MPa

SCHEME 3.14

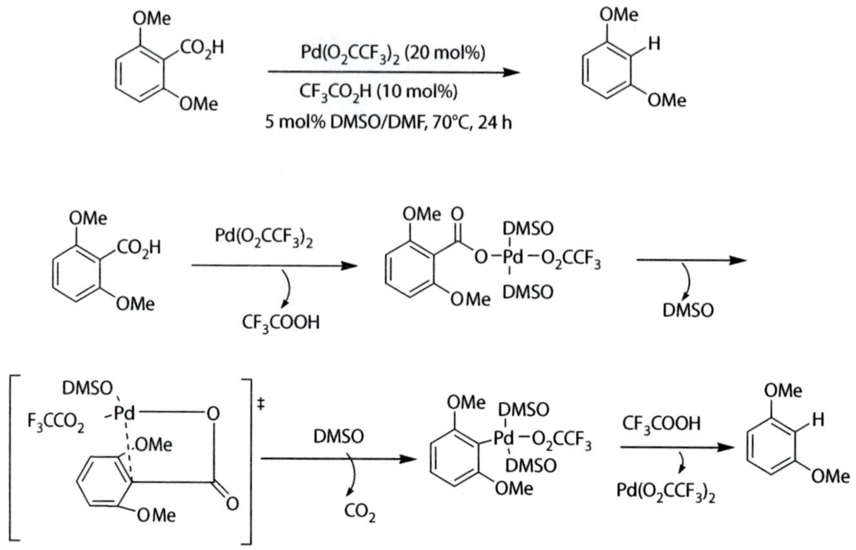

SCHEME 3.15

This method is also extended to decarboxylation of electron-rich aromatic compounds in the presence of trifluoroacetic acid as proton source (Dickstein et al., 2007) (Scheme 3.15).

3.3.6 Barton Decarboxylation

Decarboxylation is usually performed by radical methods such as the Kolbe electrolysis and the Barton decarboxylation. The Barton decarboxylation (Barton et al., 1983) is a radical reaction in which a carboxylic acid is first converted to a thiohydroxamate ester (commonly referred to as a Barton ester). The product is then heated in the presence of a radical initiator and a suitable hydrogen donor to complete the reductive decarboxylation of the initial carboxylic acid. The reaction is initiated by homolytic cleavage of a radical initiator, in this case 2,2′-azobisisobutyronitrile (AIBN), upon heating, a hydrogen is then abstracted from tri-*n*-butyltin hydride to leave a tri-*n*-butyltin radical that attacks the sulphur atom of the thiohydroxamate ester. The N–O bond of the thiohydroxamate ester undergoes homolysis to form a carboxyl radical which then undergoes decarboxylation and carbon dioxide (CO_2) is lost. The remaining alkyl radical (R·) then abstracts a hydrogen atom from remaining tri-*n*-butyltin hydride to form the reduced alkane (RH) (see Scheme 3.2). The tributyltin radical enters into another cycle of the reaction until all thiohydroxamate ester is consumed (Schemes 3.16 and 3.17).

N–O bond cleavage of the Barton ester can also occur spontaneously upon heating or by irradiation with light to initiate the reaction. In this case, a radical initiator is not required but a hydrogen-atom (H-atom) donor is still necessary to form the RH. Alternative H-atom donors to tri-*n*-butyltin hydride include tertiary thiols and organosilanes.

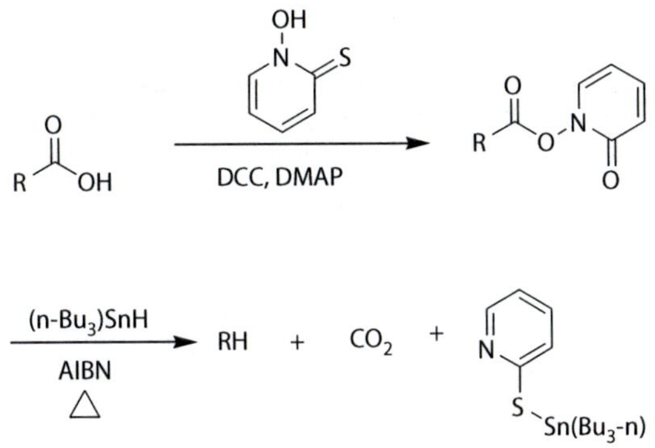

DCC, DMAP

$(n\text{-}Bu_3)SnH$, AIBN, △ → RH + CO_2 + $Sn(Bu_3\text{-}n)$

SCHEME 3.16

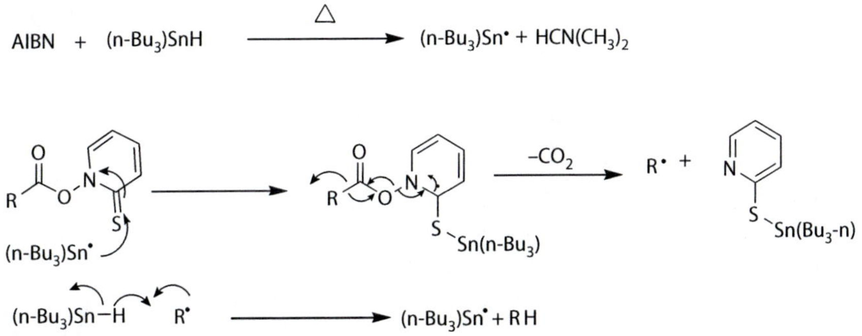

$AIBN + (n\text{-}Bu_3)SnH \xrightarrow{\triangle} (n\text{-}Bu_3)Sn^{\bullet} + HCN(CH_3)_2$

$(n\text{-}Bu_3)Sn^{\bullet}$ → $Sn(n\text{-}Bu_3)$ $\xrightarrow{-CO_2}$ $R^{\bullet}$ + $Sn(Bu_3\text{-}n)$

$(n\text{-}Bu_3)Sn{-}H \;\; R^{\bullet} \longrightarrow (n\text{-}Bu_3)Sn^{\bullet} + RH$

SCHEME 3.17

The relative expense, smell and toxicity associated with tin, thiol, or silane reagents can be avoided by carrying out the reaction using chloroform as both solvent and H-atom donor (Ko et al., 2011) (Scheme 3.18).

3.3.7 Greener Protocol for Transformation of Substituted Cinnamic Acid

Decarboxylation and oxidative transformation of aromatic olefinic compound by hydrogen peroxide or molecular hydrogen in aqueous media, which is a green protocol, were published by Fodran and his research group in 2008. From gas chromatography–mass spectrometry (GC/MS) analysis, they proved that hydrogen peroxide addition mainly produced the corresponding carbonyl compounds by oxidative decarboxylation of substituted cinnamic acids through radical mechanism (Scheme 3.19).

The reaction mechanism involves superoxide anion radicals $O_2^{\bar{\cdot}}$, produced from L-cysteine Fe(II) or L-cysteine Co(II) complexes, which has an important role to attack on the carbonyl carbon and formed corresponding peroxoacid anions or peroxoacid intermediates which give oxidative, non-oxidative decarboxylated substituted cinnamic acid as well as some cyclized benzofuran. But for ferulic acid, no cyclized product was formed due to positive inductive effect of methoxy group in the benzene ring.

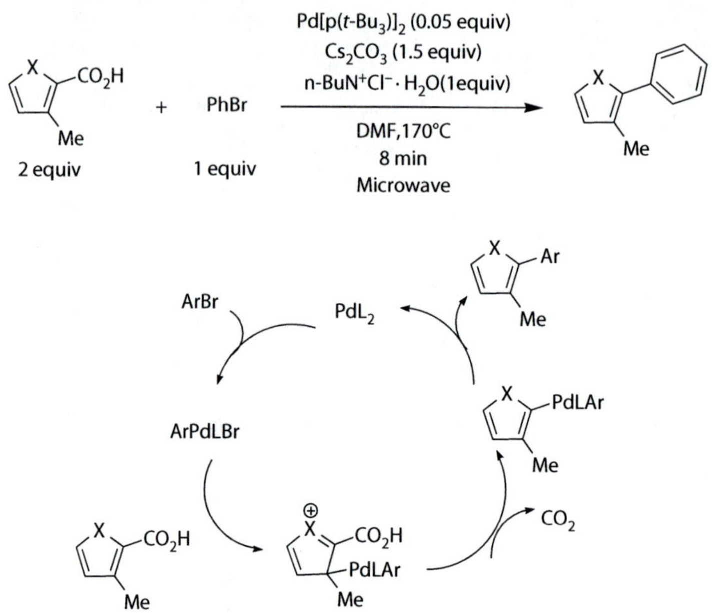

$Pd[p(t\text{-}Bu_3)]_2$ (0.05 equiv)
Cs_2CO_3 (1.5 equiv)
n-$BuN^+Cl^- \cdot H_2O$(1equiv)
DMF,170°C
8 min
Microwave

X, CO_2H, Me — 2 equiv
+ PhBr — 1 equiv
X, Me

X, Ar, Me
ArBr
PdL_2
ArPdLBr
X, PdLAr, Me
X, CO_2H, Me
⊕X, CO_2H, PdLAr, Me
CO_2

SCHEME 3.18

O, O̲, R_2, R_1
Oxygen
cysteine-Fe(II) or
cystein-Co(II)
complex
O, OO̲, R_2, R_1
R_2, R_1
O, O̲, R_2, R_1
Hydrogen peroxide
cysteine-Fe(II) or
cystein-Co(II)
complex
CHO, R_2, R_1
O, R_2, R_1

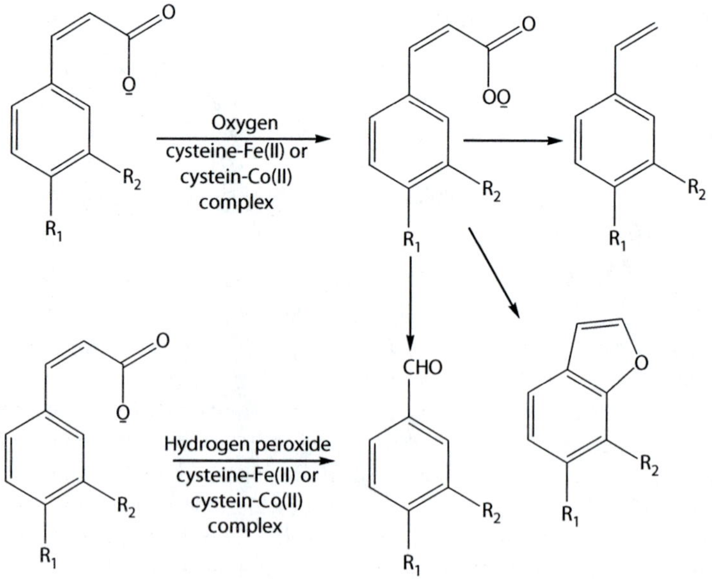

SCHEME 3.19

3.4 DECARBOXYLATION FOR GENERATION OF VINYLPHENOLS FROM FOOD SOURCES

It is well known that hydroxycinnamic acids in food sources such as coffee, whole grains and vegetables contribute to taste and aroma. The taste-active compounds are formed by phenolic degradation and other complex chemistry. It is also well accepted that the fate of hydroxycinnamic acids during thermal processing is determined by reaction conditions and that decarboxylation and oxidative reactions can occur during thermal processing. Some of these phenolic degradation products have aroma properties which directly contribute to food flavour. For example, ferulic acid can be thermally degraded to generate aroma compounds such as 4-vinylguaiacol (4-VG), guaiacol and vanillin. The procedure used to synthesize 4-vinylphenols (4-VP) involves the decarboxylation of cinnamic acids such as *p*-coumaric acid, ferulic acid, sinapic acid and caffeic acid. These compounds are commercially available and present in food sources such as barley (Hao and Trust, 2012), wheat bran (Zhou et al., 2004), sunflower seeds (Dabrowski and Sosulski, 1984) and rapeseed meal (Vuorela et al., 2004).

During the winemaking process, volatile phenols formed via decarboxylation of hydroxycinnamic acids have been reported. These volatile phenols have implications on flavour and aroma, as the literature reports the aroma threshold value of these volatile phenols in wine (Curtin et al., 2005). The effect of hydroxycinnamic acids and volatile phenols on beer quality has also been extensively investigated (Iyuke et al., 2008; Vanbeneden et al., 2008). At 90°C, 4-VG appears to be formed by decarboxylation. 4-Vinylsyringol, another volatile phenol known to have organoleptic characteristics of smoked, burned with a threshold in beer (mg/L) 0.50 (Callemien and Collin, 2009). These volatile phenols are mainly vinyl derivatives such as vinylcatechol, 4-VG and vinylphenol. They have also been associated with the formation of further products vinylphenol malvidin adducts (Schwarz et al., 2003, 2007; Pozo-Bayón et al., 2004; Morata et al., 2006). The formation of vinylphenolic pyroanthocyanin pigments was shown to be affected by the type of yeasts supplemented with hydroxycinnamic acids (Morata et al., 2007). The same study explained how vinylphenols, formed from the decarboxylation of hydroxycinnamic acids, combine with grape anthocyanins (malvidin-3-*O*-glucoside) to form vinylphenolic pyranoanthocyanins. These vinyl derivatives all play a role in the characteristic aroma of red wines and beers such as Belgian white beers, German Weizen beers and Rauch beers. Hydroxycinnamic acids, ferulic acid and *p*-coumaric acid, along with native barley enzymes, are implicated in the decarboxylation and release of the flavour-active compounds, especially the vinyl derivatives during brewing and wort fermentation. Thermal decarboxylation of ferrulic acid is known to take place during high-temperature treatments during the malt and beer production process like kilning, wort boiling, whirlpool holding, wort transfer times and beer pasteurization. Mashing temperatures are inadequate for the thermal decarboxylation of ferulic acid and hence no 4-VG can be detected in unboiled wort. But during wort boiling, the liberation of 4-VG and other phenolic flavour molecules will increase with increasing boiling times and the amount of the levels of precursor molecules (McMurrough et al., 1996; Coghe et al., 2004).

3.4.1 Temperature-Sensitive Production of Vinylphenols

When heat was applied on camelina (*Camelina sativa*) seeds in an electrical oven at three different temperatures 80°C, 120°C and 160°C for 30 min, thermal decarboxylation of polyphenolic carboxylic acids were observed by Abramovic and his group in 2011. 4-Vinyl derivatives of hydroxycinnamic acids (i.e., 4-VP), 4-vinylcatechol (4-VC) and 4-vinylsyringol (4-VS) are prepared by thermal decarboxylation of *p*-coumaric acid, ferulic acid, caffeic acid and sinapic acids, respectively, present in camelina seeds. Among the 4-vinyl derivatives of hydroxycinnamic acid, 4-VS was by far the most abundant in camelina seeds. The free 4-VG increased with increasing temperature up to 120°C but decreased notably at 160°C. This suggested that 4-VG was more heat sensitive than other 4-vinyl derivatives. When thermal treatment was performed on the whole seeds, an increased amount of 4-vinyl derivatives was obtained compared to the cake of heated seeds crushed before heating. The loss of these highly volatile compounds during heating might be prevented to a greater extent when using the whole grain. Thus, the physical form of the seed might be of great influence for the production of vinyphenol.

3.4.2 Decarboxylation for Generation of Substituted Vinylphenols (Canolol) from Substituted Cinnamic Acid

In the past few years, microwave-assisted chemical synthesis has been used extensively as an environmental-friendly, rapid and high-yielding technique. Nomura et al. (2005) reported a base-catalysed decarboxylation and amide-forming reaction of substituted cinnamic acids via microwave heating.

Decarboxylation reaction of aromatic acids (especially substituted cinnamic acid) occurred in the presence of a base and microwave heating by following mechanism (Nomura et al., 2005). Aliphatic amines are used as base for these reaction purposes. Para hydroxyl group produced good yield as compared to the acid group. The progress of the reaction also depends upon the pK_a value of the base in the reaction mixture (Schemes 3.20 and 3.21).

In 2007, Bernini et al. reported another decarboxylation reaction in the presence of 1,8-diazabicycloundec-7-ene (DBU) and aluminium oxide as solid support during microwave heating. They used the DBU as base because diazabicycloalkenes are efficient bases for the decarboxylation of acid at a pK_a is greater than 7. It was

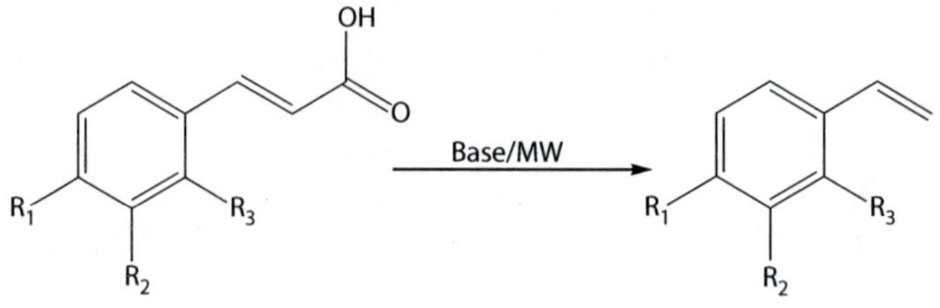

SCHEME 3.20

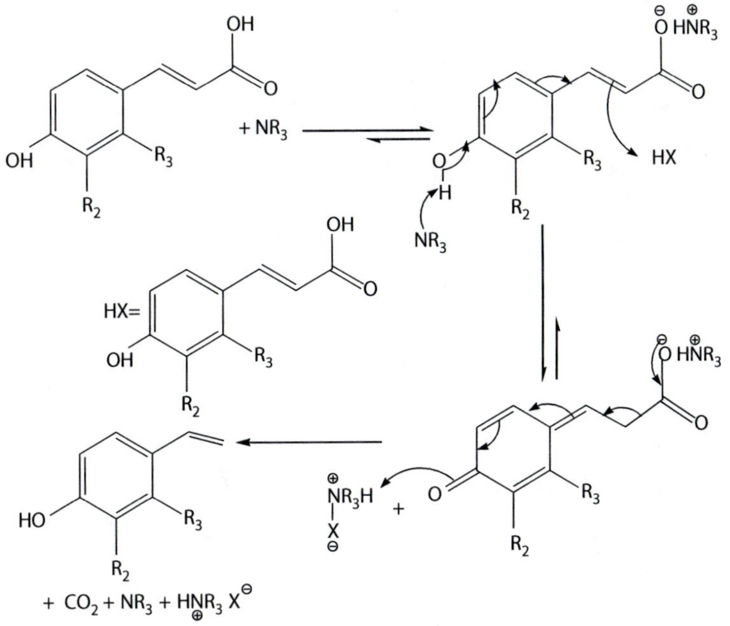

SCHEME 3.21

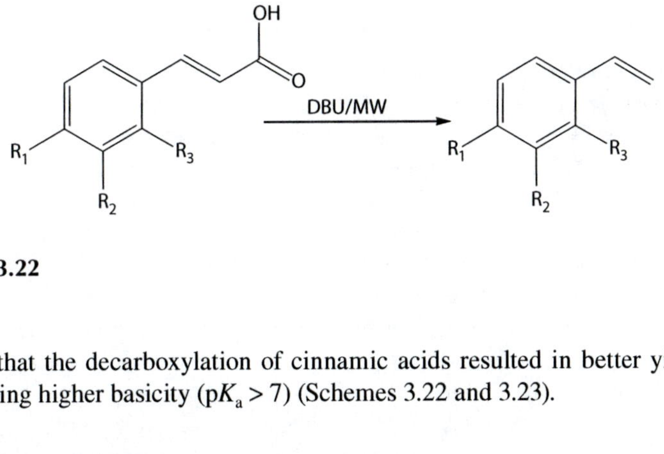

SCHEME 3.22

reported that the decarboxylation of cinnamic acids resulted in better yields with bases having higher basicity (p$K_a > 7$) (Schemes 3.22 and 3.23).

3.4.3 Decarboxylation Involving Enzymes

There are many examples for decarboxylation reactions using different chemicals, but it was reported that an enzyme can also exhibit the decarboxylase property and can produce decarboxylated products from substituted cinnamic acid by using its active site for the particular functional group. Rodriguez et al. (2008, 2010) published two papers on the production of vinylphenols using *p*-coumaric acid decarboxylases (PDCs), which catalyse the non-oxidative decarboxylation of hydroxycinnamic acids to generate to the corresponding vinyl derivatives. The study highlighted that Glu71

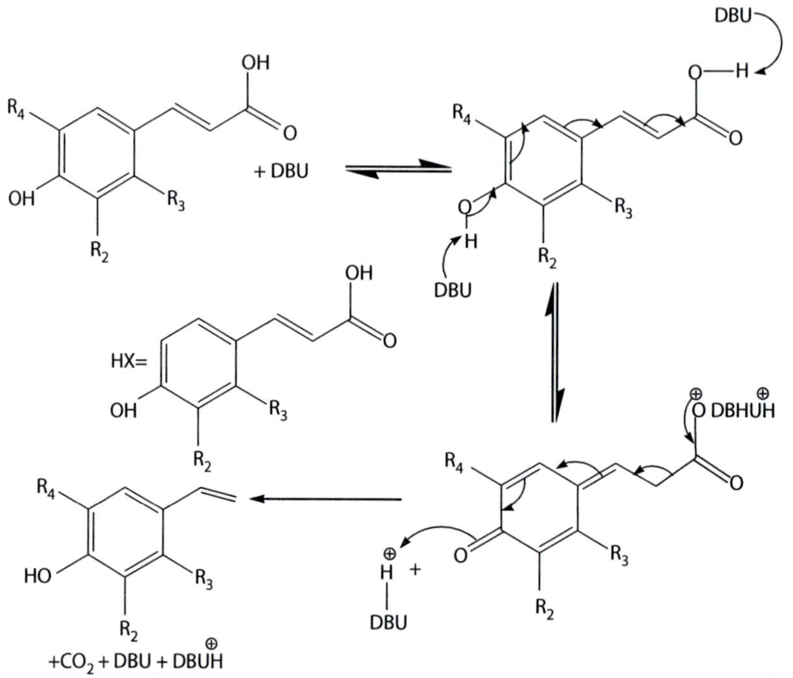

SCHEME 3.23

is involved in proton transfer, and Tyr18 and Tyr20 are involved in the proper substrate orientation and in the release of the CO_2 product.

Kinetic analysis showed that the enzyme has a 14-fold higher K_M value for *p*-coumaric and caffeic acids than for ferulic acid. PDC catalyses the formation of the corresponding 4-vinyl derivatives (vinylphenol and vinylguaiacol) from *p*-coumaric and ferulic acids, respectively, which are valuable food additives that have been approved as flavouring agents (Scheme 3.24).

Fiddler et al. (1967) while studying the thermal decomposition of ferulic acid observed decomposition at 200°C onwards, while at temperatures exceeding 340°C, unsubstituted 4-methyl- and 4-ethylguaiacol were formed. In the air atmosphere, vanillin, acetovanillon and vanillic acid, known to be oxygenated products of 4-VG, were also formed (Vanbeneden, 2007). During the process of either thermal or enzymic decarboxylation of specific yeast strains, these hydroxycinnamic acids, more specifically *p*-coumaric acid and ferulic acid, can be transformed into the highly flavour-active volatile phenols 4-VP and 4-VG. Vanbeneden et al. (2008) reported that at mashing temperatures of 90°C and 100°C, 4-VG was formed and the concentrations increased with the increase in heating time, while Fiddler et al. reported that, in dry air, ferulic acid only starts to degrade at 200°C, indicating that the thermal decarboxylation is greatly enhanced under aqueous reaction conditions.

It has been known that the bacteria *Erwinia uredovora* attacks uredospores and uredia of *Puccina graminis*, which causes leaf blight diseases of higher plants; thus,

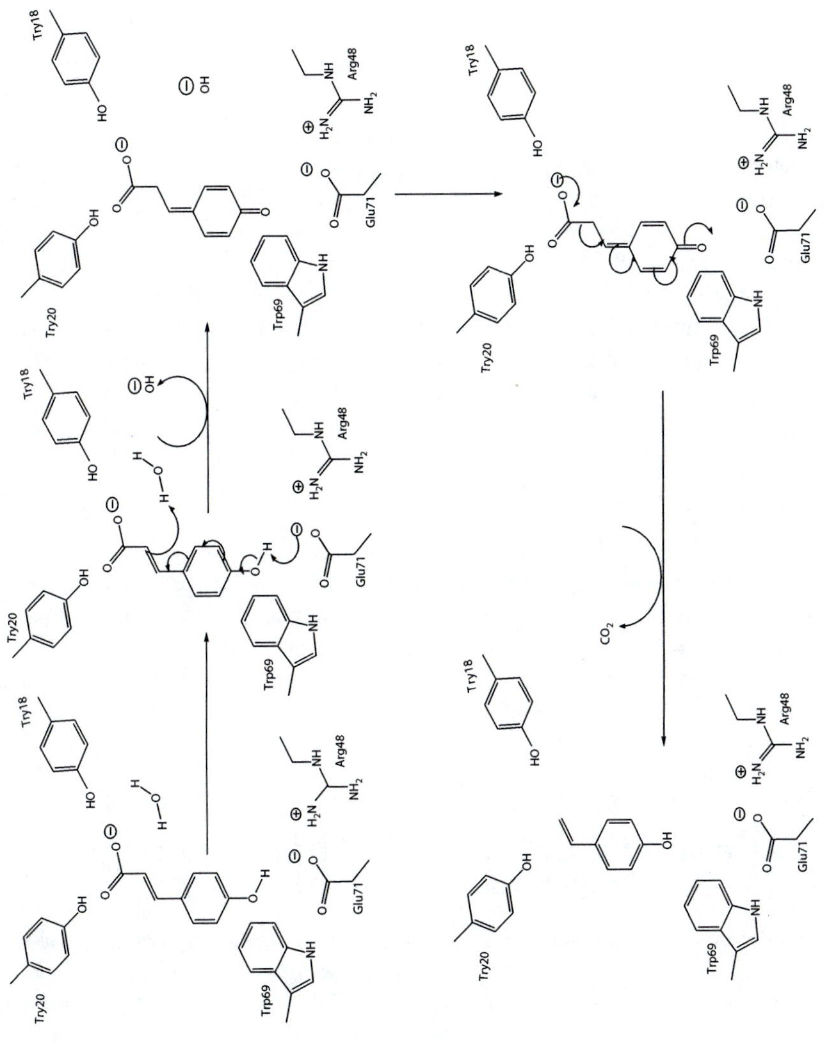

SCHEME 3.24

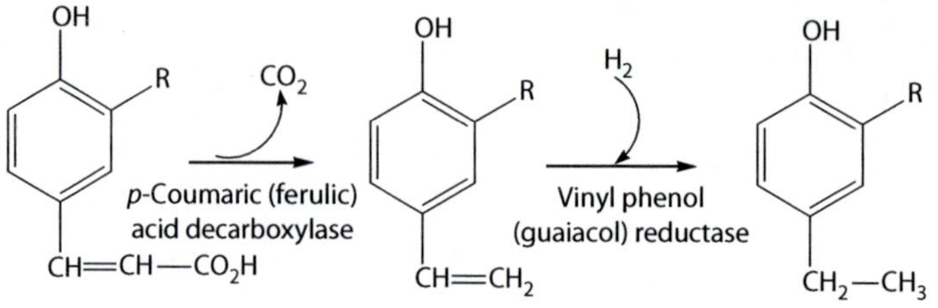

OH, R, $CH{=}CH{-}CO_2H$ → (CO_2) *p*-Coumaric (ferulic) acid decarboxylase → OH, R, $CH{=}CH_2$ → (H_2) Vinyl phenol (guaiacol) reductase → OH, R, $CH_2{-}CH_3$

SCHEME 3.25

epiphytic bacterium as a candidate for biopesticide. In 1993, Yoshida et al. isolated two bacteria, family of Enterobacteriaceae, *Klebsiella oxytoca* and *Erwinia uredovora* from *Polymnia sonchifolia* leaf, that have decarboxylation activity towards hydroxycinnamic acid to vinylphenol. Both are common gram-negative epiphytic bacteria which are widely distributed on the leaf surfaces of several plants. They also reported that crude protein from the bacterial cells had the decarboxylation activity, but the cultured media devoid of the cells did not show any decarboxylation ativity. Thus, hydroxycinnamate decarboxylase of these two bacteria was found to be substrate inducible, and the enzyme did not diffuse outside the cell.

Priest et al. (2000) isolated seven strains of *Lactobacillus* (*Lactobacillus brevis, L. crispatus, L. fermentum, L. hilgardii, L. paracasei, L. pentosus* and *L. plantarum)* from malt whisky fermentation that contained genes for hydroxycinnamic acid (*p*-coumaric acid) decarboxylase (Scheme 3.25).

With the exception of *L. hilgardii*, these bacteria decarboxylated *p*-coumaric acid and/or ferulic acid, with the production of 4-VP and/or 4-VG, respectively, although the relative activities on the two substrates varied between strains. The addition of *p*-coumaric acid or ferulic acid to cultures of *L. pentosus* in MRS broth induced hydroxycinnamic acid decarboxylase mRNA within 5 min, and the gene was also induced by the indigenous components of malt wort.

Gramatica et al. (1981) applied decarboxylation to cinnamic acids using *saccharomyces cerevisiae.*

3.5 DECARBOXYLATION AND PRODUCTION OF CANOLOL BY THERMAL TREATMENT

The canolol content of canola and rapeseed can be increased by decarboxylation of sinapic acid via roasting treatments. Roasting conditions enhanced the canolol content by a factor of 120 (Spielmeyer et al., 2010) compared to the unroasted sample proving canolol was generated during roasting consistent with our findings (Mayengbam et al., 2010). Canolol is formed by the elevated temperatures arising during the pressing (Koski et al., 2003) or roasting of seeds (Wakamatsu et al., 2005). Zacchi and Eggers (2008) reported the effect of temperature on the concentration of minor compounds (polyphenols) during thermal conditioning of pretreated seed, and its influence on the oil and the oxidative stability. Because of its potent bioactive potential, the increase of canolol content in rapeseed oil would theoretically produce oil with enhanced food value as well as longer shelf life (Spielmeyer et al., 2009). Recently, Harbaum-Piayda et al. (2010) demonstrated the possibility of such new compounds (4-VS) dimer and trimer in commercial rapeseed oils, as well as in the deodistillate. The canolol dimer was present in the deodistillate of processed rapeseed oil in significant amounts (approximately 3.50 g/kg), which implicates decarboxylation conditions to be important for generating these active vinylphenols.

A patent by Shigeru et al. (2003) (Patent 2003030888) disclosed a method for obtaining 4-VS as a methanolic extract from crude rapeseed oil. In this method, crude rapeseed oil was treated with alcohols or aqueous alcohols and a concentration of the vinylphenols prepared by distillation. Sinha et al. (2006) (US patent 6989,467 B2) invented a microwave-induced process for the preparation of substituted 4-VP from 4-hydroxyphenylaldehydes and malonic acid in the presence of organic acid and organic base.

During a study aimed at the effect of conventional oven heating (120–200°C) and microwave heating (either with steam or without steam), Mayengbam et al. (2010) found that following heat and microwave treatments, the content of sinapic acid derivatives as well as total phenolics are affected. This study indicated that when commercial canola seed was subjected to conventional hot air oven (120–200°C) and microwave heat treatment (1300 W), the level of canolol in the oil increased. The same study also discussed that the generation of canolol, as a result of decarboxylation, varied with the degree of temperature and time period. During this study, sinapoyl glucose was found to decrease significantly when treatment time increased except at 140°C in conventional oven. It became more pronounced when the temperature of treatment was elevated. There was no significant change in sinapine content below 200°C; however a significant decrease in sinapine content was observed in microwave heating with increase in time. Sinapic acid content was found to increase up to 160°C when treatment time increased. However, it started degrading with increase in time of treatment (10, 20 min as opposed to 5 min) at temperatures above 180°C. A similar pattern of increase in sinapic acid followed by a sudden decrease after a certain point of temperature was observed in microwave toasting also. There was no significant increase in canolol content at the lower temperature (120°C), although it increased dramatically starting from 140°C. This was consistent with our studies suggesting that temperatures below 90°C appeared inadequate for the thermal decarboxylation of sinapic acid as no canolol or only traces were formed. Increase in canolol over 2000-fold when toasted at 200°C for 20 min (6588.96 μg/g) compared to the control (3.09 μg/g) in the conventional oven and a more than 1600-fold in the microwave oven persisted. Maximum canolol was detected at the range of 180–200°C with a toasting time of 10–20 min in the conventional oven. In conclusion, the study by Mayengbam et al. (2010) indicated that toasting significantly increases the canolol content in the oil while phenolics in the meal decrease. It is speculated that high yields of canolol above this temperature could be associated with the various phenolics present in the seed matrix during the toasting. The decrease in total phenols and sinapic acid derivatives (SADs) is being further examined as the mechanisms underlying the temperature-dependent decrease in total phenols and SADs need to be elucidated.

REFERENCES

Abramovic, H., Terpinc, P., Polak, T., Ulrih, N. P. 2011. Effect of heat treatment of camelina (Camelina sativa) seeds on the antioxidant potential of their extracts. *J Agric Food Chem.* 59(16): 8639–8645.

Barton, D. H. R., Crich, D. and Motherwell, W. B. 1983. New and improved methods for the radical decarboxylation of acids. *J. Chem. Soc., Chem .Commun.* 17: 939–941.

Bernini, R., Mincione, E., Barontini, M., Provenzano, G. and Setti, L. 2007. Obtaining 4-vinylphenols by decarboxylation of natural 4-hydroxycinnamic acids under microwave-irradiation. *Tetrahedron.* 63: 9663–9667.

Callemien, D. and Collin, S. 2009. Structure, organoleptic properties, quantification methods, and stability of phenolic compounds in beer. *Food Rev. Int.* 26: 1–84.

Coghe, S., Benoot, K., Delvaux, F., Vanderhaegen, B. and Delvaux, F. R. 2004. Ferulic acid release and 4-vinylguaiacol formation during brewing and fermentation indications for feruloyl esterase activity in *Saccharomyces cerevisiae. J. Agric. Food Chem.* 52: 602–608.

Cohen, T., Berninger, R. W. and Word, J. T. 1978. Products and kinetics of decarboxylation of activated and unactivated aromatic cuprous carboxylates in pyridine and in quinoline. *J. Org. Chem.* 43: 837–848.

Cornella, J., Sanchez, C., Banawa, D. and Larrosa, I. 2009. Silver-catalyzed protodecarboxylation of carboxylic acids. *Chem. Commun.* 45: 7176–7178.

Curtin, C. D., Bellon, J. R., Coulter, A. D., Cowey, G. D., Robinson, E. M. C., de Barros Lopes, M. A., Godden, P. W., Henschke P. A. and Pretorius, I. S. 2005. The six tribes of 'Brett' in Australia—Distribution of genetically divergent *Dekkera bruxellensis* strains across Australian winemaking regions. *Aus. Wine Ind.* J. 20: 28-36.

Dabrowski, K. J. and Sosulski, F. 1984. Composition of free and hydrolyzable phenolic acids in defatted flours of ten oilseeds. *J. Agric. Food Chem.* 32: 128–130.

Dickstein, J. S., Mulrooney, C. A., O'Brien, E. M., Morgan, B. J. and Kozlowski, M. C. 2007. Development of a catalytic aromatic decarboxylation reaction. *Org. Lett.* 9: 2441–2444.

Fiddler, W., Parker, W. E., Wasserman, A. E. and Doerr, R. C. 1967. Thermal decomposition of ferulic acid. *J. Agric. Food Chem.* 15: 757–761.

Fodran, P., Moravčíková, P., Kolek, E. and Brezová, V. 2008. Transformation of substituted cinnamic acids using L-cysteine metal complexes in aqueous media. *Food Res. Int.* 41: 429–432.

Goossen, L. J., Linder, C., Rodrıguez, N., Lange, P. P. and Fromm, A. 2009a. Silver-catalyzed protodecarboxylation of carboxylic acids. *Chem. Commun.* 7173–7175.

Goossen, L. J., Manjolinho, F., Khan, B. A. and Rodrıguez, N. 2009b. Microwave-assisted Cu-catalyzed protodecarboxylation of aromatic carboxylic acids. *J. Org. Chem.* 74: 2620–2623.

Goossen, L. J., Thiel, W. R., Rodrıguez, N. and Linder, C. 2007. Copper-catalyzed protodecarboxylation of aromatic carboxylic acids. *Adv. Synth. Catal.* 349: 2241–2246.

Goossen, L. J., Rodriguez, N., Melzer, B., Linder, C., Deng G. and Levy, L. M. 2007. *J. Am. Chem. Soc.* 129: 4824.

Gramatica, P., Ranzi, B. M. and Manitto, P. 1981. Decarboxylation of cinnamic acids by *Saccharaomyces cerevisiae. Bioorg. Chem.* 10: 14–21.

Hao, M. and Trust, B. 2012. Qualitative and quantitative analysis of the major phenolic phenolic compounds as antioxidants in barley and flaxseed hulls using HPLC/MS/MS. *J. Sci. Food Agric.* DOI: 10.1002/jsfa.5582.

Harbaum-Piayda, B., Oehlke, K., Sönnichsen, F. D., Zacchi, P., Eggers, R. and Schwarz, K. 2010. New polyphenolic compounds in commercial deodistillate and rapeseed oils. *Food Chem.* 123: 607–615.

Iyuke, S. E., Madigoe, E. M. and Maponya, R. 2008. The effect of hydroxycinnamic acids and volatile phenols on beer quality. *J. Inst. Brew.* 114(4): 300–305.

Jones, G. B. and Chapmann, B. J. 1993. Decarboxylation of indole-2-carboxylic acid: Improved procedures. *J. Org. Chem.* 58: 5558–5559.

Sinha, A. K., Joshi, B. P. and Sharma, A. 2006. Microwave induced process for the preparation of substituted 4-vinylphenols. *US Patent 6989467.*

Ko, E. J., Savage, G. P., Williams, C. M. and Tsanaktsidis, J. 2011. Reducing the cost, smell, and toxicity of the Barton reductive decarboxylation: Chloroform as the hydrogen source. *Org. Lett.* 13: 1944–1947.

Koski, A., Pekkarinen, S., Hopia, A., Wahala, K. and Heinonen, M. 2003. Processing of rapeseed oil: Effects on sinapic acid derivative content and oxidative stability. *Eur. Food Res. Technol.* 217: 110–114.

Lu, P., Sanchez, C., Cornella, J. and Larrosa, I. 2009. Silver-catalyzed protodecarboxylation of heteroaromatic carboxylic acids. *Org. Lett.* 11: 5710–5713.

Morata, A., Gómez-Cordovés, M. C., Calderón, F. and Suárez, J. A. 2006. Effects of pH, temperature and SO_2 on the formation of pyranoanthocyanins during red wine fermentation with two species of *Saccharomyces. Int. J. Food Microbiol.* 106(2): 123–129.

Morata, A., González, C. and Suárez-Lepe, J. A. 2007. Formation of vinylphenolic pyranoanthocyanins by selected yeasts fermenting red grape musts supplemented with hydroxycinnamic acids. *International Journal of Food Microbiology.* 116: 144–152.

March, J. 1985. *Advanced Organic Chemistry: Reactions, Mechanisms, and Structure* (3rd ed.), New York: Wiley, ISBN 0-471-85472-7.

Matsubara, S., Yokota, Y. and Oshima, K. 2004. Palladium-catalyzed decarboxylation and ecorbonylation under hydrothermal conditions. Decarboxylative deterioration. *Org. Lett.* 6: 2071–2073.

Mayengbam, S., Khattab, R. Y. and Thiyam-Hollander, U. 2010. In annual project report submitted to NSERC, Canola Council of Canada and Syngenta Inc.

McMurrough, I., Madigan, D., Donnelly, D., Hurley, J., Doyle, A-M., Hennigan, G., McNllty, N. and Smyth, R. M. 1996. Control of ferulic acid and 4-vinyl guaiacol in brewing. *J. Inst. Brew.* 102: 327–332.

Moseley, J. D. and Gilday, J. P. 2006. The mercury-mediated decarboxylation (Pesci reaction) of naphthoic anhydrides investigated by microwave synthesis. *Tetrahedron.* 62: 4690–4697.

Nomura, E., Hosoda, A., Mori, H. and Taniguchi, H. 2005. Rapid base-catalyzed decarboxylation and amide-formation reaction of substituted cinnamic acids via microwave heating. *Green Chem.* 7: 863–866.

Pozo-Bayón, M. Á., Monagas, M., Polo, C. M. and Gómez-Cordovés, C. 2004. Occurrence of pyranoanthocyanins in sparkling wines manufactured with red grape varieties. *J. Agric. Food Chem.* 52(5): 1300–1306.

Priest, F. G. and Beek, S. V. 2000. Decarboxylation of substituted cinnamic acids by lactic acid bacteria isolated during malt whisky fermentation. *Appl. Environ. Microbiol.* 66(12): 5322–5328.

Rodrıguez, H., Angulo, I., de Las, B., Rivas, B., Campillo, N., Paez, J. A., Munoz, R. and Manchen, J. M. 2010. *p*-Coumaric acid decarboxylase from *Lactobacillus plantarum*: Structural insights into the active site and decarboxylation catalytic mechanism. *Protein: Struct. Funct. Bioinform.* 78(7): 1662–1676.

Rodriguez, H., Landete, J. M., Curiel, J. A., de Las Rivas, B., Mancheno, J. M. and Munoz, R. 2008. Characterization of the p-coumaric acid decarboxylase from *Lactobacillus plantarum* CECt 748(T). *J. Agric. Food Chem.* 56(9): 3068–3075.

Schwarz, M., Wabnitz, T. C. and Winterhalter, P. 2003. Formation of anthocyanin–vinylphenol adducts and related pigments in red wines. *J. Agric. Food Chem.* 51: 3682–3687.

Schwarz, M., Wabnitz, T. C. and Winterhalter, P. 2007. Pathway leading to the formation of vinylphenolic pyranoanthocyanins by selected yeasts. *J. Agric. Food Chem.* 51(12): 3682–3687.

Shepard, A. F., Winslow, N. R. and Johnson, J. R. 1930. The simple halogen derivatives of furan. *J. Am. Chem. Soc.* 52: 2083–2090.

Shigeru, M., Kenji, K., Hiroshi, M., Fumi, Y., Daisuke, W., Jun, T. and Chiaki, N. 2003. Antiradicals and fat compositions, foods, drinks, drugs or feeds containing the antiradicals. WO 2003030888.

Spielmeyer, A. and Pohnert, G. 2010. Direct quantification of dimethylsulfoniopropionate (DMSP) with hydrophilic interaction liquid chromatography/mass spectrometry. *J. Chromatogr. B*, 878: 3238–3242.

Spielmeyer, A., Wagner, A. and Jahreis, G. 2009. Influence of thermal treatment of rapeseed on the canolol content. *Food Chem.* 112(4): 944–948.

Vanbeneden, N. 2007. Release of hydroxycinnamic acids and formation of flavour-active volatile phenols during the beer production process, PhD Thesis, Faculteit Bioingenieurswetenschappen, Katholieke Universiteit Leuven.

Vanbeneden, N., Saison, D., Delvaux, F. and Delvaux, F. 2008. Release of phenolic flavour precursors during wort production: Influence of process parameters and grist composition on ferulic acid release during brewing. *Food Chem.* 111: 83–91.

Vuorela, P., Leinonen, M., Saikku, P., Tammela P., Rauha, J. P., Wennberg, T. and Vuorela, H. 2004. Natural products in the process of finding new drug candidates. *Cur. Med. Chem.* 11: 1375–1389.

Wakamatsu, D., Morimura, S., Sawa, T., Kida, K., Nakai, C. and Maeda, H. 2005. Isolation, identification, and structure of a potent alkyl-peroxyl radical scavenger in crude canola oil, canolol. *Biosci. Biotechnol. Biochem.* 69: 1568–1574.

Wiley, R. H. and Smith, N. R. 1963. m-Nitrostyrene. *Org. Synth. Coll.* 4: 731.

Yoshida, T., Hashidoko, Y., Mimako, U. and Mizutani, J. 1993. Decarboxylative conversion of hydrocinnamic acid by *Klebsiella oxytoca Erwinia uredovora*, Epiphytic bacteria of *Polymnia sonchifolia* leaf, possibly with formation of microflora on the damaged leaves. *Biosci. Biotech. Biochem.* 57(2): 215–219.

Yoshimi, Y., Hayashi, S., Nishikawa, K., Haga, Y., Maeda, K., Morita, T., Itou, T., Okada, Y., Ichinose, N. and Hatanaka, M. 2010. Influence of solvent, electron acceptors and arenes on photochemical decarboxylation of free carboxylic acids via single electron transfer (SET). *Molecules.* 15(4): 2623–2630.

Zacchi, P. and Eggers, R. 2008. High-temperature pre-conditioning of rapeseed: A polyphenol-enriched oil and the effect of refining. *Eur. J. Lipid Sci. Technol.* 110(2): 111–119.

Zhou, K., Su, L. and Yu, L. 2004. Phytochemicals and antioxidant properties in wheat bran. *J. Agric. Food Chem.* 52(20): 6108–6114.

4 Processing of Canola Proteins
A Review

L. Xu and Levente L. Diosady

CONTENTS

4.1 Introduction 59
4.2 Canola proteins 62
4.3 Canola Protein Processing 65
  4.3.1 Meal 65
  4.3.2 Protein Concentrates 68
  4.3.3 Protein Isolates 70
References 76

4.1 INTRODUCTION

Although having its root in rapeseed, canola refers only to those varieties containing low levels of erucic acid (<2%) and glucosinolates (<30 μmol/g meal), which were developed in Canada using traditional plant breeding methods in the early 1970s [1]. In the following 20 years, numerous 'double zero' canola cultivars were reported [2], thanks to the ever-improving breeding technology. However, due to the close genetic links between rapeseed and canola, researchers tend not to differentiate them when studying and discussing their protein characteristics and both terms are often used interchangeably. The world production of canola and rapeseed has been growing steadily in the last four decades and now ranks second, only after that of soyabean (Table 4.1), with Canada and China being the largest producers (Table 4.2). As the demand for vegetable oils continues to increase, the production of rapeseed/canola was forecast to exceed 60 million tons in 2010/2011 [3].

The proximate composition of canola/rapeseed varies among varieties as a result of both genetic makeup and growing conditions. As summarized in Table 4.3 [4], the oil content of canola is about twice that of soyabeans and contains much more fibre than soyabeans. The protein content of oil-free canola meal is only slightly lower than that of soyabeans. Canola is processed primarily for its oil, which makes up some 40% of the seed mass. It has an ideal fatty acid composition for human consumption, with a linoleic-to-linolenic acid ratio of approximately 2. After oil removal, the meal contains more than 40% protein with well-balanced amino acid composition. The essential amino acid composition, given in Table 4.4, indicates that canola protein is superior

TABLE 4.1
World Production of Major Oilseeds (in Million Tonnes)

Oilseed	2008/2009	2009/2010
Soyabean	212	258
Canola/rapeseed	57.9	59.4
Cottonseed	41.3	39.9
Peanut	34.5	31.5
Sunflowerseed	33.8	30.6
Palm kernel	11.9	12.5

Source: From Foreign Agricultural Service. USDA. 2010. Oilseed: World Markets and Trade. http://www.fas.usda.gov/currwmt.asp. With permission.

TABLE 4.2
Canola/Rapeseed Production (in Thousand Tonnes)

Country/Region	2008/2009	2009/2010
EU-27	18,996	21,454
Canada	12,643	11,825
China	12,100	13,200
India	6700	6400
Other	7438	6553

Source: From Foreign Agricultural Service. USDA. 2010. Oilseed: World Markets and Trade. http://www.fas.usda.gov/currwmt.asp. With permission.

TABLE 4.3
Comparison of Proximate Compositions of Canola and Soyabeans

Component	Canola (%)	Soyabean (%)
Moisture	6–9	11–14
Oil[a]	38–50	16–22
Protein[b]	36–44	45–60
Fibre	11–16	6[c]
Ash[b]	7–8	3.3–6.4

Source: From Salunkhe, D. K. et al. 1992. *World Oilseeds: Chemistry, Technology and Utilization*. Van Nostrand Reinhold, New York. pp. 59. With permission.

[a] Moisture-free basis.

[b] Moisture- and oil-free basis.

[c] Dehulled.

TABLE 4.4
Essential Amino Acid Content of Canola and Soyabean Protein (g/100 g Protein)

Essential Amino Acid	Canola	Soyabean
Isoleucine	4.2	4.2
Leucine	7.3	7.0
Lysine	5.8	5.8
Methionine	2.3	1.1
Phenylalanine	4.1	4.5
Threonine	4.5	3.8
Tryptophan	1.4	1.3
Valine	5.2	4.3

Source: From Ohlson, R. and Anjou, K. 1979. *JAOCS.* 56:431–437. With permission.

to soy protein in methionine and threonine and they are comparable in the others [5]. The protein quality measured by the determination of protein efficiency ratio and net protein utilization was found to be similar to that of casein [6]. Therefore, canola has great potential to be utilized as a source of food-grade protein to meet the need of the world's fast-growing population. However, the presence of many undesired components precludes the utilization of canola meal for human consumption. These major antinutritional compounds are glucosinolates [7], phytates [8], crude fibre and phenolic compounds [9]. Upon hydrolysis, glucosinolates form isothiocyanates and oxazolidinethiones, which are both toxic and can cause thyroid problems. Although the genetically improved canola varieties have low levels of glucosinolates, <20 μmol/g meal, their meals are still not acceptable for incorporation into food. In India and China, where the original rapeseed varieties are grown, the glucosinolate content of defatted meal could still be over 100 μmol/g. Canola meal also contains between 5% and 6% phytates [5], levels much higher than typical oilseeds. Phytates are excellent chelating agents and strongly bind Zn and Fe, making these essential micronutrients unavailable for metabolism. Defatted canola meal has an unappealing dark colour and an unpleasant taste that may be characterized by bitterness and astringency. These are known to be a result of oxidation of phenolic compounds in the seeds, which include phenolic acids and tannins. The total phenolic acid content in the meal is typically about 1–2% [10,11] and the predominant phenolic acid is sinapine, a choline ester of sinapic acid. Most tannins in canola are condensed tannins and they are flavanoid-based polyphenols. Shahidi and Naczk (1989) reported condensed tannin content in excess of 500 mg catechin equivalent per 100 g meal for most canola meals. It is obvious that all of these compounds must be removed or reduced to acceptable levels before canola protein can be used for food purpose. Currently canola meal is only used for animal feed and in some countries that do not grow the low glucosinolate varieties, it can be used only as a fertilizer.

During the past four decades, there has been continued research interest in making food-grade proteins from canola/rapeseed. Much of the effort was directed to meal processing, involving mechanical processes, aqueous and alcoholic solvent extraction, some of which also incorporated enzymatic treatments. By treating the meal, various protein products with different protein concentration and functional properties may be obtained. Due to the poor product quality and high-processing cost, these processes remain commercially unviable so far. In the meantime, inspired by the great strides made in soy protein technology and the realization that soy proteins are strong allergens for a significant fraction of the consumers, a great deal of work has been done to attempt the production of high-quality canola protein isolates. It is hoped that these products will likely command much higher prices in the market than either the meal or protein concentrates and should offset their relatively high-processing cost.

4.2 CANOLA PROTEINS

Like other seed and grain proteins, canola proteins are considered to have structural, catalytic and storage functions. Structural proteins are usually membrane components while proteins with catalytic activity are various enzymes either membrane-bound or free. Given that only small amounts of enzyme proteins are involved in enzymatic reactions, the major portion of canola proteins represents storage proteins with no enzymatic activity [13], and these proteins are located in protein bodies. Based on protein fractionation studies, most canola proteins are classified as albumins and globulins [13–16], making up more than 70% of total canola proteins. A combination of gel permeation and ion exchange isolate a basic protein named A-IV-S with a molecular weight of 14,000, corresponding to a sedimentation coefficient of 2S [14], and at least eight other peaks were observed on the chromatograms, which may represent pure or mixtures of proteins, accounting for 35% of the sodium pyrophosphate soluble nitrogen. A major component with a large molecular weight corresponding to a sedimentation coefficient of 12S appeared homogeneous in alkaline solution, but dissociated into subunits with the sedimentation coefficients 3S and 7.2S under acidic conditions. This fraction, denoted B-I, was salt soluble, but precipitated upon dialysis against distilled water; hence it is a globulin by classical nomenclature. It accounted for about 35% of rapeseed proteins. Molecular sieve chromatography revealed a great number of proteins in rapeseed with molecular weights in the range from 13,000 to 320,000 [17]. This complex composition certainly gave rise to the unique functional properties of rapeseed proteins, especially the solubility, which is very important in determining the use of a protein. Gillberg and Törnell (1976) studied the dissolution behaviour of defatted rapeseed meal [18]. The solubility of proteins was found to vary in a complicated manner with the pH of extraction, with two minimum solubility points covering a relatively wide pH range between 4.5 and 8 (Figure 4.1), corresponding to the multiple isoelectric points of canola proteins. As phytates in rapeseed may interact with the proteins to form complexes, these undesired compounds could be extracted with the proteins. Their findings on the extractability profile of phosphorus seemed to suggest that the binding of phytic acid to rapeseed proteins varied significantly with pH. It has since been reported that binary protein–phytic acid complexes tend to form at pH below the isoelectric points of

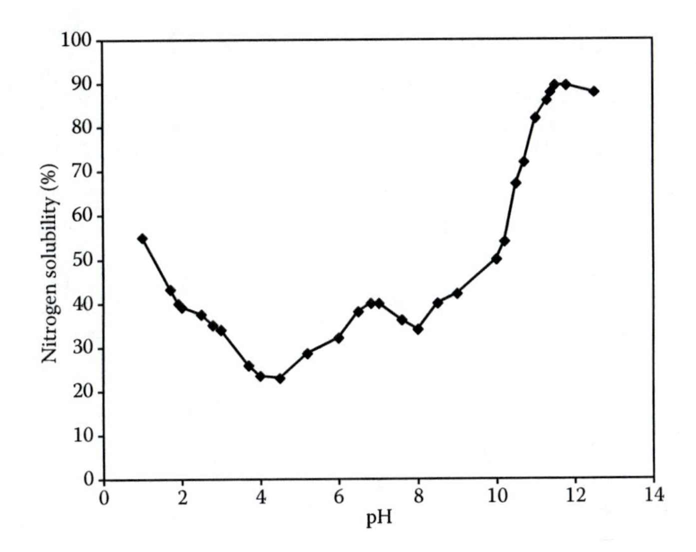

FIGURE 4.1 Effect of pH on nitrogen (protein) solubility of rapeseed. (From Gillberg, L. and Törnell, B. 1976. *J. Food Sci.* 41:1063–1069. With permission.)

rapeseed proteins, while ternary protein–metal–phytate complexes may occur in the neutral and mildly alkaline pH range [19]. Naczk et al. (1985) examined the solubility of canola meals obtained by various means [20], and also observed two minima on the solubility curves of most meals. They achieved protein solubilities greater than 70% from nontoasted meals at pH > 10. Commercial meal, however, only exhibited one minimum solubility between pH 4 and 5 and was much less soluble at high pH than other meals, likely due to excessive heating during toasting. Dissolution of canola proteins was a reversible process in a sense that the proteins dissolved at high pH could be reprecipitated when the pH was brought down to the isoelectric range. The same research group examined the precipitation profiles of canola proteins dissolved at pH 8.2 and 11.1, respectively [18]. A broad precipitation maximum was observed with the pH 11.1, covering a much wider pH range than that of the pH 8.2 extract, likely due to a much higher amount of proteins extracted at pH 11.1. It can be seen from Figure 4.1 that approximately 80% of the total protein was extracted at pH 11, as compared to only about 40% at pH 8. Apparently the pH 11.1 extract contained a wide variety of proteins with different molecular weights and isoelectric points. Using a similar method of extraction and precipitation in combination of membrane processing, Xu and Diosady (1994) obtained two protein products from rapeseed meal with completely different solubility profiles [21]. As seen in Figure 4.2, the precipitated protein isolate (PPI) exhibited a high solubility in both basic and acidic media, but was least soluble between pH 6 and 8. It probably consisted mainly of the 12S globulins. The soluble protein isolate (SPI) likely containing most of the 2S albumins was, on the other hand, highly soluble over almost the entire pH range, thus having great potential for applications in the beverage industry.

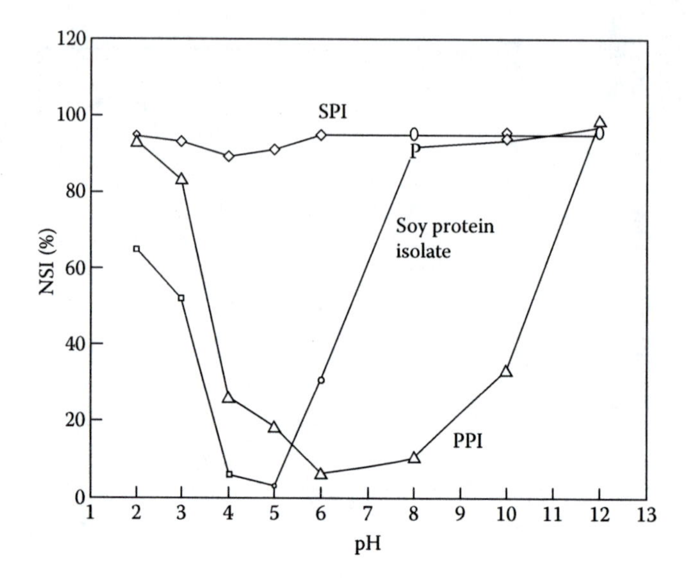

FIGURE 4.2 Effect of pH on nitrogen solubility index of rapeseed protein isolates. PPI—precipitated protein isolate; SPI—soluble protein isolate. (From Xu, L. and Diosady, L. L. 1994. *J. Amer. Oil Chem. Soc.* 71:935–939. With permission.)

TABLE 4.5
Functional Properties of Canola Protein Products

Product	Water Absorption (%)	Water-Olding Capacity (mL/g)	Fat Absorption (%)	Emulsifying Activity (%)	Overrun (%)
Precipitated protein isolate (PPI)	219	1.98	256	56.1	275
Soluble protein isolate (SPI)	Not applicable	Not applicable	514	10.8	281
Chinese rapeseed meal	273	2.48	194	51.3	237
Canola meal (Legend)[a]	287	2.61	233	50.2	205
Canola meal (Tower)[a]	363	3.46	280	60.8	80
Soyabean protein isolate	461	4.99	147	72.0	252
Soyabean meal	311	2.38	105	50.0	80

Source: From Naczk, M., Diosady, L. L. and Rubin, L. J. 1985. *J. Food Sci.* 50:1685–1688; Xu, L. and Diosady, L. L. 1994. *J. Food Sci.* 59:1127–1130. With permission.

[a] Meal extracted with methanol containing 10% ammonia and 5% water and hexane.

Besides solubility, other functional properties determining the use of protein as food include water- and oil-binding properties, emulsification and foaming properties. Water- and oil-binding properties of a protein indicate its ability of interaction with water and oil, respectively, and canola protein products usually had both high water absorption and oil absorption (Table 4.5), thus leading to good emulsification capacity for almost all products [20,22], except the SPI, which showed a poor emulsion activity despite a high fat absorption [21]. The mechanism of fat adsorption relies mostly on the physical entrapment of fat by capillary attraction. In the case of solvent-treated meals for glucosinolate removal, increase in fat adsorption was observed, which may be a result of the unfolding of protein by the solvent to expose hydrophobic groups on the surface of protein molecules. Foaming properties of all canola protein products were better than that of their soy counterparts. The protein isolates were superior to the meals in both overrun and foam stability, and their foams lasted well over 2 h.

4.3 CANOLA PROTEIN PROCESSING

4.3.1 MEAL

Containing more than 35% protein with a well-balanced amino acid composition and desirable functionalities, canola meal certainly qualifies as a protein product. Due to the low levels of glucosinolates in the meal, it is a suitable feedstuff for livestock and poultry. Based on its nutrient content, canola meal is worth 70–75% of the value of soyabean meal for feeding poultry and about 75–80% of the same for feeding swine and ruminants, while the cost of canola meal was historically much less than 70% of that of soyabean meal [23].

Canola meal is a byproduct of oil extraction, and the technology used is typical of high-oil-content seed processing, consisting of prepressing and solvent extraction (Figure 4.3), which has been practised for commercial manufacturing for decades [24]. The seeds are first cleaned and then cracked using flaking rolls. The cracked seeds are 'cooked' at 100–120°C by contacting with live steam in a cooker to rupture intact cells and inactivate myrosinase that hydrolyzes glucosinolates to produce toxic compounds. The cooked seeds are then immediately pressed to separate oil by screw presses. Pressing typically removes two-thirds of the oil so that the prepressed cake still contains 15–22% oil. This cake is flaked and conditioned before solvent extraction. In a solvent extractor, large volumes of solvent percolate the flakes in multiple stages and separate the solids from the oil-containing miscella. After oil extraction, the solids (marc) are transported to a desolventizer-toaster, where the residual solvent is removed by steam heating the meal at 130°C. It is then dried and cooled. In the meantime oil is recovered in solvent evaporators and strippers. The meal is granulated or pelletized for storage. Nowadays it is widely used in Canada and other countries as an inexpensive protein supplement, generally as a replacement for soy meal in formulated animal feeds.

As efficient as the above process is in oil extraction, both prepressing and toasting inflict much damage to the meal quality. The organic solvents used for defatting require sophisticated extraction and recovery equipment, and they pose health, fire and environmental hazards. Therefore, alternative methods have been sought

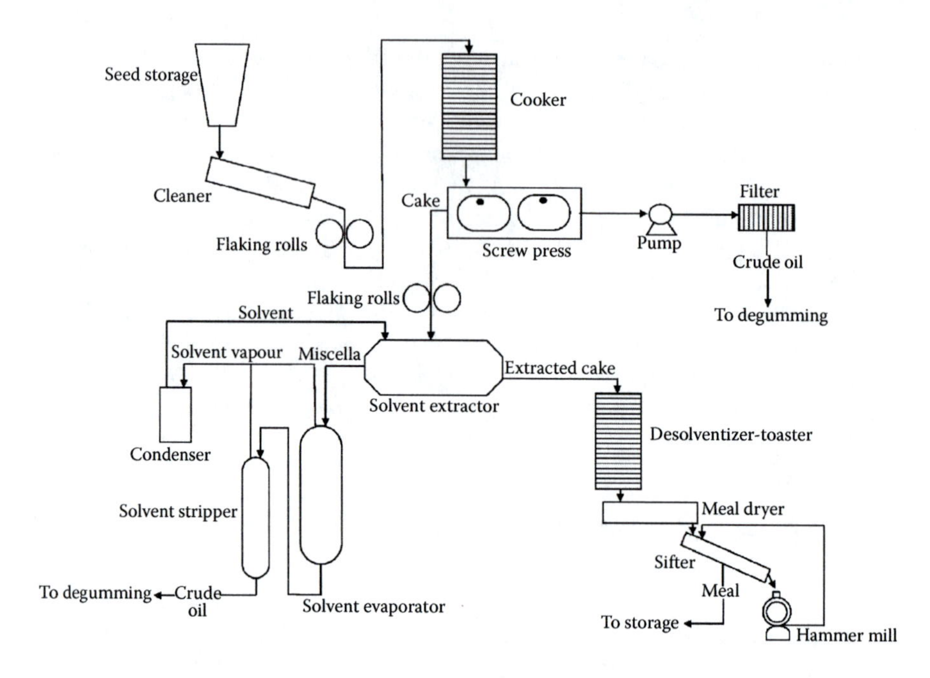

FIGURE 4.3 Commercial canola processing. (From Xu, L. and Diosady, L. L. 2003. *Extraction Optimization in Food Engineering.* Marcel Dekker, Inc., New York, New York. pp. 181. With permission.)

to produce high-quality oil and protein products. Aqueous processing, which uses mainly water to extract oil, is particularly promising due to its potential advantages of simplicity and safety. Aqueous processes are environmentally benign, so they have been extensively studied with various oilseeds. Key steps in aqueous processing include milling, extraction, solids separation, defatting and protein recovery. Unlike in solvent extraction, where oil is dissolved in a miscible solvent, in aqueous processing, oil is released by dissolving the seed matrix and the freed oil forms emulsions. It is then recovered by breaking the emulsion by techniques such as creaming, sedimentation, phase inversion, ripening and coalescence. Oil in canola seeds is contained in small oil bodies (<1 μm), which consist of an oil droplet enclosed in a membrane made up from oleosins and phospholipids. Oleosins, a group of amphiphilic proteins embedded on the membranes of oil-bodies of oilseeds, tend to form stable emulsions with the oil, thus making oil separation very difficult. Therefore, additional means are always necessary in order to break emulsions. Centrifuging, one of the most commonly used defatting methods based on forced creaming and coalescence, originated in the diary industry. Since both heating and freezing can destabilize emulsions by promoting coalescence, they can be used to facilitate defatting. Employing these techniques, Embong and Jelen (1977) investigated the technical feasibility of an aqueous process for rapeseed extraction [25], which consisted of grinding, boiling, stirring and centrifuging (Figure 4.4). The finely dried ground rapeseed was added slowly and with stirring to boiling water and boiled for 5 min. After cooling, the slurry was adjusted to pH 7.3 with NaOH, ground again and blended for 15 min.

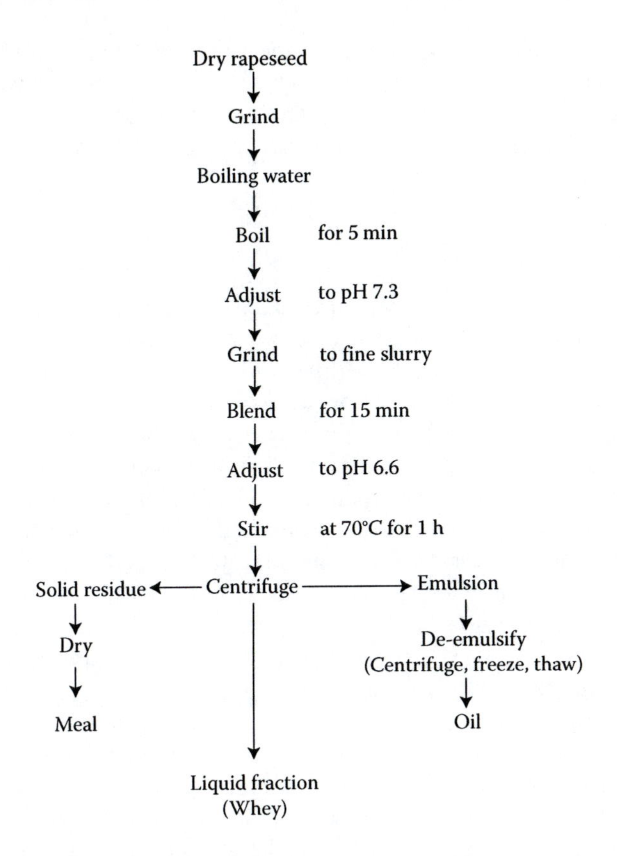

FIGURE 4.4 Aqueous processing of rapeseed. (From Embong, M. B. and Jelen, P. 1977. *J. Inst. Can. Sci. Technol. Aliment.* 10:239–243. With permission.)

The pH was adjusted to 6.6, and the slurry was stirred at an elevated temperature in a water bath. Finally, the slurry was centrifuged for 10 min. This process resulted in the formation of some free oil, an emulsion layer, an aqueous fraction and a solid residue. The emulsion was frozen in a freezer, thawed in an oven at 90°C and centrifuged into oil and aqueous fractions. Variables including solid-to-water ratio, pH, temperature of stirring and centrifuging speed were examined and optimized to maximize the oil yield. More than 90% of the oil was obtained under the optimal conditions of pH 6.6, solid-to-water ratio of 3 and stirring temperature of 75°C. The oil was of high quality in terms of free fatty acids, phospholipids and sulphur content. The solid residue after drying produced a meal containing 38% protein with a low amount of residual oil. It was, however, not known what became of the aqueous fraction. This process involved many steps, some of which could take quite long, to make rapeseed oil and meal of medium-to-low price range in the market, making it hard to compete with the existing technology economically. It was, nevertheless, one of the more successful early examples of aqueous processing, and if the process could be extended to yield a high-end protein isolate, its economics may be substantially improved. Sometimes proteolytic enzymes such as alcalase and papain were used to aid oil separation as the hydrolysis of the oil-binding proteins would favour the coalescence of oil droplets. The use of enzymes will, of course, increase the cost of processing and is therefore fit only for high-valued products. For the production of commodity items like canola oil and meal, where cost is still a major concern, simple and inexpensive processes are favoured.

4.3.2 Protein Concentrates

While soy protein products, namely concentrates and isolates are well established in the market, similar products based on other vegetable origins have long been sought as soy cannot be grown in many regions, and soy products have some problems with allergenicity and flavour reversion. Since the 1970s, there have been extensive research and development efforts to utilize canola proteins. Various approaches to make protein concentrates and isolates were investigated in an effort to develop commercially viable processes. Canola protein concentration is typically achieved by washing the meal with solvents to remove impurities to the maximum degree while retaining the protein in the solid phase. Two examples of such processing stand out in terms of technical novelty and product quality. Jones and Holme (1979) developed a process for producing a detoxified protein concentrate from defatted rapeseed high in glucosinolates and phenolic compounds [26], in which the seeds were first dehulled, and defatted with hexane to be used as the starting material. The flour thus obtained was treated with an aqueous alcohol such as isopropanol that contained potassium metabisulphite to prevent oxidation of phenolics and to inhibit enzymic degradation of glucosinolates (Figure 4.5). The concentration of isopropanol was varied from 100% to 60% (v/v) to examine the effect, and multiple consecutive extractions were performed, each at a solvent-to-flour ratio of 4. The washed meal was then dried at a temperature below 60°C. After five washings with 60% isopropanol containing 300 ppm SO_2, a protein concentrate was obtained with a protein content of nearly 70% and a protein recovery of 90%. It was essentially glucosinolate- and phenolic-free, and had an almost white colour. The intensive alcohol treatment, however, may have some undesired bearing on the functional properties of the products, especially their protein solubility, thus affecting their use in food. Furthermore, the large volumes of solvent used result in high-processing cost and make this process uneconomical. Consequently, it has not been commercially implemented.

In the 1980s, Diosady et al. (1989) used a two-solvent system to extract rapeseed [27], where the seeds were ground with methanol containing ammonia and water to produce a slurry. It was then pumped through a counter-current Karr liquid–liquid extraction column which was fitted with perforated Teflon plates evenly spaced along the shaft, as shown in Figure 4.6. A variable speed motor on the top of the column drives the vertical motion of the shaft and in turn pushes the plates up and down to agitate the liquids in the column. A second solvent immiscible with the first one and having a different density, usually hexane, was passed countercurrently to the slurry in the same column. The column performance was optimized by varying agitation, total throughput and feed ratio. Better results were achieved with polar phase as the continuous phase and hexane being the dispersed phase. Under the optimal conditions, both oil and meal of high quality were produced from this two-solvent-phase

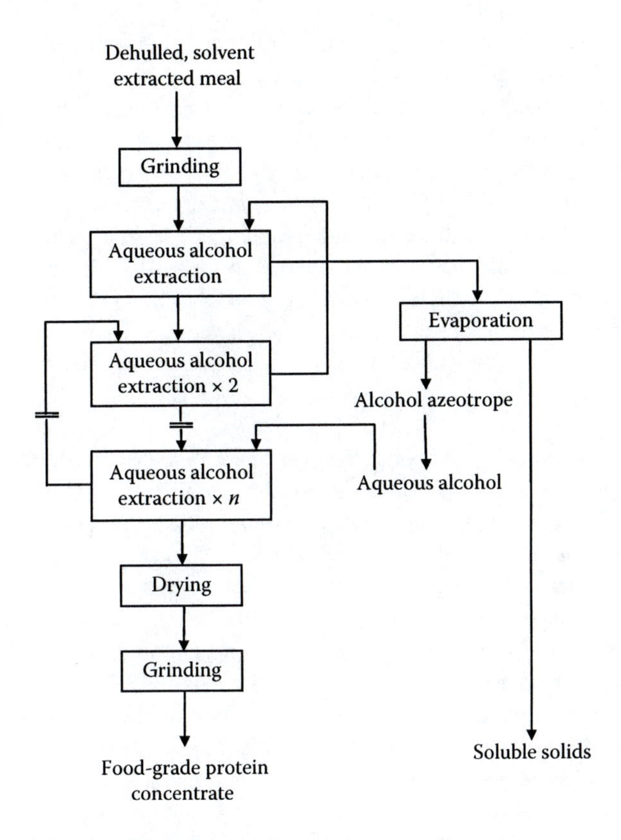

FIGURE 4.5 Process for production of detoxified protein concentrate from defatted rapeseed. (From Jones, J. D. and Holme, J. 1979. US Patent 4,158,656. With permission.)

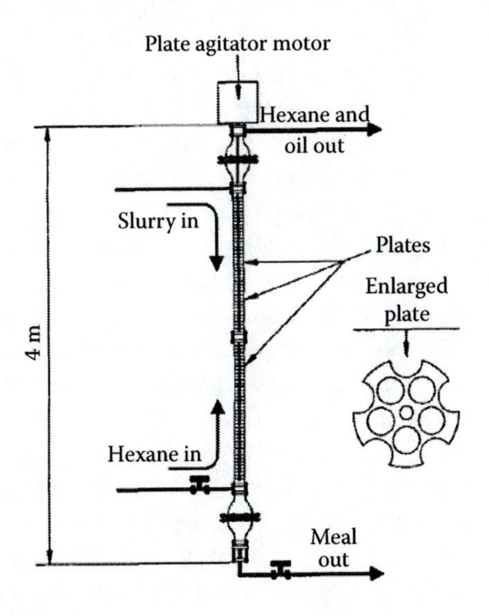

FIGURE 4.6 The Karr column.

column operation. The polar phase, methanol containing ammonia and water, not only effectively removed many undesired seed components from both the meal and the oil, but also partially denatured the proteins of oil-bodies, thus facilitating the release of oil from the cells. The oil produced was essentially degummed and low in free fatty acids, simplifying subsequent refining. The meal contained <0.5% residual oil and had a protein content of about 50% with glucosinolate levels below the detection limit. As this system extracts oil and treats the meal simultaneously in one unit, it could save much of the pre- and posttreatment, thus offering a unique alternative to the existing technology. Understandably the main challenge to its implementation is a huge capital investment and the use of two solvents.

4.3.3 Protein Isolates

Protein isolation takes an opposite approach to protein concentration, wherein the protein is dissolved while most of the impurities remain in the solids. Process development to make canola protein isolates started in the early 1970s, and continued well into the 21st century. Much of the work is still ongoing. Many of the earlier processes were based on soy protein technology, comprising two major stages of operation: aqueous extraction and protein precipitation. Alkaline extraction with dilute NaOH solutions has been extensively used to solubilize as much as 90% of the total protein in various laboratory-prepared meals [18,28,29]. These meals were usually hexane extracted and desolventized at low temperatures so the proteins remained largely intact. Water use was usually 15–20 times the amount of meal as further increase in water did not improve protein solubility. The amount NaOH added was determined by either targeted molarity (M) or pH. Both a concentration of 0.1 M and a pH above 11.0 were able to achieve protein extractabilities of 90% in these meals. With commercial meal as starting material, the extractabilities were much lower due, no doubt, to desolventizing/toasting at 130°C, which denatured the protein to a significant degree. The protein of meal treated with alcohols was also less extractable as a result of partial protein denaturation [29,30]. During alkaline extraction, extremely high pH (>12) should be avoided as undesirable chemical modifications of the protein may occur, such as the formation of harmful lysinoalanine [31]. To increase the yield, multistage extraction was employed to achieve extractability >90% [32,33]. Nockrashy et al. (1977) adopted a four-stage countercurrent extraction procedure for protein extraction from hexane defatted meal. At each stage, the supernatant from one sample was used to extract the next sample, and the final extracts from all four stages were combined to deliver an overall extractability of 94%, the highest ever reported [32]. Since their trials were conducted on a small scale of only 5 g per sample extracted with 125 mL of 0.02 N NaOH each time, the amount of product was insufficient for functionality tests after all proximate analyses. The process therefore needed proper scale-up to further demonstrate its efficiency and feasibility. The alkaline extract of canola protein, however, has an unappetizing dark brown colour. Product colour has been a concern of researchers working on the development of canola proteins for food use. Some reducing and oxidizing agents were tested for the decolourization of canola proteins [34,35], such as hydrogen peroxide and sodium sulphite. Keshavarz et al. (1977)

found that the addition of 2% sodium sulphite significantly reduced the colour of the final product [35], and unlike hydrogen peroxide, it did not affect the quality of the protein in terms of amino acid composition.

To take advantage of the characteristics of canola globulins, many researchers explored dilute NaCl solutions (saline) with concentrations from 0.2 N to 2.0 N for canola protein extraction [36–39]. Salt solutions typically extracted less protein than alkaline media, and the recovery of saline-extracted protein is often complicated by the need to remove the salt by dialysis. Although Lo and Hill (1971) reported an exceptionally high nitrogen solubility of 83.5% from hexane-defatted rapeseed meal, they used a brine solution of 10% NaCl and a high water-to-meal ratio of 30. To desalt the protein extract, dialysis was done with running tap water for 3 days [6]. Combined use of alkali and salt solution was never reported, possibly because there are some antagonistic effects between the two solutes on protein extraction. It has been known that polyphosphates are effective complexing agents for proteins. Their use in protein extraction could improve the yield significantly. Thompson et al. (1976) employed a 2% sodium hexametaphosphate (SHMP) solution to extract rapeseed protein from dehulled flour at pH 7 [40]. Their two-step procedure with an initial solution-to-flour ratio of 10 and a second ratio of 6 gave a total extraction yield of 97%. Tzeng et al. (1988) also studied the effect of SHMP concentration on the protein extraction of rapeseed meal [41]. They attained >70% extractability with only 1% SHMP at neutral pH from hexane-defatted meal. With the methanol–ammonia–water/hexane extracted meal, however, only about 10% of the protein was soluble in SHMP solution, likely due to protein denaturation by the polar solvent. Based on the findings on protein solubility, they developed a process to produce rapeseed protein isolate, where the extracted protein was concentrated and purified by ultrafiltration and diafiltration. The freeze-dried product had not only a protein content close to 90%, but also an unacceptable phytic acid content (>6%). Only after ion exchange at a solution-to-resin ratio of 4 was the phytic acid and phosphorus content reduced to below 1%. The high resin use made the process less attractive from an economical point of view.

Like soy proteins, extracted canola proteins were typically recovered by isoelectric precipitation. The precipitates, after being washed and dried, constitute the protein isolate. Due to the complex protein compositions and varietal differences among canola strains, a wide range of isoelectric points was observed, at each of which only a specific fraction of the extracted protein was precipitated, therefore protein recovery of single-step isoelectric precipitation was usually low. The highest ever reported was 65.7% of the amount of protein extracted at pH 11, obtained at pH 3.6 [32]. Moderate increase in protein yield was achieved by the same researchers with multi-isoelectric precipitation at different pH. Therefore, the further improvement in overall protein output hinges on the recovery of fractions that were not precipitated, and these proteins, due to their high solubility, are ideal for many food applications.

Since canola proteins are large molecules with molecular weights >10,000, membrane technology was investigated as an effective means for their recovery. Ultrafiltration uses semi-permeable membranes to selectively pass or retain solutes of interest, thus achieving isolation or concentration and purification. Work in this area has been inspired by a wide variety of applications of membrane technology in the food industry, especially the diary and soyabean sectors and the great strides in improving the properties, reliability and manufacturing techniques of membranes. Membrane separation is, however, relatively new and still in the trial stage for canola protein isolation. In addition to the separation of solutes of different molecular weights, its other advantages include mild operating conditions, low energy consumption and essentially no pH change and no phase changes are required. Membranes are made of different materials including modified cellulose, polymers, porous metals and ceramic materials and come in various configurations such as hollow fibres, spiral-wound and tubular to suit different applications. Membrane processing can be driven by pressure, chemical, or electric potential differences. Food processing applications are usually pressure driven since it is able to produce a desirable permeate flux for large-scale operations. Based on the membrane pore size, which limits the size of material passing into the permeate, pressure-driven membrane processes are classified as microfiltration (MF), ultrafiltration (UF), nanofiltration (NF) and reverse osmosis (RO), in order of decreasing pore size. The pore sizes of UF membranes are similar to the molecular sizes of macromolecules, thus being most suitable for protein processing. Each UF membrane is characterized by the molecular weight cut-off (MWCO)—the size of the largest molecule that can pass through it. The schematic diagram of batch ultrafiltration is shown in Figure 4.7. The feed solution is pumped from a tank and pushed through a prefilter to remove all fine solids before the solution enters the membrane module. Inside the module, small molecules and solvent such as water are driven through a porous membrane as the permeate while high-molecular-weight solutes are retained in the retentate and pumped back to the feed tank. As the feed solution is recirculated in the system, its volume is reduced and large molecules are thus concentrated as well as purified. During the process, as water passes through the membrane, macromolecules left behind are deposited on the surface of the membrane, thus building up a gel layer, which brings about most

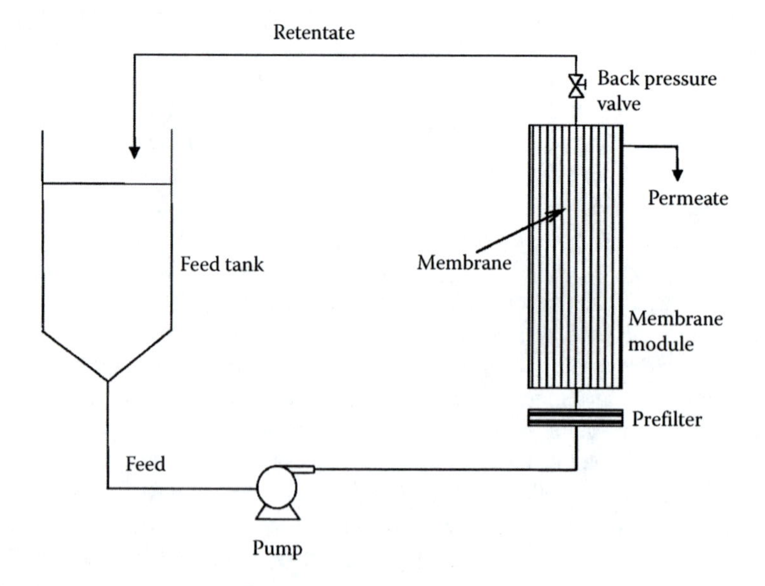

FIGURE 4.7 Schematic diagram of batch ultrafiltration.

of the resistance to permeation. In order to minimize the gel layer, ultrafiltration is usually conducted in a cross-flow manner as it is able to maximize the turbulence at the membrane surface, thus shearing away much of the deposit and preventing the formation of a thick gel layer. In UF, the concentration of small molecules remains constant, although their total mass is decreased proportionally to the solvent removal. The concentration of small molecules can be decreased by diafiltration (DF), in which solvent removed by the membrane is replaced with fresh solvent so the volume of solution and the concentration of large molecules remain constant, while the concentration of small ingredients steadily decreases. The combined use of both UF and DF can minimize the impurities in the system and produce macromolecular materials such as proteins of high purity and concentration.

So far, two processes involving membrane separation for canola protein isolation are considered promising, and both are currently under commercial development. Researchers at the University of Toronto developed a membrane-based process for canola protein isolation from defatted meal [29,42], in which, after precipitation, the soluble proteins were ultrafiltered to be concentrated and diafiltered for purification. Two protein isolates were produced: precipitated and soluble, with a combined protein recovery of more than 70% of total meal protein. Both products were high in protein (>85%), low in phytates (<1%), essentially free of glucosinolates (<2 μmol/g) and had desirable functional properties comparable to those of soy protein. While the methionine content of both protein isolates was similar to the reported values, the soluble product was found to have a higher level of lysine than any canola proteins obtained before, and the precipitated protein isolate was, on the other hand, further enriched with leucine [43]. This amino acid composition makes them suitable for use in infant formulae (Table 4.6). Despite their excellent nutritive quality,

TABLE 4.6
Essential Amino Acid Composition of Products of Membrane-Based Canola Protein Isolation (g/100 g Protein)

Essential Amino Acid	Meal	Meal Residue	Precipitated Protein Isolate	Soluble Protein Isolate	FAO/WHO/UNU Suggested Pattern for Infants
Isoleucine	4.5	5.0	5.2	3.5	4.6
Leucine	7.5	7.7	9.2	7.2	9.3
Lysine	6.6	6.6	5.9	7.3	6.6
Methionine	2.2	2.1	2.4 (3.4)[a]	2.4 (6.6)[a]	(4.2)[a]
Phenylalanine	4.7	4.5	5.2 (9.4)[b]	4.0 (6.5)[b]	(7.2)[b]
Threonine	4.8	6.5	5.8	4.2	4.3
Valine	5.7	6.8	5.8	4.7	5.5

Source: From Tzeng, Y. M. 1987. Process development for the production of high-quality rapeseed (canola) protein isolates using membrane technology. Ph.D. Thesis. University of Toronto, Toronto, Canada. With permission.

[a] Values in parentheses are sums of those of methionine and cystine.

[b] Values in parentheses are sums of those of phenylalanine and tyrosine.

the sensory properties of these protein products were, however, less than ideal likely due to the substantial levels of phenolic compounds in them. It was found that these compounds tend to bind to the proteins by different mechanisms [44]. Therefore, the University of Toronto's process was later improved with additional membrane processing in combination with heat treatment prior to precipitation, and polyvinylpyrrolidone (PVP) treatment after precipitation as shown in Figure 4.8, in order to remove phenolic compounds [45,46]. As a result, both colour and taste of the products were significantly improved, thus making them more attractive. The high quality of these canola protein isolates has generated much interest, and commercial

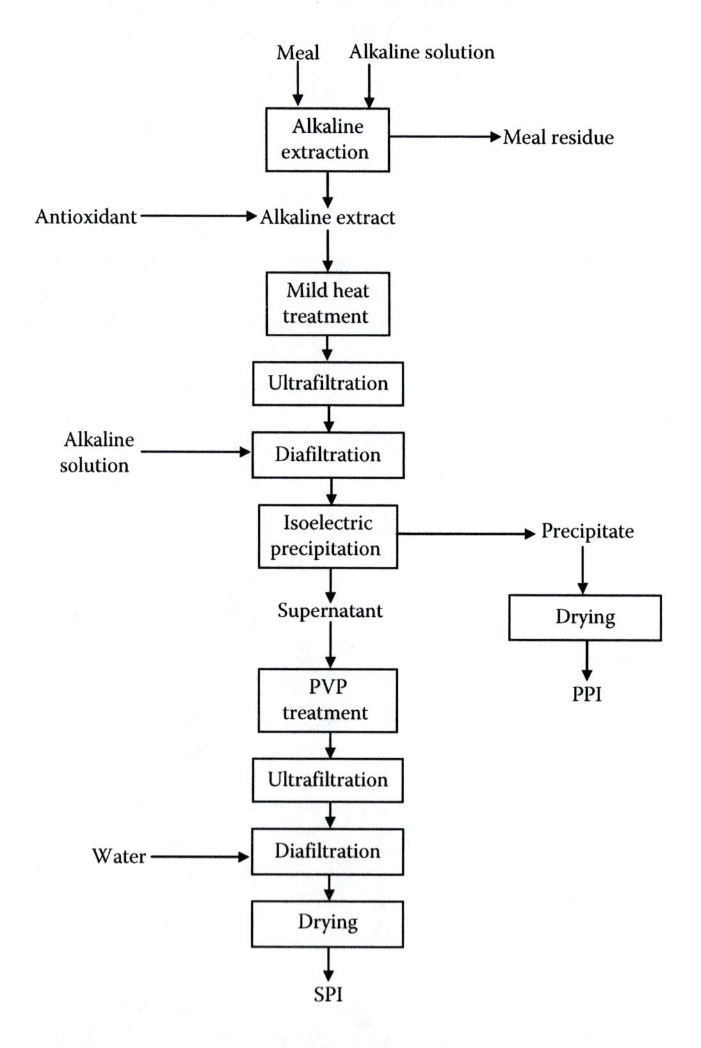

FIGURE 4.8 Membrane-based process for canola protein isolation. (From Jones, J. D. and Holme, J. 1979. Oilseed processing. US Patent 4,158,656; Diosady, L. L., Xu, L. and Chen, B. K. 2005. Production of high-quality protein isolates from defatted meals of Brassica seeds. US Patent 6,905,713. With permission.)

trials are being conducted at Baltmere, a venture capital company based in Estonia, which uses the meals of European rapeseed varieties.

Burcon NutraScience Corporation, a venture capital company founded at the turn of the century and specialized in the commercialization of canola proteins, adopted a unique process based on salt extraction [47]. Saline of 0.15 M was used as the extractant. As shown in Figure 4.9, after extraction the resulting protein solution was concentrated by ultrafiltration to a concentration in excess of 200 g/L, and then diluted with chilled water at a temperature below 15°C to form a protein micellar mass (PMM), which accounted for 40–60% extracted protein, depending on the initial protein concentration and dilution ratio. PMM was settled, separated from supernatant and dried to obtain a protein isolate with a protein content over 100% (N × 6.25). The supernatant was processed to recover additional proteins by further

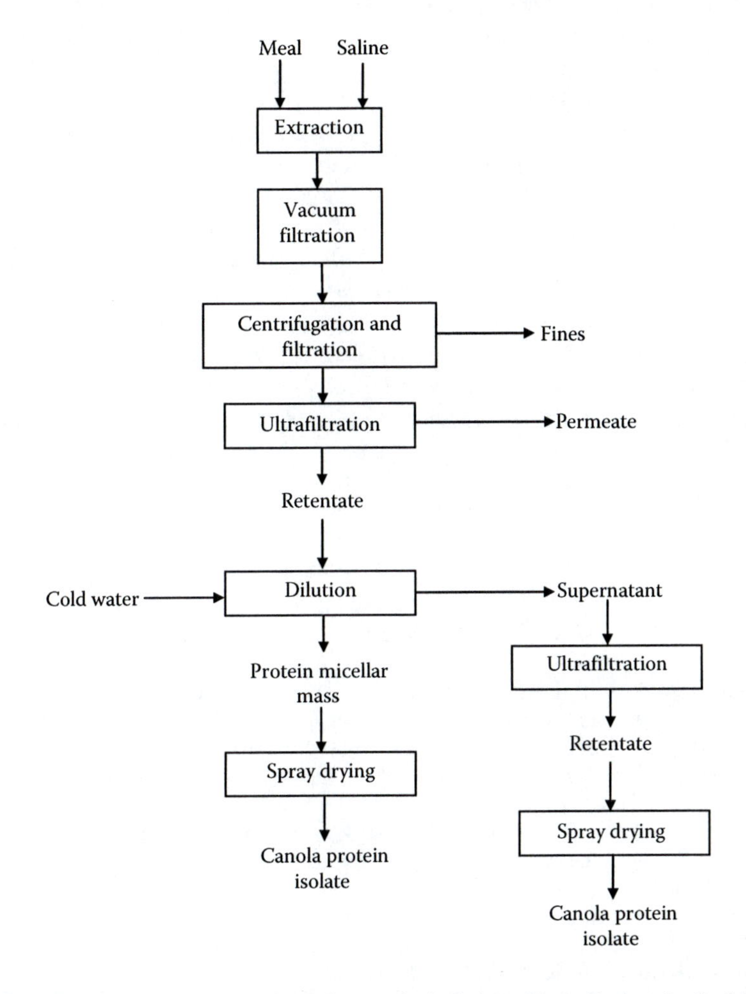

FIGURE 4.9 Burcon's process of canola protein isolation. (From Barker, L. D., Martens, R. W. and Murray, E. D. 2010. Production of oil seed protein isolate. US Patent 7,687,087 B2. With permission.)

concentration with another ultrafiltration step. The concentrated supernatant was dried to produce another protein isolate containing more than 90% protein. The two protein isolates were tested for a variety of food applications from baked goods, and processed meat products to beverages, according to their functional properties. As their technology is intensively membrane-based, requiring protein concentration >20%, which is very viscous, ultrafiltration permeate flux would be very low, especially during continuous operation, which may result in high surface area requirements or pumping costs.

Recently, BioExx Specialty Proteins Ltd, another commercial canola protein developer, used their own patented technology to successfully turn out two canola protein products, with the trade names Isolexx and Vitalexx, respectively. Isolexx is termed a protein isolate while Vitalexx contains fully hydrolyzed protein, that is claimed to be completely soluble in water across a wide pH range. Although little is disclosed to the public about their process, it is known that they use an inert fluorocarbon solvent to extract the oil from canola at very low temperatures to ensure minimum impact on the meal protein quality, thus maximizing protein solubility prior to extraction. The published data on nutritional value and functionalities indicated that these products were comparable to whey and soy proteins in amino acid composition, solubility, foaming, emulsification and gelling ability, thus suitable for application in nutritional drinks, energy snacks, snacks, baked goods, dressings and toppings.

The extensive research and development of canola proteins in both academia and industry have resulted in remarkable progress in all aspects from nutritional quality to functional characteristics, sensory properties and processing technology, although hurdles still remain to full commercial acceptance. The quickly growing demand for alternatives to soy proteins is providing an added impetus to the commercialization of canola proteins, which is proceeding at a much faster rate than before, encouraged further by the dramatic rise in the price of soyabean in the last decade. Accordingly, it is realistic to expect commercial penetration of the food protein market by a variety of canola protein products within the next 10 years.

REFERENCES

1. Daun, J. K. 1986. Glucosinolate levels in western Canadian rapeseed and canola. *JAOCS*. 63:639–643.
2. Eskin, N. A. M., McDonald, B. E., Przybylski, R., Malcolmson, L. J., Scarth, R., Mag, T., Ward, K. and Adolph, D. 1996. Canola oil. In *Bailey's Industrial Oil and Fat Products,* ed. F. Shahidi. 5th ed. John Wiley & Sons Inc., New York. pp. 1–95.
3. Foreign Agricultural Service. USDA. 2010. Oilseed: World Markets and Trade. http://www.fas.usda.gov/currwmt.asp
4. Salunkhe, D. K., Chavan, J. K., Adsule, R. N. and Kadam, S. S. 1992. Rapeseed. In *World Oilseeds: Chemistry, Technology and Utilization*. Van Nostrand Reinhold, New York. pp. 59.
5. Ohlson, R. and Anjou, K. 1979. Rapeseed protein products. *JAOCS*. 56:431–437.
6. Lo, M. T. and Hill, D. C. 1971. Evaluation of protein concentrates prepared from rapeseed meal. *J. Sci. Food Agric.* 22:128–130.
7. VanEtten, C. H. 1969. Daxenbichler, M. E. and Wolff, I. A. 1969. Natural glucosinolates in foods and feeds. *J. Agric. Food Chem.* 17:483–491.

8. Uppström, B. and Svensson, R. 1980. Determination of phytic acid in rapeseed meal. *J. Sci. Food Agric.* 31:651–656.
9. Sosulski, F. W. 1979. Organoleptic and nutritional effects of Phenolic compounds on oilseed protein products: A review. *JAOCS.* 56:711–714.
10. Krygier, K., Sosulski, F. and Hogge, L. 1982. Free, esterified, and insoluble-bound phenolic acids. 2. Composition of phenolic acids in rapeseed flour and hulls. *J. Agric. Food Chem.* 30:334–336.
11. Xu, L. and Diosady, L. L. 1997. Rapid method for total phenolic acid determination in rapeseed/canola meals. *Food Res. Intern.* 30:571–574.
12. Shahidi, F. and Naczk, M. 1989. Effect of processing on the content of condensed tannins in rapeseed meals. *J. Food Sci.* 54:1082–1083.
13. Appelqvist, L. A. 1972. Chemical constituens in rapeseed. In *Rapeseed: Cultivation, Composition, Processing and Utilization*, ed. L. A. Appelqvist and R. Olson. Elsevier Publishing Co., Amsterdam, Holland. pp. 123.
14. Bhatty, R. S., McKenzie, S. L. and Finlayson, A. J. 1968. The proteins of rapeseed (*Brassica napus* L.) soluble in salt solutions. *Can. J. Biochem.* 45:1191–1197.
15. Schwenke, K. D., Raab, B., Linow, K. J. and Uhlig, J. 1981. Isolation of the 12S globulin from rapeseed (*Brassica napus* L.) and characterization as a neutral protein on seed proteins, part 13. *Nahrung* 28:271–280.
16. Raab, B. and Schwenke, K. D. 1984. Simplified isolation procedure for 12S globulin and the albumin fraction fro rapeseed (*Brassica napus* L.). *Nahrung* 28:863–866.
17. Lönnerdal, B., Gillberg, L. and Törnell, B. 1977. Preparation of rapeseed protein isolates: A study of rapeseed protein isolates by molecular sieve chromatography. *J. Food Sci.* 42:75–78.
18. Gillberg, L. and Törnell, B. 1976. Preparation of rapeseed protein isolates: Dissolution and precipitation behaviour of rapeseed proteins. *J. Food Sci.* 41:1063–1069.
19. Cheryan, M. and Rackis, J. J. 1980. Phytic acid interactions in food systems. *Crit. Rev. Food Sci. Nutr. 13:297–335.*
20. Naczk, M., Diosady, L. L. and Rubin, L. J. 1985. Functional properties of canola meals produced by a two phase solvent extraction system. *J. Food Sci.* 50:1685–1688.
21. Xu, L. and Diosady, L. L. 1994. Functional properties of Chinese rapeseed protein isolates. *J. Food Sci.* 59:1127–1130.
22. Ghodsvali, A., Haddad Khodaparast, M. H., Vosoughi, M. and Diosady, L. L. 2005. Preparation of canola protein materials using membrane technology and evaluation of meals functional properties. *Food Res. Int.* 38:223–231.
23. Miller, W. J. 1988. Canada's canola. Canola Council of Canada.
24. Xu, L. and Diosady, L. L. 2003. Fats and oils from plant materials. In *Extraction Optimization in Food Engineering*, ed. C. Tzia and G. Liadakis. Marcel Dekker, Inc., New York, New York. pp. 181.
25. Embong, M. B. and Jelen, P. 1977. Technical feasibility of aqueous extraction of rapeseed oil—A laboratory study. *J. Inst. Can. Sci. Technol. Aliment.* 10:239–243.
26. Jones, J. D. and Holme, J. 1979. Oilseed processing. US Patent 4,158,656.
27. Diosady, L. L., Rubin, L. J. and Tar, C. G. 1989. Extraction of particulate materials. US Patent 4,859,371.
28. Finlayson, A. J., Bhatty, R. S. and McKenzie, S. L. 1976. The effects of extraction solvents on the yields and structures of *Brassica* sp. meal proteins. *Can. Inst. Food Sci. Technol. J.* 9:212–215.
29. Tzeng, Y. M., Diosady, L. L. and Rubin, L. J. 1990. Production of canola protein materials by alkaline, extraction, precipitation, and membrane processing. *J. Food Sci.* 55:1147–1151.
30. Igor, S. O., Diosady, L. L. and Rubin, L. R. 1993. Catalytic deamidation of canola proteins. *Acta Alimentaria.* 22:325–336.

31. Pfaender, P. 1983. Lysinoalanine—A toxic compound in processed proteinaceous food. *World Rev. Nutr. Diet.* 41:97–109.
32. El Nockrashy, A. S., Mukherjee, K. D. and Mangold, H. K. 1977. Rapeseed protein isolates by countercurrent extraction and isoelectric precipitation. *J. Agric. Food Chem.* 25:193–197.
33. Blaicher, F. M., Elstner, F., Stein, W. and Mukherjee, K. D. 1983. Rapeseed protein isolates: Effect of processing on yield and composition of protein. *J. Agric. Food Chem.* 31:358–362.
34. Kodagoda, L. P., Yeung, C. Y., Nakai, S. and Powrie, W. D. 1973. Preparation of protein isolates from rapeseed flour. *Can. Inst. Food Sci. Technol. J.* 6:135–138.
35. Keshavarz, E., Cheung, R. K. M., Liu, R. C. M. and Nakai, S. 1977. Adaptation of the three extraction stage process to rapeseed meal for preparation of colorless protein extracts. *Can. Inst. Food Sci. Technol. J.* 10:73–77.
36. Owen, D. F. 1973. Detoxification and isolation of rapeseed protein by aqueous saline extraction and isoelectric protein precipitation. US Patent 3,758,452.
37. Siy, R. D. and Talbot F. D. F. 1981. Preparation of low-phytate rapeseed protein by ultrafiltration: II. Membrane development and testing. *JAOCS.* 58:1021–1023.
38. Finnigan, T. J. A. and Lewis, M. J. 1985. Nitrogen extraction from defatted rapeseed, with particular reference to United Kingdom commercial rapeseed meal. *J. Sci. Food Agric.* 36:520–530.
39. Murray, E. D., Maurice, T. J., Barker, L. D. and Myers, C. D. 1980. Process for isolation of proteins using food grade salt solutions at specified pH and ionic strength. US Patent 4,208,323.
40. Thompson, L. U., Poon, P. and Procope, C. 1976. Isolation of rapeseed protein using sodium hexametaphosphate. *Can. Inst. Food. Sci. Tech. J.* 9:15–19.
41. Tzeng, Y. M., Diosady, L. L. and Rubin, L. J. 1988. Preparation of rapeseed protein isolate by sodium hexametaphosphate extraction, ultrafiltration, diafiltration and ion-exchange. *J. Food Sci.* 53:1537–1541.
42. Xu, L. and Diosady, L. L. 1994. The production of Chinese rapeseed protein isolates by membrane processing. *JAOCS.* 71:935–939.
43. Tzeng, Y. M. 1987. Process development for the production of high-quality rapeseed (canola) protein isolates using membrane technology. Ph.D. Thesis. University of Toronto, Toronto, Canada.
44. Xu, L. and Diosady, L. L. 2000. Interactions between canola proteins and phenolic compounds in aqueous media. *Food Res. Int.* 33:725–731.
45. Xu, L. and Diosady, L. L. 2002. Removal of phenolic compounds in the production of high-quality canola protein isolates. *Food Res. Int.* 35:23–30.
46. Diosady, L. L., Xu, L. and Chen, B. K. 2005. Production of high-quality protein isolates from defatted meals of Brassica seeds. US Patent 6,905,713.
47. Barker, L. D., Martens, R. W. and Murray, E. D. 2010. Production of oil seed protein isolate. US Patent 7,687,087 B2.

5 Future of Omega-9 Oils

Asim Syed

CONTENTS

5.1 Introduction 79
5.2 Omega-9 Fatty Acids 80
5.2.1 Sources of Oleic Acid 80
5.2.2 North American Oilseeds Situation 81
5.2.3 Dow Agrosciences' Omega-9 Canola Programme 83
5.3 Comparative Fatty Acid Profile and Oxidative Stability Indices 83
5.4 Food Applications of Omega-9 Oils 85
5.4.1 Frying 85
5.4.1.1 Fry Life 85
5.4.1.2 A Case Study: Comparison of Several Fry Oils in Rotational Deep Frying 86
5.4.2 Spray Oil Application 91
5.4.3 Shortening Applications 92
5.4.4 Doughnut Frying 93
5.5 Removing Trans Fat from North American Menus 95
5.6 Health Benefits of Omega-9 oils 95
5.7 Canola Health Claim and Labelling 95
5.8 Canola Oil and Consumers 96
5.9 In Line with US Dietary Guidelines 97
5.10 Next Generation of Omega-9 Oils 97
5.10.1 Ultra Low-Saturated Fat Sunflower Oil 97
5.10.2 Omega-9 Canola Oil-DHA Blend 97
5.11 Summary 98
Acknowledgements 98
References 98

5.1 INTRODUCTION

Since the beginning of the global effort to reduce or eliminate *trans* fats from the food systems in the early 1990s, there has been a consistent effort by the industry to develop high stability vegetable oils that would eliminate the need for hydrogenation for the purpose of oxidative stability. Although oils such as palm and coconut oils have been in use in the food industry and are very stable, their stability comes at the cost of very high levels of saturated fats. High levels of saturated fats have been linked to health issues and are generally deemed undesirable by the consumers as well as the health professionals. Process innovations such as inter esterification (or transesterification) are also used to product functional shortenings with reduced levels of saturated fat and no or very low levels of trans fats. This process provides valuable functional properties for some food applications. However, it does carry the label of terms such as 'interesterified' or 'modified', among other limiting factors.

One of the solutions that is gaining wide acceptance in the industry has been what is referred to as 'high oleic', 'high oleic low linolenic' or 'high stability' oils (canola, sunflower, soya, etc.).

5.2 OMEGA-9 FATTY ACIDS

Omega-9 fatty acids are a family of fatty acids which include a major fatty acid called oleic acid. It is mono-unsaturated. Oleic acid is one of the most abundant fatty acids found in nature and is contained in the primary oil produced by skin glands of animals.

Omega-9 fatty acids (also referred to as n–9 or ω–9 fatty acids) are a group of unsaturated fatty acids which have in common a final carbon–carbon double bond in the n–9 position; that is, the ninth bond from the non-carboxyl end of the fatty acid (Table 5.1).

Omega-9 fatty acids are common components of animal fats and vegetable oils. Two omega-9 fatty acids important in industry are

- Oleic acid (C18:1), which is a main component of olive and canola oils.
- Erucic acid (C22:1), which is found in rapeseed and mustard seed.

From the perspective of nutrition and the food industry in general, oleic acid is the only omega-9-type fatty acid abundant in foods. The author is taking the liberty of using the term 'omega-9' for 'oleic' acid.

5.2.1 Sources of Oleic Acid

Some of the most common food sources of omega-9 fatty acids are listed below, in the order of omega-9 fatty acid content:

- Omega-9 sunflower oil (86% oleic acid)
- Omega-9 canola oil (72% oleic acid)

TABLE 5.1
List of Omega-9 (n–9) Fatty Acids

Common Name	Lipid Name	Chemical Name
Oleic acid	18:1 (n–9)	9-Octadecenoic acid
Eicosenoic acid	20:1 (n–9)	11-Eicosenoic acid
Mead acid	20:3 (n–9)	5,8,11-Eicosatrienoic acid
Erucic acid	22:1 (n–9)	13-Docosenoic acid
Nervonic acid	22:1 (n–9)	15-Tetracosenoic acid

TABLE 5.2
Food Sources of Oleic Acid (MFA 18:1), Listed in Descending Order by Percentages of Their Contribution to Intake

Rank	Food Item	Contribution to Intake (%)	Cumulative Contribution (%)
1	Grain-based desserts	8.9	8.9
2	Chicken and chicken-mixed dishes	7.6	16.6
3	Sausage, franks, bacon and ribs	5.9	22.5
4	Nuts/seeds and nut/seed mixed dishes	5.5	27.9
5	Pizza	5.4	33.3
6	Fried white potatoes	4.9	38.2
7	Mexican-mixed dishes	4.6	42.8
8	Burgers	4.1	46.9
9	Beef and beef-mixed dishes	3.9	50.8
10	Eggs and egg-mixed dishes	3.5	54.3
11	Regular cheese	3.3	57.5
12	Potato/corn/other chips	3.2	60.7
13	Pasta and pasta dishes	3.1	63.8
14	Salad dressing	2.6	66.4
15	Dairy desserts	2.3	68.7
16	Yeast breads	2.2	70.9

Source: http://riskfactor.cancer.gov/diet/foodsources/fatty_acids/table1.html.

- Olive oil (70% oleic acid)
- Canola oil (63% oleic acid)
- Peanut oil (48% oleic acid)
- Lard (44% oleic acid)
- Sesame seed oil (40% oleic acid)
- Palm oil (40% oleic acid)

Table 5.2 lists some of the manufactured food products as the sources of omega-9 fatty acid, based on the percentage of their contribution to the intake of oleic acid. The data are taken from the National Health and Nutrition Examination Survey 2005–2006.

5.2.2 North American Oilseeds Situation

The North American oilseeds complex is undergoing a significant transformation, driven by changing needs of the food industry and the adoption of renewable fuel mandates in the United States. Table 5.3 highlights the main drivers, impacts and outcomes. The result is a significant shift in oilseed cropping patterns and vegetable oil production, as shown in Table 5.4.

The US Renewable Fuel Mandate (RFM) took effect in January 2009 and will require 1 B gallons of biodiesel production by 2012. The RFM also calls for a minimum of 1 B gallons annually of biodiesel to be produced annually from 2012 to 2022.

TABLE 5.3
Drivers, Impacts and Outcomes for Changing Oilseeds Complex

Driver	Impact	Outcomes
Healthier eating	Remove trans fats	Replace hydrogenated oils
	Reduce saturated fats	Low saturate oils
	Natural ingredients	Naturally stable oils
Biofuel mandates	Biodiesel	Soya oil use as biodiesel feedstock
	Ethanol	Increased corn acres/decreased soya acres

TABLE 5.4
US Food Industry Oil Consumption (Pounds in billions)

	Year				
	02/03	04/05	06/07	08/09	10/11
Soyabean	17.1	17.4	18.7	16.3	17.2
Food	17.0	16.9	15.9	14.2	14.3
Biodiesel	0.12	0.49	2.8	2.0	2.9
Canola	1.34	1.68	1.95	2.80	3.27
Palm	0.38	0.71	1.46	2.12	2.34
Corn	1.62	1.65	1.83	1.57	1.86
Sunflower	0.29	0.23	0.60	0.45	0.56
Cotton	0.64	0.93	0.71	0.50	0.60

Source: Adapted from Informa Economics Inc, *Vegetable Oil Consumption in the USA*, June 2011.

It is presumed to consume more than 4 B pounds of soyabean oil. Soyabean oil use in food is decreasing, reflecting the demand for biodiesel and the significant decline in the use of hydrogenated soyabean oil, which was once the food industry standard.

Expansion of corn oil production is very limited as corn oil is a byproduct from the wet milling process, and there is no forecast for capacity expansion. Fractionation of corn oil from the ethanol production stream previously was forecast to increase supply, but with poor ethanol economics, bankruptcies and tight credit markets, the capital investment is unlikely to materialize.

Sunflower production has fallen to around 2 MM planted acres of oil types from the high of 5 MM acres. Although sunflower is a high oil crop with excellent sensory and functionality traits, it is more costly and difficult to produce as compared to Roundup Ready soyabeans. Soyabean varieties with earlier maturity have reached the traditional sunflower production region, competing with them for acres.

Lastly, cottonseed production has increased slightly, but ending stocks of oil continue to decline and are at the lowest levels in recent years. Cottonseed oil is a market controlled by very few processors.

5.2.3 Dow AgroSciences' Omega-9 Canola Programme

The term 'Omega-9 Oil' is referred to by the food industry as an identifier for the high oleic low linolenic canola and sunflower oils developed from Dow AgroSciences' NEXERA™ canola and sunflower seeds.

In 1996, Dow AgroSciences (DAS) started their Omega-9 (high oleic) canola breeding programme. The programme was designed to create high-yielding canola varieties that consistently produce a 'high oleic + low linolenic' fatty acid profile. The business first commercialized varieties in the late 1990s with a programme at Japan. The programme was launched into the North American market in 2004 as trans-fat labelling began.

The programme is solely focused on breeding canola with the Omega-9 fatty acid profile. Omega-9 canola varieties from DAS are yield competitive with elite commodity canola varieties. They are available in both Roundup Ready® (a registered trademark of Monsanto) and Clearfield® (a registered trademark of BASF) versions to give grower production choices and flexibility.

5.3 COMPARATIVE FATTY ACID PROFILE AND OXIDATIVE STABILITY INDICES

The fatty-acid profile of Omega-9 Oils is typically high in oleic, low in linolenic and relatively low in saturated fat. This allows for both a 'low-saturated fat' and 'trans-fat free' (per serving size of 15 mL) label claim in the United States.

Table 5.5 shows the fatty acid profile of several oils and the corresponding OSI numbers (OSI being Oxidative Stability Index, AOCS Cd 12b-92). As the OSI data suggest, the Omega-9 oils are the stablest liquid oils in the mix, not too far from Palm oil, which contains more than 50% saturated fat. Although conventional canola oil is similar to Omega-9 oils in saturated fat content, but it is only third of Omega-9 oils in terms of oxidative stability. Low linolenic soyabean oil with 25% saturated fat is less than half as stable than Omega-9 canola.

TABLE 5.5
Fatty Acid Profile and OSI of Omega-9 Oils Relative to Other Oils

	OSI (110C) Stability Index	Oleic C18:1	Linoleic C18:2	Linoleic C18:3	Total Saturated
Omega-9 canola	17	70–74	18	2	7
Omega-9 sunflower	20	84–86	5	0	8
Commodity canola	7	61	21	9	7
NuSun	10	60	28	0	11
Corn	10	27	57	1	14
Low linolenic soyabean	8	25	55	3	16
Soyabean	6	23	54	8	17
Palm olein	17	47	11	2	40

Source: Date based on Dow Agro Sciences Analytical Lab.

TABLE 5.6
Physical and Chemical Properties of Omega-9 Oils

Oils	IV Unit	OSI (110F) Hours	Sap Value Unit	Unsap Matter %	Lecithin %	Acid Value mgKOH/g
n–9 Canola oil	94	17	192	0.97	0.003	<0.1
n–9 Sunflower oil	84	20	193	0.96	0.003	<0.1

Oils	*n*–9 Canola Oil	*n*–9 Sunflower Oil
Smoke point (°F)	>450	>520
Flash point (°F)	>250	>250
Titer (°C)	14	15
Specific gravity at 25°F	0.9136	0.9120
Pour point (°C)	16	17
Cloudy point (°C)	15	15
Viscosity (cps at 70°F)	14.5	14.7

Source: Data based on testing at Dow Agro Sciences' internal and contracted analytical labs.

The combination of high oleic acid and low linoleic acid, with the conventionally low-saturated fatty acid content, is the key to the very measurable benefits of the Omega-9 oils for the food industry, that is, improved oxidative stability resulting in longer shelf life, and longer fry life, as well as clean and bland taste profile. Table 5.6 shows some physical and chemical properties of these oils.

In converting to non-hydrogenated oils, one big challenge that the food industry has faced is the gradual and progressive build up of a hardened layer of polymerized oil on the surface of production equipment, over a period of time. This is especially true in the operations involving high heat applications like frying, spraying and so on. These polymers are formed as a result of the continuous breakdown of the polyunsaturated fatty acids, especially the linoleic acid.

Owing to high levels of monounsaturated fat and low levels of polyunsaturated fats in Omega-9 oils, they resist polymerization better than any natural liquid oils.

Dow AgroSciences' analytical lab has conducted extensive testing to understand the phenomenon of oil polymerization. In an accelerated lab test, different oils were kept at certain high temperature in a high oxygen environment to induce accelerated polymerization.

Figure 5.1 shows the comparative propensity of different vegetable oils to polymerize at fixed conditions of temperature and oxygen concentration. Soluble polymer build up started at approximately 1 h and progressively increased in concentration till it got too dense and dropped out of the solution. Low linolenic soyabean oil polymerized the fastest, followed by corn oil.

The four oils most resistant to polymerization were Omega-9 canola, partially hydrogenated soyabean oil, Omega-9 sunflower and the ultra low-saturated fat Omega-9 sunflower oil.

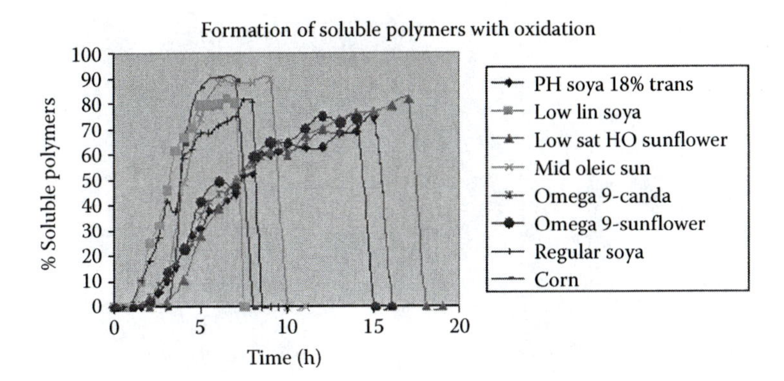

FIGURE 5.1 Comparative polymerization chart of several oils.

5.4 FOOD APPLICATIONS OF OMEGA-9 OILS

Omega-9 oils are suitable for use in a number of food applications. These include bottled oil for home cooking, frying (both restaurant and industrial frying), spray oil for crackers and chips, as industrial shortening in combination with hard fats, and so on.

5.4.1 FRYING

A good-quality frying oil must have the following essential functionalities: clean and bland taste, high oxidative stability, high smoke point and a healthy fatty acid profile (low in saturated and trans fats).

Omega-9 oils are considered high quality frying oils because they fulfill all of the above-mentioned characteristics. They are naturally low in saturated fat (7%), high in oleic acid (>72%) and low in polyunsaturated fatty acids (<18% linoleic acid and <2% linolenic acid). This fatty acid profile provides high oxidative stability (17 h OSI) and a high smoke point (>450°F).

Omega-9 oils can also blend with other liquid oils (corn, conventional canola, etc.) to attain the desired qualities of the fatty acid profile, oxidative stability, taste and cost. Figure 5.2 shows the difference in the saturated and trans fats in French fries when fried in partially hydrogenated soyabean oil and Omega-9 canola oil.

5.4.1.1 Fry Life

In general, fry life is defined as the number of days that the oil can be used in the frying operation—without any noticeable change in the taste and texture of the finished food—before the oil has to be discarded. There are several metrics available to measure the fry life of the oils, including total polar material, free fatty acids, colour of the oil, colour of the food, oil viscosity, oil smell and taste and so on.

However, it could be argued that there is no single best method to measure fry life of oils in all operations. This is because the degradation of the used frying oil depends upon several factors such as the quality of the fresh oil, kind of food being fried, moisture and fat content in food, condition of the fryer, filtration and replenishing practices, as well as the temperature and duration of batches during frying.

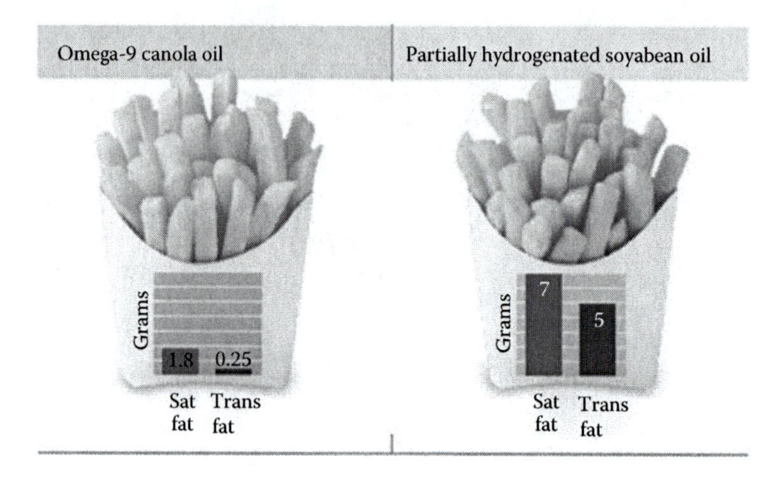

FIGURE 5.2 In 100 g serving size, there is significant reduction of saturated and trans fat in French fries (20% fat uptake), as compared to a standard partially hydrogenated soyabean oil (20% trans, 35% sat fat).

In a commercial restaurant, the measurement tools need to be fast, consistent and simple enough for the fryer operators to be able to handle properly. Obviously, the most logical end point of oil is when the fried food starts showing signs of deterioration in sensory attributes (taste, appearance or texture). The challenge is that sensory attributes are somewhat subjective and not easy to measure in an objective and consistent way by multiple operators. The quality and skill level of the staff and operators can also become a limiting factor in terms of managing the oils to their full potential.

In most controlled frying studies, total polar material (TPM) has proven to be a reliable measure of the oil quality. At least TPM has shown to be more consistent than free fatty acids, per oxide value, colour or oil viscosity. In some EU countries, 24% TPM is considered to be the end point of the fry oils. However, it cannot be stated conclusively that in all frying operations TPM above 24% will result in less than acceptable quality of the fried food. In addition, several companies sell fast reacting 'dip strips' which prove helpful in some operations but not others.

In view of above, the technical management of the frying operation should keep these factors in mind and devise the best methods to determine the end point of the frying oil in their specific operations. Below is a case study that provides the actual test data on a fry test.

5.4.1.2 A Case Study: Comparison of Several Fry Oils in Rotational Deep Frying

The following case study was conducted by Dr. Roman R. Przybylski, Department of Chemistry and Biochemistry, University of Lethbridge in 2007.

5.4.1.2.1 Materials

Oils and Fats: The following industrially processed oils were used in the frying experiments: conventional canola (Canola), low linolenic canola (LLCan), Omega-9 canola (HOLLCan), hydrogenated canola (HydCan), soyabean oil (SOY), hydrogenated soyabean oil (HydSoy), low linolenic soyabean (LLSoy), mid oleic sunflower (MidSUN), Omega-9 sunflower (HOSUN) and Palm olein (Palmolein).

5.4.1.2.2 Analytical Methods

Polar Components: Content of polar components formed during frying was analysed by the AOCS column chromatography method Cd 20–91; gravimetric method. From chromatography two fractions were collected: (1) non-polar components eluted with 1% diisopropyl ether in hexane; (2) fraction of polar components eluted with diisopropyl ether.

Fatty acid: Composition of fatty acids was analysed using AOCS procedure Ce 1–62.

5.4.1.2.3 Test method

Frying: For each frying series, four vegetable oils were used simultaneously. Oils were placed in four GE institutional fryers. These fryers mechanical temperature controllers were replaced with electronic controllers to get temperature control within ±2°C and to have faster temperature recovery when frozen product was placed into fryer. Products were fried at 185°C for: chicken strips—8 min; fish strips—7 min; French fries—5 min. One frying cycle covered three products fried in sequence one after another. Par-fried frozen French fries, chicken strips and fish strips were fried in nine cycles per day, 400 g of each product per cycle.

5.4.1.2.4 Results

5.4.1.2.4.1 Fatty Acid Profiles of the Oils Tested The fatty acid profile of the oils tested is shown in Table 5.7.

5.4.1.2.4.2 Sensory Evaluation Figure 5.3 shows the mean acceptance scores obtained for French fries, chicken and fish sticks fried in different oils. Consumer panel is a subjective type of measurement because panellists are not trained and assessment is based on previous experience of each panellist. Here some skewed results are acceptable because experience of each panellist is different within particular group of assessors. Main oil on the market will make consumers familiar to its characteristics and cause acceptance at the higher level, whereas consumers for which type oil is not known have tendency to score lower. For example, it can be canola oil for Canadians and for Americans soyabean oil.

Chicken sticks received the lowest acceptance scores when fried in hydrogenated canola and soyabean frying shortening, Palmolein and soyabean oil. The latter can be interpreted as effect of unfamiliarity with this oil for Canadian consumer; however, we have Canadian soyabean oil which is slightly different from the American variety.

Products fried in the HOLLCan, MOSUN and HOSUN oils received the highest acceptance scores for French fries and chicken strips. Fish sticks were scored at lower level than other two products, the main negative characteristics described by panellists for this product were: oily, off-flavour and stale. Due to the different coating used in this product, amount of absorbed oil was about two times higher than in other products. Generally, French fries and chicken sticks were rated at higher acceptance level than fish sticks.

TABLE 5.7
Fatty Acid Profiles of the Oils Used in the Study

Fatty Acid	HOLLCan	LLCan	Canola	HYDCan	Soyabean	HYDSoy	LLSoy	MIDSUN	HOSUN	Palmolein
C12:0										0.30
C14:0										1.03
C15:0										0.04
C16:0	3.83	4.18	4.18	4.65	10.19	10.76	10.40	4.30	3.50	39.23
C16:1	0.22	0.24	0.23	0.17	0.09	0.10	0.09	0.09	0.10	0.19
C17:0	0.19	0.15	0.14	0.09	0.11	0.12	0.11	0.05	0.04	0.10
C18:0	1.49	1.77	1.85	4.23	4.38	6.09	4.45	3.71	3.02	4.15
C18:1t	0.02	0.15	0.13	26.68	0.00	14.81	0.18	0.38	0.28	0.10
C18:1	71.36	61.86	60.64	51.89	22.57	33.35	27.41	59.56	83.56	42.73
C18:2t	0.24	0.34	0.37	7.87	0.56	6.60	0.29	0.30	0.16	0.28
C18:2	18.20	24.97	19.58	2.64	53.62	25.02	53.65	29.14	7.14	10.89
C18:3t	0.27	0.44	1.60	0.40	0.91	0.89	0.11	0.07	0.13	0.07
C18:3	1.69	2.91	8.49	0.14	6.71	1.16	2.61	0.68	0.20	0.20
C20:0	0.53	0.67	0.63	0.63	0.34	0.32	0.32	0.30	0.28	0.35
C20:1	1.38	1.42	1.30	1.08	0.17	0.17	0.16	0.26	0.28	0.14
C22:0	0.31	0.45	0.35	0.35	0.35	0.34	0.32	0.79	0.82	0.06
C24:0	0.14	0.19	0.15	0.16	0.12	0.10	0.09	0.26	0.32	0.07
C24:1	0.15	0.26	0.20	0.17	0.00	0.10	0.03	0.04	0.06	0.04
Group										
C18:1trans	0.02	0.15	0.13	26.68	0.00	14.81	0.18	0.38	0.28	0.10
C18:2trans	0.24	0.34	0.37	7.87	0.56	6.60	0.29	0.30	0.16	0.28
C18:3trans	0.27	0.44	1.60	0.40	0.91	0.89	0.11	0.07	0.13	0.07
Trans	0.53	0.93	2.10	34.95	1.47	22.30	0.58	0.75	0.57	0.45
SAT	6.47	7.40	7.29	10.13	15.49	17.73	15.68	9.42	7.98	45.32
MUFA	73.12	63.78	62.36	53.31	22.83	33.72	27.68	59.96	84.00	43.11
PUFA	19.88	27.88	28.07	2.78	60.33	26.18	56.26	29.82	7.34	11.08
n–3	1.69	2.91	8.49	0.14	6.71	1.16	2.61	0.68	0.20	0.20
n–6	18.20	24.97	19.58	2.64	53.62	25.02	53.65	29.14	7.14	10.89

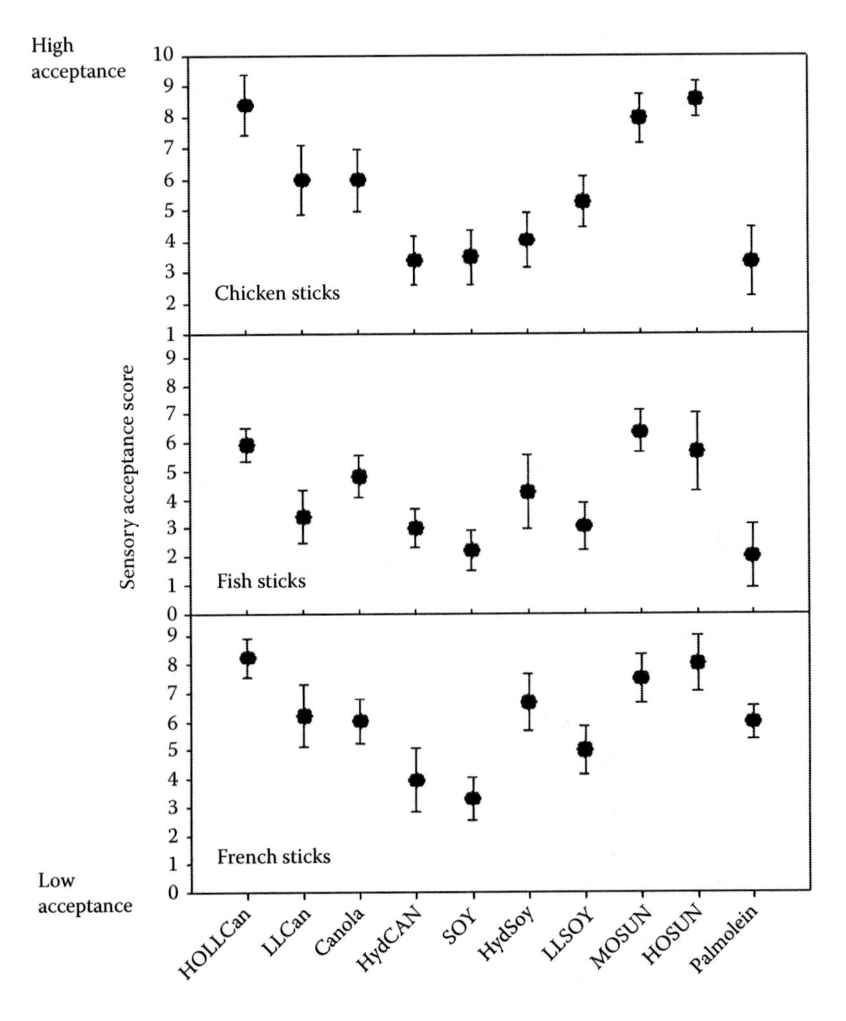

FIGURE 5.3 Average acceptance sensory scores for fried foods in different oils.

5.4.1.2.5 Polar Components

The amount of polar components provides direct measurement of oxidative degradation of unsaturated fatty acids and other endogenous oil and food components. The main factor in this degradation is the presence of oxygen and susceptibility to oxidation of oil and food components. Unsaturated fatty acids, tocopherols and sterols in oil are the main components involved in oxidative degradation. While in fried food, major ingredients such as proteins, carbohydrates and lipids are oxidized and interact with oil degradation products to form complex mixture of components with dislocated charge forming polar components. Faster rate of polar components formation is a cumulative indication of oxidative and interactive degradation of the oil and food components. Slope of the polar components curves indicate rate of formation, steeper slope represents faster formation and usually higher amount of

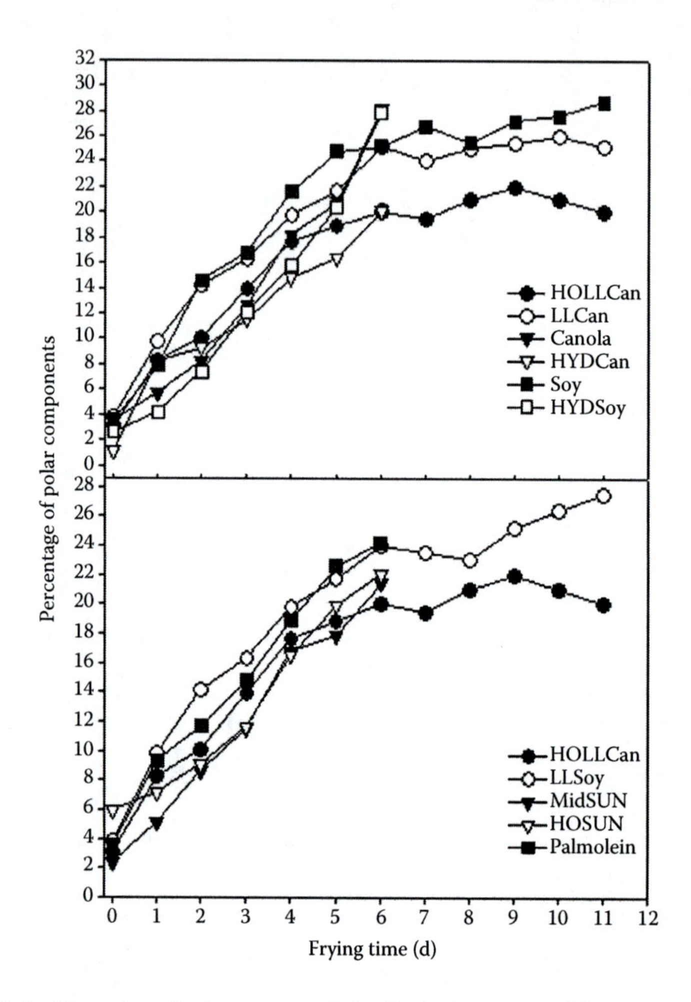

FIGURE 5.4 Formation of polar compounds in oils during rotational frying.

these components (see chart below). HOLL, MOSUN and HYD Can showed similar rate of polar components formation. Canola, soyabean and LLSoy and HYDSoy oils showed the fastest accumulation of polar components, breaking European limit of 24% after day 5 of frying (Figure 5.4). Generally, amount of polar components formed was at the lower end, probably because high ratio of the amount of fried food to the volume of oil, and polar components were removed by foods, this can be observed in the accumulation of polar components in fried foods discussed below.

5.4.1.2.6 Free Fatty Acids

The main cause for FFA formation is hydrolysis, water present in fried products and elevated temperature stimulate this process. Usually, with frying time the amount of FFA increase, similar data were observed in this project (see chart below; Figure 5.5). Relatively low levels of FFA were observed in frying using different oils. Pattern of FFA formation was similar to other parameters measured, where HOLLCan was

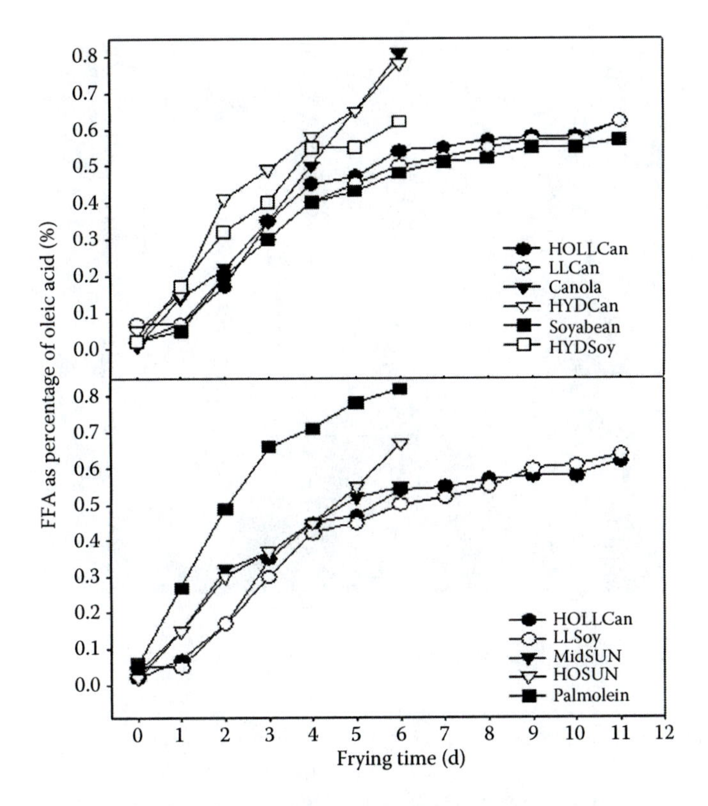

FIGURE 5.5 Formation of free fatty acids in oils during rotational frying.

found in the middle but at the lower end, indicating better resistance to degradation by hydrolysis. Due to the formation of small amounts of FFA, this measurement is not a good indicator of quality, because assessing is not important during oil degradation process. Today's food coating, food products preparation and par-frying are the main factors limiting hydrolytic degradation of oils during frying.

5.4.2 Spray Oil Application

Some baked products such as crackers or chips are sprinkled with spices and flavouring like cheese, pepper or other flavoured powders. A fine mist of heated oil is sprayed on the surface of the crackers right before the spices are added (Figure 5.6). The oil helps the spices to adhere on the food. So essentially the oil acts as a glue. Different kinds of oils are used as spray oils, including coconut, partially hydrogenated soyabean oil and so on. Some of the critical attributes of good-quality spray oils include high oxidative stability, fluidity and neutral taste. Oxidative stability is important because of the immense surface area (and thus oxygen) that the oil droplets are exposed to. Fluidity is important because the spray nozzles can get clogged if the oil viscosity is inconsistent or if it contains waxes or polymers. This can result in inconsistent misting of the spray oil on the cracker, which affects the adherence of the spices. A neutral or bland taste is important because it affects the flavour perception of the spices.

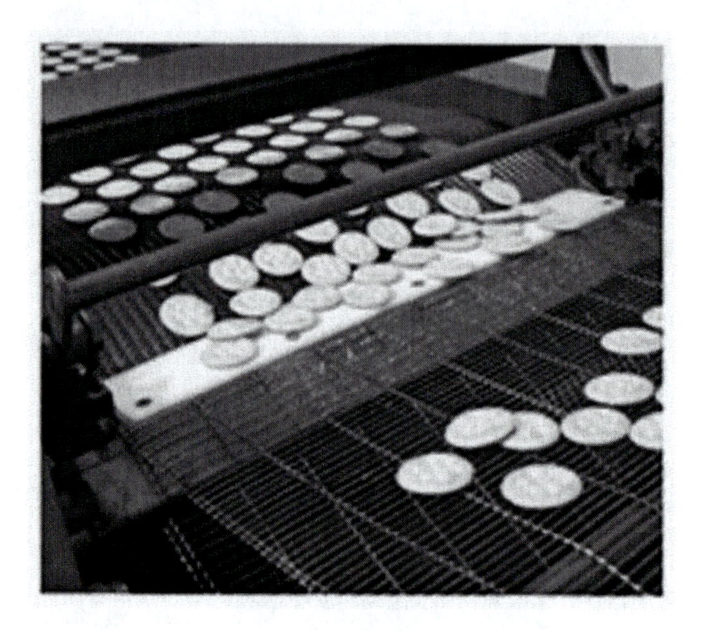

FIGURE 5.6 A spray oil line spraying oil in crackers.

Omega-9 oils are well suited for this application because of high oxidative stability, resistance to polymerize and low-saturated fat making it possible to operate without heating the spray nozzles, as it is liquid at room temperature.

5.4.3 Shortening Applications

Most of the shortenings designed for baking (and in some cases, for frying) are essentially combinations of liquid oil and a hard fat like partially hydrogenated soyabean oil, fraction of palm oil, palm kernel oil, fully hydrogenated soyabean or cottonseed oil, etc. The combination is designed so as to attain a specific melt profile, expressed as SFI (solid fat index) or SFC (solid fat content) curve.

SFI measures by volume, the ratio of crystalline (solid) phase verses liquid phase in the fat sample. It is performed manually using a glass dilatometer, and measures the increase in volume as the fat sample expands upon heating, starting with frozen sample. Density measurements are taken at a series of standardized temperature check points.

SFC is measured using NMR (nuclear magnetic resonance) and it gives an accurate measure of the solid versus liquid phase by weight%, at certain temperatures.

Practicing oil scientists have different opinions as to which method is more helpful in formulating a shortening blend. Both methods are equally useful. It is more a matter of personal experience, convenience and cost. Over all, the industry is moving towards SFC.

Both SFI and SFC curves provide valuable information about the expected functionality or behaviour of the fat blend at different processing temperatures,

TABLE 5.8
Melting Points of Individual Fatty Acids

Common Name	Carbon Chain	Melt Point (°C)
Lauric acid	12:0	44.0
Myristic acid	14:0	55.0
Palmitic acid	16:0	63.0
Stearic acid	18:0	71.0
Oleic acid	18:1	13.0
Linoleic acid	18:2	–5.0
Linlenic acid	18:3	–11.0
Elaidic (trans) acid	18:1	46.0

Source: http://www2.chemistry.msu.edu/faculty/reusch/VirtTxtJml/lipids.htm.

as well as the melting qualities in the mouth, which directly affects the taste perception.

As Table 5.8 shows, different fatty acids have different melt points. Although fatty acids in triglyceride form behave differently from their free fatty acid state, still the above table helps in understanding the melt characteristics of the triglyceride as a whole, especially when comparing two oils.

As Omega-9 oils are liquid at room temperature, they do not have a fat crystal functionality of their own, needed for most shortenings for baking, creaming or other such applications. The solid functionality (machineability and creamy mouth feel) primarily come from the solid fat in the shortening blend.

The best way to formulate an Omega-9 shortening is to replace the liquid oil portion of the existing shortening blend by Omega-9 oil, keeping the solid fat portion intact. This will provide a good starting point for further optimization. SFC or SFI should be measured and the blend should be optimized as to achieve the target melting curve. However, if the goal is to further reduce the amount of saturated fat, then solid portion should be replaced with Omega-9 oil, keeping in mind that there will be a limit to how much liquid oil can be incorporated without affecting functionality of the shortening and the taste perception of the finished product.

Generally, by replacing the liquid portion of the original shortening by Omega-9 oil, saturated fat can be reduced significantly (depending upon the starting oils) without affecting functionality and machine-ability. Omega-9 shortening does provide a longer shelf life due to higher oxidative stability (Table 5.9).

5.4.4 Doughnut Frying

Doughnut is intrinsically a very sensitive product (Figure 5.7). Any formulation or process inconsistencies, either in the formulation or the frying procedures can have drastic effects on the sensory attributes as well as shelf life.

The shortening used to fry doughnut needs to have a melt profile somewhat close to butter, in order to produce crispy and soft doughnuts. Historically, partially

TABLE 5.9
Example of an Omega-9 Shortening #11 vs. An All Purpose Shortening and Palm Oil

	Commercial (PH Soyabean + Cottonseed Oil)	Omega-9 (#11 Omega-9 Shortening)	Palm Fraction
Trans fat	31	1	<1.0
Saturated fat	23	23–25	54
Total	54	24–26	54
Polyunsaturated	5	20	9
Monounsaturated (Omega-9)	41	55	37

Note: #11 is a blend of palm oil and Omega-9 canola oil.

hydrogenated soyabean oil has been used as the fry shortening. In the last 5 years, manufacturers have started switching to alternate shortening formulations, to reduce trans fats and saturated fat. Those alternates often are some blends of palm oil fraction and one or more liquid oils.

A typical Omega-9 oil-based doughnut shortening will consist of 30–60% of palm oil, the rest being Omega-9 canola or sunflower oils or a combination there of. Exactly what fraction of palm oil, what blends of Omega-9 oils and what ratio of palm oil versus the liquid oil will depend upon the specific product goals (sensory preference, desired shelf, nutritional label, ingredient statement, cost, etc.). A partially hydrogenated soyabean oil-based doughnut shortening could have up to 45% trans fat and 35% saturated fat. An Omega-9 canola oil-based shortening would have <1% trans fat and close to 35% saturated fat.

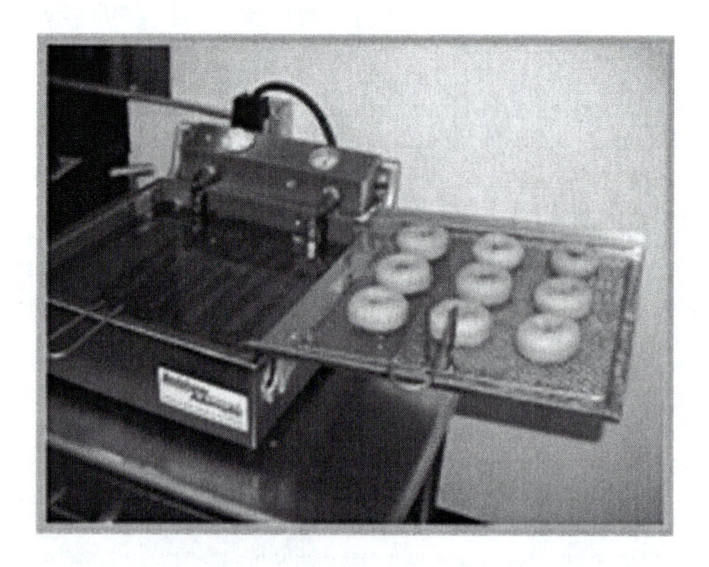

FIGURE 5.7 A typical lab scale doughnut fryer.

5.5 REMOVING TRANS FAT FROM NORTH AMERICAN MENUS

Owing to mounting medical evidence and public concern about trans fat-laden hydrogenated oils, restaurants are now switching to healthier oils to eliminate trans fat from their menus. In a 2006 article on the health impact of trans fat in the *New England Journal of Medicine*, researchers found that trans fat substantially increased the risk of heart disease, even when consumed in small amounts. Since then, a growing number of studies link trans fat and saturated fat to an increased risk of heart disease.

As a result, states like California and cities such as New York City, Boston and Philadelphia have passed a legislation to ban trans fat in restaurants. Since 2006, the US Food and Drug Administration (FDA) requires that all food labels must include the amount of trans fat found in foods.

Since 2006, restaurants that have converted into Omega-9 oils have removed nearly 700 million pounds of trans fat and 200 million pounds of saturated fat from the North American diet. This means almost 1 billion pounds of saturated and trans fats have been eliminated from our diets.

5.6 HEALTH BENEFITS OF OMEGA-9 OILS

Omega-3, omega-6 and omega-9 fatty acids all serve different functions in the body. There is evidence that incorporating balanced proportions of both essential and non-essential fatty acids is necessary for maintaining overall heart health and general wellness.

Below is an excerpt from the abstract of a recent study published in the *British Journal of Nutrition* by Gillingham and coworkers at the University of Manitoba in 2011 (p. 1):

> Recently, novel dietary oils with modified fatty acid profiles have been manufactured to improve fatty acid intakes and reduce CVD risk. Our objective was to evaluate the efficacy of novel high-oleic rapeseed (canola) oil (HOCO), alone or blended with flaxseed oil (FXCO), on circulating lipids and inflammatory biomarkers v. a typical Western diet (WD). Using a randomized, controlled, crossover trial, thirty-six hypercholesterolaemic subjects consumed three isoenergetic diets for 28 d each containing approximately 36% energy from fat, of which 70% was provided by HOCO, FXCO or WD. Dietary fat content of SFA, MUFA, PUFA n-6 and n-3 was 6, 23, 5, 1% energy for HOCO; 6, 16, 5, 7.5% energy for FXCO; 11.5, 16, 6, 0.5% energy for WD. After 28 d, compared with WD, LDL-cholesterol was reduced 15.1% ($P < 0.001$) with FXCO and 7.4% ($P < 0.001$) with HOCO. Total cholesterol (TC) was reduced 11% ($P < 0.001$) with FXCO and 3.5% ($P = 0.002$) with HOCO compared with WD. Endpoint TC differed between FXCO and HOCO ($P < 0.05$). FXCO consumption reduced HDL-cholesterol by 8.5% ($P < 0.001$) and LDL:HDL ratio by 7.5% ($P = 0.008$) v. WD.

5.7 CANOLA HEALTH CLAIM AND LABELLING

In 2006, FDA approved a Qualified Health Claim for canola oil stating 'limited and not conclusive scientific evidence suggests that eating about 1(1/2) tablespoons (19 g) of canola oil daily may reduce the risk of coronary heart disease due to the unsaturated fat content in canola oil. To achieve this possible benefit, canola oil is to replace a similar amount of saturate fat and not increase the total number of calories you eat in a day' (http://www.fda.gov/Food/).

5.8 CANOLA OIL AND CONSUMERS

Canola is perceived by consumers as one of the healthiest oils available. In 2007, the nutritionists from *Cooking Light* magazine made canola oil their recommended oil for consumers due to its healthful fatty acid profile and light, clean taste.

Substituting canola oil for other common fats in Americans' diets would improve compliance with recommended intakes of healthy fats, according to a modelling study published in the October 2007 issue of the *Journal of the American Dietetic Association*. The study looked at the effect of substituting canola oil for selected vegetable oils and canola oil-based margarine for other margarines and butter in the diets of 9000 people.

'The findings are provocative because they suggest that fairly simple recipe modifications can result in product meeting dietary guidelines for saturated fat intake and achieving adequate intakes of unsaturated fats', writes Jennifer Nettleton, assistant professor of cardiovascular disease epidemiology, University of Texas Health Sciences Center, in a JADA editorial (paragraph 4). 'Substituting canola oil for other common oils has the potential to reduce the substantial burden of coronary heart disease in the United States' (Canola Council, 2007).

Consumers are seeking to increase consumption of canola more than any other crop oil, as evidenced in Figure 5.8. Consumers indicate that they are making efforts to avoid fats containing high levels of saturated fat like lard and butter, and are trying to consume more of the oils containing unsaturated fatty acids, like olive and canola oils.

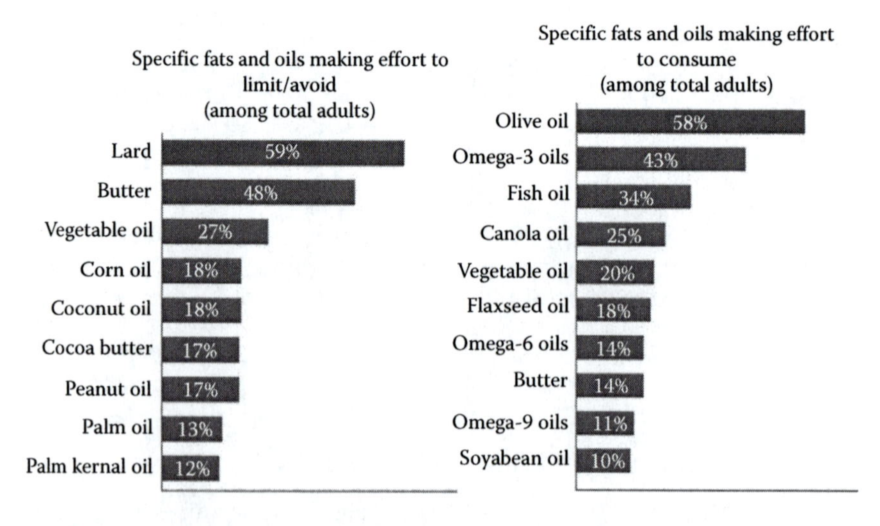

FIGURE 5.8 Fats and oils to consume and those to avoid (2010 Gallup Study of Healthy Fats and Oil).

Consumers are becoming increasingly concerned with their health and are avoiding foods containing bad fats. In fact, '64 percent of Americans are actively trying to consume less saturated fat and 64 percent are actively trying to consume less trans fat' (IFIC, 2010, p. 1).

5.9 IN LINE WITH US DIETARY GUIDELINES

The Dietary Guidelines for Americans (USDA, 2010) was released in February 2011. The Key Recommendations in the Executive Summary, under Food and Food Components to Reduce the section include:

- Consume <10% of calories from saturated fatty acids by replacing them with monounsaturated and polyunsaturated fatty acids.
- Keep trans fatty acid consumption as low as possible by limiting foods that contain synthetic sources of trans fats, such as partially hydrogenated oils, and by limiting other solid fats.
- Reduce the intake of calories from solid fats and added sugars.
- Limit the consumption of foods that contain refined grains, especially refined grain foods that contain solid fats, added sugars and sodium.

5.10 NEXT GENERATION OF OMEGA-9 OILS

There are several new oil seed varieties being developed right now. Two of those are worth mentioning, as their launch time is within the next 2–3 years

- Ultra low-saturated fat Omega-9 sunflower oil
- DHA-Omega-9 canola oil blend

5.10.1 Ultra Low-Saturated Fat Sunflower Oil

The current Omega-9 sunflower oil contains ~86% oleic acid and ~8% saturated fatty acids (stearic and palmitic). Due to its fatty acid profile, this oil has proved to be the most stable of all natural liquid oils in the market today.

The new 'Ultra Low Sat Omega-9 Sunflower Oil' is one step further than the current Omega-9 sunflower oil in terms of oxidative stability, saturated fat, taste and resistance to polymerization. This oil contains more than 92% oleic acid, <3.3% saturated fat, has OSI stability of 23 h, vs. 21 for palm oil. It was developed using non-transgenic breeding, and is expected to be commercialized in 2013 in EU and 2014 in the United States. This oil is under development and is going through rigorous characterization and application testing as we speak, and is expected to be ready for initial testing by food industry in 2012.

5.10.2 Omega-9 Canola Oil-DHA Blend

Dow AgroSciences has partnered with Martek Biosciences Corporation to develop a blend of Omega-9 canola oil with algal DHA (docosahexaenoic acid). DHA is a long-chain polyunsaturated omega-3 fatty acid and is important for brain, eye and heart health throughout the lifecycle (Martek Biosciences Cooperation, 2012).

The DHA blend will offer Omega-9 canola oil's high stability oil background with the known health benefits of omega-3 DHA fatty acid.

This oil blend will have application in the bottled oil, margarines and spreads, as well as other food applications requiring low-to-moderate heating.

Shelf-life studies as well as food applications studies are under way. The Omega-9 canola-DHA blend is expected to be available to food manufacturers before or around 2012.

5.11 SUMMARY

In the food industry, omega-9 fatty acid is synonymous to oleic acid.

- Omega-9 fatty acids are abundantly present in animal fats and vegetable oils.
- 'Omega-9 Oil' is an identifier for the high oleic low linolenic canola and sunflower oils developed by Dow AgroSciences.
- Of all natural liquid oils, Omega-9 Oils have the lowest levels of saturated fat, are the most stable and are most resistant to thermal polymerization.
- Hard fats can be blended with Omega-9 oils to formulate Omega-9 shortenings.
- Omega-9 oils are suitable for such food applications as restaurant and industrial frying, spraying, as shortening for baking and doughnut frying and so on.
- About 1 billion pounds of saturated and trans fats have been removed from our diets by Omega-9 oils so far.
- Consumers perceive olive and canola as healthy oils.
- Omega-9 oils fit the 2010 USDA Dietary Guidelines and recommendations with their uniquely high levels of monounsaturated fat.
- There is a robust pipeline of innovative next generation oil seeds scheduled to be launched in the near future.

ACKNOWLEDGEMENTS

I would like to thank my colleagues, Thomas Patterson, Josh Flook, Mary Evanson, John Keller, Frank Orthoefer (consultant at Dow), Jo-Anne Frank, Steven Wensing, Erin Hull and David Dzisiak, at Dow AgroSciences, for conducting all the tests, developing the data and providing me with all the information needed to prepare this chapter.

REFERENCES

Canola Council. 2007. http://www.canola-council.org/canola_ink_october_12_2007.aspx
FDA. 2006. http://www.fda.gov/Food/LabelingNutrition/LabelClaims/QualifiedHealthClaims/ucm073992.htm#canola

Gillingham L.G., Gustafson J.A., Han S.Y., Jassal D.S., Jones P.J. 2011. High-oleic rapeseed (canola) and flaxseed oils modulate serum lipids and inflammatory biomarkers in hyper-cholesterolaemic subjects. *Br. J. Nutr.* 105: 417–427.

IFIC. 2010. 'Consumer & Opinion Leader Research.' Food Safety, Healthy Eating and Nutrition Information. Web. 17 Nov. 2010. http://www.foodinsight.org/Resources/Survey-Research.aspx.

Informa Economics Inc, *Vegetable Oil Consumption in the USA*, June 2011.

Martek Biosciences Cooperation. 2012. http://www.martek.com/About/Martek-Products.aspx, 2012.

Unsaturated Fatty Acids from Canola Oil and Reduced Risk of Coronary Heart Disease, Docket No. 2006Q-0091 10/06/2006 enforcement discretion letter. http://www.fda.gov/Food/

USDA. 2010. http://www.cnpp.usda.gov/Publications/DietaryGuidelines/2010/PolicyDoc/ExecSumm.pdf

6 Modification of Seed Oil Formation in *Brassica* Oilseed Species

Crystal L. Snyder and Randall J. Weselake

CONTENTS

6.1 Introduction ... 101
6.2 Seed Oil Formation Pathways in BOS ... 102
6.3 Modification of BOS Seed Oil Composition ... 106
6.3.1 High-Oleic, Low-Alpha-Linolenic BOS Oils ... 106
6.3.2 BOS Oils with Altered Saturated Fatty Acid Content ... 107
6.3.3 Production of BOS Oils with Very-Long-Chain Polyunsaturated Fatty Acids ... 109
6.3.4 Production of BOS Oils with Very-Long-Chain Monounsaturated Fatty Acids ... 111
6.4 Modification of BOS Seed Oil Content ... 112
6.5 Conclusions and Future Directions ... 115
Acknowledgements ... 116
References ... 116

6.1 INTRODUCTION

The genus *Brassica* is the most economically important in the Brassicaeae tribe, containing both vegetable and oilseed species that are grown for both human consumption and industrial applications (Rakow, 2004). The most widely cultivated *Brassica* oilseed species (BOS) are *B. napus*, *B. rapa*, *B. juncea* and *B. carinata*, with *B. napus* and *B. rapa* representing most of the *Brassica* oilseed trade worldwide (Scarth and Tang, 2006). These BOS are an important source of both edible and industrial oils, and are one of the most important sources of vegetable oils worldwide after palm and soyabean (Canola Council of Canada, 2007). *B. napus* and *B. rapa* alone account for nearly $14 billion per year in economic activity across Canada (Canola Council of Canada, 2008), and it is anticipated that in Canada alone, a 50–75% increase in production will be required to keep pace with the growing demand for vegetable oil (Weselake et al., 2009). As a result, there is considerable interest in increasing seed oil content in BOS through breeding and biotechnology.

Expanding markets for both edible and industrial oils have also driven the development of speciality oils possessing fatty acid (FA) profiles suitable for specialized nutritional or industrial applications. The functional and nutritional characteristics of a vegetable oil are determined in large part by its FA composition, making modification of the FA profile a major target for oilseed breeders and biotechnologists aiming to produce 'designer' oils for specific applications. Among BOS, the level of erucic acid ($22{:}1^{\Delta 13}$) is one of the most important functional considerations; while low-erucic-acid varieties are preferred for edible applications, high-erucic-acid varieties are highly desirable for industrial applications. Much of the reduction in erucic acid and glucosinolate content for edible oil BOS has been achieved through traditional breeding (Scarth and Tang, 2006), resulting in *B. napus* and *B. rapa* cultivars that are enriched in oleic acid ($18{:}1^{\Delta 9}$) and low in saturated fatty acids (SFAs), allowing 'canola' oil to be branded as a heart-healthy oil (Canola Council of Canada, 2010).

Many other FA modifications have been targeted in BOS, including further enrichment of oleic acid for high-stability frying applications (Orthoefer, 2005), alteration of SFA content (Stoll et al., 2005) and introduction of very-long-chain polyunsaturated fatty acids (VLCPUFA), which are essential for human health and nutrition (Venegas-Caleron et al., 2010). Industrial oil targets include enrichment of erucic acid and its downstream products (Fobert et al., 2008) and production of unusual FAs such as medium-chain saturated FAs (Stoll et al., 2005) or hydroxy FAs (Cahoon et al., 2007).

There are several approaches for modifying the seed oil content and composition of BOS. Increasingly, biotechnological methods complement traditional breeding and mutagenesis strategies, while also providing an avenue to achieve modifications not possible through traditional approaches alone. Genetically engineered (GE) BOS carrying herbicide resistance traits have been widely adopted, representing more than 75% of the Canadian canola crop (Canola Council of Canada, 2010), but so far, the only modified BOS oil trait in commercial production is high-oleic, low-linolenic canola that was developed though breeding and mutagenesis (Scarth and Tang, 2006). Aside from the regulatory burden associated with introducing new GE traits, a common obstacle to commercialization of transgenic plants with modified oil traits is the relatively low accumulation of the desired FA(s) (Cahoon et al., 2007), or unacceptable loss of agronomic performance resulting from disruptions in normal lipid metabolism. Nevertheless, the development of GE varieties with modified oil traits is ongoing, often serving as a basis for increasing our understanding of the underlying molecular and biochemical mechanisms which need to be targeted in order to achieve commercially viable fatty acid profiles.

This chapter will introduce seed oil formation pathways in BOS and describe major advancements in the development of BOS with increased seed oil content or modified oil profiles designed to meet specific nutritional or industrial needs.

6.2 SEED OIL FORMATION PATHWAYS IN BOS

Seed oil in BOS is primarily composed of triacylglycerol (TAG). TAG formation in developing oilseeds can be conceptualized in two stages, with the first stage resulting in the *de novo* synthesis of FAs and *sn*-glycerol-3-phosphate, and the second stage involving the assembly of these building blocks into TAG. Although TAG assembly is often described as a series of sequential acylations of *sn*-glycerol-3-phosphate, the overall process is supported by several 'acyl-editing' reactions, which facilitate modification of acyl groups (i.e., elongation or desaturation) and incorporation of these modified acyl groups into TAG. A generalized scheme illustrating these pathways is depicted in Figure 6.1. Readers are also encouraged to consult reviews by Harwood (2005), Weselake (2005) and Weselake et al. (2009) for additional information.

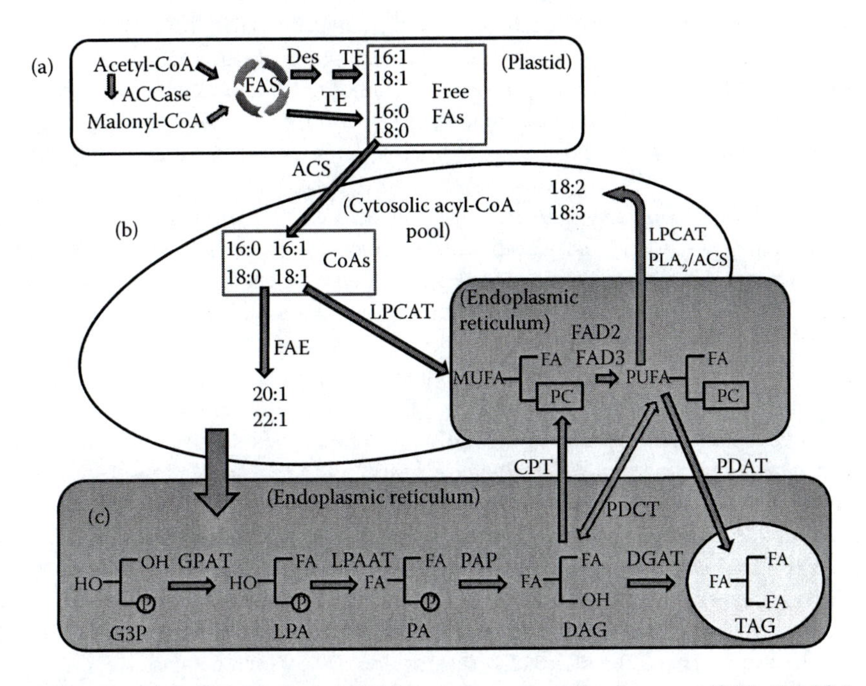

FIGURE 6.1 Seed oil biosynthesis in BOS is a compartmentalized process. (a) Plastidial fatty acid (FA) biosynthesis in BOS results in the formation of saturated or monounsaturated free FAs 16–18 carbons in length, with oleic acid (18:1) as the major product. These newly formed FAs are exported to the cytosol and become activated to acyl-CoAs, which can be channelled towards elongation or desaturation through various 'acyl-editing' reactions (b), or towards the sequential *sn*-glycerol-3-phosphate (G3P) pathway leading to TAG (c). Pathways for FA biosynthesis and TAG assembly are based on information from Harwood et al. (2005) and Weselake et al. (2009), with revisions to the acyl-editing pathways based on information from Bates et al. (2009) and Lu et al. (2009). Note that this diagram does not reflect information about the flux through various reactions; readers are referred to Bates et al. (2009) for a detailed description of acyl fluxes in developing soyabean embryos. Other abbreviations: ACCase: acetyl-CoA carboxylase; ACS: acyl-CoA synthetase; CPT: diacylglycerol:cholinephosphotransferase; DAG, *sn*-1, 2-diacylglycerol; Des: desaturase (in this case, an acyl-ACP desaturase); DGAT: diacylglycerol acyltransferase; FAD: fatty acid desaturase; FAE: fatty acid elongase; FAS: fatty acid synthase complex; GPAT: *sn*-glycerol-3-phosphate acyltransferase; LPA: lyosphosphatidic acid; LPAAT: lysophosphatidic acid acyltransferase; LPCAT: lysophosphatidylcholine acyltransferase; PA: phosphatidic acid; PAP: phosphatidic acid phosphatase; PC: phosphatidylcholine; PDAT: phospholipid:diacylglycerol acyltransferase; PDCT: phospholipid:diacylglycerol cholinephosphotransferase; PLA_2: phospholipase A_2; PUFA: polyunsaturated fatty acid; TE: thioesterase.

FA biosynthesis occurs in the plastid, beginning with the ATP-dependent formation of malonyl-CoA from acetyl-CoA and bicarbonate, catalysed by the plastidial acetyl-CoA carboxylase (ACCase) (Sasaki and Nagano, 2004). *De novo* FA biosynthesis is catalysed by the fatty acid synthase (FAS) complex, through the repeated incorporation of two-carbon units from malonyl-CoA into the nascent FA chain, which remains tethered to the FAS complex by covalent attachment to acyl carrier protein (ACP). In BOS, chain elongation continues until the FA reaches 16 or 18 carbons in length, at which point the FA may be released from ACP through the action of an acyl-ACP thioesterase, yielding palmitic acid (16:0) or stearic acid (18:0). Alternatively, the first double bond may be introduced by an acyl-ACP desaturase prior to its release, leading to the formation of palmitoleic acid ($16{:}1^{\Delta 9}$) or oleic acid. The free FAs are then activated to acyl-CoAs by an acyl-CoA synthetase on the outer envelope of the plastid, prior to being exported into the cytosol (Schnurr et al., 2002).

From the cytosolic acyl-CoA pool, nascent acyl groups can be utilized by one of several pathways. Acyl-CoAs can be further elongated through the action of a fatty acid elongase (FAE), in a process analogous to that catalysed by FAS, but drawing on a cytosolic malonyl-CoA pool as a source of donor carbon (Schwender et al., 2006). In many BOS, this leads to the formation of eicosenoic ($20{:}1^{\Delta 11}$) and erucic acid; however, in low-erucic-acid BOS, a single amino acid substitution in the elongase enzyme results in almost complete loss of function, limiting the accumulation of very-long-chain FAs (Katavic et al., 2002). In canola-type oils, such as *B. napus* and *B. rapa*, the inactivation of the elongase results in the accumulation of oleic acid, while in *B. carinata*, it appears that a larger proportion of the resulting oleic acid is further desaturated to linoleic acid (LA; $18{:}2^{\Delta 9,12}$) and alpha-linolenic acid (ALA; $18{:}3^{\Delta 9,12,15}$) (Cheng et al., 2010).

Formation of these polyunsaturated fatty acids (PUFAs) occurs primarily at the *sn*-2 position of phosphatidylcholine (PC) and involves two desaturase enzymes, a Δ12 desaturase (FAD2) and a Δ15 desaturase (FAD3), which catalyse the formation of LA and ALA, respectively. Acyl-CoAs can be channelled towards desaturation through the forward reaction for lysophosphatidylcholine acyltransferase (LPCAT), which catalyses the acyl-CoA-dependent acylation of the *sn*-2 position of lysophosphatidylcholine to form PC (Stymne and Stobart, 1984b). LPCAT can also catalyse the reverse reaction, facilitating the release of desaturated moieties back into the acyl-CoA pool (Stymne and Stobart, 1984a). Although the forward reaction is heavily favoured, most of the cytosolic acyl-CoA pool exists in a bound form with acyl-CoA-binding protein (ACBP), which has been suggested to stimulate the reverse reaction of LPCAT by helping to maintain a very low free acyl-CoA concentration in the cytosol (Yurchenko et al., 2009). Other enzymes, such as phospholipase A_2, may also play a role in releasing desaturated acyl groups from PC, but while some studies have shown that phospholipases can remove unusual groups from membrane phospholipids (Stahl et al., 1995), it remains unclear to what extent phospholipases contribute to 'acyl-editing' in the context of normal lipid metabolism.

In the 'sequential' TAG bioassembly pathway (reviewed by Weselake, 2005), *sn*-glycerol-3-phosphate undergoes a series of acylations catalysed by acyl-CoA-dependent acyltransferases. The first acylation is catalysed by *sn*-glycerol-3-phosphate acyltransferase (GPAT), which typically introduces a saturated or monounsaturated moiety at the *sn*-1 position to form lysophosphatidic acid. In BOS, lysophosphatidic acid acyltransferase (LPAAT) introduces mainly unsaturated acyl groups at the *sn*-2 position to form phosphatidic acid, which is dephosphorylated by phosphatidic acid phosphatase (PAP or lipin) to form diacylglycerol (DAG). DAG can then be utilized in the *de novo* synthesis of PC, catalysed by diacylglycerol:cholinephosphotransferase (Vogel and Browse, 1996), or can undergo a final acyl-CoA-dependent acylation catalysed by diacylglycerol acyltransferase (DGAT) to form TAG (Lung and Weselake, 2006).

Several developments over the past decade have suggested that this view of TAG bioassembly in oilseeds is incomplete, and that TAG biosynthesis in plants does not rely exclusively on acyl-CoA-dependent pathways as previously believed. Phospholipid:diacylglycerol acyltransferase (PDAT), which catalyses the transfer of an acyl group from the *sn*-2 position of PC to the *sn*-3 position of DAG, was discovered in yeast and plants, and was proposed to play a role in membrane maintenance by sequestering unusual acyl groups in TAG (Dahlqvist et al., 2000; Stahl et al., 2004). This enzyme was shown to play a major role in TAG accumulation in yeast (Oelkers et al., 2002), but there have been conflicting reports on its role in seed oil biosynthesis. Mhaske et al. (2005) reported that *Arabidopsis* mutants deficient in PDAT activity suffered no reduction in oil content and exhibited no changes in FA composition, suggesting a marginal role for PDAT in TAG accumulation. More recently, however, it was demonstrated that double mutants deficient in both DGAT1 and PDAT activity suffered a 70–80% reduction in oil content, compared to 20–40% in DGAT1 single mutants, and the double mutants also exhibited abnormal pollen and embryo development (Zhang et al., 2009). PDAT was also highly expressed in developing seeds of species that accumulate unusual FAs, but was expressed at low levels in soyabean and *Arabidopsis* (Liu et al., 2010), which further supports a role for PDAT in TAG biosynthesis in some species. Although it has not yet been studied, it is reasonable to speculate that expression of *PDAT* in BOS would follow a similar pattern as *Arabidopsis*, based on the presence of only common FAs in the seed oil.

A second major development that supports a more complex pathway for seed oil biosynthesis is the work of Bates et al. (2009), which suggests that the sequential acylation of *sn*-glycerol-3-phosphate accounts for only a small proportion of TAG synthesis in developing soyabean embryos. Instead, a large proportion of nascent acyl groups are first cycled through membrane phospholipids by various ‘acyl-editing’ mechanisms (including, e.g., the forward and reverse reactions of LPCAT). Likewise, only a small proportion of *de novo*-synthesized DAG is utilized directly for TAG bioassembly; most of the DAG used for TAG synthesis originates from PC, suggesting that interconversion of DAG and PC plays a much greater role in lipid metabolism than previously thought (Bates et al., 2009). This model was further supported by the recent discovery of an enzyme, phosphatidylcholine:diacylglycerol cholinephosphotransferase (PDCT), which catalyses the headgroup exchange to convert PC to DAG and vice versa (Lu et al., 2009). *Arabidopsis* mutants deficient in PDCT displayed a ‘reduced oleate desaturation’ phenotype, suggesting this enzyme plays a major role in channelling newly desaturated acyl groups from PC to DAG, which is subsequently used to form TAG (Lu et al., 2009).

Although studies of these mechanisms in BOS are lacking, these discoveries may shed considerable light on some of the problems that have been encountered in the biotechnological manipulation of seed oil composition in BOS. As we will discuss in some detail later, many attempts to introduce unusual FAs into oilseed crops have been hampered by the apparently inefficient exchange of unusual acyl groups between PC and the acyl-CoA pool (Cahoon et al., 2007). The discovery of PDAT and PDCT indicate there are multiple fates for acyl groups on PC other than exchange with the acyl-CoA pool, and as a result, overcoming limitations on acyl-exchange may require biotechnological manipulation of several enzymes.

6.3 MODIFICATION OF BOS SEED OIL COMPOSITION

Biotechnological modification of BOS seed oil composition has focussed mainly on the production of FAs or FA profiles possessing specialized functional or nutritional properties ideal for specific edible or industrial applications. With regard to modifying BOS oils, it should be noted that while the official definition of 'canola-quality' oil is based on maximum allowable levels of erucic acid and glucosinolates (Canola Council of Canada, 2010), drastic alterations to the rest of the FA profile may result in a product that could no longer be strictly classified or marketed as 'canola' oil. For the purposes of this chapter, we will nevertheless use the term 'canola' in reference to studies in low-erucic-acid, low-glucosinolate BOS, so that they are readily distinguishable from studies performed in high-erucic-acid, high-glucosinolate cultivars, regardless of the nature of the modification.

6.3.1 High-Oleic, Low-Alpha-Linolenic BOS Oils

Oxidative stability is a major consideration for vegetable oils intended for use in baking and frying applications since the accumulation of lipid oxidation products can result in undesirable flavours. Since oxidative stability decreases as the degree of unsaturation increases, food processors have traditionally opted to minimize the PUFA content of vegetable oils through the use of partially hydrogenated oils. Over the past decade, however, it has been widely recognized that *trans*-FAs, generated as a by-product of the hydrogenation process, have a severe, detrimental impact on cardiovascular health (Willett, 2006). As a result, there has been a focus on developing high-stability oils that are low in PUFA and are suitable for baking and frying applications without the need for hydrogenation.

High-oleic, low-linolenic (HOLL) oils have been generated in several oilseeds, including soyabean (Buhr et al., 2002), canola (Hu et al., 2006; Peng et al., 2010; Stoutjesdijk et al., 2000) and other BOS (Sivaraman et al., 2004; Velasco et al., 2003). All of these modified oils have been produced using a similar strategy of suppressing the activity of the FAD2, which reduces the formation of LA and therefore its subsequent desaturation to ALA. In some cases, such as soyabean, the palmitoyl thioesterase, which catalyses the release of 16:0 from ACP, was also down-regulated as a means of increasing the proportion of oleic acid formed through plastidial FA synthesis (Buhr et al., 2002).

Although the molecular target was similar in all cases, several different approaches have been applied to manipulate *FAD2* activity. A *B. napus* mutant with high oleic acid content was found to have a single nucleotide substitution in the *fad2* gene, which resulted in the production of a truncated, non-functional polypeptide; this discovery led to the development of an allele-specific marker for *fad2* that could be used in marker-assisted selection for increased oleic acid content (Hu et al., 2006). Similarly, HOLL *B. carinata* germplasm was obtained through a traditional breeding strategy whereby high-oleic mutants were crossed with low-linolenic mutants, resulting in lines with up to 83% oleic acid (Velasco et al., 2003). Various biotechnological strategies, such as co-suppression, antisense suppression and RNA interference, have also been used to generate BOS with HOLL phenotypes (Peng et al., 2010; Sivaraman et al., 2004; Stoutjesdijk et al., 2000). To date, however, the only HOLL canola oil in commercial production was developed using mutagenesis and traditional breeding techniques.

6.3.2 BOS Oils with Altered Saturated Fatty Acid Content

Although canola oil boasts the lowest saturated fat content of any commodity vegetable oil at <7%, research aimed at further reducing the SFA content of canola oil is ongoing. Lowering the SFA content of canola oil to below 3.5% would allow the product to be labelled as 'free of saturated fat' (Shah and Weselake, 2009), which is a significant marketing advantage given that negative perceptions surrounding dietary saturated fat persist among consumers. Additional pressure to reduce SFA content in canola is coming from the development of low-SFA soyabean varieties (Cardinal et al., 2007), which are poised to challenge canola's position as the lowest-SFA vegetable oil on the market.

In canola, the major saturated FAs are palmitic acid (~4%) and stearic acid (~2%). There are several possible strategies for reducing the total SFA content by manipulating these two FAs. In soyabean, down-regulation of ACP-thioesterase was used to increase oleic acid content (Buhr et al., 2002); this increase in oleic acid occurred at the expense of palmitic acid since more of the palmitic acid was channelled towards further elongation and desaturation on ACP. Bondaruk et al. (2007) targeted desaturation of palmitic acid directly, by introducing a palmitoyl-specific ACP desaturase from *Macfadyena unguis-cati* into *B. napus* and *Arabidopsis*. This resulted in increased conversion of 16:0 to palmitoleic acid ($16{:}1^{\Delta 9}$), but this was compensated for by an increase in 18:0, and no net reduction in SFA content was observed. Furthermore, in *Arabidopsis*, the resulting 16:1 was elongated to $18{:}1^{\Delta 11}$ and $20{:}1^{\Delta 13}$, suggesting that the palmitoleic acid was not rapidly consumed by reactions involved in TAG assembly, but rather persisted in the acyl-CoA pool long enough to undergo multiple elongations. The authors hypothesized that the substrate specificity or selectivity of the acyltransferases may limit the incorporation of palmitoleic acid into TAG. The same group was recently issued a patent for the production of canola with <4% SFA using a cyanobacterial glycerolipid desaturase (Shah and Weselake, 2009). Recently, Nguyen et al. (2010) achieved up to 43% palmitoleic acid in *Arabidopsis* using a stepwise approach that included expression of both ACP and acyl-CoA desaturases coupled with suppression of β-keto-acyl-ACP synthase (KAS) II (which elongates 16:0 to 18:0) and the FAE that elongates 18:1. Although this study achieved much higher levels of palmitoleic acid than those reported by Bondaruk et al. (2007), there was also substantial accumulation of $18:1^{\Delta 11}$ (up to 24%), while overall saturated FA content ranged from 12% to 30% with various constructs, compared to around 16% in the wild type.

While reduced SFA oils are being pursued to extend canola's marketing advantage as a 'heart-healthy' product for human consumption, there has also been work directed towards increasing the SFA content, to develop non-hydrogenated oils with desirable physiochemical characteristics for specific applications, such as spreadable margarines and shortenings. Increasing the proportion of stearic acid in the seed oil would provide the required functionality without the need for hydrogenation and the associated formation of *trans* fats, and high-stearic oils could potentially be used in place of tropical oils such as palm oil. Unlike palmitic acid, stearic acid has little impact on lipoprotein cholesterol, and is thus considered to be less atherogenic (Grundy, 1994).

An early approach to increase stearic acid content in *B. napus* and *B. rapa* involved the use of an antisense construct to suppress the expression of the gene encoding stearoyl-ACP desaturase, which resulted in reduced conversion of stearic acid to oleic acid (Knutzon et al., 1992). This strategy was successful with regard to increasing stearic acid content, generating *B. rapa* and *B. napus* lines with up to 32% and 40% stearic acid, respectively. Unfortunately, high stearic acid accumulation in *B. rapa* was associated with poor germination and reduced oil content. High stearic *B. napus* lines exhibited normal germination, but had variable oil content (Knutzon et al., 1992). Despite this success in achieving high levels of the desired FA, the associated loss of agronomic performance was likely a formidable barrier to commercialization.

In another approach, Facciotti et al. (1999) used site-directed mutagenesis to increase the stearoyl specificity of an acyl-ACP thioesterase from *Garcinia mangostana* that was previously found to increase the stearic acid content in transgenic *B. napus* (Hawkins and Kridl, 1998). Substitution of two amino acids (S111A/V193A) resulted in a 13-fold increase in specific activity towards stearoyl-ACP *in vitro*, and *B. napus* expressing this modified thioesterase accumulated up to 20% stearic acid in seed oil, compared to ~10% in lines expressing the unmodified *G. mangostana* thioesterase (Facciotti et al., 1999). It should be noted that these values are based on first-generation, segregating seeds, and it is possible that single seed analysis would have revealed individuals exhibiting greater increases in stearic acid content.

Thioesterase activity has also been targeted as a means of producing medium-chain saturated fatty acids (MCFA) in BOS. MCFA, such as lauric acid (12:0), are widely used for industrial applications, including cosmetics and surfactants, as well as for certain food applications such as confectionary. In most BOS, including canola, the endogenous acyl-ACP thioesterase exhibits a preference for 18-carbon FAs. Production of MCFA required the introduction of a thioesterase with appropriate medium-chain specificity, such as the 12:0 ACP-thioesterase from the California bay laurel (*Umbellularia californica*) (Voelker et al., 1996). Although the expression of this enzyme in canola resulted in a relatively high accumulation of lauric acid, further analysis revealed that it was limited to the *sn*-1 and *sn*-3 positions of the TAG molecule, likely a consequence of the *B. napus* LPAAT discriminating against saturated acyl-CoA substrates. This was overcome by co-expressing the cDNA encoding a thioesterase with a cDNA encoding LPAAT from coconut (*Cocus nucifera*) that could utilize 12:0-CoA (Knutzon et al., 1999). Similarly, cDNAs encoding thioesterases from other MCFA-containing species, such as cuphea (*Cuphea lanceolata*), nutmeg (*Myristica fragrans*) and elm (*Ulmus americana*) have been successfully expressed in BOS to produce oils with various MCFA, including caprylic (8:0), capric (10:0) and myristic (14:0) acids (Dehesh et al., 1996; Stoll et al., 2005). Although no difficulties with germination were reported with these MCFA-producing lines, the high-MCFA lines tended to exhibit slightly lower oil content (Knutzon et al., 1999; Larson et al., 2002).

A different strategy for producing MCFA in transgenic BOS targets the condensing enzyme of the FAS complex, KAS. There are several isoforms of KAS which differ in their substrate specificity, for example, KAS III catalyses the initial condensation in *de novo* FA synthesis while subsequent condensations from 4:0 to 16:0 are catalysed by KAS I (Stoll et al., 2005). Co-expression of a cDNA-encoding medium-chain specific KAS IV with a cDNA-encoding medium-chain thioesterase resulted in the accumulation of 8:0, 10:0 and 12:0 in transgenic *Brassica* (Dehesh et al., 1998).

6.3.3 Production of BOS Oils with Very-Long-Chain Polyunsaturated Fatty Acids

VLCPUFA, such as eicosapentaenoic acid (EPA; $20{:}5^{\Delta5,8,11,14,17}$) and docosahexaenoic acid (DHA; $22{:}6^{\Delta4,7,10,13,16,19}$) are essential for human health and nutrition (Riediger et al., 2009). Many animals, including humans, have a limited capacity to produce VLCPUFA from vegetable oils containing LA and ALA; thus, direct dietary consumption of EPA and DHA is recommended for optimal health. A variety of marine microorganisms naturally produce VLCPUFA, and these FAs bioaccumulate in fish occupying higher levels of the food chain. Fish oils currently represent a major source of dietary VLCPUFA for humans, either directly through the consumption of wild fish, or through the consumption of farmed fish which rely heavily on fish oil and fish meal as a source of VLCPUFA in their diets. Indeed, aquaculture is currently the fastest-growing food production sector and is the world's largest consumer of fish oil and meal; by 2030, it is expected that there will be a 40 million tonne shortfall in the availability of fish oil to support the industry's needs (Miller et al., 2008). Declining global fish stocks and increasing concerns over the presence of environmental toxins in fish have highlighted an urgent need to develop a sustainable land-based source of VLCPUFA.

Transgenic plants are a promising alternative for VLCPUFA production, since most common seed oils contain high levels of the precursors, LA and ALA, which can be converted to VLCPUFA via one of two transgenic pathways (Figure 6.2). Each of these pathways requires the introduction of multiple transgenes, making VLCPUFA production one of the most complex challenges in plant lipid biotechnology to date.

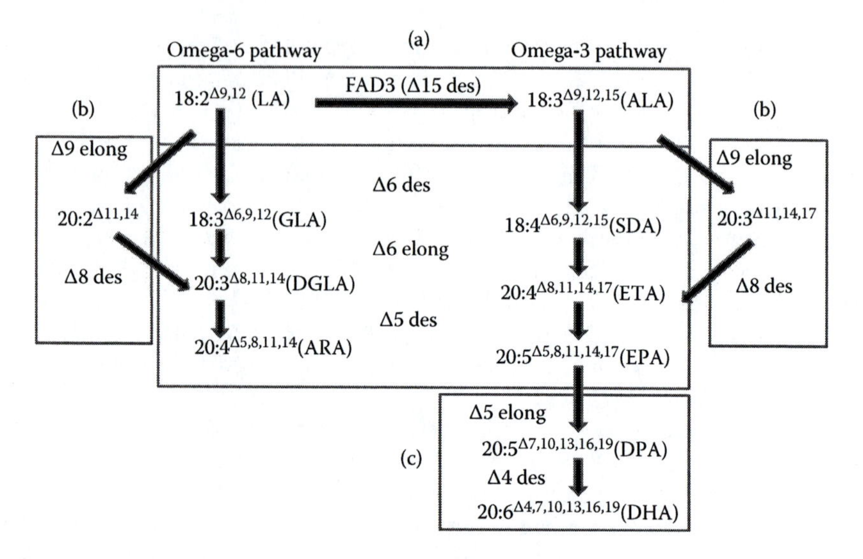

FIGURE 6.2 Pathways for very-long-chain polyunsaturated fatty acid (VLCPUFA) synthesis in transgenic oilseeds. In transgenic oilseeds, the omega-6 and omega-3 pathways for VLCPUFA synthesis begin with the endogenous precursors linoleic acid (LA) and alpha-linolenic acid (ALA), respectively. The Δ6 desaturation pathway (a) involves sequential Δ6 desaturation, Δ6-elongation and Δ5 desaturation steps to generate arachidonic acid (ARA) and eicosapentaenoic acid (EPA) in the omega-6 and omega-3 pathways, respectively. This pathway has been introduced into several BOS. (Adapted from Cheng, B. et al. 2010. *Transgenic Res.* 19: 221–229; Wu, G. et al. 2005. *Nat. Biotechnol.* 23: 1013–1017.) Alternatively, the Δ9 elongation pathway (b) results in the elongation of LA and ALA, followed by two desaturation steps (Δ8 and Δ5) to generate ARA and EPA; this pathway has been demonstrated in *Arabidopsis* leaves (Adapted from Qi, B. et al. 2004. *Nat. Biotechnol.* 22: 739–745.), but not transgenic BOS. The conversion of EPA to docosahexaenoic acid (DHA) (c) requires two additional steps catalysed by a Δ5 elongase and Δ4 desaturase, respectively. (Adapted from Wu, G. et al. 2005. *Nat. Biotechnol.* 23: 1013–1017.) In each case, the desaturation steps utilize phospholipid substrates while the elongation steps utilize acyl-CoA substrates. Other abbreviations: DPA: docosapentaenoic acid; DGLA: dihomo-gamma-linolenic acid; ETA: eicosatetraenoic acid; GLA: gamma-linolenic acid; SDA: stearidonic acid.

Preliminary studies focussed on the introduction of a single gene encoding a Δ6-desaturase, to produce gamma-linolenic acid (GLA; $18{:}3^{\Delta 6,9,12}$) or stearidonic acid (SDA; $18{:}4^{\Delta 6,9,12,15}$) from LA and ALA, respectively. Since the Δ6-desaturation step is the rate-limiting step in humans, it was suggested that consumption of SDA would be sufficient to overcome the limited synthesis of EPA and DHA in the human body (James et al., 2003). Insertion of the Δ6-desaturase into *B. juncea* yielded up to 40% GLA and about 8% SDA (Hong et al., 2002). Similar levels of GLA were obtained in *B. napus* co-expressing a *Δ6-DESATURASE* and *Δ12-DESATURASE* (Liu et al., 2001). Overexpression of the *B. napus Δ15-DESATURASE* along with introduction of fungal Δ6- and Δ12-desaturases resulted in substantially higher accumulations of SDA (up to 23%) in transgenic *B. napus* (Ursin, 2003). More recently, an omega-3 specific Δ6-desaturase has been identified which produces SDA without co-production of GLA, but so far, studies with this enzyme have not been extended to BOS (Ruiz-Lopez et al., 2009).

The production of longer-chain VLCPUFA has presented more of a challenge, and appears to be limited by the efficiency of the elongation steps. Abbadi et al. (2004) successfully engineered the production of arachidonic acid (ARA; $20{:}4^{\Delta 5,8,11,14}$) and EPA in tobacco and flax through the introduction of the Δ6-desaturation pathway; however, they obtained very low levels of 20-carbon PUFA (~5%) compared to around ~30% of the Δ6-desaturated 18-carbon intermediates (GLA and SDA). Further analysis revealed that GLA and SDA did not accumulate in the acyl-CoA pool and were therefore unavailable for elongation. Since desaturation occurs on the *sn*-2 position of PC and elongation utilizes acyl-CoA substrates, the authors suggested that inefficient exchange of acyl groups between these substrate pools resulted in 'substrate dichotomy', which limited VLCPUFA accumulation (Abbadi et al., 2004). This was further supported by the accumulation of up to 7% ARA and 3% EPA in *Arabidopsis* leaves expressing the Δ8-desaturation pathway, where LA and ALA are elongated prior to desaturation (Qi et al., 2004). Nevertheless, the Δ6-desaturation pathway has since been introduced into a number of different species, including soyabean (Kajikawa et al., 2008), *B. juncea* (Cheng et al., 2010; Wu et al., 2005) and *B. carinata* (Cheng et al., 2010).

Wu et al. (2005) obtained up to 25% ARA in *B. juncea* using a five-gene construct containing a Δ6-desaturase, two Δ6-elongases, a Δ5-desaturase and a Δ12-desaturase to increase the availability of LA feeding into the pathway. The further addition of an omega-3 desaturase, to convert ARA to EPA resulted in accumulation of up to 11% EPA. A nine-gene construct was eventually used to obtain low levels of DHA as a proof of concept, but accumulation of DHA was limited by inefficient elongation, presumably due to substrate dichotomy (Wu et al., 2005).

Zero-erucic-acid *B. carinata* was recently demonstrated to be an excellent host for VLCPUFA production, accumulating up to 25% EPA compared to an average of 5% EPA in zero-erucic-acid *B. juncea* (Cheng et al., 2010). Interestingly, it appears that zero-erucic-acid *B. carinata* accumulates high levels of LA and ALA rather than oleic acid, as is the case with low-erucic *B. napus* and *B. juncea*; this source of LA and ALA is almost completely depleted with the introduction of the VLCPUFA pathway in *B. carinata* (Cheng et al., 2010). These results suggest that *B. carinata* may have a very efficient acyl-exchange mechanism that could shed insight into the substrate dichotomy problem observed in other species.

6.3.4 Production of BOS Oils with Very-Long-Chain Monounsaturated Fatty Acids

Although considered undesirable in edible oils, erucic acid is an extremely useful FA for industrial applications, with over 1000 related patents issued for industrial applications of this FA (Scarth and Tang, 2006). As a result, there has been considerable work towards producing BOS with ultra-high erucic acid content. In high-erucic-acid rapeseed (HEAR *B. napus*), the inability of the endogenous LPAAT and LPCAT enzymes to utilize erucoyl-CoA imposed a theoretical limit of 66% erucic acid in the seed oil, based on the exclusion of erucic acid from the *sn*-2 position of TAG (Bernerth and Frentzen, 1990). This limitation may be partially relieved by the introduction of LPAAT activities from other species, such as *Limnanthes alba* and *Trapaeolum majus*, which could utilize erucoyl-CoA (Lassner et al., 1995; Taylor et al., 2010). Interestingly, *B. oleracea* L. var. *botrytis* cv Sesam was found to possess an LPAAT that could utilize erucoyl-CoA; this is apparently the first known *Brassica* LPAAT capable of inserting 22:1-CoA at the *sn*-2 position of TAG (Taylor et al., 1995).

Other enzymes have also been targeted as a means of increasing erucic acid content in BOS. Down-regulation of *FAD2* to prevent the desaturation of oleic acid was shown to be an effective strategy for increasing the accumulation of 22:1 and other very-long-chain FAs in *B. carinata* (Jadhav et al., 2005). Combining this strategy with overexpression of a crambe (*Crambe abyssynica*), *FAE1* resulted in a further increase in erucic acid in *B. carinata*, from around 40% in the wild type to 55% in the transgenic lines (Mietkiewska et al., 2008). Likewise, overexpression of the rapeseed *FAE* along with expression of *Limnanthes douglasii LPAAT* led up to 72% erucic acid in transgenic HEAR (Nath et al., 2009).

Further elongation of erucic acid results in the formation of nervonic acid ($24{:}1^{\Delta 15}$), which is an important component of the myelin in brain and nerve tissue (Martinez and Mougan, 1998). It has been suggested that dietary consumption of nervonic acid could support the synthesis and function of myelin (Sargent et al., 1994), which could be relevant therapeutically for individuals suffering from demyelinating disorders. Like erucic acid, nervonic acid also has a number of potential industrial uses, for example, as a lubricant or a feedstock for polyester synthesis (Taylor et al., 2009a).

One strategy for the production of nervonic acid in BOS is to introduce a condensing enzyme (3-keto-acyl-CoA synthase; KCS) capable of elongating erucic acid to nervonic acid. Several plants, such as borage, hemp and the 'money plant' (*Lunaria annua*) are capable of producing nervonic acid in their seed oils, with the latter accumulating up to 20% nervonic acid (Guo et al., 2009). Expression of an *L. annua KCS* gene in *B. carinata* resulted in up to 30% nervonic acid in the seed oil. The residual erucic acid content, however, was too high for human consumption. The same group subsequently isolated a *KCS* gene from *Cardamine graeca*, a plant exhibiting a high nervoic acid/erucic acid ratio, and expressed this gene in *B. carinata* and *B. napus* (Taylor et al., 2009a). Using this approach, they were able to produce about 42% nervonic acid in *B. carinata*, with only about 5% residual erucic acid. In *B. napus*, however, they obtained around 30% nervonic acid with more than 20% residual erucic acid (Taylor et al., 2009a). Such studies once again underscore the importance of selecting an appropriate BOS host for seed oil modification, and highlight the need for further comparative biochemical investigations of lipid metabolism in various BOS.

6.4 MODIFICATION OF BOS SEED OIL CONTENT

Seed oil content is a complex trait in BOS, controlled by multiple quantitative trait loci (QTL) (Barker et al., 2007; Delourme et al., 2006; Yan et al., 2009), and influenced by a variety of environmental factors (Champolivier and Merrien, 1996; Gunasekera et al., 2006). Despite this complexity, many groups are actively working towards the development of BOS with increased seed oil content, driven by the ever-increasing global demand for vegetable oil to satisfy both food and non-food applications. In Canada, it has been estimated that an absolute increase of 1% in canola oil content would be worth $90 million to the oilseed extraction and processing industry (Canola Council of Canada, 2009).

There are several biotechnological approaches to increasing BOS seed oil content. Many studies have focussed on increasing the activity of acyltransferases involved in TAG assembly (Taylor et al., 2009b; Weselake et al., 2008), reviewed by Snyder et al. (2009), while others have targeted enzymes involved in the synthesis of the TAG building blocks, *sn*-glycerol-3-phosphate (Vigeolas et al., 2007) and FAs (Roesler et al., 1997). More recently, transcription factors have emerged as a target for altering carbon metabolism and lipid biosynthesis at a higher level (Liu et al., 2010; Mu et al., 2008).

In *B. napus*, top-down metabolic control studies have indicated that the enzymes involved in TAG bioassembly exert greater overall control over TAG synthesis than those involved in FA biosynthesis (Weselake et al., 2008). Nevertheless, some studies targeting FA biosynthesis were effective in increasing seed oil content in *B. napus*. For example, Roesler et al. (1997) expressed a cytosolic homomeric acetyl-CoA carboxylase from *Arabidopsis* in the plastids of *B. napus*, resulting in a relative increase in seed oil content of about 5%. In another study, antisense suppression of mitochondrial pyruvate dehydrogenase kinase (PDHK), which negatively regulates the mitochondrial pyruvate dehydrogenase complex, resulted in increased seed oil content in *Arabidopsis* (Marillia et al., 2003). The pyruvate dehydrogenase complex catalyses the production of acetyl-CoA from pyruvate, and it was suggested that some of the acetyl-CoA could move into the plastid as acetate, where it could be re-converted to acetyl-CoA to support plastidial FA synthesis. Comparisons of near isogenic *B. napus* lines differing in oil content (Li et al., 2006) also supported this hypothesis. The gene encoding mitochondrial *PDHK* was down-regulated in the high-oil line (Li et al., 2006). Subsequent studies on mitochondrial metabolism in *B. napus*, however, have suggested that mitochondrial metabolism is not a major contributor to plastidial FA synthesis, and that the plastid imports a limited amount of mitochondrial-derived carbon in the form of pyruvate (Schwender et al., 2006). Plastidial pyruvate kinase has been shown to be important for FA biosynthesis in *Arabidopsis* (Andre et al., 2007; Baud et al., 2007), which would also support the conclusion that the plastid maintains its own source of pyruvate to support FA synthesis. Li et al. (2006) also reported higher pyruvate kinase expression in the high-oil *B. napus* line; this gene was identified based on homology with an *Arabidopsis* pyruvate kinase gene (At5g52920) that was subsequently shown to encode a plastidial form of pyruvate kinase (Baud et al., 2007).

Increasing the production of glycerol backbones for TAG synthesis was also effective for increasing overall seed oil content in *B. napus*. Vigeolas and Geigenberger (2004) found that direct injection of exogenous glycerol into developing *B. napus* seeds stimulated TAG synthesis, and there was a strong positive correlation between the *sn*-glycerol-3-phosphate content and TAG synthesis in developing seeds. Based on these findings, Vigeolas et al. (2007) subsequently expressed an *sn*-glycerol-3-phosphate dehydrogenase from yeast in *B. napus*, which led to a relative increase in oil content of up to 40%.

Among acyltransferases, GPAT, LPAAT and DGAT have all been targeted as a means of increasing seed oil content (Snyder et al., 2009; Weselake et al., 2009), although to date, only LPAAT and DGAT have been targeted specifically in BOS. Expression of a yeast *sn*-2 *ACYLTRANSFERASE* (*SLC1-1*) in high-erucic-acid *B. napus* led to relative increases in seed oil content of up to 48% under greenhouse conditions (Zou et al., 1997) and up to 13.5% in the field (Taylor et al., 2001). Recently, the expression of a *B. napus* microsomal *LPAAT* in *Arabidopsis* resulted in an average relative increase in oil content of 11% (Maisonneuve et al., 2010).

DGAT has received considerably more attention as a target for increasing seed oil content, since several lines of evidence suggest that the DGAT-catalysed reaction represents a 'bottleneck' in TAG biosynthesis. DGAT activity was found to be the lowest of the three acyltransferase involved in the sequential TAG assembly pathway (Perry et al., 1999), and DAG, the substrate for DGAT, was shown to accumulate during seed development (Perry et al., 1999; Perry and Harwood, 1993). In developing seeds of *B. napus*, DGAT activity peaks during the rapid phase of TAG synthesis, then declines sharply (Weselake et al., 1993). We now know that most plants have at least two forms of DGAT (DGAT1 and DGAT2), which share no homology and appear to have non-redundant roles in plant lipid metabolism (Shockey et al., 2006). A third DGAT, DGAT3, has been identified in peanut and is quite distinct from other DGATs in that it is a soluble enzyme (Saha et al., 2006); little is known at this point about its role in overall TAG synthesis. Overexpression of *DGAT1* from *Arabidopsis* or *B. napus* in various *B. napus* cultivars resulted in increased seed oil content under greenhouse and field conditions (Taylor et al., 2009b; Weselake et al., 2008), and metabolic control analysis in transgenic *B. napus* indicated that overexpression of *DGAT1* led to a more equitable distribution of control between FA synthesis and TAG assembly (Weselake et al., 2008). Overexpression of a *Trapaeolum majus DGAT1* in high-erucic-acid *B. napus* or *Arabidopsis* also resulted in relative increases in seed oil content of up to 30% (Xu et al., 2008). This study also achieved an 80% increase in DGAT activity *in vitro* through site-directed mutagenesis of a single residue in TmDGAT1, highlighting the potential for engineering DGAT enzymes with enhanced activity. Recently, a yeast-based system for high-throughput screening of mutagenized *B. napus DGAT1* cDNA libraries has been developed (Siloto et al., 2009a,b), which may facilitate the identification of such catalytically enhanced DGAT variants.

So far, in our own laboratory, we have been unable to functionally express *B. napus* or *Arabidopsis DGAT2* in yeast (Liu, 2011); however, overexpression of a fungal *DGAT2* in soyabean led to increased oil content under field conditions (Lardizabal et al., 2008). Several studies on DGAT2 from other species have suggested that this enzyme may play an important role in the incorporation of unusual FAs into TAG (Kroon et al., 2006; Li et al., 2010; Shockey et al., 2006); thus, there has been more interest in exploiting these enzymes to enhance the accumulation of unusual FAs in transgenic plants (Burgal et al., 2008; Mavraganis et al., 2010).

Over the past few years, the widespread availability of tools for functional genomics and transcriptomics in plants has led to the identification of several transcription factors (TFs) that act as higher-level regulators of carbon metabolism or lipid biosynthesis (reviewed in Weselake et al., 2009). Much of the work involving TFs has been performed in *Arabidopsis*, including several studies utilizing TFs from BOS. The *Arabidopsis wrinkled1* (*wri1*) mutant was found to have up to an 80% reduction in seed oil content (Focks and Benning, 1998), and *WRI1* was subsequently shown to encode a TF regulating lipid metabolism (Cernac and Benning, 2004). Recently, overexpression of two *B. napus WRI1* orthologues in *Arabidopsis* resulted in larger seeds and a 10–20% increase in oil content (Liu et al., 2010). Similarly, overexpression of two *B. napus* orthologues of *Arabidopsis LEAFYCOTYLEDON1 (LEC1)* resulted in increased oil content in *Arabidopsis* (Mu et al., 2008). *LEC1* was found to be a key regulator of lipid metabolism, activating several other TFs, including *WRI1* (Mu et al., 2008).

GLABRA2 is another transcription factor that was found to affect seed oil content in *Arabidopsis*, with the knockout mutant exhibiting an 8% increase in seed oil content (Shen et al., 2006), but the mechanism underlying this increase is yet unknown. Four orthologues of *GLABRA2* have been identified from *B. napus* (AC-genome), *B. rapa* (A genome) and *B. oleracea* (C genome), with the *B. napus* orthologue (*BnaC.GL2.b*) exhibiting the greatest similarity to *Arabidopsis GLABRA2* (Chai et al., 2010). As with the *Arabidopsis* knockout mutant, suppression of *BnaC.GL2.b* in *Arabidopsis* resulted in increased seed oil content, but surprisingly, some of the lines overexpressing *BnaC.GL2.b* also exhibited increases in seed oil content (Chai et al., 2010). Clearly, further studies are needed to clarify the mechanism by which this TF exerts its influence on oil content.

6.5 CONCLUSIONS AND FUTURE DIRECTIONS

Over the past two decades, considerable progress has been made towards the development of BOS with speciality oil profiles and increased seed oil content. Although no GE BOS expressing modified oil phenotypes have yet reached commercial production, proof-of-concept has been demonstrated for a wide range of traits that are of potential commercial interest. These studies have not only revealed a great deal about the basic genetic and biochemical regulation underlying oilseed lipid metabolism, but have also uncovered many new questions. The challenges encountered in the production of unusual FAs in transgenic oilseeds, for example, have shed light on the importance of acyl-editing mechanisms in the overall process of seed oil biosynthesis.

The identification of new enzymes, such as DGAT2, PDAT and PDCT, is exciting breakthroughs in plant lipid biochemistry, and will undoubtedly serve as a basis for future biotechnological modification of BOS oils. While enzymes such as DGAT2 and PDAT appear to play an important role in acyl-trafficking in species which naturally accumulate unusual FAs (Kroon et al., 2006; Li et al., 2010), less is known about their contribution to seed oil biosynthesis in conventional oilseeds. Furthermore, it is not well understood how modifying seed oil composition influences the behaviour of these enzymes in oilseeds that do not otherwise accumulate unusual FAs.

Another area that is in need of ongoing investigation, particularly in relation to BOS, is a comparative study of closely related species which differ in various aspects of their lipid metabolism. For example, *B. carinata* has emerged as a promising host for the transgenic production of very-long-chain FAs (Cheng et al., 2010; Taylor et al., 2009a), and appears to be more efficient than other BOS in producing these FAs, even when the genetic constructs are otherwise identical. A systematic comparison of acyl-trafficking patterns and gene expression related to lipid metabolism between various BOS species may reveal important differences which could lead to the development of novel strategies for BOS seed oil modification.

In addition, further studies on the role of certain TFs in the global regulation of seed oil biosynthesis in BOS are needed. The abundant genomic resources available for the model plant, *Arabidopsis*, have provided a wealth of information that is relevant to the study of lipid metabolism in BOS; however, studies in agronomically important BOS are required to move beyond the proof-of-concept stage and evaluate the commercial potential of various oil modification strategies.

Finally, in light of the increasing interest in development of BOS oils for speciality applications, it is important for BOS breeders and biotechnologists to seek an understanding of the potential downstream needs related to oil processing and functionality. Many industrial processes, for example, are optimized for very homogeneous feedstocks, while seed oils, for the most part, exhibit a heterogeneous composition, which can be affected by factors such as agronomic practices and environmental conditions. The development of commercially viable speciality BOS oils for such applications could be advanced through multidisciplinary approaches which recognize the needs of each participant in the value-added chain.

ACKNOWLEDGEMENTS

The authors wish to thank the following agencies and institutions for their support (to RJW) of research focussed on the biochemistry and biotechnology of *Brassica* oilseed species: Alberta Advanced Education and Technology, the Alberta Canola Producers Commission, the Alberta Crop Industry Development Fund, Alberta Innovates-BioSolutions, AVAC, Ltd., BASF Plant Science, the Canada Foundation for Innovation, the Canada Research Chairs Program, Genome Alberta, Genome Canada, the Natural Sciences and Engineering Research Council of Canada and the University of Alberta.

REFERENCES

Abbadi, A., Domergue, F., Bauer, J., Napier, J.A., Welti, R., Zahringer, U., Cirpus, P. and Heinz, E. 2004. Biosynthesis of very-long-chain polyunsaturated fatty acids in transgenic oilseeds: Constraints on their accumulation. *Plant Cell.* 16: 2734–2748.

Andre, C., Froehlich, J.E., Moll, M.R. and Benning, C. 2007. A heteromeric plastidic pyruvate kinase complex involved in seed oil biosynthesis in *Arabidopsis. Plant Cell.* 19: 2006–2022.

Barker, G.C., Larson, T.R., Graham, I.A., Lynn, J.R. and King, G.J. 2007. Novel insights into seed fatty acid synthesis and modification pathways from genetic diversity and quantitative trait loci analysis of the *Brassica* C genome. *Plant Physiol.* 144: 1827–1842.

Bates, P.D., Durrett, T.P., Ohlrogge, J.B. and Pollard M. 2009. Analysis of acyl fluxes through multiple pathways of triacylglycerol synthesis in developing soybean embryos. *Plant Physiol.* 150: 55–72.

Baud, S., Wuilleme, S., Dubreucq, B., de Almeida, A., Vuagnat, C., Lepiniec, L., Miquel, M. and Rochat, C. 2007. Function of plastidial pyruvate kinases in seeds of *Arabidopsis thaliana. Plant J.* 52: 405–419.

Bernerth, R. and Frentzen, M. 1990. Utilization of erucoyl-CoA by acyltransferases from developing seeds of *Brassica napus* L. involved in triacylglycerol biosynthesis. *Plant Sci.* 67: 21–28.

Bondaruk, M., Johnson, S., Degafu, A., Boora, P., Bilodeau, P., Morris, J., Wiehler, W., Foroud N., Weselake, R. and Shah S. 2007. Expression of a cDNA encoding palmitoyl-acyl carrier protein desaturase from cat's claw (*Doxantha unguis-cati* L.) in *Arabidopsis thaliana* and *Brassica napus* leads to accumulation of unusual unsaturated fatty acids and increased stearic acid content in the seed oil. *Plant Breed.* 126: 186–194.

Buhr, T., Sato, S., Ebrahim, F., Xing, A.Q., Zhou, Y., Mathiesen, M., Schweiger, B., Kinney, A., Staswick, P. and Clemente, T. 2002. Ribozyme termination of RNA transcripts down-regulate seed fatty acid genes in transgenic soybean. *Plant J.* 30: 155–163.

Burgal, J., Shockey, J., Lu, C.F., Dyer, J., Larson, T., Graham, I. and Browse, J. 2008. Metabolic engineering of hydroxy fatty acid production in plants: RcDGAT2 drives dramatic increases in ricinoleate levels in seed oil. *Plant Biotechnol. J.* 6: 819–831.

Cahoon, E.B., Shockey, J.M., Dietrich, C.R., Gidda, S.K., Mullen, R.T. and Dyer, J.M. 2007. Engineering oilseeds for sustainable production of industrial and nutritional feedstocks: Solving bottlenecks in fatty acid flux. *Curr. Opin. Plant Biol.* 10: 236–244.

Canola Council of Canada. Canola: Growing Great 2015. 2007. http://www.canolacouncil.org/uploads/canola_growing_great_2015.pdf (Accessed: 20-10-2010).

Canola Council of Canada. Canola Socio-Economic Value Report. 2008. http://www.canolacouncil.org/uploads/Canola_in_Canada_Socio_Economic_Value_Report_January_08.pdf (Accessed: 18-10-2010).

Canola Council of Canada. Strategy. Science. Success. Research Strategy for the Canola Industry. 2009. http://www.canolacouncil.org/uploads/Research%20Strategy%20for%20the%20Canola%20Industry.pdf (Accessed: 20-10-2010).

Canola Council of Canada. Canadian Canola Industry. 2010. http://www.canolacouncil.org/ind_overview.aspx (Accessed: 18-10-2010).

Cardinal, A.J., Burton, J.W., Camacho-Roger, A.M., Yang, J.H., Wilson, R. and Dewey, R.E. 2007. Molecular analysis of soybean lines with low palmitic acid content in the seed oil. *Crop Sci.* 47: 304–310.

Cernac, A. and Benning, C.2004. *WRINKLED1* encodes an AP2/EREB domain protein involved in the control of storage compound biosynthesis in *Arabidopsis. Plant J.* 40: 575–585.

Chai, G.H., Bai, Z.T., Wei, F., King, G.J., Wang, C.G., Shi, L., Dong, C.H., Chen, H. and Liu, S.Y. 2010. *Brassica GLABRA2* genes: Analysis of function related to seed oil content and development of functional markers. *Theor. Appl. Genet.* 120: 1597–1610.

Champolivier, L. and Merrien, A. 1996. Effects of water stress applied at different growth stages to *Brassica napus* L. var. *oleifera* on yield, yield components and seed quality. *Eur. J. Agron.* 5: 153–160.

Cheng, B., Wu, G., Vrinten, P., Falk, K., Bauer, J. and Qiu, X. 2010. Towards the production of high levels of eicosapentaenoic acid in transgenic plants: The effects of different host species, genes and promoters. *Transgenic Res.* 19: 221–229.

Dahlqvist, A., Stahl, U., Lenman, M., Banas, A., Lee, M., Sandager, L., Ronne, H. and Stymne S. 2000. Phospholipid:diacylglycerol acyltransferase: An enzyme that catalyzes the acyl-CoA-independent formation of triacylglycerol in yeast and plants. *Proc. Natl. Acad. Sci. USA*. 97: 6487–6492.

Dehesh, K., Edwards, P., Fillatti, J., Slabaugh, M. and Byrne J. 1998. KAS IV: A 3-ketoacyl-ACP synthase from *Cuphea* sp. is a medium chain specific condensing enzyme. *Plant J.* 15: 383–390.

Dehesh, K., Jones, A., Knutzon, D.S. and Voelker T.A. 1996. Production of high levels of 8:0 and 10:0 fatty acids in transgenic canola by overexpression of *Ch FatB2*, a thioesterase cDNA from *Cuphea hookeriana. Plant J.* 9: 167–172.

Delourme, R., Falentin, C., Huteau, V., Clouet, V., Horvais, R., Gandon, B., Specel, S. et al. 2006. Genetic control of oil content in oilseed rape (*Brassica napus* L.). *Theor. Appl. Genet.* 113: 1331–1345.

Facciotti, M.T., Bertain, P.B. and Yuan, L. 1999. Improved stearate phenotype in transgenic canola expressing a modified acyl-acyl carrier protein thioesterase. *Nat. Biotechnol.* 17: 593–597.

Fobert, P.R., Smith, M.A., Zou, J., Mietkiewska, E., Keller, W.A. and Taylor, D.C. 2008. Developing Canadian seed oils as industrial feedstocks. *Biofuel Bioprod. Bior.* 2: 206–214.

Focks, N. and Benning, C. 1998. *wrinkled1*: A novel, low-seed-oil mutant of Arabidopsis with a deficiency in the seed-specific regulation of carbohydrate metabolism. *Plant Physiol.* 118: 91–101.

Grundy, S.M. 1994. Influence of stearic acid on cholesterol metabolism relative to other long-chain fatty acids. *Am. J. Clin. Nutr.* 60: S986–S990.

Gunasekera, C.P., Martin, L.D., Siddique, K.H.M. and Walton G.H. 2006. Genotype by environment interactions of Indian mustard (*Brassica juncea* L.) and canola (*Brassica napus* L.) in Mediterranean-type environments: II. Oil and protein concentrations in seed. *Eur. J. Agron.* 25: 13–21.

Guo, Y.M., Mietkiewska, E., Francis, T., Katavic, V., Brost, J.M., Giblin, M., Barton, D.L. and Taylor D.C. 2009. Increase in nervonic acid content in transformed yeast and transgenic plants by introduction of a *Lunaria annua* L. 3-ketoacyl-CoA synthase (KCS) gene. *Plant Mol. Biol.* 69: 565–575.

Harwood, J.L. 2005. Fatty acid biosynthesis. *Plant Lipids: Biology, Utilization and Manipulation*, Murphy D.J., ed. Blackwell Publishing: Oxford. pp. 27–66.

Hawkins, D.J. and Kridl, J.C. 1998. Characterization of acyl-ACP thioesterases of mangosteen (*Garcinia mangostana*) seed and high levels of stearate production in transgenic canola. *Plant J.* 13: 743–752.

Hong, H., Datla, N., Reed, D.W., Covello, P.S., MacKenzie, S.L. and Qiu, X. 2002. High-level production of gamma-linolenic acid in *Brassica juncea* using a delta6 desaturase from *Pythium irregulare. Plant Physiol.* 129: 354–362.

Hu, X.Y., Sullivan-Gilbert, M., Gupta, M. and Thompson, S.A. 2006. Mapping of the loci controlling oleic and linolenic acid contents and development of *fad2* and *fad3* allele-specific markers in canola (*Brassica napus* L.). *Theor. Appl. Genet.* 113: 497–507.

Jadhav, A., Katavic, V., Marillia, E.F., Giblin, E.M., Barton, D.L., Kumar, A., Sonntag, C., Babic, V., Keller, W.A. and Taylor D.C. 2005. Increased levels of erucic acid in *Brassica carinata* by co-suppression and antisense repression of the endogenous *FAD2* gene. *Metab. Eng.* 7: 215–220.

James, M.J., Ursin, V.M. and Cleland, L.G. 2003. Metabolism of stearidonic acid in human subjects: Comparison with the metabolism of other n-3 fatty acids. *Am. J. Clin. Nutr.* 77: 1140–1145.

Kajikawa, M., Matsui, K., Ochiai, M., Tanaka, Y., Kita, Y., Ishimoto, M., Kohzu, Y. et al. 2008. Production of arachidonic and eicosapentaenoic acids in plants using bryophyte fatty acid Delta6-desaturase, Delta6-elongase, and Delta5-desaturase genes. *Biosci. Biotechnol. Biochem.* 72: 435–444.

Katavic, V., Mietkiewska, E., Barton, D.L., Giblin, E.M., Reed, D.W. and Taylor D.C. 2002. Restoring enzyme activity in nonfunctional low erucic acid *Brassica napus* fatty acid elongase 1 by a single amino acid substitution. *Eur. J. Biochem.* 269: 5625–5631.

Knutzon, D.S., Hayes, T.R., Wyrick, A., Xiong, H., Davies, H.M. and Voelker T.A. 1999. Lysophosphatidic acid acyltransferase from coconut endosperm mediates the insertion of laurate at the *sn*-2 position of triacylglycerols in lauric rapeseed oil and can increase total laurate levels. *Plant Physiol.* 120: 739–746.

Knutzon, D.S., Thompson, G.A., Radke, S.E., Johnson, W.B., Knauf, V.C. and Kridl, J.C. 1992. Modification of *Brassica* seed oil by antisense expression of a stearoyl-acyl carrier protein desaturase gene. *Proc. Natl. Acad. Sci. USA*. 89: 2624–2628.

Kroon, J.T.M., Wei, W.X., Simon, W.J. and Slabas, A.R. 2006. Identification and functional expression of a type 2 acyl-CoA: diacylglycerol acyltransferase (DGAT2) in developing castor bean seeds which has high homology to the major triglyceride biosynthetic enzyme of fungi and animals. *Phytochemistry* 67: 2541–2549.

Lardizabal, K., Effertz, R., Levering, C., Mai, J., Pedroso, M.C., Jury, T., Aasen, E., Gruys, K., and Bennett, K. 2008. Expression of *Umbelopsis ramanniana* DGAT2A in seed increases oil in soybean. *Plant Physiol.* 148: 89–96.

Larson, T.R., Edgell, T., Byrne, J., Dehesh, K. and Graham, I.A. 2002. Acyl-CoA profiles of transgenic plants that accumulate medium-chain fatty acids indicate inefficient storage lipid synthesis in developing oilseeds. *Plant J.* 32: 519–527.

Lassner, M.W., Levering, C.K., Davies, H.M. and Knutzon, D.S. 1995. Lysophosphatidic acid acyltransferase from meadowfoam mediates insertion of erucic acid at the *sn*-2 position of triacylglycerol in transgenic rapeseed oil. *Plant Physiol.* 109: 1389–1394.

Li, R.J., Wang, H.Z., Mao, H., Lu, Y.T. and Hua, W. 2006. Identification of differentially expressed genes in seeds of two near-isogenic *Brassica napus* lines with different oil content. *Planta*. 224: 952–962.

Li, R.Z., Yu, K.S. and Hildebrand, D.F. 2010. *DGAT1*, *DGAT2* and *PDAT* expression in seeds and other tissues of epoxy and hydroxy fatty acid accumulating plants. *Lipids*. 45: 145–157.

Liu, Q. 2011. Functional and topological analysis of acyl-CoA:diacylglycerol acyltransferase 2 from *Saccharomyces cerevisiae*. Ph.D. Thesis, University of Alberta, Edmonton, Alberta, Canada.

Liu, J., Hua, W., Zhan, G.M., Wei, F., Wang, X.F., Liu, G.H. and Wang, H.Z. 2010. Increasing seed mass and oil content in transgenic *Arabidopsis* by the overexpression of *wri1-like* gene from *Brassica napus*. *Plant Physiol. Biochem.* 48: 9–15.

Liu, J.W., DeMichele, S., Bergana, M., Bobik, E., Hastilow, C., Chuang, L.T., Mukerji, P. and Huang, Y.S. 2001. Characterization of oil exhibiting high gamma-linolenic acid from a genetically transformed canola strain. *J. Am. Oil Chem. Soc.* 78: 489–493.

Lu, C.F., Xin, Z.G., Ren, Z.H., Miquel, M. and Browse, J. 2009. An enzyme regulating triacylglycerol composition is encoded by the *ROD1* gene of *Arabidopsis*. *Proc. Natl. Acad. Sci. USA*. 106: 18837–18842.

Lung, S.C. and Weselake, R.J. 2006. Diacylglycerol acyltransferase: A key mediator of plant triacylglycerol synthesis. *Lipids* 41: 1073–1088.

Maisonneuve, S., Bessoule, J.J., Lessire, R., Delseny, M. and Roscoe T.J. 2010. Expression of rapeseed microsomal lysophosphatidic acid acyltransferase isozymes enhances seed oil content in *Arabidopsis*. *Plant Physiol.* 152: 670–684.

Marillia, E.F., Micallef, B.J., Micallef, M., Weninger, A., Pedersen, K.K., Zou, J.T. and Taylor, D.C. 2003. Biochemical and physiological studies of *Arabidopsis thaliana* transgenic lines with repressed expression of the mitochondrial pyruvate dehydrogenase kinase. *J. Exp. Bot.* 54: 259–270.

Martinez, M. and Mougan I. 1998. Fatty acid composition of human brain phospholipids during normal development. *J. Neurochem.* 71: 2528–2533.

Mavraganis, I., Meesapyodsuk, D., Vrinten, P., Smith, M. and Qiu, X. 2010. Type II diacylglycerol acyltransferase from *Claviceps purpurea* with ricinoleic acid, a hydroxyl fatty acid of industrial importance, as preferred substrate. *Appl. Environ. Microb.* 76: 1135–1142.

Mhaske, V., Beldjilali, K., Ohlrogge, J. and Pollard, M. 2005. Isolation and characterization of an *Arabidopsis thaliana* knockout line for phospholipid: Diacylglycerol transacylase gene (At5g13640). *Plant Physiol. Biochem.* 43: 413–417.

Mietkiewska, E., Hoffman, T.L., Brost, J.M., Giblin, E.M., Barton, D.L., Francis, T., Zhang, Y. and Taylor, D.C. 2008. Hairpin-RNA mediated silencing of endogenous *FAD2* gene combined with heterologous expression of *Crambe abyssinica FAE* gene causes an increase in the level of erucic acid in transgenic *Brassica carinata* seeds. *Mol. Breed.* 22: 619–627.

Miller, M.R., Nichols, P.D. and Carter, C.G. 2008. n-3 Oil sources for use in aquaculture—Alternatives to the unsustainable harvest of wild fish. *Nutr. Res. Rev.* 21: 85–96.

Mu, J.Y., Tan, H.L., Zheng, Q., Fu, F.Y., Liang, Y., Zhang, J.A., Yang, X.H. et al. 2008. *LEAFY COTYLEDON1* is a key regulator of fatty acid biosynthesis in *Arabidopsis. Plant Physiol.* 148: 1042–1054.

Nath, U.K., Wilmer, J.A., Wallington, E.J., Becker, H.C. and Mollers, C. 2009. Increasing erucic acid content through combination of endogenous low polyunsaturated fatty acids alleles with *Ld-LPAAT* plus *Bn-fae1* transgenes in rapeseed (*Brassica napus* L.). *Theor. Appl. Genet.* 118: 765–773.

Nguyen, H.T., Mishra, G., Whittle, E., Bevan, S.A., Owens-Merlo, A., Walsh, T.A. and Shanklin, J. 2010. Metabolic engineering of seeds can achieve levels of {omega}-7 fatty acids comparable to the highest levels found in natural plant sources. *Plant Physiol.* 154: 1897–1904.

Oelkers, P., Cromley, D., Padamsee, M., Billheimer, J.T. and Sturley, S.L. 2002. The *DGA1* gene determines a second triglyceride synthetic pathway in yeast. *J. Biol. Chem.* 277: 8877–8881.

Orthoefer, F.T. 2005. Performance of *trans*-free vegetable oils in shortenings and deep-fat frying. *Lipid Technol.* 17: 101–106.

Peng, Q., Hu, Y., Wei, R., Zhang, Y., Guan, C., Ruan, Y. and Liu, C. 2010. Simultaneous silencing of *FAD2* and *FAE1* genes affects both oleic acid and erucic acid contents in *Brassica napus* seeds. *Plant Cell Rep.* 29: 317–325.

Perry, H.J., Bligny, R., Gout, E. and Harwood, J.L. 1999. Changes in Kennedy pathway intermediates associated with increased triacylglycerol synthesis in oil-seed rape. *Phytochemistry* 52: 799–804.

Perry, H.J. and Harwood, J.L. 1993. Changes in the lipid content of developing seeds of *Brassica napus. Phytochemistry* 32: 1411–1415.

Qi, B., Fraser, T., Mugford, S., Dobson, G., Sayanova, O., Butler, J., Napier, J.A., Stobart, A.K. and Lazarus, C.M. 2004. Production of very long chain polyunsaturated omega-3 and omega-6 fatty acids in plants. *Nat. Biotechnol.* 22: 739–745.

Rakow, G. 2004. Species origin and economic importance of *Brassica.* In *Biotechnology in Agriculture and Forestry, Vol 54*, Pua E.C., Douglas C.J., eds. Springer-Verlag: Berlin Heidelberg. pp. 3–7.

Riediger, N.D., Othman, R.A., Suh, M. and Moghadasian, M.H. 2009. A systemic review of the roles of n-3 fatty acids in health and disease. *J. Am. Diet. Assoc.* 109: 668–679.

Roesler, K., Shintani, D., Savage, L., Boddupalli, S. and Ohlrogge, J. 1997. Targeting of the *Arabidopsis* homomeric acetyl-coenzyme A carboxylase to plastids of rapeseeds. *Plant Physiol.* 113: 75–81.

Ruiz-Lopez, N., Haslam, R.P., Venegas-Caleron, M., Larson, T.R., Graham, I.A., Napier, J.A. and Sayanova, O. 2009. The synthesis and accumulation of stearidonic acid in transgenic plants: A novel source of 'heart-healthy' omega-3 fatty acids. *Plant Biotechnol. J.* 7: 704–716.

Saha, S., Enugutti, B., Rajakumari, S. and Rajasekharan, R. 2006. Cytosolic triacylglycerol biosynthetic pathway in oilseeds. Molecular cloning and expression of peanut cytosolic diacylglycerol acyltransferase. *Plant Physiol.* 141: 1533–1543.

Sargent, J.R., Coupland, K. and Wilson, R. 1994. Nervonic acid and demyelinating disease. *Med. Hypotheses*. 42: 237–242.

Sasaki, Y. and Nagano, Y. 2004. Plant acetyl-CoA carboxylase: Structure, biosynthesis, regulation, and gene manipulation for plant breeding. *Biosci. Biotechnol. Biochem.* 68: 1175–1184.

Scarth, R. and Tang, J. 2006. Modification of *Brassica* oil using conventional and transgenic approaches. *Crop Sci.* 46: 1225–1236.

Schnurr, J.A., Shockey, J.M., de Boer, G.J. and Browse, J.A. 2002. Fatty acid export from the chloroplast. Molecular characterization of a major plastidial acyl-coenzyme A synthetase from *Arabidopsis. Plant Physiol.* 129: 1700–1709.

Schwender, J., Shachar-Hill, Y. and Ohlrogge, J.B. 2006. Mitochondrial metabolism in developing embryos of *Brassica napus. J. Biol. Chem.* 281: 34040–34047.

Shah, S. and Weselake, R.J. 2009. Transgenic plants with reduced level of saturated fatty acids and methods for making them. European Application No. 04802331.1.

Shen, B., Sinkevicius, K.W., Selinger, D.A. and Tarczynski, M.C. 2006. The homeobox gene *GLABRA2* affects seed oil content in *Arabidopsis. Plant Mol. Biol.* 60: 377–387.

Shockey, J.M., Gidda, S.K., Chapital, D.C., Kuan, J.C., Dhanoa, P.K., Bland, J.M., Rothstein, S.J., Mullen, R.T. and Dyer, J.M. 2006. Tung tree DGAT1 and DGAT2 have nonredundant functions in triacylglycerol biosynthesis and are localized to different subdomains of the endoplasmic reticulum. *Plant Cell.* 18: 2294–2313.

Siloto, R.M.P., Truksa, M., Brownfield, D., Good, A.G. and Weselake, R.J. 2009a. Directed evolution of acyl-CoA:diacylglycerol acyltransferase: Development and characterization of *Brassica napus DGAT1* mutagenized libraries. *Plant Physiol. Biochem.* 47: 456–461.

Siloto, R.M.P., Truksa, M., He, X.H., McKeon, T. and Weselake, R.J. 2009b. Simple methods to detect triacylglycerol biosynthesis in a yeast-based recombinant system. *Lipids* 44: 963–973.

Sivaraman, I., Arumugam, N., Sodhi, Y.S., Gupta, V., Mukhopadhyay, A., Pradhan, A.K., Burma, P.K. and Pental, D. 2004. Development of high oleic and low linoleic acid transgenics in a zero erucic acid *Brassica juncea* L. (Indian mustard) line by antisense suppression of the *fad2* gene. *Mol. Breed.* 13: 365–375.

Snyder, C.L., Yurchenko, O.P., Siloto, R.M., Chen, X., Liu, Q., Mietkiewska, E. and Weselake, R.J. 2009. Acyltransferase action in the modification of seed oil biosynthesis. *Nat. Biotechnol.* 26: 11–16.

Stahl, U., Banas, A. and Stymne, S. 1995. Plant microsomal phospholipid acyl hydrolases have selectivities for uncommon fatty acids. *Plant Physiol.* 107: 953–962.

Stahl, U., Carlsson, A.S., Lenman, M., Dahlqvist, A., Huang, B., Banas, W., Banas, A. and Stymne, S. 2004. Cloning and functional characterization of a phospholipid:diacylglycerol acyltransferase from *Arabidopsis. Plant Physiol.* 135: 1324–1335.

Stoll, C., Luhs, W., Zarhloul, M.K. and Friedt, W. 2005. Genetic modification of saturated fatty acids in oilseed rape (*Brassica napus*). *Eur. J. Lipid Sci. Technol.* 107: 244–248.

Stoutjesdijk, P.A., Hurlestone, C., Singh, S.P. and Green, A.G. 2000. High-oleic acid Australian *Brassica napus* and *B. juncea* varieties produced by co-suppression of endogenous Delta 12-desaturases. *Biochem. Soc. Trans.* 28: 938–940.

Stymne, S. and Stobart, A.K. 1984a. Evidence for the reversibility of the acyl-CoA: Lysophosphatidylcholine acyltransferase in microsomal preparations from developing safflower (*Carthamus tinctorius* L.) cotyledons and rat liver. *Biochem. J.* 223: 305–314.

Stymne, S. and Stobart, A.K. 1984b. The biosynthesis of triacylglycerols in microsomal preparations of developing cotyledons of sunflower (*Helianthus annuus* L.). *Biochem. J.* 220: 481–488.

Taylor, D.C., Barton, D.L., Giblin, E.M., MacKenzie, S.L., Vandenberg, C.G.J. and McVetty, P.B.E. 1995. Microsomal lysophosphatidic acid acyltransferase from a *Brassica oleracea* cultivar incorporates erucic acid into the *sn*-2 position of seed triacylglycerols. *Plant Physiol.* 109: 409–420.

Taylor, D.C., Francis, T., Guo, Y.M., Brost, J.M., Katavic, V., Mietkiewska, E., Giblin, E.M., Lozinsky, S. and Hoffman, T. 2009a. Molecular cloning and characterization of a KCS gene from *Cardamine graeca* and its heterologous expression in *Brassica* oilseeds to engineer high nervonic acid oils for potential medical and industrial use. *Plant Biotechnol. J.* 7: 925–938.

Taylor, D.C., Francis, T., Lozinsky, S., Hoffman, T., Giblin, M. and Marillia, E.F. 2010. Cloning and characterization of constitutive *Lysophosphatidic Acid Acyltransferase 2 (LPAT2)* gene from *Tropaeolum majus* L. *Open Plant Sci. J.* 4: 7–17.

Taylor, D.C., Katavic, V., Zou, J.-T., MacKenzie, S.L., Keller, W.A., An, J., Friesen, W. et al. 2001. Field-testing of transgenic rapeseed cv. Hero transformed with a yeast *sn*-2 acyltransferase results in increased oil content, erucic acid content and seed yield. *Mol. Breed.* 8: 317–322.

Taylor, D.C., Zhang, Y., Kumar, A., Francis, T., Giblin, M.E., Barton, D.L., Ferrie, J.R. et al. 2009b. Molecular modification of triacylglycerol accumulation by over-expression of *DGAT1* to produce canola with increased seed oil content under field conditions. *Botany* 87: 533–543.

Ursin, V.M. 2003. Modification of plant lipids for human health: Development of functional land-based omega-3 fatty acids. *J. Nutr.* 133: 4271–4274.

Velasco, L., Nabloussi, A., De Haro, A. and Fernandez-Martinez, J.M. 2003. Development of high-oleic, low-linolenic acid Ethiopian-mustard (*Brassica carinata*) germplasm. *Theor. Appl. Genet.* 107: 823–830.

Venegas-Caleron, M., Sayanova, O. and Napier, J.A. 2010. An alternative to fish oils: Metabolic engineering of oil-seed crops to produce omega-3 long chain polyunsaturated fatty acids. *Prog. Lipid Res.* 49: 108–119.

Vigeolas, H. and Geigenberger, P. 2004. Increased levels of glycerol-3-phosphate lead to a stimulation of flux into triacylglycerol synthesis after supplying glycerol to developing seeds of *Brassica napus* L. in planta. *Planta* 219: 827–835.

Vigeolas, H., Waldeck, P., Zank, T. and Geigenberger, P. 2007. Increasing seed oil content in oilseed rape (*Brassica napus* L.) by over-expression of a yeast glycerol-3-phosphate dehydrogenase under the control of a seed-specific promoter. *Plant Biotechnol. J.* 5: 431–41.

Voelker, T.A., Hayes, T.R., Cranmer, A.M., Turner, J.C. and Davies, H.M. 1996. Genetic engineering of a quantitative trait: Metabolic and genetic parameters influencing the accumulation of laurate in rapeseed. *Plant J.* 9: 229–241.

Vogel, G. and Browse, J. 1996. Cholinephosphotransferase and diacylglycerol acyltransferase—Substrate specificities at a key branch point in seed lipid metabolism. *Plant Physiol.* 110: 923–931.

Weselake, R.J. 2005. Storage lipids. In *Plant Lipids: Biology, Utilization and Manipulation*, Murphy D.J., ed. Blackwell Publishing: Oxford. pp. 162–221.

Weselake, R.J., Pomeroy, M.K., Furukawa, T.L., Golden, J.L., Little, D.B. and Laroche, A. 1993. Developmental profile of diacylglycerol acyltransferase in maturing seeds of oilseed rape and safflower and microspore-derived cultures of oilseed rape. *Plant Physiol.* 102: 565–571.

Weselake, R.J., Shah, S., Tang, M., Quant, P.A., Snyder, C.L., Furukawa-Stoffer, T.L., Zhu, W. et al. 2008. Metabolic control analysis is helpful for informed genetic manipulation of oilseed rape (*Brassica napus*) to increase seed oil content. *J. Exp. Bot.* 59: 3543–3549.

Weselake, R.J., Taylor, D.C., Rahman, M.H., Shah, S., Laroche, A., Mcvetty, P.B.E. and Harwood J.L. 2009. Increasing the flow of carbon into seed oil. *Biotechnol. Adv.* 27: 866–878.

Willett, W.C. 2006. Trans fatty acids and cardiovascular disease—Epidemiological data. *Atherosclerosis Supp.* 7: 5–8.

Wu, G., Truksa, M., Datla, N., Vrinten, P., Bauer, J., Zank, T., Cirpus, P., Heinz, E. and Qiu, X. 2005. Stepwise engineering to produce high yields of very long-chain polyunsaturated fatty acids in plants. *Nat. Biotechnol.* 23: 1013–1017.

Xu, J., Francis, T., Mietkiewska, E., Giblin, E.M., Barton, D.L., Zhang, Y., Zhang, M. and Taylor D.C. 2008. Cloning and characterization of an acyl-CoA-dependent diacylglycerol acyltransferase 1 (DGAT1) gene from *Tropaeolum majus*, and a study of the functional motifs of the DGAT protein using site-directed mutagenesis to modify enzyme activity and oil content. *Plant Biotechnol. J.* 6: 799–811.

Yan, X.Y., Li, J.N., Fu, F.Y., Jin, M.Y., Chen, L. and Liu, L.Z. 2009. Co-location of seed oil content, seed hull content and seed coat color QTL in three different environments in *Brassica napus* L. *Euphytica.* 170: 355–364.

Yurchenko, O.P., Nykiforuk, C.L., Moloney, M.M., Stahl, U., Banas, A., Stymne, S. and Weselake, R.J. 2009. A 10-kDa acyl-CoA-binding protein (ACBP) from *Brassica napus* enhances acyl exchange between acyl-CoA and phosphatidylcholine. *Plant Biotechnol. J.* 7: 602–610.

Zhang, M., Fan, J., Taylor, D.C. and Ohlrogge, J.B. 2009. *DGAT1* and *PDAT1* Acyltransferases have overlapping functions in *arabidopsis* triacylglycerol biosynthesis and are essential for normal pollen and seed development. *Plant Cell.* 21: 3885–3901.

Zou, J., Katavic, V., Giblin, E.M., Barton, D.L., MacKenzie, S.L., Keller, W.A., Hu, X. and Taylor, D.C. 1997. Modification of seed oil content and acyl composition in the Brassicaceae by expression of a yeast *sn*-2 acyltransferase gene. *Plant Cell.* 9: 909–923.

7 Measurement of Oil Content by Rapid Analytical Techniques

Véronique J. Barthet

CONTENTS

7.1 Introduction 125
7.2 Pulse NMR 127
7.3 NIR Analysis 130
    7.3.1 Oil and Protein Measurements 136
    7.3.2 Chlorophyll Measurement 138
    7.3.3 α-Linolenic Acid Measurement 139
Acknowledgements 140
References 141

7.1 INTRODUCTION

Canola is the most important oilseed produced in Canada. Since 2009, over 10 million tons of canola have been produced by Canadian growers annually and is the main vegetable oil consumed by Canadians. The seeds are crushed to produce meal (about 55% of the seed) and oil (about 45% of the seed) but canola is mainly marketed for its oil. In oilseeds (canola), oil could be defined as a storage material that contains aliphatic compounds such as triacylglycerols (triglycerides, TAG) (Gunstone and Herslöl, 2000). Oil is the main parameter to assess the canola quality and to market it. It is therefore important to measure all seed components that will affect both the quantity and the quality of canola oil. To have all stakeholders involved in the canola (oilseed) trade satisfied, it is important (a) to have rapid analytical methods that give the real content of the seed components, such as oil and (b) to have these methods standardized.

Since canola is sold for crushing, the oil content analysis should give an estimate of the amount of oil that could optimally be obtained by a crushing plant (crushing plant with solvent extraction). World trade is usually overseen by organizations to help buyers, sellers, producers, exporters, importers and users to conduct their business. The Federation of Oils, Seeds and Fats Associations (FOSFA, http://www.fosfa.org/) is an international organization involved exclusively with the international trade of oilseeds, oils and fats. It is considered that FOSFA contracts/standards manage about 85% of the international trade of oilseeds, oils and fats. FOSFA is using standards issued by the International Organization for Standardization (ISO) to regulate the oilseed trade. The mandatory analytical method specified by FOSFA (2005) as the reference method to determine oil content is the ISO 659: 2009 method (1998). The America Oil Chemists' Society (AOCS, http://www.aocs.org) also developed a method (AOCS, Am 2-93: 2009) to analyse the oilseed oil content. Both the AOCS Am 2-93 method (2009) and the ISO 659–2009 method have been harmonized, meaning that they are equivalent methods, with the same scope and the same principle. They are solvent extraction methods with several stages of grinding and extraction; their scope is to produce an exhaustive extraction of neutral lipids. Hexane or petroleum ether could be used as the solvent for both methods. The extracted component is then estimated gravimetrically, and it is defined as crude fat or oil content. The multiple (triplicate) extractions with grinding and regrinding make the method costly due to analyst time, solvent consumption and disposal. Despite the length of the method, for the trade, it is the only recognized reference method capable of an exhaustive extraction of all nonpolar lipids. It takes 48–72 h to obtain results with this type of extraction method.

Some compounds, such as chlorophyll, have a negative impact on canola seed quality because they have damaging effects on canola oil quality. Chlorophylls are present in high levels in immature canola seeds. During processing, chlorophylls *a* and *b* from the seeds are transformed into pheophytins and pyropheophytins (Daun and Thorsteinson, 1989; Endo et al., 1992). Chlorophylls and their derivatives are extracted with the oil during crushing; they have pro-oxidant effect on canola oil. Chlorophyll derivatives are removed during oil processing at the bleaching step (Mag, 1990; Unger, 2011). Oils, from high chlorophyll samples, have also been shown to store poorly due to high levels of oxidation products formed during the bleaching step (high temperature and long-period bleaching step). High chlorophyll content also increases the canola refining cost since more bleaching clay needs to be added to remove the chlorophyll derivatives. Measuring chlorophyll content rapidly and accurately is therefore important for crushers to optimize their crushing and oil refining processes.

Protein is the most important component of canola meal, therefore protein content of the canola seed also impacts its marketing. There are two reference methods to measure the total protein content, the Kjeldahl method (AOCS Official Method Ba 4d-90) and the Dumas or combustion method (AOCS Official Method Ba 4e-93; ISO 16634–1: 2008). Both methods, very old, have been modified and automated over the years. With the combustion method, all forms of nitrogen are oxidized by combustion under oxygen, then reduced into nitrogen. After elimination of the other compounds, the nitrogen gas is measured using thermal conductivity. This is a safe and rapid method. However, all nitrogen-containing nonprotein compounds, such as glucosinolates and sinapine, are measured by this method, leading to a slight over estimation of the total nitrogen content for canola (Daun and DeClercq, 1994; Jung et al., 2003). Nitrogen content results are multiplied by a protein conversion factor to get the total protein content from the nitrogen content measurements. This protein conversion factor is still not clearly defined (Jones, 1941; Tkachuk, 1969; Mossé, 1990; Daun and DeClercq, 1994; Daun, 1999; Mariotti et al., 2008). However, for canola seed and meal, the general hypothesis that proteins contain 16% nitrogen is widely accepted to calculate protein contents from nitrogen values—protein contents are calculated from nitrogen content results by multiplying them by 100/16 or 6.25.

Vegetable oil functional and nutritional values are dependent on the nature of the different fatty acids present in the oils. In sound oilseeds, fatty acids are found almost exclusive as building blocks of the triacylglycerides with negligible amount of free fatty acids. Fatty acids are analysed by gas chromatography (GC) after being transformed into volatile compounds. Several derivatization methods could be used to prepare these volatile derivatives, however, since almost no free fatty acids are found in sound canola, base catalysed derivatization could be used to prepare the fatty acid methyl esters (FAMEs). The FAMEs are analysed by GC, the relative fatty acid composition is calculated from the sum of all fatty acids (even the unknown) present in the sample.

At the breeding level, canola quality is defined by its contents of oil, protein, glucosinolate, erucic acid and total saturates. A breeder needs to select, plant and analyse thousands of samples in a very short time for its breeding program so that he can register new lines of improved quality every year. To allow a breeder to run a successful program or a grain company to segregate the seeds they are receiving, rapid, robust and easy-to-handle methods are necessary to analyse the canola seed quality. Two techniques—near-infrared spectrophotometry (NIR) and pulse nuclear magnetic resonance (NMR)—are commonly used by the industry to measure canola quality parameters. NIR can predict several quality parameters and has been used for all kinds of materials (Daun et al., 1994; Williams and Norris, 2001) and can predict the canola quality (oil, protein, glucosinolate, chlorophyll and fatty acid composition) whereas NMR is more restrictive, it is regularly used to measure oil and moisture contents (Rubel, 1994). Both methods are secondary techniques and both instruments have to be calibrated with the appropriate calibration sets. The calibration set could contain from five samples (pulse NMR) to several thousands (NIR with neural network). These techniques also offer the advantages that once properly calibrated, they can be used for months without being recalibrated. Regardless of the technique, the results have to be accurate and repeatable and reproducible if the price is affected by the obtained results.

The complexity of some of the reference official methods affects their repeatability and reproducibility; the more steps in a method and the more sources of error could lead to result variations and high standard deviations. Our own experience in our laboratory has shown that rapid techniques such as NIR and NMR could be more repeatable than the official wet-chemistry methods. Batten (1998) reported several results agreeing with our observations.

The goal of this chapter is to present two of the rapid methods used to analyse canola quality. The particular advantages, disadvantages and limitations of each of these techniques will be discussed.

7.2 PULSE NMR

Several articles and book chapters deal with this technique (Srinivasan, 1979). Magnetic nuclear resonance is based on atom properties; hydrogen atom nuclei are made of one proton and one neutron and have an overall spin that can be used in NMR. In a pulse-NMR instrument, the molecules are placed in an electromagnetic field, the hydrogen atoms have their nucleus oriented such that their magnetic moments are aligned with or against the magnetic field. Then a second discontinuous magnetic field, a radio frequency, is applied to change the orientation of the magnetic field of the hydrogen nucleus. The excited nuclei return to their original state by exchanging their energy; this return to the relaxation state produces a signal called the free induction decay. This signal is used to measure the hydrogen present in the sample. In a solid phase, each of the hydrogen nuclei has a limited surrounding to exchange its energy leading to fast decay, whereas in a liquid environment, the immediate surrounding of the nuclei are not as restricted and the energy exchange is slower leading to a slower decay. The oilseeds' major components are oil, proteins, carbohydrates and moisture; all are sources of hydrogen in the seeds. In oilseeds, the oil is found in a liquid state (oil-bodies), the signal for the oil hydrogen decaying slower than the signal from the other hydrogen makes possible to measure it. The seed oil content is determined after the instrument has been calibrated using reference sets.

Pulse-NMR method's main advantage is the time gain compared to the extraction methods, the time of analysis is very short (a few minutes) versus a few days. Pulse-NMR instruments are easy to maintain, official methods using this technology have been published (AOCS Ak 3–94; ISO 5511:1992; ISO 10632:2000; ISO 10632:2000; AOCS Ak 4–95) making it easy to use this technology for commercial analyses. The analysis is usually conducted on whole seeds and requires minimum to no sample preparation. Pulse-NMR usually requires few samples (could be as low as five) for calibration as opposed to other spectrophotometric methods such as NIR which could require up to several thousands for calibration purposes.

As any secondary methods, to provide moisture and oil content for canola seeds, pulse-NMR instruments should be calibrated with the appropriate grain samples and the appropriate methods. Oil content can be measured by several methods, however, they are not identical and do not give equivalent results (Barthet et al., 2002; Barthet and Daun, 2004). For oil content, the method used to calibrate the instrument was what is considered by FOSFA as the reference method (FOSFA, 2005; AOCS Official Method Am-2–03). The appropriate sample set is a set of canola samples for which the oil content ranges from 39% to 50% (8.5% moisture basis) since the oil content of canola seed grown in Western Canada falls within that range. Ring tests performed for ISO 659:2009 and ISO 10565:1998 showed that repeatability and reproducibility were similar for the two methods. However, it has been suggested that repeatability and reproducibility were better with NMR than with solvent extraction. Pulse-NMR method required little sample preparation and was easy to perform whereas the triple extraction required a lot of dexterity from the operator, each step requiring meticulous sample transfer to ensure that no sample was lost. Erroneous oil content could be easily obtained if some sample was lost during transfer (lower oil content) or if some nonoil particle fell in the oil beaker (higher oil content).

The oilseed section uses a three-tiered system in order to ensure accurate results obtained with the pulse-NMR method. First, the checksamples are analysed with every analysis and the rapid method results are compared with the reference method results. Second, throughout the year, samples are randomly taken, analysed by both methods and the results compared. Finally, verification samples are made annually and analysed using both the methods. The results from the 2011 verification set comparison are shown in Table 7.1. The paired *t*-test statistical analysis showed that the results obtained by the two methods (extraction and pulse NMR) were not statistically different. When the results from the rapid method were graphed against the results of the reference method (Figure 7.1), a linear relationship was obtained with a slope and an intercept close to 1.00 ± 0.05 and 0.00, respectively. A slope of 1 indicates both methods are obtaining the same results and an intercept of zero means that there is no bias (consistent difference in results) between the two methods. Analytical results from the pulse NMR method are only deemed suitable and accurate if the regular check sample system (all three tiers) indicates equivalent performance.

TABLE 7.1
Canola Oil Content Analysis (%, at 8.5% Moisture), 2011 Verification Set (as of May 2011)

Method	ISO 659–2009/AOCS Am2–93 (2009) Extraction with Petroleum Ether	NMR Calibrated with Petroleum Ether Extraction
1	41.00	41.18
2	42.65	42.93
3	44.08	44.29
4	45.19	45.14
5	46.21	46.25
6	47.39	46.88
7	48.88	48.47
8	39.65	39.47
9	47.98	48.24
10	42.15	41.93
11	36.97	36.41
12	43.34	43.32
13	45.68	45.46
14	43.56	43.64
15	45.68	45.71
16	49.55	49.46
17	41.00	41.06
18	40.64	40.19
	Paired *t*-Test	
Mean	43.98	43.89
Sd	3.41	3.45
SEM	0.80	0.81
T	1.40	
Degree of Freedom	17	
P	0.1786	

Note: At the 0.05 level, the difference of the population mean is NOT statistically different.

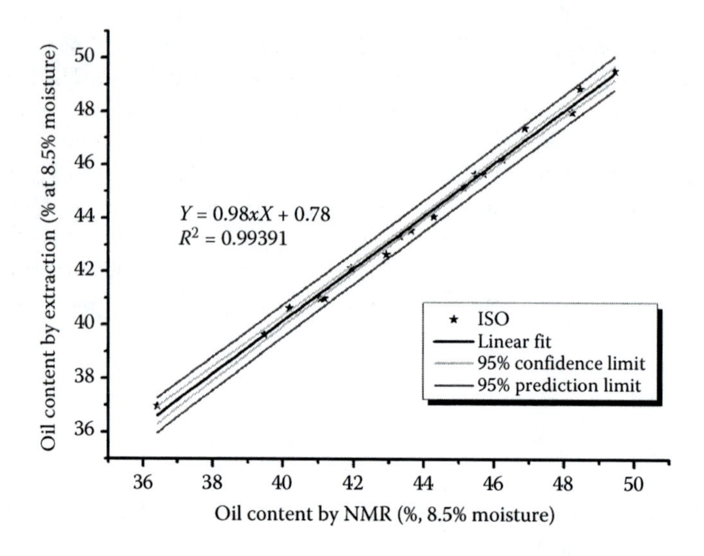

FIGURE 7.1 Oil content analysis (%, 8.5% m.b.), linear fit with confidence and prediction limits, canola oil content by ISO 659–2009 versus NMR (oil content, % at 8.5 m.b.).

7.3 NIR ANALYSIS

Near-infrared spectroscopy (NIRS) is also a rapid nondestructive technique, able to measure a large number of seed components in one rapid (about 2 min) analysis. It is a secondary technique. NIRS results are predicted as they are calculated from the calibration data sets. As for NMR or any secondary method, the chosen reference methods used to calibrate the instrument strongly affect the results obtained by the NIR method.

Some components are difficult, if not impossible, to measure because (a) the analytical errors on the reference methods are too high or because (b) their concentration in the samples is too low (Coates, 2002; Mentink et al., 2006).

For canola, oil, protein, glucosinolate and chlorophyll contents, as well as fatty acid composition, can be predicted by NIRS in less than a minute, a considerable gain of time considering the complexity and length of some of the analyses. Seeds can be analysed ground or whole, making this technique very versatile. Unfortunately, there are no official methods to analyse whole intact oilseeds by NIR and only one method is available for analysing the ground seeds (AOCS Am 1-92). The American Association of Cereal Chemists International (AACCI) has an official method, giving general information and guidelines for NIR users on how to develop a calibration model and test the performance of the calibration (AACC 39–00.01). However, it is difficult to actually develop a common official method for NIR, as an ISO standard, since there are numerous commercially available NIR instruments, each with different wavelength range and calculation model.

The infrared spectrum can be divided into three parts, wavelength ranges of 700–3000; 3000–10,000 and 50,000–1,000,000 nm for near-infrared, mid-infrared and far-infrared, respectively (ISO 20473:2007). Near-infrared (NIR) spectroscopy is based on the interactions of the NIR light with the molecules of a sample. The interactions of irradiated NIR light with the molecules produce absorption bands due to the vibration of the molecules. The wavelength at which this phenomenon happens is specific for a bond. Several guides are available detailing wavelengths and functional groups (Workman and Weyer, 2007). This spectrophotometric method is a secondary type of method, based on the use of calibration sets of samples with known composition, and the comparison of the spectra of the reference data with the spectra of the unknown sample. The calibration sets are assembled by collecting spectra from samples of known composition and constructing mathematical models to relate the NIR spectra to the concentration of the compounds of interest, using chemometric methods. Interferences (overlapped bands, baseline drifts, scattering and path-length variations) must be accommodated during the development of the mathematical models.

Several types of NIR instruments are commercially available. They could be very simple such as filter instruments with up to 20 filters of narrow wavelength ranges. These instruments can be used for oil content analysis (one 2310 nm filter) or chlorophyll analysis (two filters in the visible range 696 and 674 nm). Grating monochromators or diode array NIR spectrophotometers have large wavelength ranges, and more complicated chemometric analyses (principal component analysis and/or partial least squares regression) can be used for data processing. The interferometers, such as Fourier-Transform-NIR (FT-NIR) spectrophotometers, have also large wavelength ranges using both NIR or mid-infrared (MIR) wavelengths; the data processing uses Fourier-Transform (FT) treatment of the data. It is considered that for a filter instrument, calibration must be developed with a minimum of 15 samples per wavelength used in the model. The last two types of instruments can use several hundred if not thousands of samples in a calibration.

A typical spectra of intact canola seed samples are presented in Figure 7.2. The derivatives (Figure 7.2) are used to separate the overlapped peaks. The second derivative, in which case the absorption bands are the 'valleys', rather than peaks, showed a clearer image of the absorption bands. Depending on the instrument and the software complexity, scatter correction and the use of derivatives are usually used to develop the calibration equations. The chemometric data processing for the last two types of instruments is often carried out using partial least squares regression (PLS), a mathematical procedure which combines the spectral variance with the variance introduced by the reference data. Although fewer than 100 samples can be used to develop a PLS calibration model, PLS can handle up to 10,000 samples. Artificial neural network (ANN) calibrations are based on mathematical models inspired by the structure and function of the neurons. The ANN system usually requires more than 20,000 samples to develop a calibration model. It can produce very stable calibrations due to the large amount of variance provided by the database.

Once the calibration model has been developed, it needs to be validated. This requires another set of samples, different from the calibration sample set. Usually, it is considered that a ratio 20/80 is adequate. This means that for a certain overall population of samples 80% of these samples are used to develop the calibration model and 20% of the samples are used to validate the calibration model. After validation, it is important to keep a calibration updated by adding samples to the original

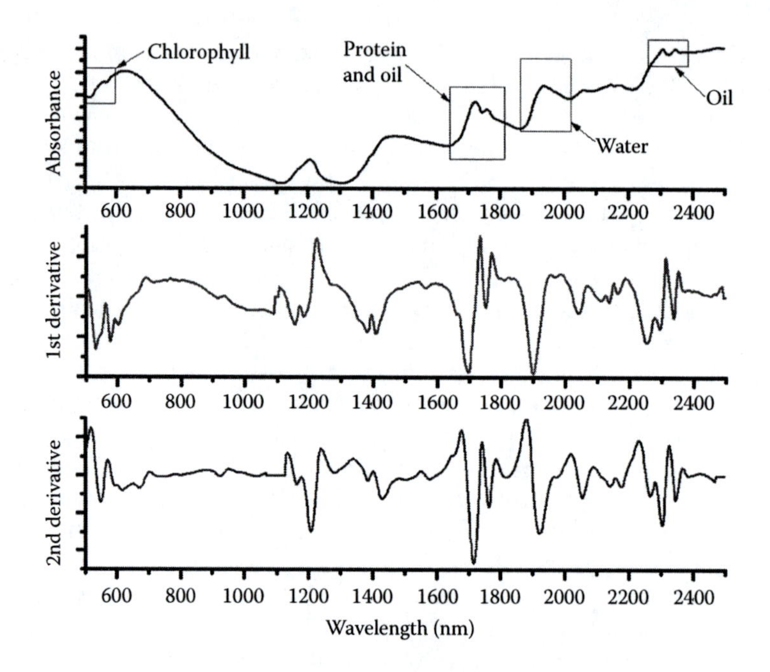

FIGURE 7.2 Spectra of intact canola seeds with the first and second derivatives. Spectra obtained by reflectance using a 6500 Foss spectrophotometer. The presented data averaged 50 scans from 450 to 2500 nm at a wavelength resolution of 2 nm. Note: There should be a big band at the 670 nm area, unless the canola was essentially chlorophyll free. The top spectrum shows a small band at about 580 nm.

calibration set. However these new samples need to add new variance, for example, from a new season, location, variety, or any other new source of variance.

Several parameters affect the NIR results, for example, are the seeds whole or ground? Grinding samples make a nonhomogenous sample more homogenous, which often improves the repeatability and reproducibility of the results. Particle size can affect NIR results, so the shape and distribution of the ground samples are important. This is particularly important for filter instruments; in monochromator and FT-NIR instruments, scatter corrections and derivatives can be used to correct for particle size differences.

Other parameters such as sample moisture, thickness, temperature, age and cleanness (free from foreign material) will affect the NIR results. It is important to note that since the NIRS analysis is using calibrations derived from a set of samples to predict chemical characteristics of another sample set, variance of both sample sets must be represented in both the sample sets.

The error of the reference method affects the error of the NIR result. The coefficient of variation (CV) of the reference method for constituents, such as oil or protein contents, should be between 1.0% and 2.0% to develop a good calibration model (Williams and Norris, 2001). Williams (Williams and Norris, 2001) described how two factors, the standard error of the predicted value or SEP and the RPD, can be used to assess NIR calibrations. The SEP is the standard deviation of the residuals of the predicted *y* values (NIR results) for each constituent, used only with the verification set. The RPD is the standard deviation of the reference values of the validation data set divided by the SEP obtained from the NIR and the reference data. He also presented RPD ranges (Table 7.2) as a guideline to how the NIR calibration will be used.

NIR technology is routinely used in our laboratory to analyse all types of grains. We use several types of NIR instruments with different wavelength ranges, different modes of operation (transmittance or reflectance), and various chemometric approaches (multiple linear regression or PLS). As with any analytical instrument, it is important to know the advantages and disadvantages of each instrument and their limitations. Our NIR 1 is a reflectance filter instrument equipped with three filters, 2310 nm for oil analysis and 674 and 696 nm for chlorophyll analysis (Tkachuk et al., 1988) using ground seeds. This is a very basic instrument that could be equipped with up to 10 filters; the mathematical prediction model is developed using multiple linear relationship between NIR response at the specific wavelength (filter) and the reference results. The NIR 2 is a transmittance spectrophotometer with a wavelength range of 570–1100 nm; the calibration models are developed using partial least squares with whole seeds. The NIR 3 is the most versatile of our NIR instruments; it is a reflectance spectrophotometer using whole seeds and with the largest wavelength range (400–2500 nm) when compared to NIR 1 and NIR 2. As with NMR, the calibrations of our instruments are tested regularly with various sample sets which have never been used to develop the calibration models. These samples are all analysed by the appropriate reference methods. After being run through the NIR instrument, the NIRS values are obtained using the appropriate calibration model data. These predicted values are then compared to the reference values. Tables 7.3 through 7.5 present a summary of various verification sets. The data were obtained with the

TABLE 7.2
Residual-Predicted Deviation Ranges Calculated from the Verification Set Results, Guide to Determine the Accuracy of the NIR Calibration

RPD Range		Comments
0–2.3	Very poor	Not recommended
2.4–3.0	Poor	Rough screening
3.1–4.9	Fair	Screening
5.0–6.4	Good	Quality control
6.5–8.0	Very good	Process control
>8.1	Excellent	Any application

Source: Adapted from Williams, P.C. 2001. *Near-Infrared Technology*, 2nd edition, American Association of Cereals Chemists. Inc., St Paul, Minnesota, USA. Chapter 8, pp. 145–169.

Note: RPD: residual-predicted deviation.

TABLE 7.3
Examples of Verification Results Obtained in Our Laboratory for the Analysis of Intact Canola Seeds by NIR 3. Verification Set, NIR-Predicted Values Obtained with NIR 3

Analysis	SEP	RPD	Linear Fit *R* Square	Linear Fit Equation	Comments
Oil content	0.50	6.68	0.9759	$1.02x - 1.14$	Process control
Protein content	0.32	8.59	0.9864	$1.00x + 0.05$	Any application

Note: SEP: standard error of the predicted value; RPD: Residual-predicted deviation.

TABLE 7.4
Examples of Verification Results Obtained in Our Laboratory for the Analysis Chlorophyll Content (mg/kg) in Canola Seed

	SEP	RPD	Linear Fit *R* Square	Linear Fit Equation	Comments
NIR 1, ground seed, filter instrument, calibration 1	6.44	2.95	0.88494	$1.41x - 14.36$	Rough screening
NIR 2, whole seed, transmission, 570–1100 nm	9.08	2.00	0.75068	$1.36x + 2.69$	Not recommended
NIR 1, ground seed, filter instrument, calibration 2	2.82	8.00	0.97796	$1.03x - 2.00$	Process control

Note: SEP: standard error of the predicted value; RPD: Residual-predicted deviation.

TABLE 7.5
Examples of Verification Results Obtained in Our Laboratory for the Analysis α-Linolenic Acid in Canola Seed (% of α-Linolenic Acid in the Oil), the Predicted Results Were Obtained with NIR 3

	N	SEP	RPD	Linear Fit *R* Square	Linear Fit Equation	Comments
Verification set all samples	2578	0.69	5.31	0.97241	$0.90x + 1.07$	Quality control
Verification set conventional canola only	2220	0.40	3.47	0.92865	$0.89x + 1.18$	Screening
Verification set low linolenic canola only	358	0.72	1.02	0.73033	$0.45x + 1.99$	Not recommended

Note: SEP: standard error of the predicted value; RPD: Residual-predicted deviation.

various instruments for different projects. The results suggested (Tables 7.3 through 7.5) that not all seed components can be predicted with the same accuracy with all the instruments. This depends partly on the instrument and its wavelength range, and on the calibration sets, the chemical structure of the analysed compound, and its concentration in the seed. Graphs obtained by plotting the reference value against the NIR value are presented in Figures 7.3 through 7.6.

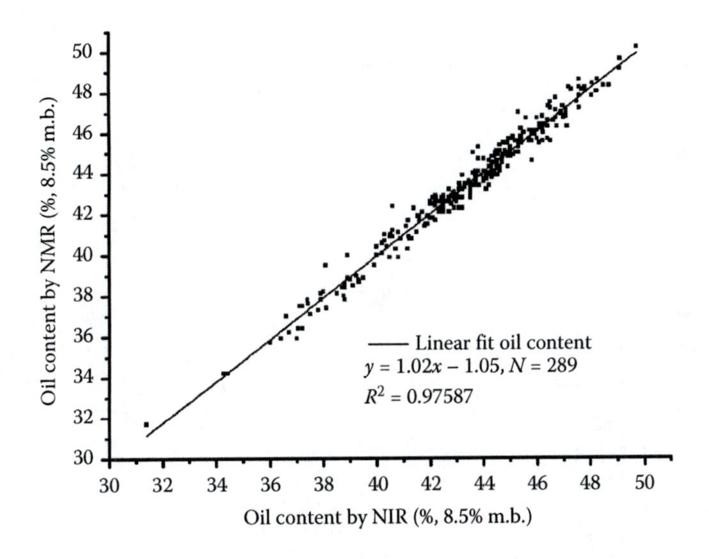

FIGURE 7.3 Oil content analysis (%, 8.5% m.b.), linear fit canola oil content by pulse-NMR (calibrated according to ISO 659–2009) versus NIR (oil content,% at 8.5 m.b.).

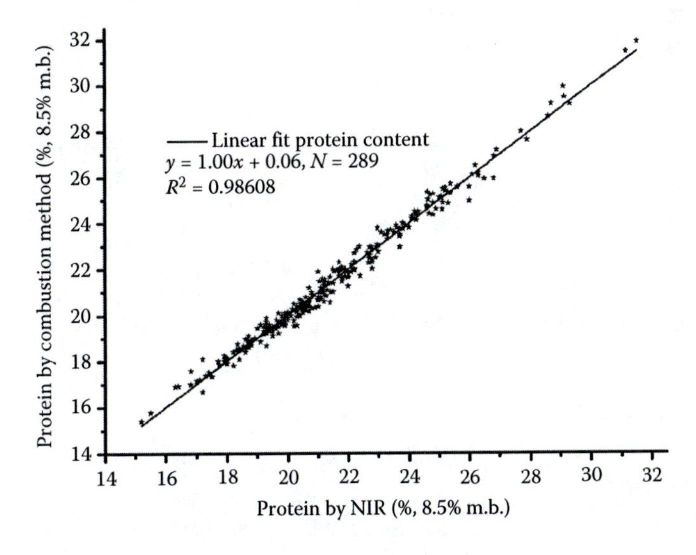

FIGURE 7.4 Protein content analysis (%, 8.5% m.b.), linear fit canola protein content by NIR versus combustion method AOCS Ba4e-93.

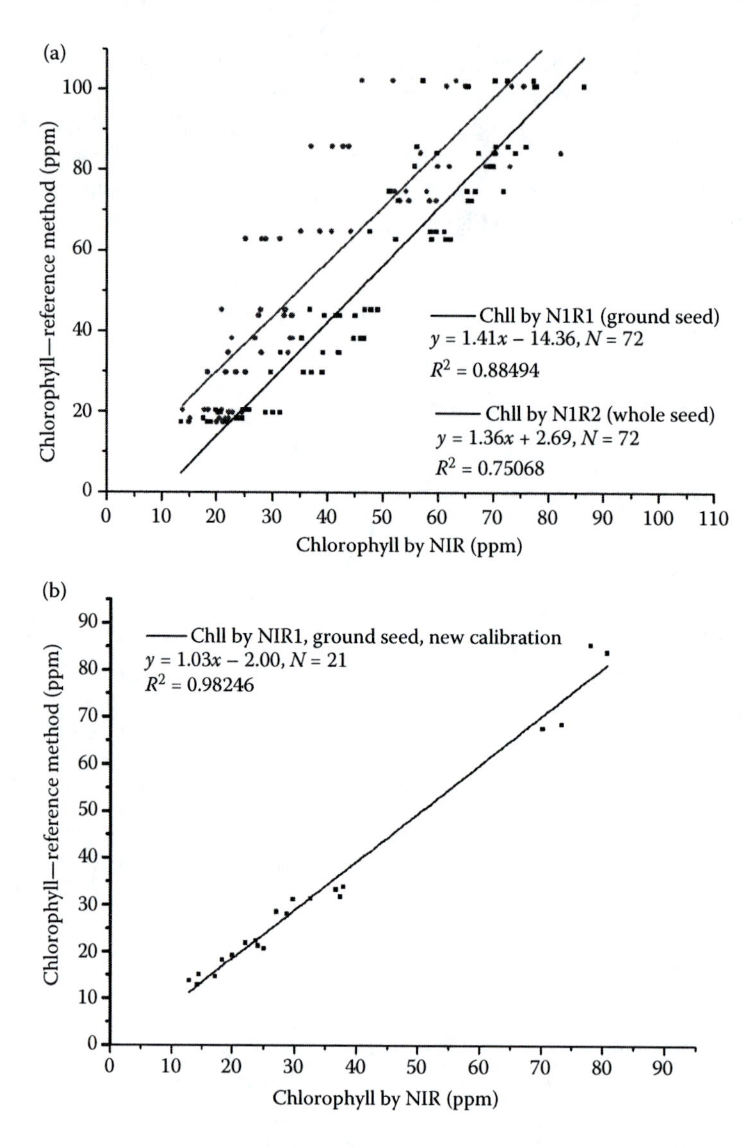

FIGURE 7.5 (a) Chlorophyll content (mg/kg), linear fit canola chlorophyll content by NIR versus ISO 10519:1997. NIR-1 and NIR-2 used ground and intact seeds, respectively. (b) Chlorophyll content (mg/kg), linear fit canola chlorophyll content by NIR-1 versus ISO 10519:1997. Results after expanding the calibration.

7.3.1 Oil and Protein Measurements

Oil content is assessed as crude oil by exhaustive extraction with petroleum ether (ISO 659:1998). In our laboratory, NMR data are used to control the NIR, since we can analyse over 50 samples in quadruplicate by NMR in the time we need to analyse six samples in duplicate by the exhaustive extraction method. We use the extraction method to control the NMR and re-analyse any sample for which the NIR

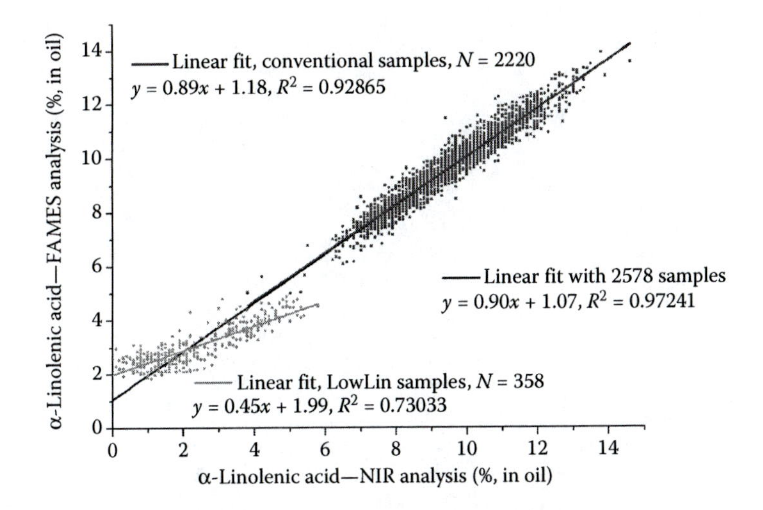

FIGURE 7.6 α-Linolenic acid content analysis (% in the oil), linear fits canola α-linolenic acid content by NIR-3 versus ISO 5508–1990. Linear fit with conventional and LowLin canola samples (*N* = 2578), linear fit with conventional canola samples only (*N* = 2220) and linear fit with LowLin canola samples only (*N* = 358).

and the NMR do not match, since the wet-chemistry method is the reference method considered to be giving the only true results. The verification set for 2010–2011 (Table 7.3, Figure 7.3) showed a very good relationship between the NIR-predicted values and the reference data. Oil had several typical absorption bands in both the low (758, 816, 928 and 1042 nm) and the high (1162, 1208, 1724, 1764, 2308 and 2346 nm) wavelength ranges making this seed component easy to analyse. However, when developing a calibration, the software selects the wavelength areas where the spectral data are most highly correlated with the reference data, and many of these 'classical' wavelengths may not be used (Hruschka, 2001). Some instruments may not use the lower wavelengths whereas others, such as transmittance instruments, will not use the higher wavelengths.

The reference method used in our laboratory to measure protein content is the combustion or Dumas method (AOAC 992–23 or ISO 16634–1:2008). It has been shown to be safer and more reproducible than the Kjeldahl method (Williams et al., 1998). The 2010–2011 verification set to control the prediction model for protein analysis by NIR (Table 7.3, Figure 7.4) showed also a very good relationship between NIR-predicted values and reference data. The linear fit is almost perfect (perfect linear equation $y = 1x$), the R-square showed that over 99% of the results were accurately predicted using the developed calibration model. The SEP (0.32) and the RPD (8.59) obtained with this protein verification set (Table 7.3) suggested that the protein model was better and more accurate than the oil NIR prediction model (SEP = 0.50, RPD = 6.8). Crude oil in canola is mainly triacylglycerides; these glycerol esters are constituted mostly of CH bonds which are present in large quantities in all biological molecules, even proteins. Proteins, on the other hand, are constituted of molecules called amino acids, bonded together by a specific bond—the peptide bond (an amide

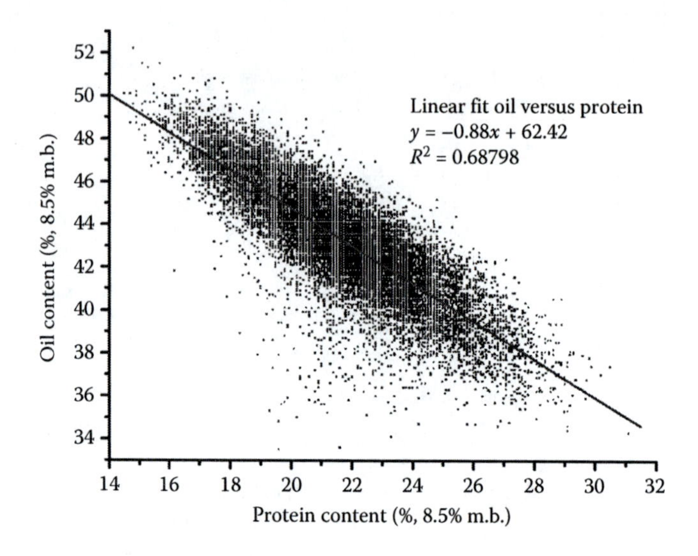

FIGURE 7.7 Relationship between oil and protein content in canola samples harvested in Western Canada from 2000 to 2010.

bond). The mathematical model developed for the NIR 3, the software used all wavelengths for which a strong relation with the compound of interest was shown. In the equation, it was observed that the wavelengths related to protein content were used in the equation model for oil content with negative multipliers. It is known that in canola seed, there is a negative relationship between oil and protein contents; the higher the oil, the lower is the protein content of the seed (Figure 7.7). In the mathematical model to predict oil content, the inverse relationship of protein content–oil content was used—wavelengths corresponding to protein (such as amide bond) were shown with a negative correlation coefficient. This could explain why the protein prediction model showed a slightly better RPD than the oil prediction model; there were about 17% of the samples that did not fit the linear relation high oil–low protein (Figure 7.7) in this particular example.

7.3.2 Chlorophyll Measurement

Chlorophyll is essential for photosynthesis in all plants. Several chlorophyll derivatives can be found, but in canola seed, the chlorophyll derivatives are chlorophyll *a* and *b*. In Canada, because of the short growing season (May to September–October), canola seed can contain high levels of chlorophyll. Seed immaturity, mainly due chlorophyll content, is a degrading factor for canola seed in Canada (http://grainscanada.gc.ca/oggg-gocg/10/oggg-gocg-10-eng.htm). Numbering distinctly green seed content gives an approximation of the level of seed immaturity in the sample. It could also provide an estimate of the chlorophyll content range; however, it does not give the true chlorophyll content (Daun, 1982, 2000, 2003). It is important to have a rapid assessment of the chlorophyll content upon delivery at processing plants, primary or terminal elevators.

The reference method for chlorophyll determination is ISO 10519:1997; chlorophyll is measured spectrophotometrically after extraction, results being expressed as mg/kg (or ppm). NIRS is a rapid method that could be used to measure the chlorophyll content. Chlorophyll content is not truly measured in the NIR range. The best wavelengths used to measure chlorophyll are in the 650–700 nm area.

Table 7.3 and Figure 7.5a and 7.5b showed the results of experiments in which two types of NIR instruments were assessed to measure chlorophyll content in canola seed in a nonlaboratory setting. The objective of these experiments was to select the type of instrument to use. The two instruments—NIR 1 and NIR 2—were calibrated with the same set of samples, ground seeds were used with NIR 1 and whole seeds were used with NIR 2. Figure 7.5a and Table 7.4 showed that NIR 1 was able to predict the chlorophyll content of the samples with a slightly better accuracy than NIR 2. Chlorophyll is not present homogenously in a canola sample (Daun, 2000, 2003). Most of the seeds in the sample could have a low chlorophyll content (below 10 ppm) with 1–2% of the seeds with a chlorophyll content as high as 400 ppm, the resulting average sample chlorophyll content could vary from 25 to 30 ppm (or higher). By using ground seeds for the analysis (with NIR 1), the nonhomogenous sample becomes homogenous, leading to a more reproducible and accurate analysis when compared to whole seed analysis. A second set of experiments, using only NIR 1, was done after upgrading the calibration (Figure 7.5b, Table 7.4) by scanning samples with higher and lower chlorophyll contents (larger range of chlorophyll contents). The sample grinding was optimized and standardized to minimize particle size and sample texture effects on the measurement. The results (Figure 7.5b, Table 7.4) showed a mathematical model when compared to the first one (Figure 7.5a). The RPD showed (Table 7.3) that the NIR 2 instrument could predict the chlorophyll content in canola samples. The results were not statistically different from those obtained by the reference method ($F = 1.078$, $p = 0.4344$). This system was used in a nonlaboratory environment (primary and terminal elevators). The results of this experiment indicated that chlorophyll could be measured accurately and easily at grain elevators using this robust type of NIR instrument.

7.3.3 α-Linolenic Acid Measurement

In canola, the most important fatty acids are oleic acid (C18:1), α-linolenic acid (ALA, C18:3), erucic acid and the sum of the total saturated fatty acids. Canola is often referred as a double low rapeseed, low in total glucosinolate—<30 μmol/g oil-free solid dry basis, and low erucic acid—<2% (http://canolacouncil.org/canola_the_official_definition.aspx). To ensure that the seeds conform to the definition of canola, it is important to analyse the erucic acid content. Nowadays monthly monitoring of Canadian canola exports showed that erucic acid content is well below the 2% mark, in fact, the erucic acid content average was below 0.15%. Canola oil has been modified in response to industry demand for an oil that allows deep-frying. It was necessary to develop an oil more stable to oxidation, to allow the high deep-frying temperatures. Low α-linolenic acid canola (LowLin) was developed. The new varieties could be grouped into low α-linolenic acid (below 5%) with an oleic acid content of around 65%, or into very low α-linolenic acid (below 3%) with a content of oleic acid higher than 70%. As a result, in canola, α-linolenic acid could range from 2% to 13% whereas oleic acid content could range from 55% to 75%. In our section, the chosen reference method to analyse the fatty acid composition of canola was the ISO 5508:1990 method.

Figure 7.6 and Table 7.5 present the comparative results between the NIR data and the results obtained from the FAMEs analysis for α-linolenic acid (ALA). The sample set contained 2220 samples of conventional canola (ALA ranging from 5% to 13%) and 358 samples of LowLin canola (ALA < 5.0% by FAMES analysis). The first statistical analysis with all the samples ($N = 2578$) showed a good RPD (5.31) and a good R-square (0.97241). This seemed to suggest that the mathematical model for ALA was a good prediction model. However, Figure 7.6 showed that the correlation plot corresponding to the conventional canola fitted this linear relationship better than the LowLin canola. When each canola population was treated as a separate verification set, the statistical analyses suggested that the model for LowLin canola was not a good prediction model. Conventional canola showed an RPD of 3.47 with an R-square 0.929 whereas LowLin canola had an RPD of 1.02 with an R-square 0.730. These results suggested that this prediction model could still be used to predict the ALA content of conventional canola whereas the actual model cannot be used to analyse ALA accurately in LowLin canola. In this particular example, the NIR prediction model can be used to analyse conventional canola and will only be useful to screen/differentiate/segregate LowLin canola samples from conventional canola samples with no or little accuracy on the ALA content of the LowLin samples. The linear fit equations using 2220 (conventional only) and 2578 samples (conventional + LowLin) suggested that the model was biased with conventional canola samples, with more influence on the equation/prediction than LowLin samples, since the lack of LowLin samples had almost no influence in the linear equation of the $N = 2220$ linear fit. This particular verification set was also biased due to the large number of conventional samples ($N = 2220$), compared to the number of LowLin samples ($N = 358$). The former will affect the linear relation more than the latter, due only to their large sample size (over six times more conventional than LowLin samples).

This example showed that the ALA composition cannot really be accurately predicted in LowLin canola by NIR. However, the NIR technique is still useful for such analyses, since it can segregate the canola seeds into high, medium and low, based on their ALA content. This is very useful at the grain elevator level where bin storage has to be decided in minutes upon delivery. It is also a very useful tool for breeders who need to analyse thousands of samples every year in their programme. However, the technique is of limited use to determine the ALA content of a sample when a precise and accurate result is needed, such as a nutrition study for example.

ACKNOWLEDGEMENTS

Thanks to Mr B. Misener for providing the fatty acid analysis, Mrs M. MacLean for providing the oil data, the Analytical Section of the Grain Research Laboratory for providing the protein data, Mr B. Siemens for providing all the NIR and the chlorophyll data and reviewing the chapter and Mr P.C. Williams for his comments. The Canada Grain Commission reference number of this book chapter is #1052.

REFERENCES

American Association Cereal Chemists International: Approved method 39–00.01: Near-Infrared Methods—Guidelines for Model Development and Maintenance. First Approval November 3, 1999, 1–5.

American Oil Chemists' Society: Official method Am 2-93. Determination of Oil Content in Oilseeds. Re-approved in 2009.

American Oil Chemists' Society: Official method Ba 4d-90. Nitrogen-ammonia-protein Modified Kjeldahl Method using Titanium dioxide + Copper sulfate Catalyst. Re-approved in 2009.

American Oil Chemists' Society: Official methods Ba 4e-93: Generic Combustion Method for Determination of Crude Protein. AOCS. Re-approved 2009.

American Oil Chemists' Society: Recommended Practice Ak 3–94. Oil Content of Oilseeds by Nuclear Magnetic Resonance. Re-approved in 2009.

American Oil Chemists' Society: Standard Procedure Ak 4–95. Simultaneous determination of oil and moisture contents of oilseeds using pulsed nuclear magnetic resonance spectroscopy. Re-approved in 2009:

American Oil Chemists' Society: Standard Procedure Am 1–92. Determination of Oil, Moisture and Volatile Matter, and Protein by Near-Infrared Reflectance. Re-approved in 2009.

Barthet, V.J. and Daun, J.K. 2004. Oil content analysis: Myths and reality. In: *Oil Extraction and Analysis—Critical Issues and Comparative Studies*, edited by Luthria, D.L. AOCS Press, Champaign, Illinois (USA), Chapter 6, pp. 100–117.

Barthet, V.J., Chornick, T.L. and Daun, J.K. 2002. Comparison of several methods to measure the oil content in soft oilseeds. *J. Oleo Sci.,* 51(9), 589–597.

Batten, G.D. 1998. Plant analysis using near infrared reflectance spectroscopy: The potential and the limitation. *Aust J Exp Agr.*, 38, 697–706.

Coates, D.B. 2002. Is near infrared spectroscopy only as good as the laboratory reference values? An empirical approach. *Spectroscopy Europe*, 14(4), 24–26.

Daun, J.K. 1999. The effect of glucosinolates on the nitrogen to protein ratio for rapeseed and canola. *GCIRC Bulletin*, 16, 58–63.

Daun, J.K. and DeClercq, D.R. 1994. Comparison of combustion and Kjeldahl methods for determination of nitrogen in oilseeds. *JAOCS*, 71(10), 1069–1072.

Daun, J.K. 2000. How green is green? Sampling and perception in assessing green seeds and chlorophyll in canola. *JAOCS*, 77(11), 1209–1213.

Daun, J.K. 2003. How green is green? Long-term relationship between green seeds and chlorophyll in canola grading. *JAOCS*, 80(2), 119–122.

Daun, J.K. 1982. The relationship between rapeseed chlorophyll, rapeseed oil chlorophyll and percentage green seeds. *JAOCS*, 59(1), 15–18.

Daun, J.K. and Thorsteinson, C.T. 1989. Determination of chlorophyll pigments in crude and degummed canola oils by HPLC and spectrophotometry. *JAOCS*, 66(8), 1124–1128.

Daun, J.K., Clear, K.M. and Williams, P. 1994. Comparison of three whole seed near-infrared analyzers for measuring quality components of canola seed. *JAOCS*, 71(10), 1063–1068.

Endo, Y., Thorsteinson, C.T. and Daun, J.K. 1992. Characterization of chlorophyll pigments present in canola seeds, meal and oil. *JAOCS*, 69(6), 564–568.

Federation of Oils, Seeds and Fats Association: International Official Method Oilseeds—Determination of Oil Content-Solvent Extraction (Reference Method) as described in F.O.S.F.A. International, Technical Manual, Part Two, Standard Contractual Methods, pp. 64–71, Federation of Oils, Seeds and Fats Association Limited, London, 2005.

Gunstone, F.D. and Herslöl, B.G. 2000. *Lipid Glossary 2, Volume 12*, The Oily Press Lipid Library, Bridgewater.

Hruschka, W.R. 2001. Data Analysis: Wavelength selection methods. In: *Near-Infrared Technology in the Agriculture and the Food Industries*, 2nd edition, edited by Williams, P. and Norris, K., American Association of Cereals Chemists. Inc., St Paul, Minnesota, USA, Chapter 3, pp. 39–58.

International Organization for Standardization: ISO 10519:1997 (E): Rapeseed: Determination of chlorophyll content–Spectrometric method.

International Organization for Standardization: ISO 5508:1990 (E): Animal and vegetable fats and oils–Analysis by gas chromatography of methyl esters of fatty acids.

International Standard Organization: ISO 10565:1998L: Oil and moisture in seeds by low field NMR spectroscopy.

International Standard Organization: ISO 10632:2000: Oilseed residues—Simultaneous determination of oil and water contents—Method using pulsed nuclear magnetic resonance spectroscopy.

International Standard Organization: ISO 16634–1:2008. Food Products—Determination of the Total Nitrogen Content by Combustion according to the Dumas Principle and Calculation of the Crude Protein Content—Part 1: Oilseeds and Animal Feeding Stuffs. Approved in 2008.

International Standard Organization: ISO 20473:2007: Optics and photonics—Spectral bands.

International Standard Organization: ISO 5511–1992. Oilseeds—Determination of Oil Content—Method using Continuous-Wave Low-Resolution Nuclear Magnetic Resonance Spectrometry (Rapid method). Re-approved in 1997.

International Standard Organization: ISO 659:1998. Oilseeds—Determination of Oil Content (Reference method). Re-approved in 2009.

Jones, D.B. 1941. Factors for converting percentages of nitrogen in foods and feeds into percentages of proteins. Circular No 183, issued August 1931, revised February 1941, United States Department of Agriculture, Washington, DC, 1–21.

Jung, S., Rickert, D.A., Deak, N.A., Aldin, E.D., Recknor, J., Johnson, L.A. and Murphy, P.A. 2003. Comparison of Kjeldahl and Dumas methods for determining protein contents of soyabean products. *JAOCS*, 80(12), 1169–1173.

Mag, T. 1990. Further processing of canola and rapeseed oils. In: *Canola and Rapeseed—Production, Chemistry, Nutrition and Processing Technology*, edited by Shahidi F., Avi Book, Van Nsotrand Reinhold, New-York, Chapter 15, pp. 251–276.

Mariotti, F., Tome, D. and Patureau Mirand, P. 2008. Converting nitrogen into protein—beyond 6.25 and Jones factors. *Crit. Rev. Food Sci. Nutr.*, 48, 177–184.

Mentink, R.L., Hoffman, P.C. and Bauman, L.M. 2006. Utility of near-infrared reflectance spectroscopy to predict nutrient composition and in vitro digestibility of total mixed rations. *J. Dairy Sci.*, 89, 2320–2326.

Mossé, J. 1990. Nitrogen to protein conversion factor for ten cereals and six legumes or oilseeds. A reappraisal of its definition and determination: variation according to species and to seed protein content. *J. Agric. Food Chem.*, 38, 18–24.

Rubel, R. 1994. Simultaneous determination of oil and water contents in different oilseeds by pulsed nuclear magnetic resonance. *JAOCS*, 71(10), 1057–1062.

Srinivasan, V.T. 1979. A comparison of different pulse sequences in the nondestructive estimation of seed oil by pulsed NMR technique. *JAOCS*, 56(12), 1000–1003.

Tkachuk, R. 1969. Nitrogen-to-protein conversion factors for cereals and oilseeds meals. *Cereal Chem.*, 46, 419–423.

Tkachuk, R., Mellish, V.J., Daun, J.K. and Macri, L.J. 1988. Determination of chlorophyll in ground rapeseed using a modified near infrared reflectance spectrophotometer. *JAOCS*, 65(3), 381–385.

Unger, E.H. 2011. Processing. In: *Canola—Chemistry, Production, Processing and Utilization*, edited by Daun, J.K., Eskin, N.A.M. and Hickling, D. AOCS Press, Urbana, Chapter 6, pp. 163–188.

Williams P.C. 2001. Implementation of near-infrared technology. In: *Near-Infrared Technology*, 2nd edition, edited by P.C. Williams and K. Norris, American Association of Cereals Chemists. Inc., St Paul, Minnesota, USA. Chapter 8, pp. 145–169.

Williams, P.C., Sobering D. and Antoniszyn, J. 1998. Protein Testing Methods at the Canadian Grain Commission. Proceedings of the Wheat Protein Symposium, Saskatoon, SK, March 9 and 10.

Workman, J. Jr. and Weyer, L. 2007. In: *Practical Guide to Interpretive Near-Infrared Spectroscopy*, edited by Workman, J. Jr. and Weyer, L., CRC Press, Taylor & Francis Group, Boca Raton, FL.

8 The Potential for Ultrasound and Supercritical Fluid Extraction for Value-Added Processing of Canola

Curtis B. Rempel and M.G. Scanlon

CONTENTS

8.1 Introduction 145
8.2 Extraction of Oils and Bioactive Components from Canola or Oilseed Rape 147
8.3 Extraction of Essential Oils 155
8.4 Extraction of Oilseed Bioactives 158
8.5 Extraction of Other Bioactives 160
8.6 Ultrasonic and SC-CO_2 Applications in Oilseed Processing 160
References 163

8.1 INTRODUCTION

The application of ultrasound energy or sonication for process enhancement of bioactive molecules or compounds from plant material is widely published (Saliová et al., 1997; Vinatoru et al., 1997; Vinatoru, 2001; Bruni et al., 2002; Melecchi et al., 2002; Albu et al., 2004; Schinor et al., 2004; Wang and Weller, 2006). A fairly recent review has summarized the scope of ultrasonic-assisted extractions (Vilkhu et al., 2008). Part of the attraction of ultrasound for extraction processes is that it is a relatively simple and inexpensive method which can be conducted at ambient temperatures using any particular solvent (Ashokkumar et al., 2008).

Ultrasound is typically classified into two categories: low-intensity ultrasound, frequently in the MHz range that is used in materials sciences and medical imaging applications, and lower frequency high-intensity ultrasound in the kHz range that is often referred to as sonication. Ultrasound for extraction of plant material typically utilizes sound waves with frequencies not much >20 kHz, which is the upper limit of human hearing. Sonication results in mechanical vibrations or pressure waves which in turn results in cavitation or the formation and collapse of microscopic bubbles that release tremendous energy as pressure, heat and mechanical shear (Chemat et al., 2004). This has the effect of mechanical disruption of cell wall material and concomitant release of plant cell contents accentuated by local heating of the contents which enhances the diffusion of the extract. Together, this results in improved mass transfer (Keil, 2007).

Ultimately, ultrasound extraction should provide greater economic return over solvent extraction alone as it can decrease extraction times, reduce solvent volumes, and it results in higher yield of bioactive compounds due in part to a unique means of disruption of plant matrices. Additional benefits can also be realized when utilizing ultrasound for the extraction of thermolabile bioactive compounds. While local heat is generated, which results in improved mass transfer, the overall operating temperature and temperature duration is relatively low when compared to other extraction methods and this can result in improved bioactivity of some compounds (Vilkhu et al., 2008).

In the late 1960s, Kurt Zosel at the Max Planck Institute for Coal Research in Mülheim recognized the potential of non-toxic and environmentally benign CO_2, used in a 'supercritical' state, for natural product extraction (McHugh and Krukonis, 1986). The principle is straightforward—beyond a specific critical temperature and pressure a gas such as CO_2 becomes a 'supercritical' fluid, a state that is neither gas nor liquid, but has properties of both. An advantage to using CO_2 as a solvent is that the critical state is reached relatively readily—at a temperature of only 31°C and a pressure of 73.8 bar (Wang and Weller, 2006). No distinct gas or liquid phase can exist above the critical point, and the supercritical phase has a unique combination of properties from both states. In a supercritical state, CO_2 exhibits low viscosity and high diffusion rates, just like a gas, and has liquid-like densities (Eckert et al., 1996; Eckert and Chandler, 1998) that provide good salvation power to the fluid.

Because supercritical fluids such as carbon dioxide have the characteristics of both liquids and gases, they have several major advantages over liquid solvents. First, supercritical fluids have a more favourable mass transfer due to their higher diffusion coefficient and lower viscosity. Second, the solvent power and selectivity of supercritical CO_2 (SC-CO_2) can be further controlled by fluid density, which can be manipulated by temperature and pressure (Leitner, 2000; DeSimone, 2002). Even small changes in temperature or pressure result in dramatic changes in the density, viscosity and dielectric properties of SC-CO_2 (Licence et al., 2003; Reverchon and De Marco, 2006; Khosravi-Darani, 2010). In addition to selective fractionation, other advantages of using SC-CO_2 for extraction include: (1) no disposal of undesirable solvents from processing or solvent residues remaining in the extracted material, potentially allowing for a 'green' label; (2) exclusion of oxygen mitigates oxidative degradation of bioactive compounds; (3) the low operating temperatures minimize thermal degradation of sensitive materials and (4) the extracts are sterile as microorganisms and their spores are not soluble in SC-CO_2 (Dillow et al., 1999; Rozzi and Singh, 2002; Spilimbergo et al., 2002; List et al., 2003; Beckman, 2004; Munshi and

Bhaduri, 2009; Arai et al., 2009). Extraction with SC-CO_2 can be employed for a variety of applications and some of these will be explored later.

8.2 EXTRACTION OF OILS AND BIOACTIVE COMPONENTS FROM CANOLA OR OILSEED RAPE

Vegetable oils, such as canola or oilseed rape, consist primarily of triglycerides, triacylglycerols of fatty acids. These as well as cholesterol, waxes and free fatty acids are quite soluble in SC-CO_2. The oil content of canola or oilseed rape ranges from 40 to 55 wt% and the composition is 97–99 wt% triglycerides with very low levels of saturated fatty acids (~6%, high levels of oleic acid (~60%)), intermediate levels of linoleic and linolenic acids (~20% and 10%, respectively) and 0.5–1 wt% minor lipids. Canola differs from oilseed rape in that they contain <2% erucic acid in their oil and <30 μg glucosinolates/g of dry meal. Solubility of triacylglycerols in supercritical CO_2 may be fairly similar, and small variations in fatty acid composition will likely not have significant impact on extraction efficiency. However, solubility in supercritical CO_2 may be sensitive to free fatty acids, mono- and diglycerides, which are present in oils, and differences may result in significant changes in oil extraction efficiency.

In 1996, a method using SFE for extraction of oil from seeds was approved by the AOCS Method Am 3-96 (1997) and this method was adopted by AOAC (Method 999.02). This method is based upon gravimetric analysis from soy, canola, sunflower and safflower. The method allows for choice of CO_2 alone or CO_2 with 15% ethanol as a modifying cosolvent. The operating parameters are standardized to 100°C, 7500 psi, with or without 15% ethanol at 2 mL/min with a total extraction time of 30 min (CO_2 alone) or 45 min (CO_2 + 15% ethanol).

Several studies have focused on the suitability of SFE using CO_2 heat and with ethanol as an analytical tool to determine fat in canola/oilseed rape and other oilseeds (Barthet and Daun, 2002; Taylor et al., 1997). Barthet and Daun (2002) compared oil extraction from canola using AOCS Method Am 3-96, with and without ethanol as a cosolvent, with exhaustive extraction using petroleum ether (FOSFA AOCS Am 2-93). Without the ethanol cosolvent, oil recoveries using SC-CO_2 were 10–15% lower than that determined using the FOSFA method. When ethanol was used as a cosolvent, the oil recoveries from canola were about 3% lower than values determined by FOSFA. Barthet and Daun (2002) concluded that temperature was a greater factor in oil extraction than pressure, as oil recovery increased with increasing temperature while pressure had no significant affect on oil yield. Two 30 min extractions resulted in significantly higher ($p = 0.009$) oil extraction yields than a single 60 min extraction. Oil recovery increased with the amount of ethanol added as a cosolvent. However, increasing ethanol concentration increased the green colouration of the canola oil, indicating greater extraction of polar compounds as ethanol concentration increased. Highest extraction yields using SC-CO_2 were obtained when a triple extraction was conducted—two 30 min extractions with CO_2 alone followed by a 60 min extraction with 15% ethanol. The FOSFA oil extraction yields were always greater than SC-CO_2, even with double extraction and addition of ethanol. The acyl lipid content in the SC-CO_2 extracted canola oil was close to 100%

when no ethanol was included. When ethanol was added as a cosolvent the acyl lipid content of the extracted oil declined by 10–15%.

Additional studies have been conducted on the extraction of triglycerides and free fatty acids using SC-CO_2 alone. Typically, an increase in pressure increases oil extraction yield and operating pressure has the greatest impact on oil yield. This is confounded by temperature. An increase in extraction temperature increases the oil extraction yield at high pressure. With lower pressure, an increase in extraction temperature lowers the oil extraction yield (Dunford and Temelli, 1997; Fattori et al., 1988). Table 8.1 summarizes selected SC-CO_2 operating parameters for extraction/fractionation of oil and components from canola and oilseed rape.

Bulley et al. (1984) observed that the oil solubility of crushed canola seeds extracted with SC-CO_2 at 35 MPa and 40°C during the initial linear was 7.2 mg oil/g CO_2 during the initial linear phase and 8.7 mg of oil/g CO_2 at a CO_2 flow rate of 0.64 g/min during the later stages of extraction. At 30 MPa and 40°C, the concentration of oil dropped to 5.4 mg oil/g CO_2 at a flow rate of 0.45 g/min and the concentration remained relatively constant during the 5 h extraction time (Bulley et al., 1984).

TABLE 8.1
Selected Supercritical CO_2 Operating Parameters for Extraction and Fractionation of Canola/Oilseed Rape

Author	Seed Moisture (%)	Temperature (°C)	Pressure (MPa)	Duration (h)	CO_2 Flow Rate
Stahl et al. (1980)	—	50	30	—	—
Bulley et al. (1984)	—	40	30, 35	5	0.45, 0.64 and 1.84 g/min
Fattori et al. (1987)	—	55	36	—	0.7 g/min
Fattori et al. (1988)		25, 40, 55, 70	10, 20, 30, 38	Up to 5	0.7 g/min
Taylor et al. (1993)	—	80	68	0.45–2	5 L/min
Temelli (1992)	—	40, 55, 70	34.5, 48, 65	5	650 mL/min and 5.8 L/min
Dunford and Temelli (1996)	—	35, 55, 75	21.4, 41.4, 62.4	1, 3, 5	2.5 g/min
Dunford and Temelli (1997)	12.7–42.5	35, 55, 75	20.7, 41.4, 62.0	3	—
Przybylski et al. (1998)	—	40	41.4	8	10 L/min
Barthet and Daun (2002)	—	80, 100, 110	51.7, 62	0.5–1	2 mL/min
Vuorela et al. (2004)	—	50	46	—	0.4 mL/min
Jenab et al. (2006)	—	40	34		1.6 L/min
Sun et al. (2008)	—	51, 56, 70	30, 40	6	1 L/min
Boutin and Badens (2009)	—	35, 55, 75	15, 30, 45	0.33, 1.1, 2	8, 13.5, 19 kg/h

One of the first papers comparing SC-CO_2 extraction as an alternative to petroleum-based solvent extraction of canola found that the highest observable oil solubility was 11 mg/g CO_2 at 36 MPa pressure and 55°C. Flow rate of CO_2 was fixed at 0.7 g/min for all of the pressure/temperature parameters investigated (Fattori et al., 1988). In a previous study by the same authors (Fattori et al., 1987), the extracted canola oil using SC-CO_2 and hexane was compared for differences in fatty acid composition. Extraction conditions of 36 MPa, 55°C and 0.7 g/min CO_2 were used. The SC-CO_2 extracted oil was found to have higher concentrations of C22 and C24 fatty acids than the hexane extracted oil. The authors also found no significant levels of phosphorus in the canola oil when extracted using SC-CO_2 alone, which differed from the hexane extracted oil and the authors suggested that since a degumming step used in hexane extract oil to remove phosphorus can be omitted when using SC-CO_2, this may provide a processing advantage. These extraction results corroborated those obtained by Stahl et al. (1980), who conducted a study to determine whether oil extraction yields with SC-CO_2 were comparable to hexane extraction. SC-CO_2 extraction at 300 bar, 50°C resulted in 39% rapeseed oil yield while hexane resulted in a 40% oil extraction yield (w/w).

A study modelling the influence of different parameters of SC-CO_2 on the oil extraction yield utilized three different operating pressures, three temperatures, three extraction times and three CO_2 flow rates (see Table 8.1) (Boutin and Badens, 2009). The highest oil recovery yield was 90% (wt%) using the lowest pressure (45 MPa), highest temperature (75°C), longest (120 min) extraction time and highest CO_2 flow rate (19 kg/h). The quantity of oil recovered ranged from 0.2 to 14.4 g oil per kg of CO_2 used. Extraction pressure, extraction time and CO_2 flow rate were highly significant. Four interactions were also significant—pressure × temperature, pressure × extraction time, pressure × CO_2 flow rate and extraction time × CO_2 flow rate. Similar to studies described so far, operating pressure has the greatest influence on oil extraction yield.

Interactions between SC-CO_2 operating pressure and temperature on oil extraction efficiency of oilseed rape have been further modelled (Boutin et al., 2011). Increasing the extraction pressure from 30 to 34 MPa increased the oil extraction efficiency, especially at 20 min extraction time. Increasing the temperature from 50°C to 70°C decreased the extraction efficiency due in part to a decrease in CO_2 density. The authors concluded that small variations in temperature and pressure could lead to significant differences in extracted oil yield especially during the initial phase of the extraction.

Increasing the CO_2 rate decreased the extraction time. The effect of temperature, pressure and CO_2 flow rate were more pronounced during the first half of the extraction and differences in oil yield were similar after 4 h of extraction time regardless of the operating parameters. The authors postulated that the increase in CO_2 flow rate resulted in increased internal mass transfer rate with concomitant increase in extraction efficiency. The model identified a clear trade-off between CO_2 flow rate and extraction duration. Higher CO_2 flow rates increase oil extraction but the efficiency diminishes over time while the cost of the extraction increases due to time and CO_2 costs. High CO_2 flow rates with short duration appear to be the most efficient.

Moisture content of seed affects oil solubility and mass transfer kinetics as high moisture content acts as a barrier to the diffusion of CO_2 into the sample matrix and oil out of the sample matrix. Conventional hexane extraction of canola utilizes preheating and cooking of flaked canola to inactivate enzymes, remove moisture and further rupture cell structure to enhance extraction efficiency. Dunford and Temelli (1997) examined impact of seed moisture and pre-heat/cooking treatment as well as SC-CO_2 extraction parameters on canola oil yield and composition. Canola seeds were flaked, pre-heated to 40°C in <5 min and then cooked at 90°C for 15 min. Moisture content of the feed material was adjusted to 12.7–42.5% (w/w moisture- and oil-free basis). Amount of moisture lost from the samples during SC-CO_2 extraction increased significantly with temperature and moisture content of feed material and decreased with pressure. Heat pre-treatment, pressure, temperature, moisture content of feed material and pressure × temperature interaction effects on final moisture content of residual material were significant ($p < 0.05$). Consistency and cloudiness of extracted oil was correlated with moisture loss from feed material. Extracted oil yield was typically higher with increasing feed material moisture content, and further increased with increasing temperature and pressure. The exception was 20.7 MPa where oil yield decreased with increasing temperature. Moisture contents of 37.8% and 42.5% in feed material did not impact oil yield or composition significantly. Moisture content and pre-heating/cooking had less impact than during SC-CO_2 extraction parameters on oil yield and composition. Free fatty acid content (FFA) increased with decreasing pressure due to a decrease in triglyceride solubility. Oleic and linolenic acids had the highest concentrations in the FFA fractions of the oil extracts.

In a more recent study, samples of crushed and cooked canola seeds were extracted with SC-CO_2 and a commercial organic solvent (AW406 with *n*-hexane content ~30%, total hexane content ~70%) (Jenab et al., 2006). In this study, the oil solubility was 7.1 mg oil/g CO_2 (during SC-CO_2 parameters of 34 MPa, 40°C and CO_2 flow rate of 1.6 L/min). These results are in agreement with Bulley et al. (1984) but are lower than that reported by Fattori et al. (1988).

Under these extraction conditions, the extracted oil yield using SC-CO_2 was 20% (wt/wt dry based) while the Soxhlet extraction using AW406 organic solvent was 36%. Fatty acid composition of the oils extracted by SC-CO_2 and solvent also varied. The linoleic acid concentration was higher in the oil extracted with SC-CO_2 while the erucic acid and behenic acid levels were lower when compared to solvent extraction. Mass transfer rates of fatty acids in SC-CO_2 are controlled by their chain length and saturation level of chemical bonds (Jenab et al., 2006; Reverchon and Marrone, 2001). In the early phase of the extraction, the triacylglycerols high in polyunsaturated fatty acids are extracted at higher rates than those containing long-chain fatty acids such as behenic acid (Fattori et al., 1987; Jenab et al., 2006). Both high- and low-molecular weight triacylglycerols are equally soluble in hexane and consequently no selective extractions can be performed when using organic solvents for oil extraction (Fattori et al., 1987; Jenab et al., 2006).

The concentration of chlorophyll in the SC-CO_2 extracted oil was significantly lower than the solvent extracted oil. This is due, in part, to the lower solubility and/or mass transfer rate of polar compounds in SC-CO_2. However, these polar compounds can be extracted at higher CO_2 volumes when other oil components have already been extracted (Przybylski et al., 1998). No significant differences were observed between amounts of unsaponifiable material in SC-CO_2 and solvent extracted oils. These results are different than those obtained by Przybylski et al. (1998).

Some of the minor lipids, such as phospholipids, are insoluble in pure SC-CO_2. Addition of a cosolvent during SC-CO_2 has been shown to increase phospholipid recovery (Temelli, 1992). This was the first report on the recovery of phospholipids from canola oil using SC-CO_2 extraction. Triglycerides and phospholipids were extracted with SC-CO_2 in two subsequent steps, using canola flakes and press cake as starting material with 0%, 5%, 10% and 15% ethanol, respectively. Several SC-CO_2 operating parameters were evaluated. Maximum yield of lipids was achieved with operating parameters of 70°C, 62 MPa and 5% ethanol. Oil yields were greater when flakes were used as starting feed material rather than press cake. This was due, in part, to packing of the crumbled press cake relative to the flakes, which tended to be more uniform in size. Solubility isotherms for lipid extracts containing phospholipids indicated an increase in solubility as pressure increased at constant temperatures. There was a crossover of the iostherms at 27.6 MPa and this is consistent with other reports (Fattori et al., 1988; Dunford and Temelli, 1997).

Oleic, linoleic and linolenic acids were the major fatty acids in the extracted canola oil. There was a decrease in relative concentrations of oleic (C18:1 ω-9) and linolenic acid when ethanol was added as a cosolvent while oleic (C18:1 ω-7) and linolenic acid concentrations increased significantly ($p < 0.01$). Use of ethanol resulted in extraction of C16:1 which is not present when SC-CO_2 is used alone. Longer chain fatty acids (C20:0, C22:0 and C22:1) were not present in the SC-CO_2 extracts when canola flakes were used as the starting feed material. However, these longer chain fatty acids were present in the extracted oil when ethanol was included as a cosolvent and press cake was the feed material. The extraction of phospholipids using ethanol as a cosolvent, without need for degumming, provides opportunity for the cosmetics and food industry that has yet to be fully exploited.

The composition of canola press cake or meal is also extremely important as it is an excellent source of protein and other compounds for animal feed. Typically, the meal requires toasting at temperatures up to 130°C to remove residual solvent that is used to extract oil in commercial processing. The toasting process denatures proteins present in the meal, which may lower the functionality of the meal. Canola meals extracted with SC-CO_2, with and without ethanol as cosolvent, have been compared to those extracted with hexane (Sun et al., 2008). The SC-CO_2 extracted meal had significantly higher ($p < 0.05$) levels of phosphorus/phospholipids than the hexane extracted meal. As predicted, use of ethanol as a cosolvent extracted more phospholipid than SC-CO_2 alone. The highest protein meal (42%) was the SC-CO_2 + ethanol extraction. The nitrogen solubility index is an important indicator of protein denaturation. The nitrogen solubility index of the SC-CO_2 (33%) and SC-CO_2 + ethanol (31%) extracted canola meals were significantly lower than that of the hexane extracted meal (41%). The SC-CO_2 extracted meal had lower glucosinolate content than hexane extracted meal. The phenolic acid contents of hexane and SC-CO_2 were similar but higher than meals extracted with SC-CO_2 + ethanol. The authors concluded that canola meals extracted with SC-CO_2 and SC-CO_2 + ethanol were similar to hexane extracted meals in both chemical composition and functionality (Sun et al., 2008).

In addition to high-quality protein, canola/rapeseed meal also contains minerals, vitamins including tocopherols and phenolic compounds including phenolic acids, flavones and flavonols (vinylsyringol, sinapin, etc.) (Vuorela et al., 2004). These researchers conducted a study to determine the effectiveness of different methods for the isolation of food-grade rapeseed phenolics. The isolation methods included aqueous ethanol, hot water, enzyme-assisted (ferulic acid esterase) and SC-CO_2. No sinapin and very low levels of synapic acid phenolics were isolated from rapeseed meal using SC-CO_2. While yields of phenolic compounds were low using SC-CO_2, the extracted phenolics significantly inhibited the oxidation of low-density lipoprotein (LDL) particles. SC-CO_2 was the only method that isolated vinylsyringol from rapeseed meal.

Li et al. (2010) investigated the effects of SC-CO_2 operating parameters on extraction yield of oil and recovery of phenolic compounds from canola meal when compared to traditional solvent extraction. These investigators found that when canola meal samples were extracted using SC-CO_2, they obtained a comparable oil level to that obtained when extracting with *n*-hexane. The study also showed that the lowest residual oil levels remaining in the canola meal were achieved with SC-CO_2 operating parameters that are attainable in most SC-CO_2 extraction systems. However, yield of phenolic compounds such as sinapine and sinapic acid were significantly lower with SC-CO_2 extraction than yields obtained from *n*-hexane extraction. Using a cosolvent such as ethanol influences the retention of phenolic compounds and optimization of operating parameters for the ethanol cosolvent requires further investigation.

One of the first studies examining the oxidative stability of canola oil extracted with SC-CO_2 was conducted by Przybylski et al. (1998). Flaked canola seeds were extracted with SC-CO_2 at 40°C and 41.4 MPa and the oil collected as fractions dependent upon the volume of CO_2 used. Fraction I used 400 L of CO_2, fraction II was the oil collected from 400 to 1600 L, fraction III was the oil collected from 1600 to 2800 L, and fraction IV was the oil collected from 2800 to 4800 L CO_2. Collected fractions comprised 20%, 58%, 15% and 7% of the total oil extracted from flaked seeds.

Triglycerides with unsaturated fatty acids were extracted more efficiently at the beginning of the extraction. The first fraction contained the highest levels of polyunsaturated fatty acids (PUFA). The composition of saturated and monounsaturated increased when the volume of CO_2 used for the extraction increased and thus were found in higher concentrations in fractions 3 and 4. As the volume of CO_2 increased, the amount of linolenic acid in the fractions decreased from 11.4% to 9.3%. Free fatty acid content declined from 2.0% to 0.7% from fraction I to fraction IV.

The amount of phospholipids increased from 0.35 mg/kg in fraction I to 9.95 mg/kg in fraction IV. Tocopherols were present in equal amounts in all fractions. The oil extracted in fraction IV contained higher amounts of phospholipids and unsaponifiable material and exhibited better oxidative stability as measured by peroxide value (AOCS Method Cd8-53). The lowered oxidative stability of fraction I is a result of higher PUFA content, increased level of FFA and absence of phospholipids. In fraction IV, the tocopherol and phospholipid contents were the highest, the levels of PUFA and FFA were the lowest.

Beta-sitosterol brassicasterol and campesterol were found to be the major sterol compounds in the oil fractions. Beta-sitosterol represented 60% of the total sterol content of the flaked seeds. The total amounts of sterols extracted increased by 51% in fraction IV compared to fraction I. The brassicasterol was present in highest amounts in fraction II. The levels of pigments extracted from the seeds increased when the volume of CO_2 used was increased, that is, with increasing extraction duration.

Glucosinolates are another group of bioactive compounds found in canola/oilseed rape. They are not toxic until hydrolysed and then are associated with goitrogenicity and antinutritional effects in animals which consume the meal as feed. In humans, the glucosinolates may have a positive health benefit due to anticarcinogenic activity. As mentioned earlier, in order to be classified as canola, the dry meal must contain <30 μg glucosinolates/g.

Crushing canola disrupts cell membranes and brings the glucosinolates in close proximity with myrosinase enzyme, and some hydrolysis occurs until the enzyme is inactivated by heat during commercial oil extraction operations. The effect of SC-CO_2 extraction conditions (temperature, pressure, extraction time and moisture content) on the myrosinase activity and glucosinolate hydrolysis in flaked and whole canola seeds was studied (Dunford and Temelli, 1996).

In a preliminary study, when canola flakes (7.7% moisture) were exposed to SC-CO_2 at 21.4–62.1 MPa and 35–75°C for 3 h, 85–100% of the original myrosinase activity was retained (Dunford, 1995). The effect of temperature and pressure were not significant and the residual enzyme activity following SC-CO_2 extraction was similar to the feed material.

In the subsequent study, the experiments were conducted on canola flakes containing 19% moisture, which is typical of canola seed moisture content at harvest (Dunford and Temelli, 1996). At SC-CO_2 operating temperature of 35°C, 85% of the original enzyme activity was retained. At 19% moisture and 75°C, there was a significant ($p < 0.05$) drop in enzyme at all pressures studied. At 62.1 MPa and 75°C, only 10% of the original enzyme activity remained in the canola flakes.

Significant glucosinolate degradation was observed after 5 h of extraction of low moisture (8.5% w/w) whole canola seed. In canola flakes, glucosinolate degradation was minimal at all moisture levels tested. When canola flakes were extracted at low moisture levels, myrosinase enzyme is not affected but glucosinolate degradation was minimal during the 3 h of extraction under the range of SC-CO_2 operating parameters studied. Therefore, myrosinase inactivation prior to SC-CO_2 extraction may not be necessary.

The deodorizer distillate fraction, which is a by-product of conventional vegetable oil refining, is a rich mixture of aldehydes, ketones, free fatty acids, sterols, tocopherols and other components which can be utilized for value-added products in the food, feed and nutraceutical/natural health product sectors. Semi-continuous column fractionation of canola oil deodorizer distillate using SC-CO_2 was conducted to determine feasibility of recovering components such as sterols and tocopherols (Güçlü-Üstündağ and Temelli, 2007). The effect of operating parameters including pressure (20, 25 MPa) using a temperature gradient (70–100°C), temperature (70, 100°C) and a linear temperature gradient (70–100°C at 25 MPa) was evaluated for extraction yield and separation efficiency. Total extract yield increased significantly ($p < 0.05$) with pressure. At 25 MPa, the highest yield was obtained at the lowest temperature evaluated (70°C). The use of a thermal gradient (70–100°C) in the fractionation column decreased the content of volatile compounds, free fatty acids and tocopherols while increasing the sterol content significantly ($p < 0.05$). The tocopherol content followed the order 100°C > 70–100°C > 70°C. For sterol, the order was reversed after 1.5 h.

The concentration of sterols, di- and triglycerides in the extract fractions was lower than the respective feed concentrations under all of the investigated operating parameters; the distribution of other components was affected by fractionation time, temperature and pressure. The volatiles were enriched up to a factor of 6.3, but the decrease in volatile concentration with time resulted in concentrations lower than the feed values in the latter fractions. The free fatty acids were enriched in the latter fractions relative to their concentration in the feed. Semi-continuous processing of the deodorizer distillate at 25 MPa and 70–100°C yielded a residue containing 40% sterols and this study highlights the value of using the canola deodorizer distillate as a source for the extraction of phytosterols.

Prior to extraction, canola/oilseed rape, like all oilseeds, are subject to mechanical treatment. This may be steam pressing or cold pressing, cooking, or flaking. These processes collapse the cell structure in order to increase the quantity of oil extracted. A novel approach to mimic mechanical pre-treatment has been investigated (Dong and Walker, 2008). This approach utilized rapid CO_2 depressurization or explosion to break the seed cells. This controlled explosion process was characterized based on total release time, rate of depressurization and effect of phase change on the rate of depressurization. The experiments were conducted on canola flakes and the explosions were carried out using five different temperatures (25°C, 35°C, 45°C, 55°C, 65°C) at a constant pressure of 10.3 MPa. Explosions were also conducted at four different pressures (3.4, 6.9, 10.3, 20.7 MPa) at a constant temperature of 35°C. The exploded canola flakes were then subject to SC-CO_2 extraction (34.5 MPa, 50°C, 700 mL/min CO_2 flow rate, 7 h). For the unexploded (control) canola flake, the constant extraction rate period occurred during the first 3 h until ~43% of the available oil was extracted. Following this, the extraction rate decreased at a constant rate and after 7 h, nearly 63% of the oil was extracted. The extraction curve was similar to that obtained by Pzrybylski et al. (1998) and Jenab et al. (2006). However, oil extraction rates were lower than those reported by other researchers. For the exploded canola, the extraction curve was lower than that of unexploded canola flake for the first 3 h phase and then higher during the later 4 h extraction. Oil extraction yields were improved for any explosion parameter tested when compared to the unexploded flake. Explosion at 35°C and 20.7 MPa resulted in the highest oil yield. Fatty acid composition of the oil was not affected by the different explosion conditions.

Oilseed extraction without the use of petroleum-based solvents, reduced water usage and reduced energy requirements are becoming increasingly important for environmental sustainability and SC-CO_2 as an extraction system may provide the industry with an opportunity to move to a more sustainable platform. Isolation of minor lipid components from complex lipid mixtures is receiving increased attention due to their biological activity and health benefits and SC-CO_2 has considerable potential for this purpose. The solubility of minor lipid components in SC-CO_2 and the solubility behaviour of lipids, cosolvents and SC-CO_2 have been reviewed

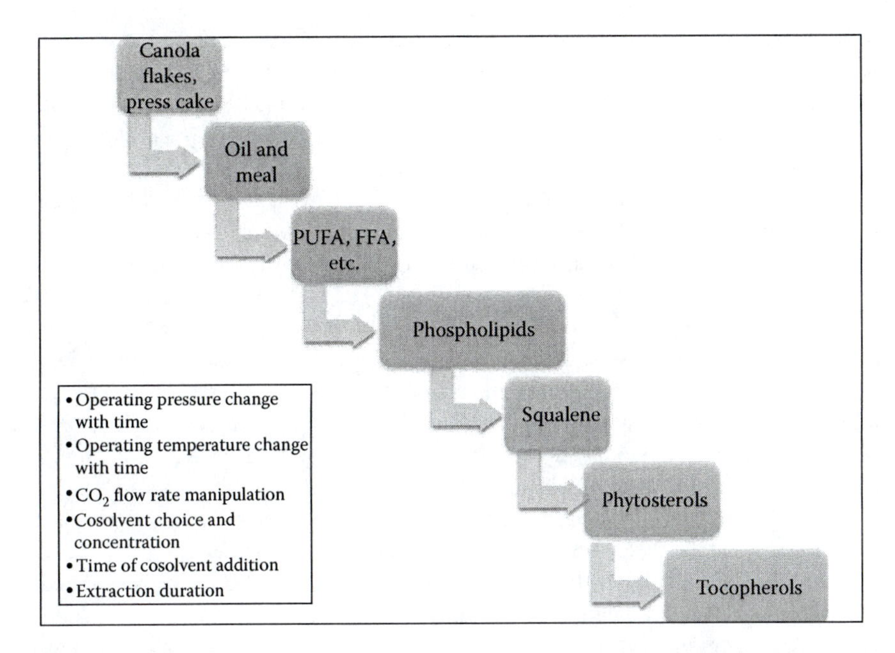

FIGURE 8.1 Theoretical manipulation of supercritical CO_2 operating parameters (pressure, temperature, CO_2 flow rate, cosolvent choice, cosolvent flow rate, extraction duration) for the extraction/fractionation of canola oil and components. *The diagram shows a step-wise extraction sequence for illustrative purpose only. The sequence of extraction need not follow this order exactly.*

and differences in the solubility behaviour of components and the effect of operating conditions on solubility can be effectively exploited for the fractionation of these complex multicomponent mixtures to isolate bioactive minor lipid components (Güçlü-Üstündağ and Temelli, 2004, 2005).

A theoretical extraction of oil and components from canola and oilseed rape, press cake/meal and/or deodizer distillate is illustrated in Figure 8.1. Manipulation of SC-CO_2 operating parameters, including cosolvent choice and concentration, results in sequential or differential fractionation of these components and relative yields as described earlier and explored in the following sections using other plants as starting material for reference.

8.3 EXTRACTION OF ESSENTIAL OILS

Ultrasound has been shown to be effective in extracting essential oils and lipids from oilseeds (Luque-García and Luque de Castro, 2004; Li et al., 2004; Zhang et al., 2008). For example, in the extraction of oil from two varieties of soyabeans using hexane, isopropanol or hexane–isopropanol mixture (Li et al., 2004), the solvents were added to ground soyabeans and the mixtures were ultrasonicated at 20 kHz for periods between 0 and 3 h at varying ultrasonic intensity levels. The mixed solvent was superior with respect to oil yield increase, resulting in a 9% increase in oil yield when compared to hexane or isopropanol, but the extraction capability of the mixed solvent was further enhanced by the application of ultrasound. The absolute oil yield was 32% after 30 min extraction and increased to 62% when used in combination with ultrasound. This oil yield was substantially higher than the yield obtained by extraction with the hexane–isopropanol solvent alone for 3 h.

Ultrasonication also dramatically decreased lipid extraction time throughput of flax (Metherel et al., 2009). In this study, ground flaxseed was extracted with a variety of organic solvents, alone or as a mixture, assisted with sonication at 20 kHz. Power was automatically varied to maintain constant amplitudes of 20%, 60% and 100% of 240 μm for sonication exposures for 5, 10, or 20 min. Results were compared to a standard 24 h, Folch-based, 2:1 chloroform:methanol extraction. Generally, longer time exposures and higher sonication amplitudes resulted in increased lipid recoveries. However, ultrasound-assisted extraction in 3:2 hexane:isopropanol for 10 min resulted in similar lipid yields as the 24 h standard method. More importantly, yields of some of the valuable fatty acids, such as 18:3 n-3, were increased with ultrasound assistance, with no loss in quality due to oxidation. The authors concluded that the ultrasound-assisted extraction of lipids with hexane:isopropanol at greatly reduced time exposure could contribute significantly to high-throughput analytical processing of samples for fatty acid determination.

Chickpea contains oil that is comprised of polyunsaturated fatty acids ranging from 6.5% to 9.0%. The effects of ultrasonic power, extraction temperature, time, extractant flow rate and solvent type on extraction efficiency and oil quality were investigated (Lou et al., 2010). Figure 8.2 shows that ultrasound-assisted extraction

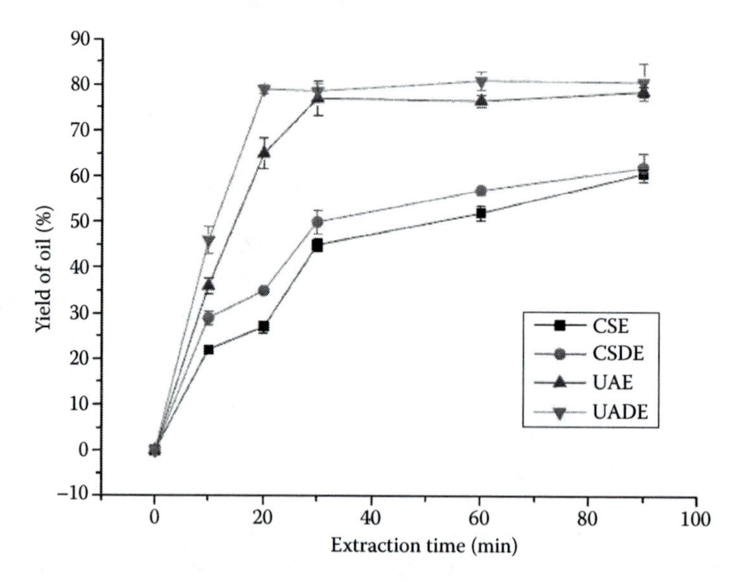

FIGURE 8.2 Effect of ultrasonication at 230 W in a dynamic system on the extraction of oil using hexane–isopropanol mixture with a solvent to solid ratio of 8.5 (mL/g). CSE, conventional solvent extraction; CSDE, conventional solvent dynamic extraction; UAE, ultrasound-assisted extraction; UADE, ultrasound-assisted dynamic extraction. (Adapted from Lou, Z. et al. 2010. *J. Food Eng.* **98**: 13–18, Figure 3.)

significantly reduced the extraction time and improved the extraction yield of oil from chickpea. The authors stated that the 'ultrasound-assisted extraction technique allowed target components to dissolve in the solvent at a higher speed thereby boosting yield (in) a shorter time'. Furthermore, the fatty acid composition of oil extracted with ultrasound-assistance was not significantly different from oil extracted by the conventional solvent method. This indicates that the nutritional profiles of the chickpea oil are not changed when ultrasound is used to enhance extraction. Utilization of ultrasound allows for reduced extraction time and higher yield without any loss of oil composition.

Ultrasound has also been used to enhance extraction of oil from oilseed rape (Wei et al., 2008). As with other studies, extraction efficiency was significantly affected by extraction time and extraction power, and then the liquid:solid ratio. A liquid:solid ratio of 1:4 (L:g), an ultrasound-assisted extraction time of 60 min, and power of 500 W were found to be optimal for extracting up to 20 mg of ground oilseed rape, when compared to a standard Soxhlet extraction method.

It should be noted that all of these studies have focused on enhancing the throughput of analytical labs or plant breeding programmes targeting oil yield and quality improvement. No study has focused specifically on using ultrasound-assisted extraction in a commercial oilseed pressing facility, although the principles of these studies are important in this context. It should also be noted that these studies involve grinding samples in contrast to expeller or cold pressing, and a time advantage may be achieved if grinding is commercially feasible when used in tandem with ultrasound.

Significant research has been conducted on extraction and fractionation of essential oils from plant and animal matrices using SC-CO_2. In the past decade, research has been published on the application of SC-CO_2 on oils from vegetables (carrot, tomato), fruit/berry (apricot, cherry, grape, sea buckthorn, citrus zest), nut (hazelnut, walnut, almond, peanut, pecan), cereal (wheat germ, oat, rice bran), pseudocereal (amaranth), specialty oilseed (borage, chia) and ethnobotanical plants (cloudberry, evening primrose, gardenia, chamomile, sage, veronica), as well as dairy fat/whey (Kakuda and Kassama, 2006; Reverchon and De Marco, 2007). These studies are applicable to the extraction of oils and phytochemicals from canola/oilseed rape and several are reviewed in greater detail here.

The extraction of borage seed oil using SC-CO_2 has been investigated (Lu et al., 2007). The effects of extraction pressure (200–300 bar), temperature (10–55°C), CO_2 solvent flow rate (7.5–12 kg/h) and bed length (0.25–0.50 m) were examined. The effects of CO_2 flow rate and bed length on extraction were smaller than those of pressure and temperature. Following extraction of 70% of the oil (approximately 0.20 kg of oil/kg of seed), the extraction rate was reduced progressively until maximum extraction of 0.31 kg of oil/kg of seed was reached. The total amount of oil recovered was identical to Soxhlet extraction using hexane. The authors further determined that SC-CO_2 extraction could be described in three distinct stages. An initial stage occurs while the accessible oil is being extracted throughout the length of the bed. When the accessible oil near the bed entrance is exhausted, the intermediate stage begins. During this time, an interface of easily accessible oil develops along the entire length with simultaneous extraction of oil from inner particles. The final stage is the one in which only less accessible oil in the flaked seed particles is extracted.

This study was conducted using pilot scale equipment with the purpose of optimizing processes for scale-up.

SC-CO_2 was employed to extract oil rich in polyunsaturated fatty acid from chia (*Salvia hispanica* L.) (Ixtaina et al., 2010). Researchers studied the impact of temperature, pressure and extraction time on oil extraction, yield, and oil composition. The highest oil yield was 93% after 300 min extraction at 450 bar. Fatty acid composition was found to vary with SC-CO_2 operating conditions. The major fatty acids included palmitic (6.8–14%), stearic (2.5–13%), oleic (3.9–11.1%), linoleic (19.6–35%) and linolenic (44.4–63.4%). There was a significant effect of extraction time on the percentage of linoleic and linolenic acids and the omega-3/omega-6 ratio. As extraction time increased the levels of linoleic acid increased. The oil obtained by SC-CO_2 with optimal operating conditions allowed a yield similar to conventional solvent extraction with *n*-hexane. As well, the acid composition with iodine and saponification values were similar to those of chia oil obtained via *n*-hexane extraction. However, the acidity and peroxide indices of the oil obtained by SC-CO_2 extractions were lower than those of oil extracted with *n*-hexane. The lower amount of free fatty acids and lower peroxide value are indicative of higher quality oil utilizing SC-CO_2.

Recently, SC-CO_2 has been utilized for the extraction of gardenia (*Gardenia jasminoides*) fruit (He et al., 2010). Gardenia has been utilized for centuries in Chinese herbal medicine and the extracts are used for their anti-inflammatory and cholagogue properties (Wang et al., 2004). The major constituents of gardenia fruits are irridoid glycosides. In this study, the total oil yield, yields of particular fatty acids such as stearic, linoleic, linolenic and eicosenoic acids as well as tocopherols were all on par with *n*-hexane extraction.

8.4 EXTRACTION OF OILSEED BIOACTIVES

Ultrasound has also been used to extract phenol-containing fractions from small samples of plant material. Using high-power ultrasound at a frequency of 30 kHz, Kadkhodaee and Hemmati-Kakhki (2007) extracted the three major constituents of saffron (picicrocine, safranal and crocin) from the flowers of *Crocus sativa* L. at 20°C. Compared to the water extraction procedure proposed by ISO, the ultrasonic method was far more efficient in extracting the active components from saffron in a much shorter time period. The extraction yield was found to increase over time as well as with the amplitude used in sonication. Sonication at short intervals proved to be far more effective than continuous sonication indicating this method is a potent alternative to water extraction. Wang et al. (2008) showed that ultrasonification was not only as effective as Soxhlet extraction for the extraction of phenolic compounds from wheat bran but also was much quicker. Using response surface methodology (RSM) optimum extraction was achieved using 64% ethanol, a temperature of 60°C and an extraction time of 25 min yielding gallic acid in milligram quantities.

Vitamin E has been shown to be an important factor in the prevention of chronic diseases including cardiovascular disease and certain cancers. Extraction and quantification of vitamin E in plant and animal tissues can be problematic. There is a need to disrupt the tissue matrix to release the vitamin E constituents. Traditionally, solvent extraction followed by saponification is utilized to extract vitamin E compounds from food and feed samples (Bramley et al., 2000). However, this methodology has limitations including incomplete recovery of tocopherols as well as excessive degradation of tocopherols. Hence a more efficient extraction process is required. Extraction yields and quantification of tocopherols from chicken liver and plasma samples were evaluated for four extraction techniques: solvent, ultrasound-assisted solvent, saponification and solvent, or saponification and ultrasound-assisted solvent (Xu, 2008). The measured value of α-tocopherol in the liver sample using ultrasound-assisted solvent extraction was 1.5–2.5 times greater than that obtained by solvent or saponification plus solvent methods. Furthermore, the reproducibility of the ultrasound-assisted solvent method was greater than any of the saponification methods. Xu (2008) concluded that compared with traditional methods, the ultrasound-assisted solvent methods could effectively and efficiently extract tocopherols from complex tissue such as livers without any chemical degradation of target material.

Supercritical CO_2 has been used to extract oil and tocopherols from wheat germ in several research studies (Ge et al., 2002; Panfili et al., 2003; Eisenmenger et al., 2006; Shao et al., 2008; Piras et al., 2009; Gelmez et al., 2009). These have focused on the effects of extraction parameters (i.e., temperature, pressure, CO_2 flow rate, cosolvent flow rate, extraction time) on oil and tocopherol yield and sterol and phospholipid content of the extracted oil. A recent study optimized the SC-CO_2 extraction for antioxidant concentration and antioxidant activity of the SC-CO_2 extracts rather than simply the oil yield (Gelmez et al., 2009). The effects of pressure (148–602 bar), temperature (40–60°C) and extraction time were modelled. The optimum extraction conditions were 336 bar, 58°C and 10 min, resulting in 5.3% tocopherol yield, 6 mg gallic acid equivalent (GAE) phenolics/g extract, 6.7 mg tocopherol/g extract and 57.3 mg scavenged DPPH/g extract. The tocopherol yield under these conditions corresponded to almost complete recovery.

Several studies have demonstrated the suitability of SC-CO_2 for the enrichment of rice bran oil with oryzols, tocols and phytosterols (Dunford et al., 2003; Perretti et al., 2003). Rice bran oil is extremely rich in bioactive phytochemicals such as γ-oryzanol (10,000–20,000 ppm), phytosterols (15,000–20,000 ppm) and tocopherol/tocotrienols (tocols) (1500–2000 ppm) with proven health benefits (Kaimal, 1999). γ-Oryzanols are unique to rice bran oil and are potent hypocholesteremic agents (Ramsay et al., 1991). The tocotrienols that comprise 70% of the tocols in rice bran oil have been shown to be powerful antioxidants with antithrombotic properties as well (Yoshino et al., 1989). The conventional method of chemical refining destroys the entire oryzanol complement and substantial amounts of tocols in addition to heavy neutral oil loss. Therefore, chemical refining is not suitable for refining rice bran oil (Gopala Krishna, 1992; Kaimal et al., 2002). Kuk and Dowd (1998) found that the quality of rice oil extracted by SC-CO_2 was superior to that of oil obtained by hexane extraction.

Recently, Balachandran et al. (2008) showed that rice bran oil extracted with SC-CO_2 had negligible phosphatides, wax and prooxidant metals (Fe and Cu) and the oil was superior in colour quality when compared to rice bran oil extracted with hexane. The total rice bran oil yield using optimal SC-CO_2 parameters was comparable to that of hexane extraction (22.5%) and the tocols, sterols and oryzol yields ranged from 1500 to 1800 ppm, 15,350 to 19,000 ppm and 5800 to 11,100 ppm, respectively. In addition to high recovery of these bioactives, significant cost savings could be realized using SC-CO_2 as there was no need for a 'degumming' process to remove phosphatides nor was bleaching of the oil required (typical with hexane extraction) when extracted with SC-CO_2.

8.5 EXTRACTION OF OTHER BIOACTIVES

The effect of ultrasound on extraction and biological activity of peptides has also been investigated (Jia et al., 2010). They investigated the use of ultrasound for the enzymatic preparation of angiotensin I-converting enzyme (ACE)-inhibitory peptides from defatted wheat germ protein. Analysis of ACE-inhibitory activity indicated that ultrasound during enzyme treatments had little effect on the ACE-inhibitory activity of the peptides, while ultrasonic pre-treatment resulted in a 21–41% increase in ACE-inhibitory activity of the hydrolysate obtained from the defatted wheat germ protein. The ultrasonic pre-treatment appears to promote the release of ACE-inhibitory peptides from the defatted wheat germ protein during enzymatic hydrolysis.

8.6 ULTRASONIC AND SC-CO_2 APPLICATIONS IN OILSEED PROCESSING

Many vegetable oils are traditionally extracted using hexane. For example, the processing of canola, sunflower and soyabean oil in North America typically involves two main processes: mechanical pressing and extraction followed by further processing to remove impurities. Owing to the high residual oil content, the press cake which is generated as a result of the mechanical pressing is further extracted, typically using *n*-hexane, to recover the residual oil. The remaining press cake is then used as a feed meal for animal or aquaculture production.

This process requires large amounts of solvent. Additional processing (desolventization/toasting) is required with an operating temperature of 100–110°C to evaporate the solvent from the meal. Some compounds with potential nutraceutical value may undergo thermal degradation from the heat or denaturation from the solvent and this economic value is lost in the processing. Additionally, the cost of evaporation of solvent from oil and meal is also significant and solvent is lost in the process, although process engineering has had a substantial impact on solvent recovery during the extraction process. Operating losses of solvents range from 0.2 to 2.0 gallons per ton of oilseed processed. The cost of hexane transport, storage and disposal are also significant due to toxicological, high flammability and environmental safety issues. Ultrasound-assisted and SC-CO_2 extraction for oilseed processing need to be evaluated in the context of environmental safety, consumer acceptance and value of co-extracted products in addition to capital and operating costs.

High-intensity ultrasound has been used successfully for applications other than the extraction of bioactive compounds which are relevant to the oilseeds processing industry including emulsification/homogenization (Canselier et al., 2002; Cucheval and Chow, 2008; Kentish et al., 2008), crystallization (Bund and Pandit, 2007; Luque de Castro and Priego-Capote, 2007; Kordylla et al., 2008; Gogate and Kabadi, 2009), viscosity alteration (Seshadri et al., 2003; Knorr et al., 2004; Iida et al., 2008) and defoaming (Dedhia et al., 2004; Gallego-Juarez, 2010; Jambrak et al., 2010).

Vilkhu et al. (2008) point out that there are limited publications which focus on pilot-scale or commercial applications and/or have included continuous ultrasonic processes for extraction purposes. As discussed earlier, many of the applications are bench-scale examinations of how ultrasound can increase the speed of extraction or improve extraction yield. However, major advances have been realized in the past several years that are not in peer-reviewed literature, but which are moving a laboratory-based prototype technology into fully operational commercial processes in Europe, Asia and the United States (Patist and Bates, 2008). Advances such as availability of high amplitude/power units suitable for large commercial operations, and improved energy efficiency of equipment have ensured that the equipment is operationally cost competitive with other extraction processes, while reduced maintenance costs, enhanced flow-cell design, and the capacity to manipulate the frequency of the ultrasonic fields improve the efficiency and the scope of the application of the technology (Patist and Bates, 2008).

Oil and oil fractions, phenols, tocopherols and peptides are all of interest to the canola/oilseed rape processing industry for their potential use in functional food products and nutraceuticals. The successful use of ultrasound-assisted extraction of these components in various plant or tissue systems demonstrates that ultrasound-assisted extraction is a viable alternative for the canola/oilseed rape industry for the recovery of value-added products from whole seeds, hulls and press cakes. However, due to limited research on pilot-scale application, it is difficult to model cost advantages of ultrasound-assisted extraction versus conventional solvent extraction when applied to commodity oilseed processing.

SC-CO_2 promises shorter extraction times, no chemical residue and a safer operating environment as a replacement for *n*-hexane extraction (Sahena et al., 2009). Several studies have shown that oil yields using SC-CO_2 are on par with solvent extraction and this is a crucial factor if SC-CO_2 is to be competitive economically with solvent extraction (Taylor et al., 1993; Perrut, 2000; Bozan and Temelli, 2002; Bravi et al., 2002; Lu et al., 2007; Ixtaina et al., 2010; Li et al., 2010). The SC-CO_2 extractions which were reviewed earlier were conducted using temperature, pressure and solvent flow rates which are readily attainable in commercial-scale systems. Many studies have been conducted on pilot-scale equipment and the extraction of valuable materials from solid substrates by means of SC-CO_2 has been carried out on a commercial scale for more than 25 years (Brunner, 2005).

It is important to note that use of SC-CO_2 for extraction/fractionation of lipids and bioactive molecules do not contribute directly to the greenhouse gas effect associated with global warming. The CO_2 which is utilized is isolated as a by-product from primary sources such as production of hydrogen or ammonia (DeSimone, 2002). Furthermore, the SC-CO_2 system can be run as a 'closed-loop' where the CO_2 is recycled. Finally, due to the low heat of vaporization of CO_2, energy costs may be significantly reduced relative to water-intensive processes which are currently necessary for conventional oilseed processing, which often require large amounts of energy to heat water for extraction and then further energy to dry the final product.

Several research studies have focused on oil yield (Fattori et al., 1988; Bozan and Temelli, 2002; Dunford and Temelli, 1997; Pradhan et al., 2010), fatty acid composition (Chang et al., 2000; Jenab et al., 2006; Soares et al., 2007) and oxidative stability of extracted oils (Przbylski et al., 1998; Jenab et al., 2006) using SC-CO_2 when compared to solvent extraction. The extraction of commodity oils is predictable. Oil extraction yields increase with increasing pressure up to a certain pressure, which depends on the extraction temperature and then the yield decreases with increasing pressure. This maximum extraction pressure, which occurs before the observed decline in oil extraction yield, increases with temperature (Jiao et al., 2008; Xu et al., 2008; Ixtaina et al., 2010).

SC-CO_2 may have an economic advantage over solvent extraction if one factor in the economic value of cardiovascular, diabetes and chemo-protective compounds such as phytosterols, tocopherols, tocotrienols and other phenolic/aromatic compounds as their recovery from the solvent 'deodorizer distillate' fraction is questionable (Temelli, 2009; Sahena et al., 2009). Many studies have shown that fractionation of these compounds is effective when SC-CO_2 is utilized (Chang et al., 2000; Sahena et al., 2009; Yang et al., 2010). Preserving bioactivity and unique flavour and aroma profiles of specialty oils during SC-CO_2 extraction is a major advantage since volatile aromatic compounds are lost during hexane evaporation in traditional processing (Sun et al., 2008).

Consider also more highly purified lecithin and other purified forms of phospholipid concentrates from oilseeds. Isolating a more purified form of lecithin using SC-CO_2 may increase the price dramatically when compared to a lower quality product. Nutraceutical-grade phospholipids (i.e., concentrated phosphatidylcholine or phosphatidylserine) concentrated using SC-CO_2 may command prices of US $1500/lb in certain markets. Such economic incentives could easily justify investment of the SC-CO_2 plant and equipment.

SC-CO_2 extraction of oil leaves a meal containing proteins and carbohydrates that can be further fractionated. The mild conditions of SC-CO_2 extraction minimizes the damage to residual proteins, resulting in enhanced functionality when compared to proteins in the meal obtained by conventional solvent extraction (Sun et al., 2008). This may have a significant impact on economic valuation of SC-CO_2 processing. A 'biorefining' model which would maximize the value of all the costreams (oil/fatty acid, protein/peptide, phospholipid, vitamin and polyphenols, etc.) generated in the SC-CO_2 extraction process may tip the economic return in favour of SC-CO_2 over conventional solvent extraction. Further research is needed to validate this 'biorefining' model.

Another factor to consider when comparing the economic value of SC-CO_2 to conventional processing is consumer acceptance. Many consumers are being drawn to 'clean' or 'green' labels which can be applied to food products as part of the product offering. Consumers were more willing to accept and purchase SC-CO_2 extracted canola oil if they were given nutritional and/or processing information regarding the benefits of SC-CO_2 technology (Mak, 2006). Furthermore, the sensory quality of SC-CO_2 extracted canola oil was found favourable by most people when tested (Mak, 2006). Brunner (2005) noted that SC-CO_2 may be useful even if its sole use was for removing the residual solvent from oil and meal fractions so that consumers could be confident that no residual solvent remained in the food product.

Mendes et al. (2002) conducted an economic evaluation for an industrial scale model pertaining to the use of SC-CO_2 to concentrate tocopherols present in the deodorizer distillate from soyabean oil processing. The SC-CO_2 experimental conditions used to concentrate the tocopherols were operating temperatures of 40°C, 60°C and 80°C and pressure of 90 and 170 bar. The deodorizer distillate had tocopherol concentrations ranging from 11% to 13%. The SC-CO_2 process concentrated the tocopherols to at least 40%. A better process efficiency was obtained at lower temperature and pressure, due in part to the solubility of tocopherols in CO_2. From this experimental data, an economic model was tested using capital or equipment costs, production costs including variable and fixed costs (prices of soyabeans, CO_2, tocopherol yield, etc.). The model also considered recycling and no recycling of the CO_2. The total return on investment was calculated to be 28% when CO_2 was recycled and 53% when CO_2 was not recycled. The break even time was 2.1 years when CO_2 was recycled and 1.2 years when CO_2 was not recycled. Costs were higher when CO_2 was recycled because compression costs of CO_2 represent 59% of the costs of a supercritical plant. The authors concluded that the model plant would be profitable even at 25% capacity.

SC-CO_2 equipment design is also evolving. Currently SC-CO_2 plants are still operating on a semi-continuous basis, by cycling through multiple extraction vessels that are filled and emptied in a batch-wise fashion (Martinez and Vance, 2008). However, industry pundits believe that continuous extraction SC-CO_2 designs will be available within the next 10 years. This is needed for the high volume throughput that the industry requires.

In summary, the potential of SC-CO_2 to replace solvent extraction as an environmentally friendly option appears promising. Economics currently favour extraction of specialty oils and bioactives but use of SC-CO_2 for commodity oil extraction/processing appears attainable as well. Ultimately, the combined extraction of ultrasound followed by supercritical CO_2 extraction may prove to be the most cost effective and efficient means of extracting oil and other bioactives in a 'biorefining' model (Glisic et al., 2011).

REFERENCES

Albu, S., Joyce, E., Paniwnyk, L., Lorimer, J.P. and Mason, T.J. 2004. Potential for the use of ultrasound in the extraction of antioxidants from *Rosmarinus officinalis* for the food and pharmaceutical industry, *Ultrason. Sonochem.* **11**: 261–265.

AOCS Official Method AM 3-96. 1997. Oil in oilseeds: Supercritical fluid extraction method, *Official Methods and Recommended Practices of the American Oil Chemists' Society*, 5th ed. (1996). AOCS Press, Champaign, IL, 1996.

Arai, K., Smith Jr, R.L. and Aida, T.M. 2009. Decentralized chemical processes with supercritical fluid technology for sustainable society. *J. Supercrit. Fluids* **47**: 628–636.

Ashokkumar, M., Sunartio, D., Kentish, S., Mawson, R., Simons, L., Vilkhu, K. and Versteeg, C. 2008. Modification of food ingredients by ultrasound to improve functionality: A preliminary study on a model system. *Innov. Food Sci. Emerg. Technol.* **9**: 155–160.

Balachandran, C., Mayamol, P.N., Thomas, S., Sukumar, D., Sundaresan, A. and Arumughan, C. 2008. An ecofriendly approach to process rice bran for high quality rice bran oil using supercritical carbon dioxide for nutraceutical applications, *Bioresour. Technol.* **99**: 2905–2912.

Barthet, V.J. and Daun, J.K. 2002. An evaluation of supercritical fluid extraction as an analytical tool to determine fat in canola, flax, solin, and mustard, *J. Am. Oil Chem. Soc.* **79**: 245–251.

Beckman, E.J. 2004. Supercritical and near-critical CO_2 in green chemical synthesis and processing, *J. Supercrit. Fluids* **28**: 121–191.

Boutin, O. and Badens, E. 2009. Extraction from oleaginous seeds using supercritical CO_2: Experimental design and products quality, *J. Food Eng.* **92**: 396–402.

Boutin, O., De Nadai, A., Perez, A.G., Ferrasse, J-H., Beltran, M. and Badens, E. 2011. Experimental and modelling of supercritical oil extraction from rapeseeds and sunflower seeds, *Chem. Eng. Res. Design* **89**: 2477–2484.

Bozan, B. and Temelli, F. 2002. Supercritical CO_2 extraction of flaxseed, *J. Amer. Oil Chem. Soc.* **79**: 231–235.

Bramley, P.M., Elmadfa, I., Kafatos, A., Kelly, F.J., Manios, Y., Roxborough, H.E., Schuch, W., Sheehy, P.J.A. and Wagner, K.H. 2000. Vitamin E, *J. Sci. Food Agric.* **80**: 913–938.

Bravi, M., Bubbico, R., Manna, F. and Verdone, N. 2002. Process optimisation in sunflower oil extraction by supercritical CO_2, *Chem. Eng. Sci.* **57**: 2753–2764.

Bruni, R., Guerrini, A., Scalia, S., Romagnoli, C. and Sacchetti, G. 2002. Rapid techniques for the extraction of vitamin E isomers from *Amaranthus caudatus* seeds: Ultrasonic and supercritical fluid extraction, *Phytochem. Anal.* **13**: 257–261.

Brunner, G. 2005. Supercritical fluids: Technology and application to food processing, *J. Food Eng.* **67**: 21–33.

Bulley, N.R., Fattori, M., Meisen, A. and Moyls, L. 1984. Supercritical fluid extraction of vegetable oil seeds, *J. Amer. Oil Chem. Soc.* **61**: 1362–1365.

Bund, R.K. and Pandit, A.B. 2007. Sonocrystallization: Effect on lactose recovery and crystal habit, *Ultrason. Sonochem.* **14**: 143–152.

Canselier, J.P., Delmas, H., Wilhelm, A.M. and Abismaïl, B. 2002. Ultrasound emulsification—An overview, *J. Dispersion Sci. Technol.* **23**: 333–349.

Chang, C.J., Chang, Y-F., Lee, H-Z., Lin, J-Q. and Yang, P-W. 2000. Supercritical carbon dioxide extraction of high-value substances from soybean oil deodorizer distillate, *Ind. Eng. Chem. Res.* **39**: 4521–4525.

Chemat, F., Grondin, I., Costes, P., Moutoussamy, L., Sing, A.S.C. and Smadja, J. 2004. High power ultrasound effects on lipid oxidation of refined sunflower oil, *Ultrason. Sonochem.* **11**: 281–285.

Cucheval, A. and Chow, R.C.Y. 2008. A study on the emulsification of oil by power ultrasound, *Ultrason. Sonochem.* **15**: 916–920.

Dedhia, A.C., Ambulgekar, P.V. and Pandit, A.B. 2004. Static foam destruction: Role of ultrasound, *Ultrason. Sonochem.* **11**: 67–75.

DeSimone, J.M. 2002. Practical approaches to green solvents, *Science* **297**: 799–803.

Dillow, A.K., Dehghani, F., Hrkach, J.S., Foster, N.R. and R. Langer, R. 1999. Bacterial inactivation by using near- and supercritical carbon dioxide, *Proc. Natl. Acad. Sci. USA* **96**: 10344–10348.

Dong, M. and Walker, T.H. 2008. Characterization of high-pressure carbon dioxide explosion to enhance oil extraction from canola, *J. Supercrit. Fluids* **44**: 193–200.

Dunford, N.T. 1995. *Use of SC-CO_2 for Edible Oil Processing*, University of Alberta, Edmonton.

Dunford, N.T., Teel, J.A. and King, J.W. 2003. A continuous countercurrent supercritical fluid deacidification process for phytosterol ester fortification in rice bran oil, *Food Res. Int.* **36**: 175–181.

Dunford, N.T. and Temelli, F. 1996. Effect of supercritical CO_2 on myrosinase activity and glucosinolate degradation in canola. *J. Agric. Food Chem.* **44**: 2372–2376.

Dunford, N.T. and Temelli, F. 1997. Extraction conditions and moisture content of canola flakes as related to lipid composition of supercritical CO_2 extracts, *J. Food Sci.* **62**: 155–159.

Eckert, C.A. and Chandler, K. 1998. Tuning fluid solvents for chemical reactions, *J. Supercrit. Fluids* **13**: 187–195.

Eckert, C.A. Knutson, B.L. and Debenedetti, P.G. 1996. Supercritical fluids as solvents for chemical and materials processing, *Nature* **383**: 313–318.

Eisenmenger, M., Dunford, N.T., Eller, F., Taylor, S. and Martinez, J. 2006. Pilot-scale supercritical carbon dioxide extraction and fractionation of wheat germ oil, *J. Amer. Oil Chem. Soc.* **83**: 863–868.

Fattori, M., Bulley, N.R. and Meisen, A. 1987. Fatty acid and phosphorus contents of canola seed extracts obtained with supercritical carbon dioxide, *J. Agric. Food Chem.* **35**: 739–743.

Fattori, M., Bulley, N.R. and Meisen, A. 1988. Carbon-dioxide extraction of canola seed: Oil stability and effect of seed treatment, *J. Amer. Oil Chem. Soc.* **65**: 968–974.

Gallego-Juarez, J.A. 2010. High-power ultrasonic processing: Recent developments and prospective advances, *Physics Procedia.* **3**: 35–47.

Ge, Y., Ni, Y., Yan, H., Chen, Y. and Cai, T. 2002. Optimization of the supercritical fluid extraction of natural vitamin E from wheat germ using response surface methodology, *J. Food Sci.* **67**: 239–243.

Gelmez, N., Kincal, N.S. and Yener, M.E. 2009. Optimization of supercritical carbon dioxide extraction of antioxidants from roasted wheat germ based on yield, total phenolic and tocopherol contents, and antioxidant activities of the extracts, *J. Supercrit. Fluids* **48**: 217–224.

Glisic, S.B., Ristic, M. and Skala, D.U. 2011. The combined extraction of sage (*Salvia officinalis* L.): Ultrasound followed by supercritical CO_2 extraction, *Ultrason. Sonochem.* **18**: 318–326.

Gogate, P.R. and Kabadi, A.M. 2009. A review of applications of cavitation in biochemical engineering/biotechnology, *Biochem. Eng. J.* **44**: 60–72.

Gopala Krishna, A.G. 1992. A method for bleaching rice bran oil with silica gel, *J. Amer. Oil Chem. Soc.* **69**: 1257–1259.

Güçlü-Üstündağ, Ö. and Temelli, F. 2004. Correlating the solubility behavior of minor lipid components in supercritical carbon dioxide, *J. Supercrit. Fluids* **31**: 235–253.

Güçlü-Üstündağ, Ö. and Temelli, F. 2005. Solubility behavior of ternary systems of lipids, cosolvents and supercritical carbon dioxide and processing aspects, *J. Supercrit. Fluids* **36**: 1–15.

Güçlü-Üstündağ, Ö. and Temelli, F. 2007. Column fractionation of canola oil deodorizer distillate using supercritical carbon dioxide, *J. Amer. Oil Chem. Soc.* **84**: 953–961.

He, W.H., Gao, Y.X., Yuan, F., Bao, Y.N. Liu, F.Z. and Dong, J.Q. 2010. Optimization of supercritical carbon dioxide extraction of gardenia fruit oil and the analysis of functional components, *J. Amer. Oil Chem. Soc.* **87**: 1071–1079.

Iida, Y., T. Tuziuti, T., Yasui, K., Towata, A. and Kozuka, T. 2008. Control of viscosity in starch and polysaccharide solutions with ultrasound after gelatinization, *Innov. Food Sci. Emerg. Technol.* **9**: 140–146.

Ixtaina, V.Y., Vega, A., Nolasco, S.M., Tomás, M.C., Gimeno, M., Bárzana, E. and Tecante, A. 2010. Supercritical carbon dioxide extraction of oil from Mexican chia seed (*Salvia hispanica* L.): Characterization and process optimization, *J. Supercrit. Fluids* **55**: 192–199.

Jambrak, A.R., Herceg, Z., Subaric, D., Babic, J., Brncic, M., Brncic, S.R., Bosiljkov, T., Cvek, D., Tripalo, B. and Gelo, J. 2010. Ultrasound effect on physical properties of corn starch, *Carbohydr. Polym.* **79**: 91–100.

Jenab, E., Rezaei, K. and Emam-Djomeh, Z. 2006. Canola extraction by supercritical carbon dioxide and a commercial organic solvent, *Eur. J. Lipid Sci. Technol.* **108**: 488–492.

Jia, J., Ma, H., Zhao, W., Wang, Z., Tian, W., Luo, L. and He, R. 2010. The use of ultrasound for enzymatic preparation of ACE-inhibitory peptides from wheat germ protein, *Food Chem.* **119**: 336–342.

Jiao, S.S., Li, D., Huang, Z.G., Zhang, Z.S., Bhandari, B., Chen, X.D. and Mao, Z.H. 2008. Optimization of supercritical carbon dioxide extraction of flaxseed oil using response surface methodology, *Int. J. Food Eng.* **4**: 42–56.

Kadkhodaee, R. and Hemmati-Kakhki, A. 2007. Ultrasonic extraction of active compounds from saffron, *Acta Hort.* **739**: 417–426.

Kaimal, T.N.B. 1999. Rice bran as a food supplement, *J. Oil Technol. Assoc. India* **31**: 25–37.

Kaimal, T.N.B., Vali, S.R., Rao, B.V.S.K., Chakrabarti, P.P., Vijayalakshmi, P., Kale, V., Rani, K.N.P., Rajamma, O., Bhaskar, P.S. and Rao, T.C. 2002. Origin of problems encountered in rice bran oil processing, *Eur. J. Lipid Sci. Technol.* **104**: 203–211.

Kakuda, Y. and Kassama, L. 2006. Supercritical fluid technology for extraction of bioactive components, in *Functional Food Ingredients and Nutraceuticals*, J. Shi, ed. CRC Press, Boca Raton, FL.

Keil, F. and Wiley InterScience (Online service). 2007. Modeling of process intensification, Wiley-VCH: John Wiley [distributor], Weinheim Chichester.

Kentish, S., Wooster, T.J., Ashokkumar, M., Balachandran, S., Mawson, R. and Simons, L. 2008. The use of ultrasonics for nanoemulsion preparation, *Innovat. Food Sci. Emer. Technol.* **9**: 170–175.

Khosravi-Darani, K. 2010. Research activities on supercritical fluid science in food biotechnology, *Crit. Rev. Food Sci. Nutr.* **50**: 479–488.

Knorr, D., Zenker, M., Heinz, V. and Lee, D-U. 2004. Applications and potential of ultrasonics in food processing, *Trends Food Sci. Technol.* **15**: 261–266.

Kordylla, A., Koch, S., Tumakaka, F. and Schembecker, G. 2008. Towards an optimized crystallization with ultrasound: Effect of solvent properties and ultrasonic process parameters, *J. Crystal Growth.* **310**: 4177–4184.

Kuk, M. and Dowd, M. 1998. Supercritical CO_2 extraction of rice bran, *J. Amer. Oil Chem. Soc.* **75**: 623–628.

Leitner, W. 2000. Designed to dissolve, *Nature* **405**: 129–130.

Li, H., Pordesimo, L. and Weiss, J. 2004. High intensity ultrasound-assisted extraction of oil from soybeans, *Food Res. Int.* **37**: 731–738.

Li, H., Wu, J., Rempel, C.B. and Thiyam, U. 2010. Effect of operating parameters on oil and phenolic extraction using supercritical CO_2, *J. Amer. Oil Chem. Soc.* **87**: 1081–1089.

Licence, P., Ke, J., Sokolova, M., Ross, S.K. and Poliakoff, M. 2003. Chemical reactions in supercritical carbon dioxide: From laboratory to commercial plant, *Green Chem.* **5**: 99–104.

List, G., King, J. and Dunford, N.T. 2003. Supercritical fluid extraction in food engineering, in *Extraction Optimization in Food Engineering*, C. Zia and G. Liadaku, eds. CRC Press, 2003.

Lou, Z., Wang, H., Zhang, M. and Wang, Z. 2010. Improved extraction of oil from chickpea under ultrasound in a dynamic system, *J. Food Eng.* **98**: 13–18.

Lu, T., Gaspar, F., Marriott, R., Mellor, S., Watkinson, C., Al-Duri, B., Seville, J. and Santos, R. 2007. Extraction of borage seed oil by compressed CO_2: Effect of extraction parameters and modelling, *J. Supercrit. Fluids* **41**: 68–73.

Luque de Castro, M.D. and F. Priego-Capote, F. 2007. Ultrasound-assisted crystallization (sonocrystallization), *Ultrason. Sonochem.* **14**: 717–724.

Luque-García, J.L. and Luque de Castro, M.D. 2004. Ultrasound-assisted Soxhlet extraction: An expeditive approach for solid sample treatment: Application to the extraction of total fat from oleaginous seeds, *J. Chromatogr. A.* **1034**: 237–242.

Mak, S.A. 2006. *Sensory and Chemical Characterization of Canola Oil Extracted by Supercritical Carbon Dioxide*, University of Alberta.

Martinez, J.L. and Vance, S.W. 2008. Supercritical extraction plants: Equipment, process and costs, in *Supercritical Fluid Extraction of Nutraceuticals and Bioactive Compounds*, J.L. Martinez, ed. CRC Press, Taylor & Francis, Boca Raton, FL. pp. 25–49.

McHugh, M.A. and V.J. Krukonis, V.J. 1986. *Supercritical Fluid Extraction: Principles and Practice*, Butterworth, Stoneham, MA.

Melecchi, M.I.S., Martinez, M.M., Abad, F.C., Zini, P.P., do Nascimento Filho, I. and Caramão, E.B. 2002. Chemical composition of *Hibiscus tiliaceus* L. flowers: A study of extraction methods, *J. Sep. Sci.* **25**: 86–90.

Mendes, M.F., Pessoa, F.L.P. and Uller, A.M.C. 2002. An economic evaluation based on an experimental study of the vitamin E concentration present in deodorizer distillate of soybean oil using supercritical CO_2, *J. Supercrit. Fluids* **23**: 257–265.

Metherel, A.H., Taha, A.Y., Izadi, H. and Stark, K.D. 2009. The application of ultrasound energy to increase lipid extraction throughput of solid matrix samples (flaxseed), *Prostaglandins, Leukot. Essent. Fatty Acids* **81**: 417–423.

Munshi, P. and Bhaduri, S. 2009. Supercritical CO_2: A twenty-first century solvent for the chemical industry, *Curr. Sci.* **97**: 63–72.

Panfili, G., Cinquanta, L., Fratianni, A. and Cubadda, R. 2003. Extraction of wheat germ oil by supercritical CO_2: Oil and defatted cake characterization, *J. Amer. Oil Chem. Soc.* **80**: 157–161.

Patist, A. and Bates, D. 2008. Ultrasonic innovations in the food industry: From the laboratory to commercial production, *Innovat. Food Sci. Emerg. Technol.* **9**: 147–154.

Perretti, G., Miniati, E., Montanari, L. and Fantozzi, P. 2003. Improving the value of rice by-products by SFE, *J. Supercrit. Fluids* **26**: 63–71.

Perrut, M. 2000. Supercritical fluid applications: Industrial developments and economic issues, *Ind. Eng. Chem. Res.* **39**: 4531–4535.

Piras, A., Rosa, A., Falconieri, D., Porcedda, S., Dessi, M.A. and Marongiu, B. 2009. Extraction of oil from wheat germ by supercritical CO_2, *Molecules* **14**: 2573–2581.

Pradhan, R.C., Meda, V., Rout, P.K., Naik, S. and Dalai, A.K. 2010. Supercritical CO_2 extraction of fatty oil from flaxseed and comparison with screw press expression and solvent extraction processes, *J. Food Eng.* **98**: 393–397.

Przybylski, R., Lee, Y-C. and Kim, I-H. 1998. Oxidative stability of canola oils extracted with supercritical carbon dioxide, *LWT—Food Sci. Technol.* **31**: 687–693.

Ramsay, M.E., Hsu, J.T., Novak, R.A. and Reightler, W.J. 1991. Processing rice bran by supercritical fluid extraction, *Food Technol.* **45**: 98–104.

Reverchon, E. and De Marco, I. 2006. Supercritical fluid extraction and fractionation of natural matter, *J. Supercrit. Fluids.* **38**: 146–166.

Reverchon, E. and De Marco, I. 2007. Essential oils extraction and fractionation using supercritical fluids, in *Supercritical Fluid Extraction of Nutraceuticals and Bioactive Compounds*, CRC Press, Boca Raton, FL. pp. 305–335.

Reverchon, E. and Marrone, C. 2001. Modeling and simulation of the supercritical CO_2 extraction of vegetable oils, *J. Supercrit. Fluids* **19**: 161–175.

Rozzi, N.L. and Singh, R.K. 2002. Supercritical fluids and the food industry, *Compr. Rev. Food Sci. Food Safety* **1**: 33–44.

Sahena, F., Zaidul, I.S.M., Jinap, S., Karim, A.A., Abbas, K.A., Norulaini, N.A.N. and Omar, A.K.M. 2009. Application of supercritical CO_2 in lipid extraction—A review, *J. Food Eng.* **95**: 240–253.

Saliová, M., Toma, S. and Mason, T.J. 1997. Comparison of conventional and ultrasonically assisted extractions of pharmaceutically active compounds from Salvia officinalis, *Ultrason. Sonochem.* **4**: 131–134.

Schinor, E.C., Salvador, M.J., Turatti, I.C.C., Zucchi, O.L.A.D. and Dias, D.A. 2004. Comparison of classical and ultrasound-assisted extractions of steroids and triterpenoids from three Chresta spp, *Ultrason. Sonochem.* **11**: 415–421.

Seshadri, R., Weiss, J., Hulbert, G.J. and Mount, J. 2003. Ultrasonic processing influences rheological and optical properties of high-methoxyl pectin dispersions, *Food Hydrocoll.* **17**: 191–197.

Shao, P., Sun, P. and Ying, Y. 2008. Response surface optimization of wheat germ oil yield by supercritical carbon dioxide extraction, *Food Bioprod. Process.* **86**: 227–231.

Spilimbergo, S., Elvassore, N. and Bertucco, A. 2002. Microbial inactivation by high-pressure, *J. Supercrit. Fluids* **22**: 55–63.

Soares, B.M.C., Gamarra, F.M.C., Paviani, L.C., Gonçalves, L.A.G. and Cabral, F.A. 2007. Solubility of triacylglycerols in supercritical carbon dioxide, *J. Supercrit. Fluids* **43**: 25–31.

Stahl, E., Schuetz, E. and Mangold, H.K. 1980. Extraction of seed oils with liquid and supercritical carbon dioxide, *J. Agric. Food Chem.* **28**: 1153–1157.

Sun, M., Xu, L., Saldaña, M. and Temelli, F. 2008. Comparison of canola meals obtained with conventional methods and supercritical CO_2 with and without ethanol, *J. Amer. Oil Chem. Soc.* **85**: 667–675.

Taylor, S.L., Eller, F.J. and King, J.W. 1997. A comparison of oil and fat content in oilseeds and ground beef—Using supercritical fluid extraction and related analytical techniques, *Food Res. Int.* **30**: 365–370.

Taylor, S., King, J. and List, G. 1993. Determination of oil content in oilseeds by analytical supercritical fluid extraction, *J. Amer. Oil Chem. Soc.* **70**: 437–439.

Temelli, F. 1992. Extraction of triglycerides and phospholipids from canola with supercritical carbon dioxide and ethanol, *J. Food Sci.* **57**: 440–457.

Temelli, F. 2009. Perspectives on supercritical fluid processing of fats and oils, *J. Supercrit. Fluids* **47**: 583–590.

Vilkhu, K., Mawson, R., Simons, L. and Bates, D. 2008. Applications and opportunities for ultrasound assisted extraction in the food industry: A review, *Innovat. Food Sci. Emerg. Technol.* **9**: 161–169.

Vinatoru, M. 2001. An overview of the ultrasonically assisted extraction of bioactive principles from herbs, *Ultrason. Sonochem.* **8**: 303–313.

Vinatoru, M., Toma, M., Radu, O., Filip, P.I., Lazurca, D. and Mason, T.J. 1997. The use of ultrasound for the extraction of bioactive principles from plant materials, *Ultrason. Sonochem.* **4**: 135–139.

Vuorela, S., Meyer, A.S. and Heinonen, M. 2004. Impact of isolation method on the antioxidant activity of rapeseed meal phenolics. *J. Agric. Food Chem.* **52**: 8202–8207.

Wang, J., Sun, B., Cao,Y., Tian, Y. and Li, X. 2008. Optimisation of ultrasound-assisted extraction of phenolic compounds from wheat bran, *Food Chem.* **106**: 804–810.

Wang, L. and Weller, C.L. 2006. Recent advances in extraction of nutraceuticals from plants, *Trends Food Sci. Technol.* **17**: 300–312.

Wang, S.C., Tseng, T.Y., Huang, C.M. and Tsai, T.H. 2004. Gardenia herbal active constituents: Applicable separation procedures, *J. Chromatogr. B Analyt. Technol. Biomed. Life Sci.* **812**: 193–202.

Wei, F., Gao, G-Z., Wang, X-F., Dong, X-Y., Li, P-P., Hua, W., Wang, X., Wu, X-M. and Chen, H. 2008. Quantitative determination of oil content in small quantity of oilseed rape by ultrasound-assisted extraction combined with gas chromatography, *Ultrason. Sonochem.* **15**: 938–942.

Xu, X., Gao, Y.X., Liu, G.M., Wang, Q. and Zhao, H. 2008. Optimization of supercritical carbon dioxide extraction of sea buckthorn (*Hippophae thamnoides* L.) oil using response surface methodology, *LWT-Food Sci. Technol.* **41**: 1223–1231.

Xu, Z. 2008. Comparison of extraction methods for quantifying vitamin E from animal tissues, *Biores. Technol.* **99**: 8705–8709.

Yang, H., Yan, F., Wu, D., Huo, M., Li, J., Cao, Y. and Jiang, Y. 2010. Recovery of phytosterols from waste residue of soybean oil deodorizer distillate, *Biores. Technol.* **101**: 1471–1476.

Yoshino, G., Kazumi, T., Amano, M., Tateiwa, M., Yamasaki, T., Takashima, S., Iwai, M., Hatanaka, H. and Baba, S. 1989. Effects of gamma-oryzanol on hyperlipidemic subjects, *Curr. Ther. Res.* **45**: 543–552.

Zhang, Z-S., Wang, L-J., Li, D., Jiao, S-S., Chen, X.D. and Mao, Z-H. 2008. Ultrasound-assisted extraction of oil from flaxseed, *Separ. Purif. Technol.* **62**: 192–198.

9 Processing of Virgin Canola Oils

Bertrand Matthäus

CONTENTS

9.1 Introduction 171
9.2 Sensory Assessment of Cold-Pressed Canola Oil 172
9.3 Influence of the Seed Material on the Quality of Cold-Pressed Canola Oil 174
9.3.1 Why Is It So Difficult to Produce High-Quality Canola Oil? 174
9.3.2 Pre-Treatment of the Seed Material before Storage 175
9.3.3 Influence of Storage Conditions 176
9.4 Influence of the Press Parameters on the Quality of Cold-Pressed Canola Oil 179
9.5 Production of Virgin Canola Oil from Dehulled Seeds 180
9.6 Purification 180
9.7 DGF Canola Oil Award 182
9.8 Conclusion 183
References 184

9.1 INTRODUCTION

Although virgin olive oil is a hot topic of discussion in many countries around the world, most of the other oils are always refined and require extensive extraction. But some countries also use other cold-pressed virgin oils like nut oils, pumpkin seed oil, or even canola oil which are becoming increasingly popular. The main reasons for this increased interest by consumers for this type of oil are the excellent nutritional properties of the oil (Trautwein et al., 1999; Junker et al., 2001). The demand by consumers for less-processed food is responsible for the increasing desire for edible oils with a natural taste and smell. Additionally, virgin oil has the image of healthier oil in comparison to refined oils. For producers, this type of oil is becoming more and more attractive because of its added value. In comparison to refined canola oil, the price for virgin oils ranges between 4 and 16 Euros per litre compared to 1 Euro. Most of the producers can economize in regional material cycles, resulting in shorter routes of transport and smaller transportation costs (Widmann, 1994a,b). They supply a manageable and quantitatively limited market in a radius of between 25 and 100 km. Only a few of them supply the oil all over the country.

For the production of virgin canola oil, the pressing process involves the extraction of raw material by a screw press, the simplest method for producing oil in small- and medium-sized facilities (Dunning, 1953; Peterson et al., 1983; Stöver et al., 1988). The oil yield, however, is much lower here than in big plants and ranges between 75% and 85%. The processing capacity of such small plants is between 0.5 and 25 t/d. After pressing, the oil obtained is purified either by filtration using different techniques or by stepwise sedimentation. No further treatment of the oil is carried out as any problems during transportation from the field to the bottle cannot be compensated. Thus it is very important to ensure the production of high quality virgin edible canola oil by carefully selecting top-quality raw materials, using a gentle pressing process, immediately cleaning the crude oil, as well as ensuring optimum storage conditions for the oil. If any of these conditions are not followed, it will result in drastic loss of quality.

9.2 SENSORY ASSESSMENT OF COLD-PRESSED CANOLA OIL

A loss of quality is noticeable by different parameters which describe the quality of the oil. The most important parameter for the evaluation of the quality of virgin oils is the sensory impression, because more than any other parameter, the appearance and the taste of a product deeply influence the buying decision of the consumer.

For the sensory evaluation of virgin canola oil, a standard method by the German Society of Fat Science (DGF), DGF-C-II 1 (07) (DGF, 2011), is available. This method evaluates the oils both descriptively and quantitatively with a minimum of four trained panelists (Figure 9.1). For good virgin canola oils from sound seeds, attributes such as *seed-like*, *nutty*, *wood-like* and *astringent* have been found useful and typical, while off-flavours are described as *rancid*, *fusty*, *musty*, *roasty*, *burnt* and *bitter* (Figure 9.2). Most of these result from the formation of volatile degradation products or the development of aroma-active compounds during faulty processing.

Date:.............

Tester:............

Sample:..............

Positive attributes	**0**	**1**	**2**	**3**	**4**	**5**
Canola seed like						
Nutty						
Adstringent						
Wood-like/strawy						
Negative attributes	**Yes**	**No**				
Roasty/burnt						
Bitter						
Rancid						
Fusty/musty						
Others						

FIGURE 9.1 Evaluation sheet for the sensory evaluation of virgin canola oil according to the DGF method DGF-C-II 1 (07). (Adapted from DGF Einheitsmethoden, 2. 2011. Auflage einschließlich 15. Akt.-Lfg. Wissenschaftliche Verlagsgesellschaft, Stuttgart.)

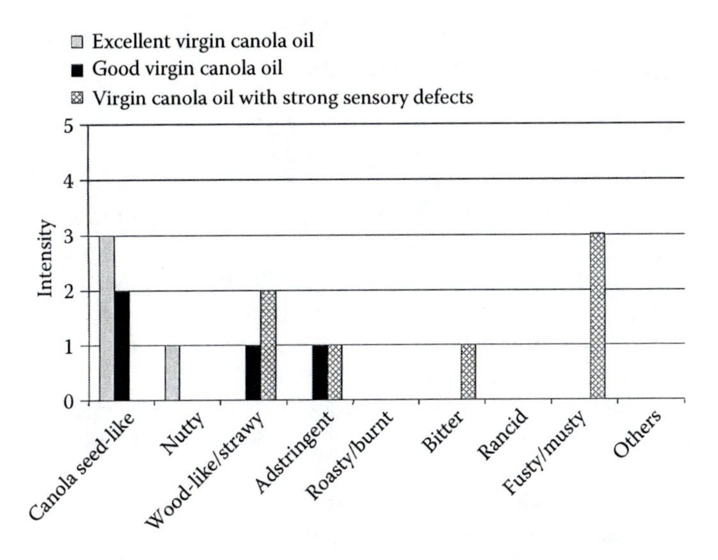

FIGURE 9.2 Sensory evaluation of different qualities of virgin canola oil.

A quantitative assessment of each positive attribute is carried out on a scale from 0 for not perceivable to 5 for very strongly perceivable. For the negative attributes only the existence is determined as "yes" or "no". From the individual results of all tasters, the median value is calculated for describing the sensory quality. The advantage of the median value, compared to the mean value, is that outliers are not influencing the results and will be excluded. For the median, all numbers are arranged in ascending order and the number in the middle is the resulting value. This method improves the reliability and repeatability of the sensory analysis. In contrast, the mean value of the results for each attribute is influenced by every single result even if there is an outlier in the data set.

However, panel testing is a time-consuming and training-intensive evaluation procedure, where skilled staff is needed. In order to support the sensory panel's evaluation, a purge and trap analysis of the volatile compounds in cold-pressed virgin canola oils has been set up. With this technique, key volatiles for some of the most common defects can be detected with an objective analysis method. For example, oils with a rancid attribute show compounds such as hexanal, heptanal, octanal, nonanal, *trans*-2-heptenal, *trans*-2-octenal, *trans*-2-nonenal, *trans*-2-decenal and *trans*-2-undecenal, and *trans*/*cis*-2,4-heptadienal and *trans*/*cis*-2,4-decadienal at elevated levels. For musty attributes, the branched alcohols 2-methylpropanol and 2- and 3-methylbutanol are characteristic key compounds. However, this method will only be able to detect known defects.

In addition to sensory evaluation, some other parameters are suitable to describe the quality of cold-pressed oils. Such characteristic features are oxidative stability (Rancimat test), tocopherol content and composition, amount of *trans*-fatty acids or stigmastadiene, showing a heat treatment during production, as well as content of chlorophyll, as a measure not only for the maturity of the raw material, but also as an indicator of improper pressing conditions.

9.3 INFLUENCE OF THE SEED MATERIAL ON THE QUALITY OF COLD-PRESSED CANOLA OIL

The most important point for the production of high-quality virgin canola oil is to start with high-quality raw material. Since no other purification of the crude oil than sedimentation or filtration follows the oil extraction, it is important to keep in mind that the quality of the virgin canola oil corresponds perfectly to the quality of the raw material used for the processing. Therefore, it is absolutely necessary not to start oil processing only with the oil extraction from the raw material, but the process has to start much earlier, at the best already on the field. The producer of this type of oil has no chance to improve the oil quality after the pressing process. Purification by sedimentation or filtration only removes turbid matter, but no components which impair the oil quality, such as free fatty acids, products of oxidative degradation, or degradation products of the metabolism of the seeds or of micro-organisms.

Although the processing of virgin canola oil, with pressing by a screw press and purification, seems to be a very easy-to-handle process, the reality on the market shows another picture. While refined oils always have the same high quality, the quality of virgin canola oils is far more variable with sensory quality showing much more differences between the very good oils with a pleasant taste and smell, but also with very bad ones that are unacceptable to consumers.

9.3.1 Why Is It So Difficult to Produce High-Quality Canola Oil?

One reason why the handling of canola seeds for the production of high-quality virgin oil is so difficult is because of the high oil content of the seeds. Canola seeds constitute up to 40% or more of the dried matter and a low content of carbohydrates compared to cereals. Oil is very susceptible to oxidation as degradation products of the oxidative process are already noticeable at very low concentrations. In addition, this effect is enhanced because oil is an excellent carrier for aroma components, which retains and concentrates volatile compounds. Therefore, the oil fraction of the raw material acts as sensory memory that remembers everything that has been done during pre-treatment and storage until the processing step.

Another important point is the low content of carbohydrates in canola seeds which results in a remarkably lower tolerance against moisture. Carbohydrates are able to bind certain amounts of moisture resulting in lower amounts of free available water, which otherwise could act in processes in the seeds as reaction partner directly or as reaction medium indirectly. Higher amounts of free available water are responsible for increasing metabolic processes and increasing the population of micro-organisms (Niewiadomski, 1990; Schumann and Graf, 2005).

This high susceptibility of canola seeds makes it difficult to maintain the good quality of the seeds after harvest until processing. Since canola seeds are processed continuously over at least 1 year, it is necessary to store them after harvest under appropriate conditions to avoid degradation. The aim of an optimal storage is to maintain the good quality of the seeds until further processing without losses in quality during storage. But the problem is that the seeds are living organisms. They have the natural desire to develop new plants, which results in the degradation of storage compounds like lipids, carbohydrates, or proteins into carbon dioxide, water and energy. This leads to a loss of mass, development of unpleasant aroma compounds, decrease of germination capacity, increase of temperature and improved conditions for micro-organisms. Water and temperature are the driving factors for the degradation processes and if there is no control of these parameters degradation will increase significantly. Improper pre-treatment and storage of the raw material after harvest can result in remarkable financial losses for the owner.

Another point is that only viable and germinable seeds are optimally storable. This means that the metabolic processes must not go to zero, otherwise the result would be the dying of the seed material. Therefore the aim of responsible storage has to be the limitation of factors favouring metabolic processes to the necessary minimum. By this, it is possible to reduce losses by respiration and consequently the formation of degradation products. Keeping a high seed quality during storage requires ventilation and cooling of the raw material and the limitation of foreign matter which often is characterized by a high moisture content and settlement by micro-organisms. Additional factors like species and state of the seeds and damaged seeds are important criteria which unfavourably influence the storage time and must be taken into consideration.

From these different points, it becomes clear that it is important for maintaining the high seed quality after harvest to do the splits between reducing the respiration rate of the seeds and keeping the seeds alive.

9.3.2 Pre-Treatment of the Seed Material before Storage

After harvesting, cleaning and, if necessary, drying of seeds are the most important pre-treatment steps. Both, the amount of foreign matter and the moisture content, are basis for the settlement of the oil mills with the farmers when seeds are delivered. In Canada, for canola seeds, a so-called Canola standard was established by the Canadian Grain Commission defining the maximum amount of foreign matter in the seeds as 2%, while the amount of moisture should be between 6% and 9%. In Germany, oil mills have similar conditions, but the moisture content has to be below 9%, otherwise the farmer has to accept deductions. In contrast, soyabeans with lower oil content and a higher content of protein and fibre are allowed to come from the field with about 13% moisture, which is considered as useful for a long-term storage.

Foreign matter such as stems, broken seeds, foreign seeds and so on often contain higher amounts of moisture, chlorophyll, free fatty acids, or a higher population of micro-organisms.

Up to 40% of the volume of stored canola seeds consists of hollows, in which an appropriate relative humidity is adjusted, depending not only on the amount of seed moisture, but also on the amount and moisture of foreign material. This humidity sets the speed of metabolism in the seeds and favours the growth of mould, yeast and bacteria on the seeds during the storage period. Therefore, a limitation of the amount of foreign matter in the raw material to 2% and also a limitation of the seed moisture is necessary to ensure that high-quality oil and meal are obtained.

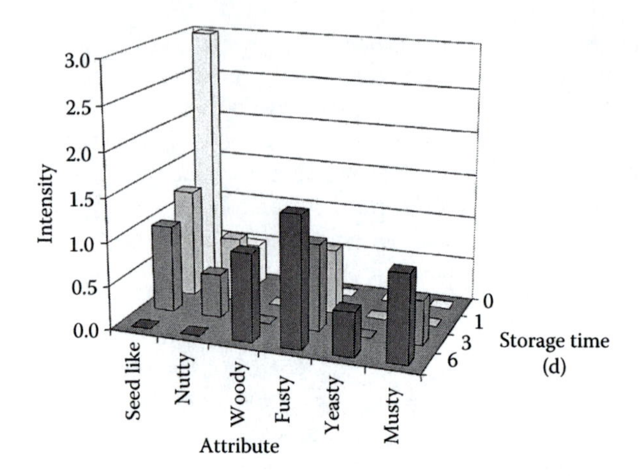

FIGURE 9.3 Influence of the presence of broken seeds during storage of canola seeds on the sensory evaluation of the resulting virgin canola oil.

It is also advisable to do the seed cleaning directly after harvest and before storage to keep a high seed quality for a longer time. Foreign matter should be removed as much as possible. In general, it is useful to clean the material to <1% foreign material if a longer storage period is required.

An amount of more than 5% foreign matter results in a straw-like aroma, because seeds of other plants such as wheat, but also parts of stems, not only from canola are pressed with the seeds resulting in an extraction of aroma-relevant compounds from these materials. With increasing foreign matter, the intensity of the attribute 'seed-like' decreases, while attributes like 'straw-like' or 'woody' remarkably increase.

In broken seeds at room temperature, but even faster at higher temperatures, enzymatic and microbial reactions take place because the substrates usually separated in the intact seeds come together. This results in degradation reactions of the appropriate substrates leading to fusty sensory attributes of the oil. During the storage of seed material with 5% broken seeds at 40°C, the attribute 'seed-like' was no longer detectable after 6 days of storage, while attributes such as 'fusty', 'woody' or 'musty' characterize the sensory impression of such a cold-pressed oil (Figure 9.3). Further, as the amount of free fatty acids increases and the composition of the volatile components changes, the sensory impression of the oils has changed negatively. Another important factor which results in a quality decrease of the oil is the drying condition of the seeds prior to storage, because this pre-treatment can cause a burnt aroma of the oil.

9.3.3 Influence of Storage Conditions

The main problem during storage is moisture because a certain amount of water is not only sufficient for the development of micro-organisms, but also for the activity of enzymes, both of which result in the deterioration of seed quality. Sources of moisture are either the seeds themselves or especially foreign matter, such as foreign seeds, pods, or stems. Additionally, the formation of water as a result of metabolic

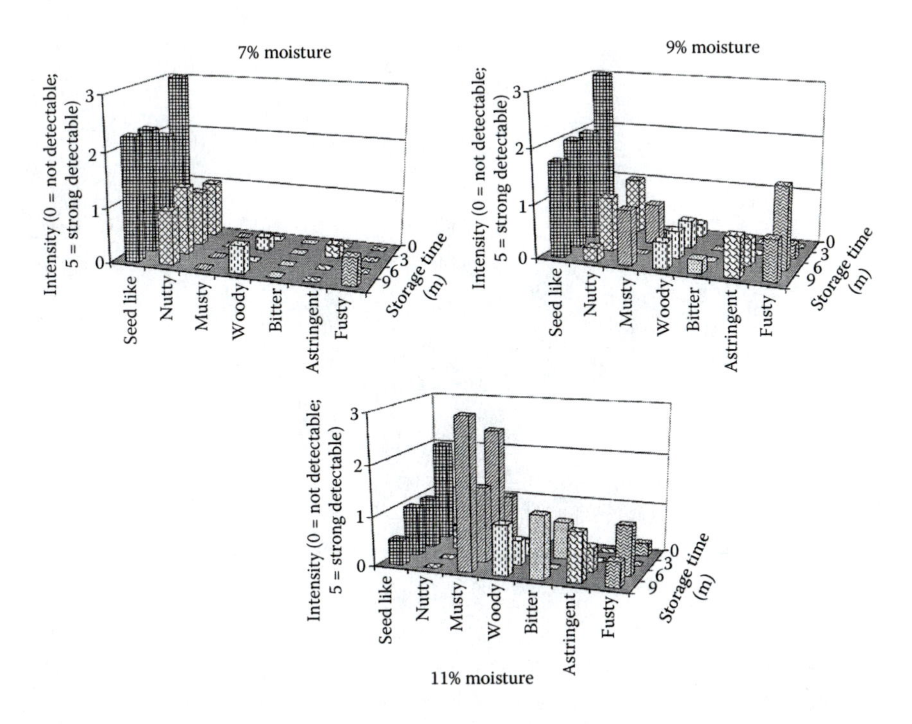

FIGURE 9.4 Influence of storage of canola seeds with different amounts of moisture over a period of 9 months on the sensory evaluation of the resulting oils.

processes is a great problem. With increasing amounts of moisture, the respiration rate of the seeds increases resulting in the degradation of storage compounds like triacylglycerols, carbohydrates and proteins and the development of volatile and non-volatile degradation products such as free fatty acids or aroma-active compounds. While the respiration rate is low up to 8% of moisture, there is a drastic increase if the moisture content increases further. Much more pronounced is this effect when seeds are settled by micro-organisms.

Therefore for the production of virgin canola oil, it is necessary to dry the seed material after harvest carefully if the moisture content is higher than 8%. Figure 9.4 shows the results of a storage experiment with canola seeds containing different amounts of moisture. The seeds were stored over a period of 9 months and at appropriate dates, the seed material was pressed under defined conditions. The resulting virgin oil was tasted by a trained sensory panel.

Seeds stored with a moisture content of 7% were stable over a period of 9 months. The resulting oils showed no decrease of the positive sensory attributes *seed-like* or *nutty* and no development of negative attributes like *fusty* or *musty*. During storage of the seeds, the resulting oil quality remained constant at a high level. The results were different, when the moisture content increased to 9%. In this case, a clear decrease of the positive attributes and an increase of negative attributes occurred, making the resulting oils inedible after 6 months. Storage of canola seeds with 11% moisture resulted even in a faster development of negative attributes while positive

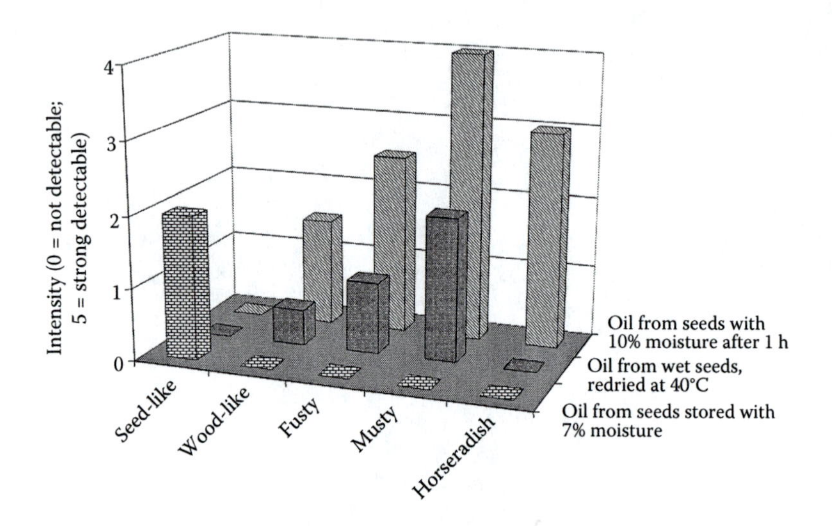

FIGURE 9.5 Influence of short-term storage of canola seeds with moisture content of 10% on the sensory evaluation of the resulting oil.

sensations were only detectable within the first month of storage. These experiments show that a limitation of the moisture content to 9%, as used by large processing plants, is adequate to ensure the quality of the refined oil but it is not sufficient for the producers of virgin canola oil. In the latter case, a maximum moisture content should be between 7% and 8%. In addition storage of canola seeds at 9% moisture or even higher over a period of 9 months resulted in a continual increase of the content of free fatty acids. No change in the content of free fatty acids was detectable in seeds stored at a moisture content of 7% (Attenberger et al., 2005).

The deterioration of canola seeds by moisture takes place very fast. Figure 9.5 shows the effect of a short-term storage of canola seeds with 10% moisture on the sensory evaluation of the resulting canola oil. While canola oil from seeds stored at 7% moisture showed the typical *seed-like* and *nutty* taste and smell, storage of canola seeds with 10% moisture resulted in the formation of unpleasant *fusty* and *musty* aroma components as well as the smell and taste for horseradish within 1 h. The smell and taste for horseradish is typical for glucosinolate degradation products like isothiocyanates. The sensory perception for *seed-like* and *nutty* typical for virgin canola oil was no longer detectable. In summary, it becomes clear that seed material stored with higher moisture content becomes unusable for the production of high-quality tasty virgin canola oil in a very short time.

Gentle drying at 40°C of wet raw material stored for 1 h was not suitable to restore the typical attributes. By drying, it was possible only to reduce the intensity of the negative attributes *musty* and *fusty* and to remove the volatile isothiocyanates responsible for the smell and taste for horseradish, but the oil was still not suitable for human consumption. This experiment shows that already very short storage times at higher moisture contents result drastically in the loss of quality. That has to be avoided absolutely after the harvest of canola seeds.

9.4 INFLUENCE OF THE PRESS PARAMETERS ON THE QUALITY OF COLD-PRESSED CANOLA OIL

During screw pressing, the parameters that can be varied include the temperature of the press head, the speed of the screw press, the diameter of the nozzle, as well as the type of the press. Not all of these parameters affect the quality of the oil to the same extent and not all parameters describing the quality of the oil are influenced by the press settings.

The press parameters have no influence on the fatty acids and tocopherols and the oxidative stability of the oil is not changed as a result of the different press settings. On the other hand, the content of chlorophyll and phosphorus as well as the amount of free fatty acids are strongly influenced by the pressing conditions. Especially an increase of the press head temperature leads to an increase of these components which are of special interest because they influence the stability of the oil. However, the diameter of the nozzle as well as the speed of the screw press has no influence on the amount of free fatty acids, but the use of a small 6 mm nozzle results in increasing amounts of chlorophyll if the speed of the screw press is reduced. The reason is that at lower speeds, the seed material remains for a longer time in the screw press and therefore the extraction of components from the seeds with the oil is more effective.

Chlorophyll, a ubiquitous plant pigment, is a photosensitizer for singlet oxygen formation under light resulting in a faster deterioration of the oil. In addition, chlorophyll is undesirable because it leads to an unpleasant green or brown colour in the oil. Phospholipids are also ubiquitous in plants and are recovered in the pressed oil to a higher extent under harsh pressing conditions. This leads to a white precipitation during storage of the oil. Consumers normally reject products with such a white precipitation. Free fatty acids are degradation products of the triacylglycerols, formed either by enzymatic treatment or by heat. They are more susceptible to oxygen, which results in a faster degradation of the free fatty acids to undesirable aroma components. Therefore, it is important to avoid the formation of these components during production to improve the quality and to prolong the shelf life of the oil.

The sensory attribute 'seed-like', typical for the taste of virgin canola oil, is hardly influenced by the pressing parameters. Only using a small nozzle with a slow speed results in a significant less-pronounced 'seed-like' impression of the oil. The press parameters have a stronger effect on the sensory attribute 'burnt'. Using a small nozzle, the intensity of this attribute increases with increasing speed of the screw press because the temperature stress of the seed material increases. A larger diameter of the nozzle leads to a less-pronounced development of this negative attribute and also an increase of the press head temperature from 60°C to 90°C results only in a small increase of the intensity of the attribute 'burnt'.

In summary, if high-quality seed material is used for the pressing process, the settings of the screw press can be varied over a wide range without running the risk of changing the quality of the resulting oil. Nevertheless, a gentle pressing process is recommended to avoid higher contents of chlorophyll, phosphorus, as well as free fatty acids in the oil impairing the stability during storage.

9.5 PRODUCTION OF VIRGIN CANOLA OIL FROM DEHULLED SEEDS

Dehulling of canola seeds is not a commonly used process, since it is expensive due to the small size of the seeds. For the production of refined oils, this type of pre-treatment is not economical, although the resulting meal has some advantages if used as animal feed and also for the extraction of protein for human consumption. Phenolic compounds and fibre are reduced in the resulting meal, which improves its quality for animals from a nutritional point of view. The use of dehulled seeds also has some advantages concerning the reduction of processing costs, because the energy effort during further processing is lower. But dehulling has the disadvantage that the amount of antinutritive compounds such as sinapine, glucosinolates and inositol phosphates is enriched in the resulting dehulled material (Matthäus, 1998).

An advantage of dehulling before screw pressing is the possibility of keeping the press temperature below 40°C, which limits the activity of seed enzymes and reduces the transfer from undesired components of the seeds into the oil (Schneider, 1979a,b; Piva et al., 1985; Schneider and Khoo, 1986). As a result of dehulling, the taste and smell of this type of oil should be milder than that of conventional virgin, cold-pressed canola oils, with a less intensity of its typical sensory attribute *seed-like*.

9.6 PURIFICATION

Purification of virgin, cold-pressed canola oil only involves the separation of solid impurities, mainly particles of the seed material. This is an important step to ensure the quality of the oil for a longer storage time. Disrupted particles of the seeds contain enzymes, but also adhered micro-organisms which can metabolize the oil to form degradation and metabolism products impairing especially the sensory quality of the oil. Depending on the settings of the screw press, speed of the rotating screw shaft, size of the press cake exit, temperature during pressing and moisture content of the seed, the amount of solid components in the oil ranges between 1% and 13%. The aim of this type of purification is the separation of the two-phase system consisting of oil (liquid phase) and seed particles (solid phase). In general, two different methods, sedimentation and filtration, are used, depending on the performance of the plant. A third method, centrifugation of the crude canola oil is not widespread, but seems to be very gentle.

Sedimentation uses the different specific density of the liquid and solid phase which leads to a slow settling of the solid particles as a result of gravity. There are two possibilities to use this method. The first one can be used as a batch system, in which a container is filled with crude oil and seed particles are allowed to sediment within 15–30 days. Since the throughput of oil of this method is strongly limited, the method is only suitable for small plants with a low production of oil up to 50 kg/h. A drawback of this type of purification is the long contact of oil with the disrupted seed material. During this long time period, enzymes and also micro-organisms from disrupted seed material start to degrade the oil. Investigations have shown that sedimentation in the batch system over a period of 21 days impairs oil quality significantly in comparison to other types of purification (Figure 9.6) (Attenberger et al., 2005).

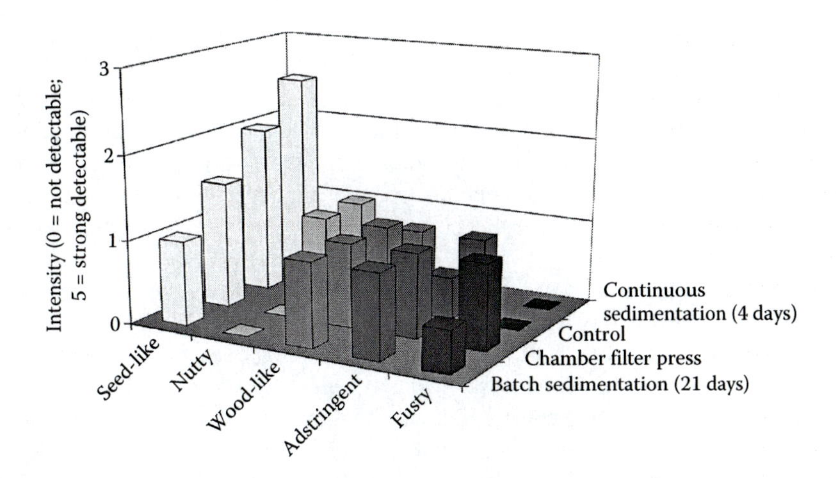

FIGURE 9.6 Influence of different cleaning procedures for the removal of turbid matter on the sensory evaluation of virgin canola oil.

From this point of view, a second method seems to be more practical. This method is working continuously using a multilevel sedimentation tank, in which addition of crude oil, removal of purified oil and elimination of enriched solid particle take place simultaneously. By this, a greater throughput of oil is possible, only limited by the number and size of the sedimentation tanks and economical aspects. Additionally, the contact time between oil and disrupted seed material is noticeably shorter, resulting in much better quality of the purified oil.

Filtration is the mechanical separation of solid and liquid phase which allows the removal of insoluble solids or suspended material from a liquid by passing it through a porous medium only permeable for the liquid phase. In small- and medium-sized plants, this is mostly achieved by means of the formation of a filter cake from the seed particles between porous filter materials within a pressure gradient. The filter cake improves the result of the filtration. Sometimes filter aids can be used to increase the effect of the filter materials. These are inert cellulose materials which improve the formation of a filter cake for the filtration process. Filtration in small- and medium-sized plants is carried out by the use of chamber filter presses or vertical pressure plate filters, which enable a much higher throughput in comparison to sedimentation. The last step of the purification process in small- and medium-sized plants is passing the oil through a fine-pored protection filter to ensure a defined clarity of the oil.

Sometimes virgin, cold-pressed canola oil used as edible oil is also on the market as natural turbid oil, which is not or only insufficiently purified. In this natural turbid oil the intensity of the sensory attribute *seed-like*, typical for virgin canola oil is stronger than in purified virgin oil. However, this type of oil has some problems with the formation of free fatty acids as a result of the formation of metabolic and degradation products from enzymes and micro-organisms located on the seed particles (Attenberger et al., 2005). Therefore, a longer storage of these oils is not advisable.

Some producers of cold-pressed edible canola oils treat the oil with hot water steam after removal of seed particles. The aim of this treatment is the removal of undesired volatile compounds, which negatively influence the sensory quality of the oil. Additionally, the storage stability of the oils should be improved. The purified oil is treated with hot water steam at temperatures between 120°C and 180°C over a period of 1–4 h in a batch system. Under these conditions, no changes in the fatty acid composition or in the composition and the amount of tocopherols are noticeable. Nevertheless, the appearance of oligomer triacylglycerols or stigmasta-3,5-diene, as degradation product of ß-sitosterol, a phytosterol, often may be good indicators for a hot water steam treatment.

As a result of this treatment, volatile compounds with a steam pressure lower than the temperature used go out of the oil. The resulting oil should be milder in taste and interfering aroma compounds which negatively influence the sensory evaluation of the oil should be removed. If the temperature is too high or the treatment time is too long the result of the steam treatment is a product without smell and taste. Another problem is that aroma compounds which are responsible for the positive sensory attribute like *seed-like* in cold-pressed canola oil are removed first, while aroma components which account for negative sensations remain in the oil. Thus, often the result of a hot water steam treatment is that the oils get a nasty taste and smell, which make them inedible.

9.7 DGF CANOLA OIL AWARD

The German Society for Fat Science (DGF) created in 2006 the DGF Canola Oil Award for virgin canola oils of excellent flavour with the aim to strengthen the consumer's trust in the quality of virgin canola oil, to improve the transparency on the market, and last but not least, to improve the awareness of the producers for the quality of their product (Matthäus et al., 2008). Especially this final point is of major importance, because without knowledge of what constitutes high-quality virgin canola oil, it is not possible for the producer to supply the consumer with such a product.

Both parties, the consumer and the producer have benefited from the award. Since successful participants are allowed to label their products with a special symbol as shown in Figure 9.7, the consumer gets the information that the producer is involved in the quality of his product. The most important quality feature of virgin canola oil is sensory perception. The motivation for the producers to take part at the Canola Oil Award is that they expect some advantages compared to the competitors in the market. The producer has the advantage to advertise his product as a high-quality one with a pleasant taste and smell. The award is a proof that he is able to deliver excellent quality oils.

After the call for the DGF Canola Oil Award in August, oils are sent to the DGF Canola oil panel in October which carries out the sensory assessment until end of November. The prerequisite for receiving the DGF Canola Oil Award is that the typical sensory sensation *seed-like* has to be perceivable at least in an intensity of 1, while off-flavours like *musty*, *fusty*, *rancid*, *roasted*, *burned* or *bitter* are not allowed. The attributes *wood-like/strawy* and *astringent* might be accepted at a low intensity. The occurrence of any of the off-flavours results in the rejection of the oil for the award. In some cases, the result of the sensory evaluation is supported by analysing the volatile compounds by an analytical method using dynamic headspace analysis (Brühl and Fiebig, 2005).

DGF-RAPSÖL-MEDAILLE
2011/2012
für ausgezeichneten
Geschmack
nativer Rapsspeiseöle

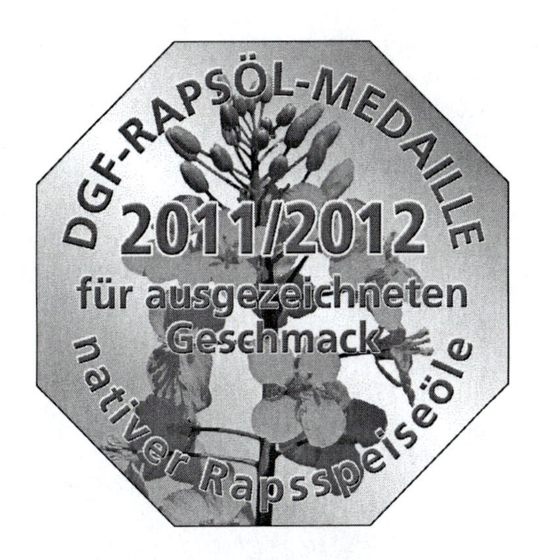

FIGURE 9.7 Medal of the DGF Canola Oil Award for excellent flavour. (Courtesy of the German Society of Fat Science, Frankfurt, Germany. With permission.)

In the first year, 26 oils were submitted and 16 samples were awarded in January 2007 in Berlin during the Green Week. After the first call, on average between 30 and 40 oils are submitted for the Award each year and between 50% and 70% of the oils receive medals from the DGF Canola Oil Award. Most of the participants are from Germany but also producers from other countries take part at the DGF Canola Oil Award.

9.8 CONCLUSION

Canola oil is distinguished by a well-balanced fatty acid composition which results in important nutritional properties. The prominent feature of cold-pressed edible canola oil is the characteristic 'seed-like' and 'nutty' smell and taste, which predetermine its use in the cold kitchen for the preparation of salads. For high-quality canola oil, a careful choice of high-quality seeds, a gentle oil pressing process, an extensive cleaning of the oil and proper storage conditions are necessary. Otherwise quality losses are inevitable. The consumer has no means to recognize which type of oil one is buying. Therefore, the producer is committed to do everything necessary to produce high-quality virgin oil.

The main factor affecting the quality of virgin rapeseed oil is the period from harvest to processing and not the processing itself. During this time, the high oil content of the seeds acts as sensory memory and everything done with the seeds comes back as taste and smell of the oil. The control of parts of foreign matter in the seeds, storage conditions and drying conditions are very important. Since producer of virgin canola oils cannot improve the quality of the oil during processing, it is absolutely necessary that they take care on the quality of the raw material and maintain the high quality of the seeds after harvest until processing. To reach this aim of producing high-quality virgin canola oil, all participants in the production chain are as critical as the pressing facility. All members of the production chain have to be sensitized for the quality of the end product (oil/press cake) and especially the storage facility is of decisive importance.

The awarding of the DGF Canola Oil Award makes it easier for the consumer to choose high-quality canola oil on the market. On the other hand, the producer can document and take a critical look at the quality of his product. The producer can show that he is capable of producing high-quality virgin canola oil. This certificate can be used for advertising their product against that produced by his competitors.

REFERENCES

Attenberger, A., Matthäus, B., Brühl, L. and Remmele, E. 2005. Research into the influencing factors on the quality of cold pressed rapeseed oil used as edible oil and determination of a quality standard. *Technologie- und Förderzentrum.* Eigenverlag, Technologie- und Förderzentrum.

Brühl, L. and Fiebig, H-J. 2005. Assistance of dynamic headspace chromatography for panel sensory evaluation. *Riv. Ital. Sostanze Gr.* **82**: 291–297.

DGF Einheitsmethoden, 2. 2011. Auflage einschließlich 15. Akt.-Lfg. Wissenschaftliche Verlagsgesellschaft, Stuttgart.

Dunning J. W. 1953. History and latest development in expeller and screw press operations on cottonseed. *J. Amer. Oil Chem. Soc.* **30**: 486–492.

Junker R., Kratz M., Neufeld M., Erren M., Nofer J. R., Schulte H., Nowak-Gottl U., Assmann G. and Wahrburg U. 2001. Effects of diets containing olive oil, sunflower oil, or rapeseed oil on the hemostatic system. *Thromb. Haemost.* **85**: 280–286.

Matthäus, B. 1998. Effect of dehulling on the composition of antinutritive compounds in various cultivars of rapeseed. *Fett/Lipid.* **100**: 295–301.

Matthäus, B., Brühl, L. and Amoneit, F. 2008. The DGF Rapeseed Oil Award—A tool to improve the quality of virgin edible rapeseed oil. *Lipid Technol.* **20**: 31–34.

Niewiadomski, H. 1990. *Rapeseed—Chemistry and Technology, Developments in Food Science*, Vol. 23. Elsevier, Amsterdam.

Peterson, C. L., Auld, D. L. and Thompson, J. D. 1983. Experiments with vegetable oil expression. In: *Transactions of the ASAE*, **26**(5): S. 1298–1302.

Piva, G., Pietri, A., Maccagni, A. and Santi, E. 1985. Fattori antinutrizionali della farina di estrazione di colza. *Riv. Ital. Sostanze Gr.* **62**: 99–103.

Schneider, F. H. 1979a. Schälung von Rapssaat durch definierte Verformung. I. Untersuchungen zur Saatanatomie. *Fette Seifen Anstrichmittel.* **81**: 11–16.

Schneider, F. H. 1979b. Schälung von Rapssaat durch definierte Verformung. II. Untersuchungen zum Schalverhalten. *Fette Seifen Anstrichmittel.* **81**: 53–59.

Schneider, F. H. and Khoo, D. 1986. Trennpressen—Versuch einer Bestandsaufnahme experimenteller Arbeiten. *Fette, Seifen, Anstrichmittel.* **88**: 329–340.

Schumann, W. and Graf, T. 2005. Anforderungen an die Rapssaat im Hinblick auf Qualitätsoptimierung. In: *Dezentrale Ölsaatenverarbeitung*, KTBL-Schrift 427. Landwirtschaftsverlag GmbH, Münster.

Stöver H.-M., Münch E.-W. and Sitzmann W. 1988. Gewinnung von Mineralölsubstituten aus Ölsaaten. *Fat Sci. Technol.* **90**: 547–550.

Trautwein E. A., Rieckhoff D., Kunath-Rau A. and Erbersdobler H. F. 1999. Replacing saturated fat with PUFA-rich (sunflower oil) or MUFA-rich (rapeseed, olive and high-oleic sunflower oil) fats resulted in comparable hypocholesterolemic effects in cholesterol-fed hamsters. *Ann. Nutr. Metab.* **43**: 159–172.

Widmann, B. A. 1994a. Verfahrenstechnische Maßnahmen zur Minderung des Phosphorgehaltes von Rapsöl bei der Gewinnung in dezentralen Anlagen. *Forschungsbericht Agrartechnik. MEG Nr. 262. Institut für Landtechnik Weihenstephan.*

Widmann, B. A. 1944b. Gewinnung und Reinigung von Pflanzenölen in dezentralen Anlagen—Einflussfaktoren auf die Produktqualität und den Produktionsprozess. *Forschungsbericht, Landwirtschaft und Forsten Bayer. Staatsministerium für Ernährung.*

10 Rapeseed Proteins
Recent Results on Extraction and Application

Frank Pudel

CONTENTS

10.1 Introduction 187
10.2 The Potential of Rapeseed Proteins 188
10.3 Why Is Rapeseed Protein Extraction More Difficult 189
  10.3.1 Storage Proteins 189
  10.3.2 Secondary Plant Substances 190
10.4 How to Design Value-Added Rapeseed Processing 190
  10.4.1 Deoiling Process 190
  10.4.2 Protein Concentrate Process 193
  10.4.3 Protein Isolate Process 193
  10.4.4 Protein Fractionation Process 193
10.5 How to Get the Best Raw Material for Protein Extraction 195
10.6 Ongoing Rapeseed Protein Application Projects 199
10.7 Conclusions 201
References 202

10.1 INTRODUCTION

There is a worldwide growing demand on plant proteins. Large amounts of plant proteins are needed for the production of animal proteins, like meat, fish, eggs or milk, taking into account that about 8 kg of oilseed meal is needed to produce 1 kg of meat. Particularly, there is a rapidly increasing shortage of proteins which are prospectively needed for aquaculture, because fishmeal production is no more to expand. Additionally, due to their nutritional and functional advantages, it is to expect that animal proteins more and more will be partially or completely replaced by proteins of vegetable origin in both certain human nutrition and industrial applications. In most cases, meals as by-products of the conventional oil mill process are not able to meet the quality requirements. Protein products of high purity, like pure protein fractions, protein isolates or concentrates are needed.

Rapeseed is a potential source for such products because it is the major crop in Europe and one of the most important oilseeds worldwide. It contains between 19% and 22% proteins. In 2008, an amount of about 8 Mio t rapeseed oil was produced in Europe, almost twice as much in 2004 (FEDIOL, 2010). The only reason for this development is the predominant use of rapeseed oil for biodiesel production. Taking into account that rapeseed contains up to 45% oil, there is an amount of about almost 10 Mio t rapeseed meal (or cake) available in Europe, which is used for animal feeding, particularly for cattles, having a comparably low price.

Rapeseed proteins possess besides their high nutritional value a distinct functional potential enabling stabilization of emulsions and foams as well as formation of gel-like and other structured systems with high water-binding capacity. Therefore, a lot of new value-added applications in human nutrition, animal feeding (like the use of rapeseed protein concentrates in aquaculture) and for different technical purposes may be expected.

Technologies for processing and application of rapeseed proteins are manifold described in the literature. However, no single commercial plant has been installed so far.

10.2 THE POTENTIAL OF RAPESEED PROTEINS

Similar to other oilseeds too, rapeseed contains not only oil, but also considerable amounts of proteins, polysaccharides, fibres and secondary plant substances. These compounds are to a different content located in the various seed compartments. After conventional oilseed processing, most of them must be enriched in the cake or meal. The protein content in rapeseed varies depending on the variety and conditions of cultivation and climate. Raw protein contents of 19–22% in rapeseeds and 31–36% in rapeseed meals can be obtained (Schwenke, 1994).

Comparing with other protein sources and with the Food and Agriculture Organization (FAO)/World Health Organization (WHO)/United Nations Organization (UNO)-suggested pattern of amino acid requirements for adults, school children and preschool children, rapeseed protein isolates exhibit favourable amino acid composition (Schwenke, 1994).

On the other hand, proteins possess very interesting functional properties. Owing to their specific structure with both hydrophilic and hydrophobic properties they can stabilize interfaces and form films. By physical, enzymatic or chemical modification the subunits can be dissociated and the polypeptide chains can be unfolded which improves the interface-stabilizing properties. And last but not the least they can form networks to build bioplastics (Figure 10.1).

On the basis of their manifold functionalities, proteins can be used both in various nutritional and technical applications: texturized proteins as meat extenders and replacers as well as fibres for textiles, protein-stabilized emulsions and foams in food dressings as well as asphalt emulsions or fire control foams, protein-based films, and coatings for fruit moisture control as well as for packaging purposes.

Most important technical application possibilities are (Krause, 2007):

- Fillers and binders for chipboards
- Binders for papers and cupboards
- Label glues and adhesives

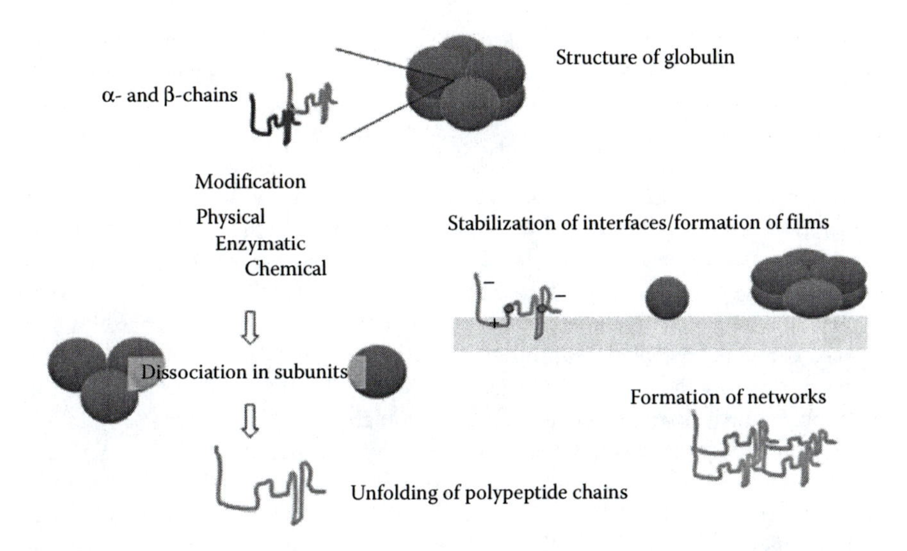

FIGURE 10.1 Correlation between structure change and surface functionality of proteins. (From Krause, J.-P., J. Kroll and H. M. Rawel. 2007. Verarbeitung von Rapssaat—Eigenschaften und Gewinnung von Proteinen. UFOP-Schriften Heft 32. Rapsprotein in der Humanernährung. UFOP: Berlin. With permission.)

- Solubilizers, dispersion agents and emulsifiers
- Surface coatings for papers and paper boards
- Packaging films
- Encapsulation of pharmaceuticals, flavouring agents and vitamins
- Detergents and cosmetics
- Xerogels
- Thermoplastics

Currently, the main problem consists of rapeseed proteins classified as 'novel food' according to the EU regulations, which does not allow its use as food or food additive before passing time and cost-consuming admission procedures.

However, besides the 'novel food' hurdle, there are also other reasons why rapeseed protein is not produced in industrial scale so far. Particularly, there are some processing difficulties in comparison with, for instance, soyabean protein.

10.3 WHY IS RAPESEED PROTEIN EXTRACTION MORE DIFFICULT

10.3.1 Storage Proteins

Rapeseed contains two major storage proteins: the 2 S albumin napin with a molar weight of 12–17 kDa and the 12 S globulin cruciferin with a molar weight of about 300 kDa. The napin cruciferin ratio depends on the rapeseed variety and is for canola-type quality about 1.1–1.3. This is significantly different to soyabean, which contains about 90% globulin (Schwenke, 1994; Natsch, 2006).

To be economic, both protein fractions have to be extracted and this requires the adjustment of different extraction parameters in a multi-step process.

10.3.2 Secondary Plant Substances

Furthermore, rapeseed contains different specific secondary plant substances. The best known are the glucosinolates. If a rapeseed cell is damaged, then the enzyme system myrosinase begins immediately to decompose the glucosinolates to more or less volatile degradation products. These breakdown products have mostly negative nutritional effects. Mainly isothiocyanates are formed being very reactive substances which react already at mild conditions with some functional groups of the proteins changing their solubility, isoelectric point (IP), and the ratio of hydrophilic/hydrophobic properties as well as their molar weight.

Polyphenols, particularly *trans* sinapic acid, create dark colour and bitter taste, and also react with proteins, in a similar way like glucosinolates breakdown products. Finally, phytic acid forms complexes both with trace metals, which lower their bioavailability, and with globulins too, which change their IP to low pH values (Kroll, 2007).

Therefore these secondary plant substances should be removed before or during protein extraction in order to secure high yield and quality of rapeseed proteins. In Table 10.1, some technological options are listed.

10.4 HOW TO DESIGN VALUE-ADDED RAPESEED PROCESSING

There are several different possibilities to design a process which produces both rapeseed oil and proteins. Each process step is able to influence yield and quality of oil and proteins as well as the final process design which strongly depends on the requirements of the targeted applications. This is important since, particularly the proteins have a wide range of functionality. There is no rapeseed-processing technology suitable for all purposes.

Therefore, a modular process design concept was developed which can fulfill various requirements. This concept consists of four processing steps:

1. Deoiling process leading to cake or meal
2. Protein concentrate process based on cake
3. Protein isolate process based on meal
4. Protein fractionation process in order to get high purified rapeseed protein fractions for special applications

10.4.1 Deoiling Process

To design a whole rapeseed oil and protein extraction process, at first it is to decide whether oil and protein are to be extracted separately (conventional oil mill process added by protein extraction) or simultaneously.

For a longer period, a lot of work has been done to develop simultaneously aqueous, aqueous alcoholic or enzymatic-assisted extraction of oil, and protein from specific

TABLE 10.1
Secondary Plant Substances of Rapeseed

	Nutritional Aspects	Effects at Protein	Detoxification
Glucosinolates and break down products 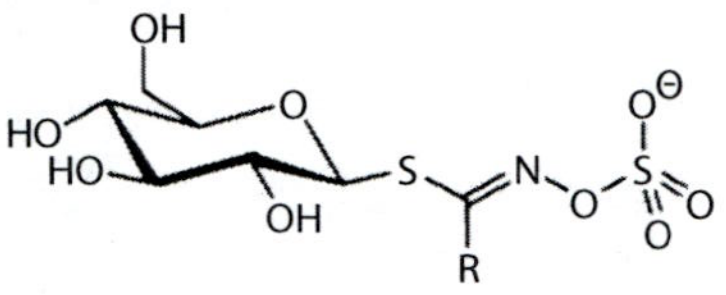	Intensive smell + taste Anticarcinogenic Antimicrobial Goitrogenic Mutagenic Cytotoxic Hepatotoxic Phytotoxic	Myrosinase hydrolyses glucosinolates Glucosinolates break-down products react with functional groups at protein (at free amino, SH and tryptophane side groups) Change of solubility, IP and hydrophobic properties Increase of molar weight	Enzyme inactivation Ethanolic extraction of glucosinolates
Polyphenols 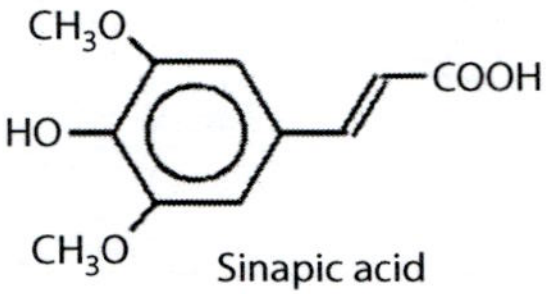 Sinapic acid	Free and esterified phenolic compounds: condensed tannins Dark colour Bitter taste Astringent effects	React with functional groups at protein, similar to isothiocyanates	Use of reducing agents to avoid oxidation Pre-extraction with alcohols Membrane processing Adsorption processing
Phytic acid 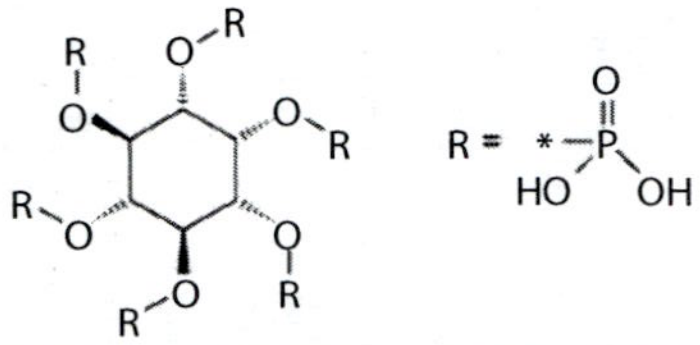	Forms complexes with Ca, Fe, Mn, Zn and lower their bioavailability but also discussed to be cancer preventing	Noncovalent interactions with proteins Forms insoluble electrostatic complexes with globulins and change their IP to low pH	Seed dehulling Pre-extraction at minimal protein solubility pH values Use of high ionic strenghts for protein isolation Ultrafiltration Phytase treatment

pre-treated seeds. An overview is given by Natsch (2006). What we know now is both oil and protein yield due to inadequate cell disruption (Heckelmann, 2010), emulsification and interactions between the secondary plant substances and proteins are at a maximum of about 80%, and therefore, too low to be economical (Natsch, 2006).

The conventional oil mill process is optimized to high oil yield. There are oil mills extracting the oil only mechanically by one or two pressing steps. Other oil mills use hexane extraction after pre-pressing.

Only pressing is cheaper, but the oil yield is lower, and the cake contains 7% oil or more. This residual oil in the expeller cake causes emulsion forming during the following aqueous protein extraction.

Pressing followed by hexane extraction leads to the highest oil yield. The meal contains only about 1% residual oil. After solvent extraction, the used hexane has to be removed from the meal which is done in desolventizer toaster (DT) systems. During this process step, the proteins within the meal are partially damaged leading to losses of functionality (Becker, 1983; Natsch, 2006; Krause, 2007).

In soyabean processing, this is quantified by the protein dispersibility index (PDI). Large PDI values stand for good solubility (in water) and high functionality. Measuring rapeseed products, PDI only covers the globulin portion of the proteins because PDI determination is carried out in aqueous solutions using distilled water at neutral pH (AOCS Standard Procedure Ba 10b-09). Nevertheless, PDI can also be useful for a first estimation of the influence of rapeseed-processing steps on the protein quality.

In our modular process design concept, the first step is conventional deoiling, improved by proper conditioning in order to inactivate the myrosinase and gentle desolventizing which keeps a high PDI in the meal and final milling (Figure 10.2).

Further improvements of this basic deoiling process could be reached by additional options.

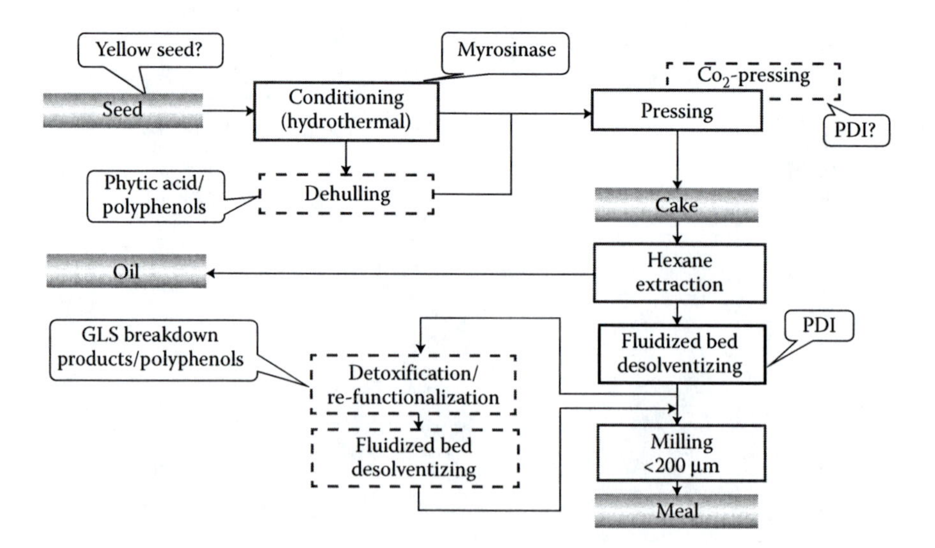

FIGURE 10.2 Deoiling process.

The use of yellow seed as well as seed dehulling could additionally lower the content of secondary plant substances, particularly phytic acid and phenolics, but yellow (winter rape) seed is not available, and dehulling is not to be used in oil mills by now.

A new crushing alternative is pressing with CO_2, proposed as HIPLEX® processed by companies such as Crown Iron Works and Harburg-Freudenberger. This leads to higher oil yield and better oil and protein quality due to the lower temperature stress in the press (Nazareth, 2009).

Finally, some detoxification and refunctionalization steps could be arranged between desolventizing and milling.

10.4.2 Protein Concentrate Process

To get protein concentrates, expeller cake can be used as raw material. After (aqueous) counter current extraction and thermo-coagulation, the proteins can be separated. The dried matter contains about 60–70% proteins. The separated by-product can be used as a fibre concentrate in animal feeding or as a feedstock for fermentation (Figure 10.3).

10.4.3 Protein Isolate Process

If the target is protein isolate with protein contents higher than 90%, defatted rapeseed meal as feedstock is required. The process is similar to the concentrated one. The protein separation is done after counter current extraction and membrane filtration (Figure 10.4).

10.4.4 Protein Fractionation Process

Highly purified rapeseed protein fractions are able to be obtained by ion-exchange chromatography. The process is comparable with the protein isolate process.

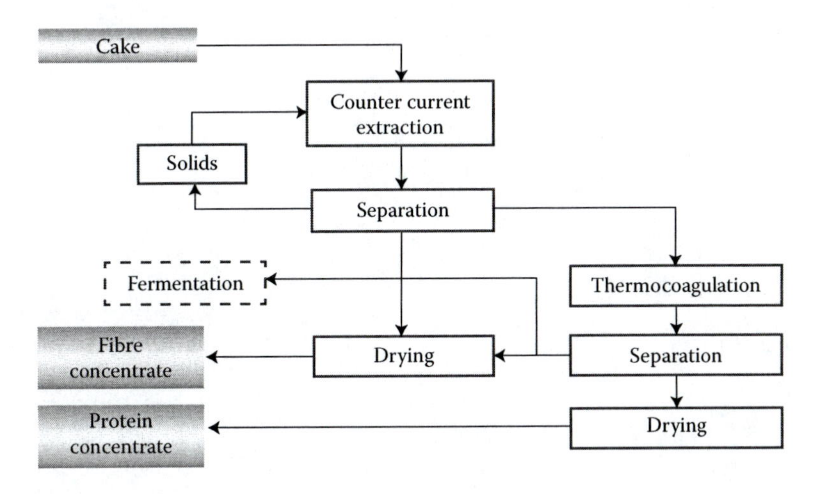

FIGURE 10.3 Protein concentrate process.

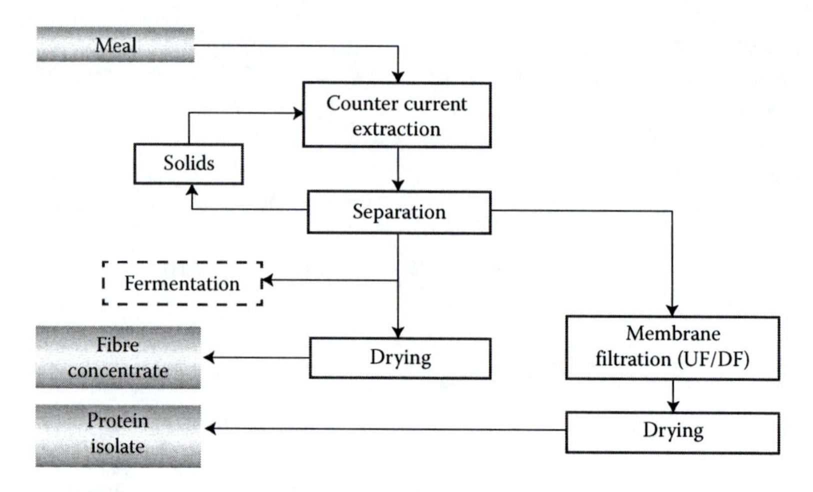

FIGURE 10.4 Protein isolate process.

A protein-rich solution recovered by counter current extraction of a gentle deodorized meal is fed into an ion-exchange chromatography column and fractionated (Figure 10.5). This process is very simple, feasible in industrial scale, has high yield, and leads to products with more than 95% purity.

Figure 10.6 shows sodium dodecyl sulphate polyacrylamide gel electrophoresis (SDS-PAGE) blots. On the left side the protein solution is shown after extraction, on the right side the fractionated proteins, pure cruciferin, and pure napin are shown. The cruciferin fraction has good emulsifying, film and gel formation properties, whereas the napin fraction is characterized by a high solubility and foam stabilization properties.

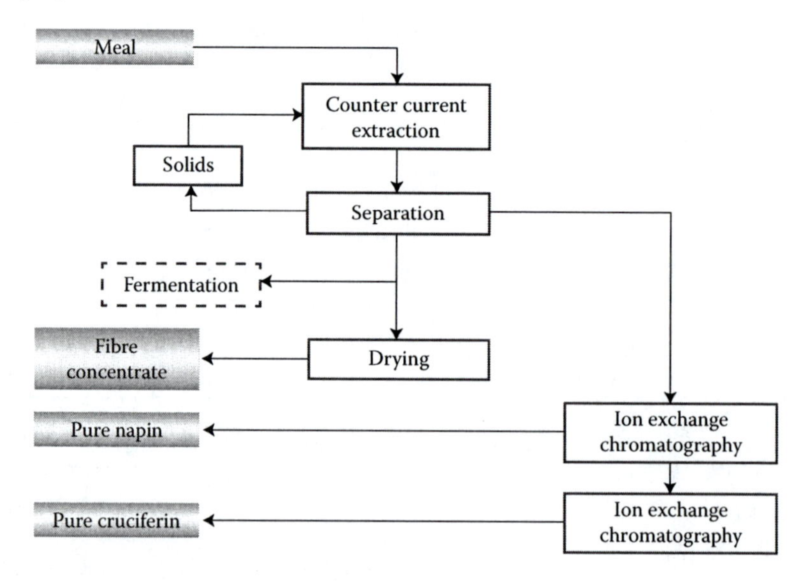

FIGURE 10.5 Protein fractionation process.

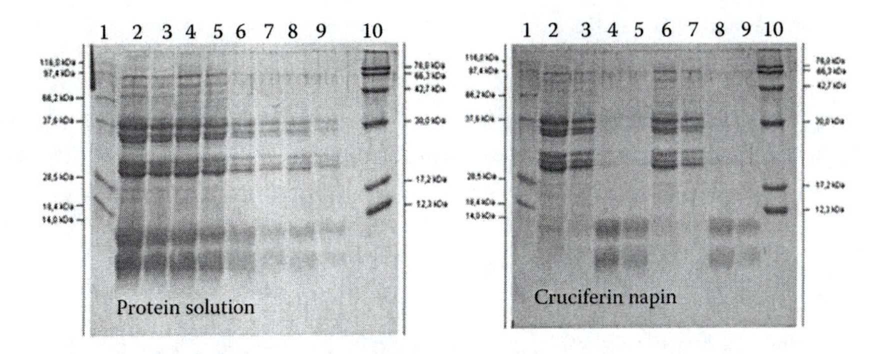

FIGURE 10.6 SDS-PAGE before and after fractionation.

10.5 HOW TO GET THE BEST RAW MATERIAL FOR PROTEIN EXTRACTION

The most important requirements for the meal from which proteins should be extracted are

- Low oil content
- Low hexane content (<300 ppm)
- Low contents of undesired components (glucosinolates, phytic acid and phenolics)
- Particle size (<200 μm)
- Minimal thermal damage, high PDI and low protein denaturation

Meal desolventizing is the most critical step regarding to the protein quality. After oil extraction, the oil content in the meal is decreased to about 1%. The hexane content is about 30% and has to be removed up to lower than 300 ppm. This is made in DT systems, consisting of pre-desolventizing, desolventizing, toasting and stripping, drying and cooling zones. Especially during desolventizing, toasting and stripping, temperatures of more than 100°C exist. The treatment takes between 1 and 2 h (De Kock, 2007). Under these conditions, the proteins will be damaged and the PDI will be reduced.

To avoid PDI decrease during desolventizing in soyabean processing, the so-called flash desolventizers (FDS) are used to produce white flakes. Flaked meal is given in a pipe, in which superheated hexane at about 85°C (or higher) is circulating with high velocity and evaporating most of the solvent from the flakes. This treatment is finished after some seconds. Subsequently residual solvent is removed from the meal by stripping with superheated steam in a flake stripper. In this way, PDI up to 85% can be reached depending on the used raw material. To fulfill other requirements, flakes PDI can be adjusted by a final flake cooking system. Cooking with addition of water, desuperheated, or saturated steam leads to PDI values between 15% and 85% (Milligan and Suriano, 1974).

Flash desolventizing is possible due to a very high heat and mass transfer surface of the flakes. Vavlitis and Milligan (1993) described that in the case of 0.23 mm thick flakes there is an active surface in the tube of about 6.700 m^2 available. But, if flakes are only a little bit thicker, this active surface will be drastically lower. Finally, spherical particles lead to a very low active surface of about 1.500 m^2 (Vavlitis and Milligan, 1993). Hexane-wetted rapeseed meal has rather a spherical shape than that of flat blanks. Therefore, a flash desolventizer system seems to be unsuitable for gentle desolventizing of rapeseed meal.

A process alternative to realize very high heat and mass transfer coefficients is the application of the fluidized-bed technology. In a joint project, PPM Pilot Pflanzenöltechnologie Magdeburg e.V., Magdeburg, Dr. Weigel Anlagenbau, Magdeburg, and Otto-von-Guericke-University of Magdeburg developed a new batch fluidized-bed desolventizer system. Figure 10.7 shows the principle of the system and Figure 10.8 shows a small pilot scale batch equipment.

A fluidized bed is a quantity of solid particles which are placed by a fluid under such conditions that the solid/fluid mixture behaves as a fluid. In our case, the fluid (superheated hexane) is fed in from the bottom and distributed by a perforated plate. It leaves the separation chamber on top. The meal is fed in from the top and fluidized by the fluid. After treatment, the distributor plate is turned, and the desolventized meal can be removed from the equipment.

The velocity of the fluid must be higher than the minimum fluidized-bed velocity. At the upper end, the velocity has to be lower than the fluctuation velocity above that the meal is discharged. Minimum fluidized-bed velocity and fluctuation velocity depend on particle size. Therefore, the operating range of a stable fluidized bed is defined by the minimum fluidized-bed velocity of the largest particles, and the fluctuation velocity of the smallest particles. In our case particles with a size <0.4 mm would begin to leave the apparatus if the fluid velocity is just high enough that particles of about 5 mm can be fluidized.

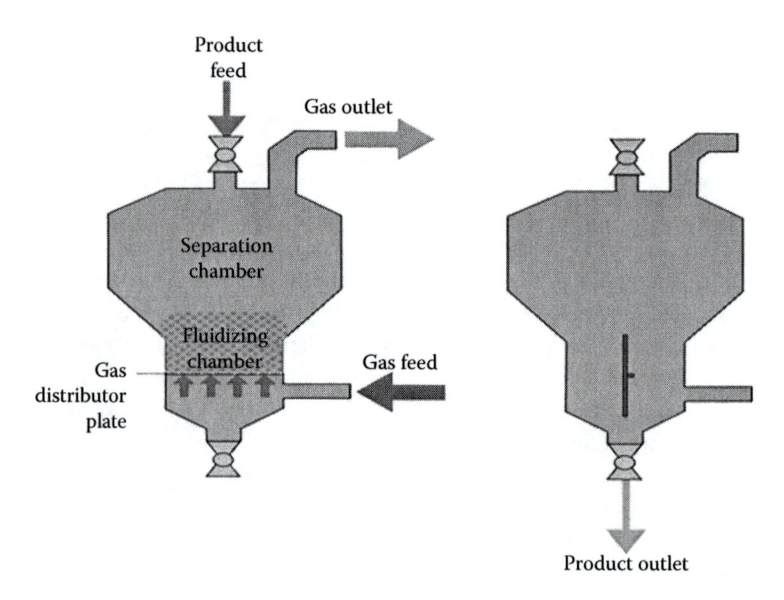

FIGURE 10.7 Scheme of fluidized-bed desolventizer system.

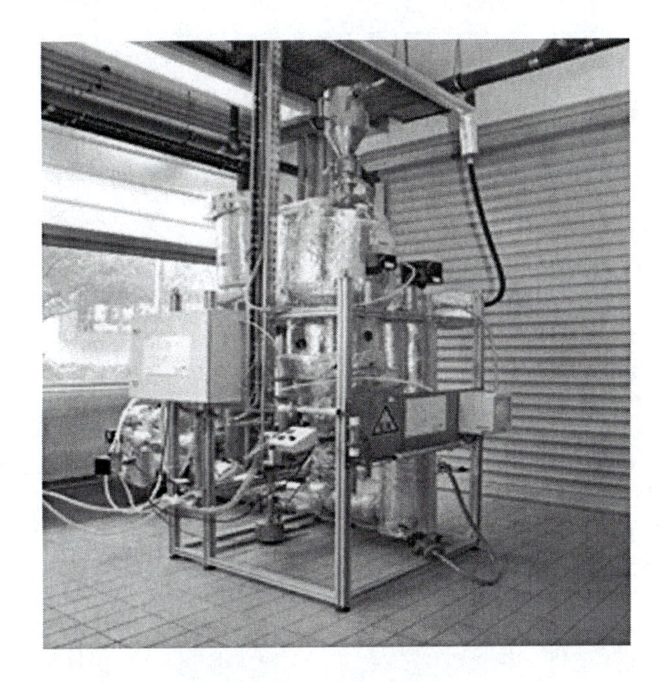

FIGURE 10.8 Small pilot-scale fluidized-bed desolventizer.

We investigated two different operating regimes shown in Figure 10.9. The first one, called total condensation, uses nitrogen as a fluid. The nitrogen is heated and fed by a blower into the fluidized-bed chamber. It removes hexane and water from the meal and then it leaves the apparatus. After filtration, the fluid is totally condensed. Hexane and water are separated, and the nitrogen is led back. The second one, called partial condensation, uses superheated hexane. The batch operation begins with

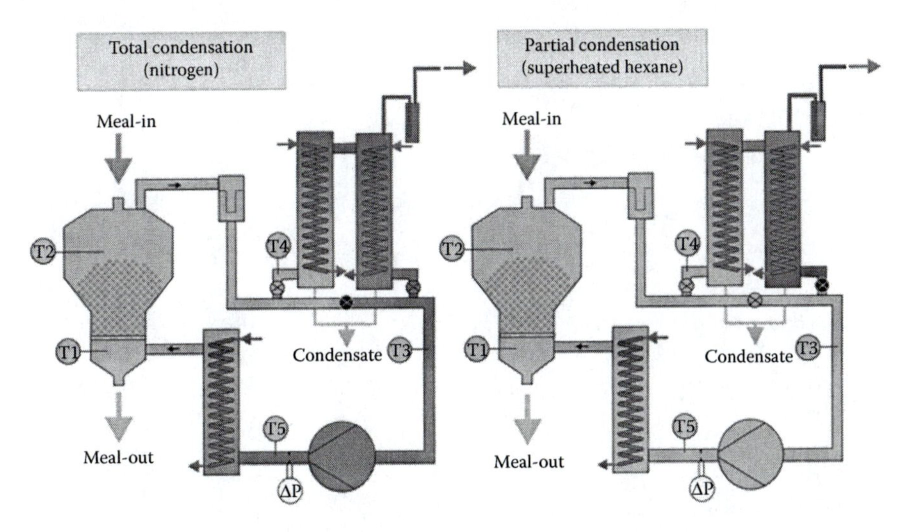

FIGURE 10.9 Operation modes of batch small pilot-scale fluidized-bed desolventizer.

TABLE 10.2
Energy Requirements of Different Operation Modes

	Total Condensation	Partial Condensation
Specific heat power (kWh/kg)	0.57	0.20
Specific cooling power (kWh/kg)	0.54	0.10
Specific electric power (kWh/kg)	0.03	0.028

nitrogen as a fluid in the same way as previously described. But after leaving the filter, the fluid is only partially condensed. In this way, the circulating fluid contains more and more hexane. The carried out experiments showed that by partial condensation mode, the targeted hexane content can be reached after a shorter time. In this case, energy requirements are quite lower than in the case of total condensation mode (Table 10.2).

Table 10.3 shows the results regarding product quality. It is compared with PDI and contents of secondary plant substances of different materials: a commercial press cake from an oil mill, a commercial meal made from this press cake in the same oil mill, two at 75°C and 95°C fluidized-bed desolventized meals, produced by extraction of the commercial press cake in our own small pilot-scale extraction facility as well as an 'air desolventized' meal. The meals desolventized in the fluidized-bed desolventizer have the highest PDI. On the other hand, there is no effect of the fluidized bed desolventizing on secondary plant substances.

Figure 10.10 shows a commercially fluidized-bed desolventized meal. It can be seen that thermal stress influences the appearance considerably.

Table 10.4 shows the main economic data for commercial batch fluidized-bed desolventizing plants shown in Figure 10.11. The 1 m diameter plant has a maximum capacity of 1.200 t per year and the 2 m plant of 6.000 t per year. Now we are going to develop a continuous one (Figure 10.12).

TABLE 10.3
Results of Fluidized-Bed Desolventizing

	PDI (%) AOCS Ba 10b-09	Glucosinolates (µmoL/g) EG 1864/90L (LUFA)	Phytic Acid (g/kg) SAA A004 (OHMI)	Sinapic Acid (g/kg) LC/MS (LUFA)
Commercial press cake (oil mill)	23.7	18.2	16.9	11.5
Commercial meal (oil mill)	13.6	7.0	16.7	8.0
Gentle desolventized meal (fluidized bed, 75°C)	33.4	20.3		13.9
Gentle desolventized meal (fluidized bed, 95°C)	32.0	18.6	14.4	13.6
'Air desolventized' meal	30.4	20.5	16.8	13.7

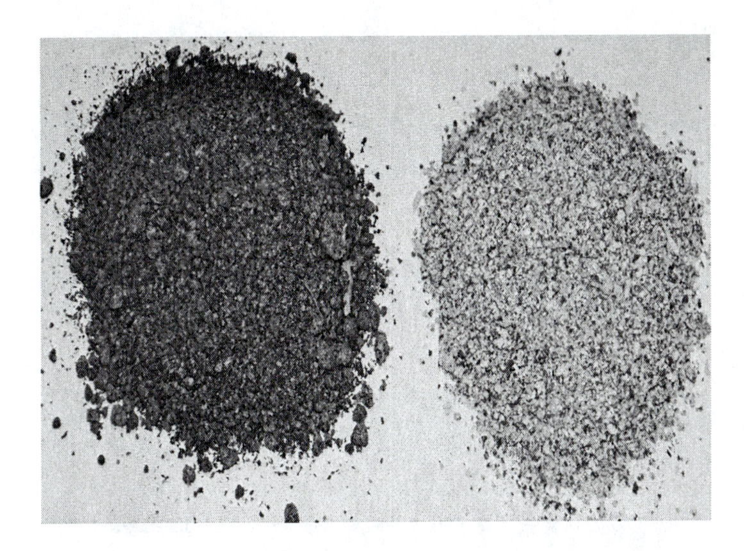

FIGURE 10.10 Commercially (left) and fluidized-bed (right) desolventized rapeseed meal.

TABLE 10.4
Economic Data of Commercial Batch Fluidized-Bed Desolventizing Plants

Fluidized bed chamber diameter:	mm	1000	2000
Capacity meal feed, wet	kg/h	200	1000
Batch size meal feed, wet	kg	100	500
Capacity meal feed, wet			
One shift utilization	kg/a	400,000	2,000,000
Two shift utilization	kg/a	800,000	4,000,000
Three shift utilization	kg/a	1,200,000	6,000,000
Electric power per kg meal feed, wet	kWh/kg	0.23	0.013
Steam per kg meal feed, wet	kg/kg	0.20	0.005
Steel construction [ca. L × B × H]	m	6 × 4 × 4.5	8 × 6 × 6
Required space [ca. L × B × H]	m	12 × 10 × 8	14 × 12 × 11
Suggested plant price (netto)	T€	587	854
Specific financing costs per kg meal feed, wet			
One shift utilization	€/kg	0.336	0.085
Two shift utilization	€/kg	0.189	0.043
Three shift utilization	€/kg	0.140	0.028

Source: Dr. Weigel Anlagenbau GmbH.

10.6 ONGOING RAPESEED PROTEIN APPLICATION PROJECTS

As described above, there are a several interesting possible applications for rapeseed proteins. At PPM, there are actually three projects in development.

The first one investigates the usability of rapeseed protein products as aquafeed. Aquaculture is the fastest-growing food sector (Figure 10.13). In 2009, half of all

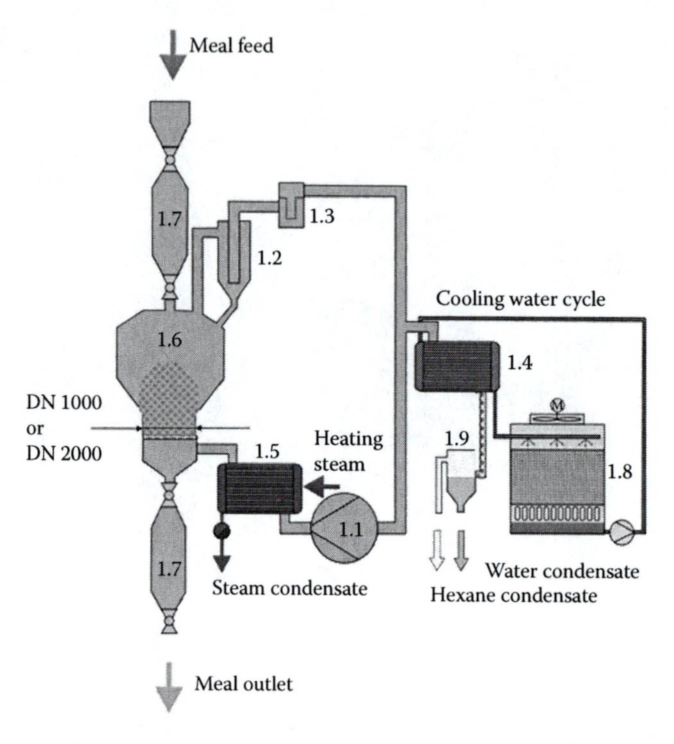

FIGURE 10.11 Design of a batch fluidized-bed desolventizer.

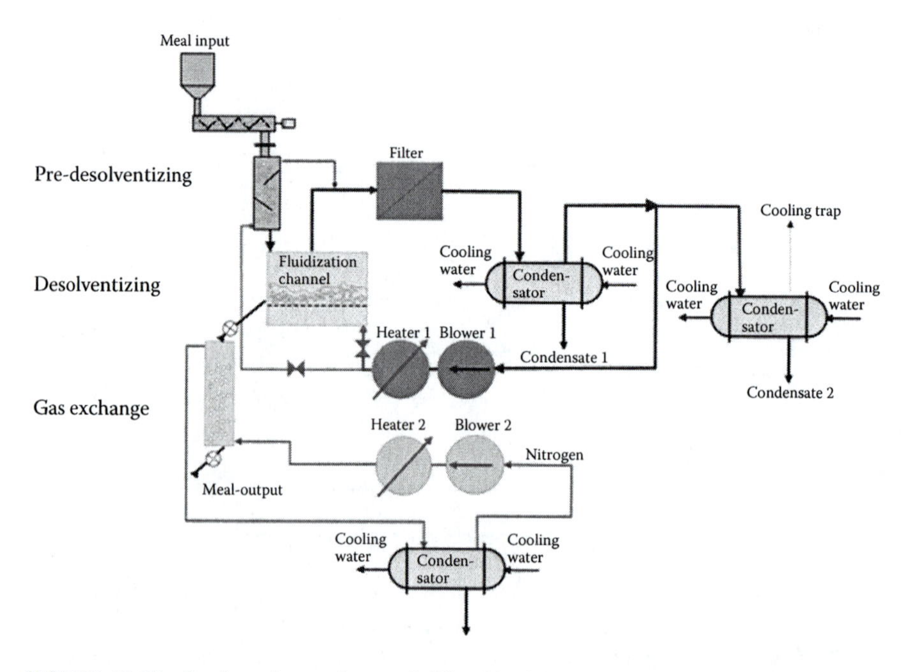

FIGURE 10.12 Design of a continuous fluidized-bed desolventizer.

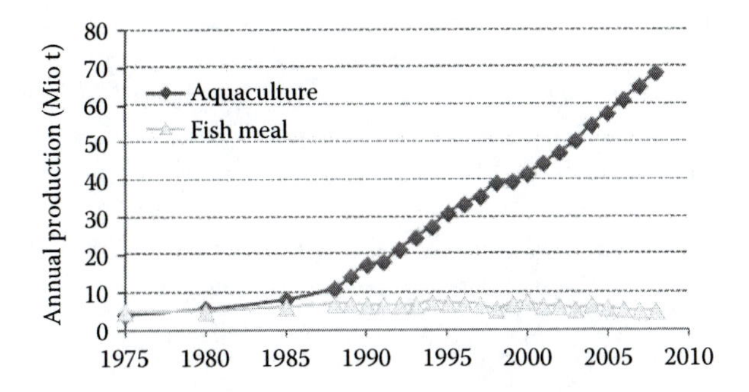

FIGURE 10.13 Development of aquaculture and fish meal production. (From Adem, H. 2011. Bewertung des ernährungsphysiologischen. Potenzials von Rapsproteinfraktionen für die Fischzucht, Projektschlussbericht, Büsum. With permission.)

fish and shellfish destined for human consumption were cultured, and production of farmed fish eclipsed that of wild caught fish. Sixty-eight percent of the worldwide fish meal consumption is used for aquaculture. However, fish meal, the most important source of protein in fish feeds, is a limited resource with an annual production volume between 5 and 6.5 Mio t. Tremendous price increases for fish meal together with environmental concerns, therefore, force the aquaculture sector to find alternative protein sources to be included in fish feeds. Presently, most relevant alternatives are protein concentrates derived from vegetables (Slawski, 2011).

Within a joint project, together with Gesellschaft für Marine Aquakultur, Büsum, Germany, rapeseed protein concentrates and isolates as fish meal replacers in the diets of common carp, turbot, wels catfish, turbot and rainbow trout were tested. The results are to be published by Slawski (2011) and Adem (2011).

The other projects are dealing with the use of rapeseed proteins as

- Additives for plastic films in order to improve vapour barrier and oxygen permeation properties.
- Paper additive in order to improve water retention and coating hold out as well as printability at reduced costs.

Additionally, there is a project running and investigating the possibilities to use the by-products from rapeseed processing (after protein extraction) as fermentation substrates.

10.7 CONCLUSIONS

Since the rapeseed contains two different major storage proteins with quite different properties and some specific secondary plant substances which react with the proteins under certain conditions, rapeseed protein extraction becomes difficult. Each single processing step influences resulting protein yield and quality. Therefore, the process design strongly depends on the targeted application of the extracted proteins.

A modular concept for value-added rapeseed processing was developed based on conventional deoiling done by oil mills. The use of a new fluidized-bed desolventizer system allows gentle solvent removal without PDI decreasing. Other technology steps, like dehulling, pressing under CO_2 atmosphere, or detoxification/refunctionalization steps may lead to further improvements.

After deoiling, rapeseed proteins can be extracted and purified in order to get concentrates, isolates, or pure albumin and cruciferin fractions which are suitable for a wide range of applications in human and animal nutrition as well as for chemical and technical purposes.

In the near future, it is necessary to identify high value and high volume applications for rapeseed proteins in order to initiate first industrial process installations.

REFERENCES

Adem, H. 2011. Bewertung des ernährungsphysiologischen. Potenzials von Rapsproteinfraktionen für die Fischzucht. Projektschlussbericht: Büsum.

Becker, K. W. 1983. Current trends in meal desolventizing. *JAOCS*, **2**, 216–219.

De Kock, J. 2007. Desolventizing and meal quality. *DGF Symposium New Trends in Oilseed Crushing*, Leipzig.

FEDIOL. http://www.fediol.be/6/index.php.

Heckelmann, A. 2010. Entwicklung eines Hochspannungsimpuls-unterstützten Verfahrens zur Verdrängungsextraktion von Ölen und funktionellen Proteinen aus Ölsaaten am Beispiel von Raps (Abschlussbericht AiF 15241 BG). Forschungskreis der Ernährungsindustrie e.V.: Bonn.

Krause, J.-P., J. Kroll and H. M. Rawel 2007. Verarbeitung von Rapssaat—Eigenschaften und Gewinnung von Proteinen. UFOP-Schriften Heft 32. Rapsprotein in der Humanernährung. UFOP: Berlin.

Kroll, J., J.-P. Krause and H. M. Rawel 2007. Native sekundäre Inhaltsstoffe in Rapssamen—Eigenschaften und Wechselwirkungen mit Proteinen. *Deutsche Lebensmittel-Rundschau.*, **4**, 149–153.

Milligan, E. D. and J. F. Suriano 1974. System for production of high and low protein dispersibility index edible extracted soybean flakes. *JAOCS*, **51**, 158–161.

Natsch, A. 2006. Untersuchung der Herstellbarkeit von Rapsproteinprodukten auf der Grundlage verschiedener Entölungsverfahren. Dissertation, TU Berlin: Berlin.

Nazareth, Z. M., A. D. Nicolas and A. J. Lawrence 2009. Functional properties of soy protein isolates prepared from gas-supported screw-pressed soybean meal. *JAOCS*, **86**, 315–321.

Schwenke, K. D. 1994. Rapeseed proteins. In: *New and Developing Sources of Food Proteins*, edited by B. J. F. Hudson. Chapman & Hall.

Slawski, H. 2011. Rapeseed protein products as fish meal replacement in fish nutrition. Dissertation, Christian-Albrechts-Universitat zu Kiel.

Vavlitis, A. and E. D. Milligan 1993. Flash desolventizing. *Proceedings of the World Conference on Oilseed Technology and Utilization*, pp. 286–289. AOCS Press: Champaign, IL, USA.

11 Frying Stability of High-Oleic, Low-Linolenic Canola Oils

Bertrand Matthäus

CONTENTS

11.1 Introduction 203
11.2 Health Aspects of the Frying Medium 204
11.3 Alternatives to Commonly Used Frying Media 205
11.4 Use of High-Oleic, Low-Linolenic Canola Oil during Frying 206
11.4.1 Frying Performance 206
11.4.2 Sensory Quality of the Frying Product 206
11.4.3 Chemical Parameters of the Frying Medium 206
11.4.4 Comparison of the Results for Different Frying Media 208
11.4.5 Results from Other Frying Trails 209
11.5 Influence of the Frying Medium on the Storage Stability of the Fried Product 210
11.6 Conclusion 215
References 215

11.1 INTRODUCTION

Frying is one of the most important methods for the preparation of foods, because it is fast and results in tasty food with a typical flavour and yellow brown colour accepted by the consumer. Consumption of deep-fried food has increased over the last decades, especially since the consumption of frozen food becomes more and more important and fast food is a growing market.

An important influence on the frying process is the frying medium, the oil. It mainly serves as a medium for the heat transfer from the heating source to the food, but additionally the oil is important as it enhances the flavour and is responsible for the typical smell and taste of fried products. Thus, the choice of the frying medium for industrial production as well as for preparation of food at home is of utmost importance for the quality and the taste of the resulting food. The main driving factors for the choice of the frying medium are economical aspects. Availability and price are very important, because the costs caused by the frying medium are a significant factor in the calculation of the total production costs. Another important aspect is the stability of the frying medium during the frying process. This is because during deep-fat frying, the oil is exposed to extreme conditions, such as elevated temperature, over a longer period of time in the presence of water from the frying product and air at the surface from the atmosphere. These extreme conditions of heating cause different chemical reactions in the oil, including hydrolysis and polymerization of unsaturated fatty acids, but also oxidation, if the oil cools down. The result is a change of the composition of the frying medium as well as the formation of volatile chain-scission products, nonvolatile oxidized derivatives and dimeric, polymeric or cyclic substances (Chang et al., 1978; Stevenson et al., 1984; Xu et al., 1999). In this process not only desired components are formed, but also compounds with adverse nutritional effects and potential hazards to human health. Therefore, the frying medium should be stable against oxidation during processing and should not diminish the shelf life of the fried product. This is especially important for snacks and convenient food such as potato crisps or preprepared Berlin doughnuts, which have to be stored over a longer period of time before consumption.

Last but not the least, it has to be taken into consideration that the frying medium becomes a significant part of the food which can significantly influence the quality of the whole product. Depending on the fried product, a lot of oil is taken up during the frying process and after frying, the fatty acid composition of the food has changed towards the fatty acid composition of the frying medium. For example, raw potatoes only contain small amounts of fat, but after frying, potato crisps comprise of nearly 40% of the frying medium. Frying with olive oil resulted in a high amount of oleic acid in the product after frying, whereas after using lard, saturated and monounsaturated fatty acids were predominate in the product (Sanchez-Muniz et al., 1992).

11.2 HEALTH ASPECTS OF THE FRYING MEDIUM

Recently, the nutritional and physiological aspects of foods with undesirable lipids have become a great concern to consumers so that the composition of the frying medium is very important for the preparation of healthier foods. Particular attention has been focussed on the presence of *trans*- and saturated fatty acids in commonly used frying media. A strong correlation between the intake of *trans*-fatty acids and the risk of coronary heart diseases has been identified (Stender et al., 1995; Precht and Molkentin, 1995). *Trans*-fatty acids increase the triacylglycerols and low-density lipoprotein (LDL) levels in blood and decrease the high-density lipoprotein (HDL) level. Thus, the Food and Drug Administration (FDA) and other organizations recommend a maximum intake of *trans*-fatty acids of one energy percent (Anonymous. 2005, 2000; Hahn et al., 2005).

The main source for *trans*-fatty acids is partially hydrogenated fat. Stender et al. (2006) reported that the content of *trans*-fatty acids differed widely in standardized fast-food meals from two well-known restaurants obtained from different countries all over the world. Although it was the same product, the content of *trans*-fatty acids was between 0.5% and 11% for one fast-food restaurant and between 0.5% and 25% for the other one. The differences in the content of *trans*-fatty acids were likely due to the different oil sources used during frying. In this connection, it has to be mentioned that the amount of *trans*-fatty acids formed during the frying process is only very small (Gertz, 2006), so that the high content of *trans*-fatty acids in fried products comes from the frying medium. Consequently, the perfect oil should result in high quality and tasty food in terms of appearance, flavour, aroma, texture and mouthfeeling. It should have a low price, high stability and some advantages with regard to health aspects. For improved oxidative stability during the deep-fat frying process, the use of fats and oils with low unsaturation is advisable, because the oxidation rate of such oils is much lower than for oils with polyunsaturated fatty acids. This fact is important because polyunsaturated fatty acids are, in general, responsible for oxidation and off-flavour development that lower the palatability of fried food (Mounts et al., 1994; Warner and Mounts, 1993; Warner et al., 1994; Warner et al., 1997).

In particular, the high amount of linolenic acid in conventional canola oil has some disadvantages resulting from its high oxidation rate. The subsequent formation of volatile compounds with a low threshold is responsible for unpleasant room-odour during deep-fat frying, a problem also associated with soyabean oil. Carré et al., (2003) showed that already a content of more than 1.1% linolenic acid resulted in significant higher intensities for fishy and paint odours. Therefore, it is recommended to use oils low in linolenic acid for deep-fat frying. On the other side, a certain amount of linolenic acid is necessary for the formation of the typical flavour of the fried products as accepted by the consumer. Nevertheless, different investigations have shown that reduced levels of linolenic acid result in improved quality and stability of the oil (Eskin et al., 1989; Xu et al., 1999).

11.3 ALTERNATIVES TO COMMONLY USED FRYING MEDIA

Today palm olein (PO), hydrogenated peanut oil or other hydrogenated oils were principally used for the industrial preparation of fried food, but also at home hydrogenated fats and oils are in use. These oils are not only characterized by a high smoke point and oxidative stability during the thermal treatment of deep-fat frying and a low amount of polyunsaturated fatty acids, but also by a high content of saturated fatty acids or *trans*-fatty acids with all the described nutritional disadvantages.

Because of the nutritional disadvantages of commonly used frying media, the search for new frying oils with better nutritional properties and comparable thermal and oxidative stability has been underway. More and more vegetable oils rich in oleic acid and zero *trans*-fatty acids have become the focus of interest, because monounsaturated fatty acid lowers LDL in blood, while increasing HDL (Trautwein et al., 1999; Kratz et al., 2002). In addition to this nutritional benefit, oils high in oleic acid are characterized by improved oxidative stability making them suitable for applications where high temperature is used.

By conventional methods and also by genetic techniques, different plants are cultivated in which seed oils contain significantly more oleic acid than the traditional varieties. Such oils, originally developed for technical applications, are also of interest for human nutrition and preparation of food. Especially the higher oxidative stability is interesting for applications where higher temperature is in use. In addition to high-oleic canola oil, high-oleic soyabean and high-oleic sunflower oils (HOSO) are also available. These oils are available with different amounts of oleic acid ranging from 75% to more than 90%. High-oleic canola varieties are available with levels of oleic acid of more than 70% and reduced amounts of linolenic acid.

11.4 USE OF HIGH-OLEIC, LOW-LINOLENIC CANOLA OIL DURING FRYING

11.4.1 FRYING PERFORMANCE

In a frying trial with French fries over a period of 72 h, the frying performance of high-oleic, low-linolenic (HOLL) canola oil was compared with palm olein (PO), high-oleic sunflower oil (HOSO) and partially hydrogenated canola oil (PHCO). For the investigation, fryers, usually applied in household, were used with a frying temperature of 175°C chosen. For the investigation, 2.0 L of the appropriate edible oil was filled into the fryer and afterwards the oil was heated up to 175°C within 10 min. After reaching the temperature of operation, the oil was held at this temperature for 1 h. Afterwards, 50 g batches of pre-fried potatoes were fried for 3.5 min with five frying operations carried out each day. Between each frying step, the fryer was held at 175°C for 1 h without frying material, resulting in a thermal load on the oil of 6 h per day. At the end of each day, the oil was cooled down, filtrated and 200 mL of oil was stored at 6°C until they were analysed. In addition, the French fries were evaluated for sensory impression directly after frying. The next day 200 mL fresh oil was added and the experiment was repeated for 11 successive days. This provided a total thermal load on the oils of 72 h.

11.4.2 SENSORY QUALITY OF THE FRYING PRODUCT

Important for the assessment of a frying process is the quality of the fried product. In addition to the taste of the French fries, the colour, crust and the inner composition of the fried potatoes were evaluated.

With the continuing frying time, the taste of the fried potatoes was judged as inferior in quality. The French fries took on rancid aroma components and the taste turned into bitter, burnt and rancid. Especially French fries deep-fried with PHCO showed a strange smell and taste, which led to a clear devaluation of the products. This is not surprising because it is known that hydrogenated frying oils impart a different type of flavour to food. For French fries obtained with HOLL canola oil, PO and HOSO, respectively, as a frying medium, the taste was still satisfactory for human consumption after 66 h of deep-fat frying (Figure 11.1). On further frying, the French fries were judged as worse. In the first 42 h of frying the assessment of French fries fried in PO and HOSO were both evaluated as better than French fries fried in HOLL canola oil. However, with further frying, the results were comparable. Examination of the other characteristics of the fried products, such as crust, inner composition or colour, showed acceptable results for all oils with respect to the colour of the French fries. The inner composition and the crust were assessed as adequate and good over a frying period of 54 h. For HOLL canola oil and PO, respectively, these parameters were even reasonable after a 66 h of frying. Only the inner composition and the crust of PHCO were evaluated as worse only after 30 h of frying.

11.4.3 CHEMICAL PARAMETERS OF THE FRYING MEDIUM

In the investigation, the amount of polar compounds increased linearly with the frying time, but the content in the oils did not reach the official limit of 24% defined

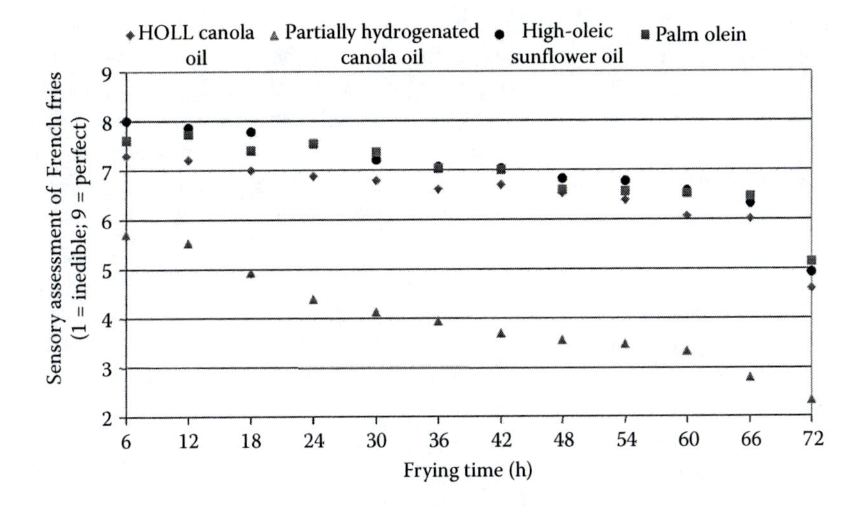

FIGURE 11.1 Sensory evaluation of French fries deep fried in different oils.

in many countries, which would lead to a rejection of the oils (Figure 11.2). The amount of polar compounds in HOLL canola oil, HOSO and PHCO was comparable, but significantly different ($P = 0.01$), with higher amounts of polar compounds in PO, as a result of the higher initial content of this oil. Nevertheless, the increase of polar compounds in PO was similar to that of the other oils, since the slope of the curves was comparable showing that the rate for the formation of polar compounds was comparable for the different oils.

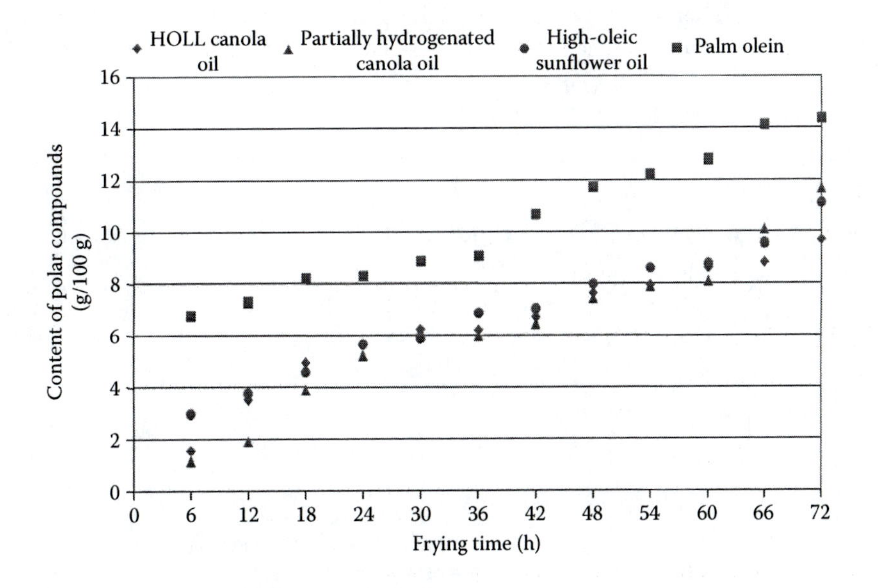

FIGURE 11.2 Polar compounds of oils during frying.

In fresh oils, the amount of oligomer triacylglycerols was below 0.3%, but during deep-fat frying, the content increased linearly with the frying time. None of the oils, however, exceeded the official limit of 12% within the period of frying of 72 h. The differences between the different oils were small, but significant ($P = 0.01$). The lowest amount of oligomer triacylglycerols was found in HOLL canola oil after a frying period of 72 h with about 6% found, whereas, the highest amount was determined in PHCO, with about 7.5% oligomer triacylglycerols. None of the oils exceeded the limit of 2% free fatty acids within a frying period of 72 h. At the beginning of the frying experiment, all oils started with a low amount of free fatty acids (<0.1%), typical for refined oils. With continuous frying, the content of free fatty acids increased in the oils nearly linearly with the frying time, although the slope of the increase was different for the different oils. While the amount of free fatty acids of HOLL canola oil rose to about 0.3%, the highest amount was found for PO with 0.6%.

11.4.4 Comparison of the Results for Different Frying Media

A summarized comparison of the used oils was carried out by the distribution of rank numbers according to the outcome of each oil at the most important parameters for the assessment of the oils after a frying time of 72 h. The oil coming out on the top got a 1 while the worst oil had a 4. After distribution of the rank numbers, the mean value was calculated for each oil. For this assessment the following parameters, oligomer triacylglycerols, polar compounds, free fatty acids as well as the sensory evaluation of the oil and the French fries were used.

Table 11.1 shows that no significant differences ($P < 0.01$) were found between HOLL canola oil, HOSO and PHCO concerning the total assessment of the results. Nevertheless it was obvious that HOLL canola oil showed clear advantages with regard to sensory evaluation, both oil and product, while PHCO revealed better results for the chemical parameters but had the worst sensory evaluation. Further on it should be pointed out that only small differences in the chemical parameters of all oils were found. Only the total result of the assessment of PO was significantly worse than the results of the other oils ($P < 0.01$).

TABLE 11.1
Summarized Results, Calculated from the Most Important Parameters

Type of Oil	Oligomer Triacyl-glycerols	Polar Compounds	Free Fatty Acids	Sensory Evaluation (Oil)	Sensory Evaluation (French Fries)	Total Result
HOLL canola oil	2	3	4	1	1	2.2
HOSO	3	1	2	4	1	2.2
PHCO	1	2	1	4	4	2.4
PO	4	4	3	4	1	3.2

Note: HOLL canola oil = High-oleic, low-linolenic canola oil; PHCO = Partially hydrogenated canola oil; HOSO = High-oleic sunflower oil; PO = Palm olein.

11.4.5 Results from Other Frying Trails

In another frying trial by Xu et al. (1999), three HOLL canola oils with different levels of linolenic acid and HOSO were compared with commercial PO. The oils were heated over a period of 80 h at 190°C by frying potato chips. Fatty acid analysis, iodine value, colour index, dielectric constant, free fatty acids and the total polar compounds were used for the assessment of the suitability of the oils. Additionally, a sensory evaluation was carried out.

The amount of polar compounds increased significantly during frying and was strongly correlated to the frying time. At the beginning of the frying trial, the amount was at 2.2–2.8% for the unusual oils and increased during 80 h of frying to a final level of 47.5% (high-linolenic canola oil), 45.8% (medium-linolenic canola oil), 44.6% (HOSO and PO), 43.7% (low-linolenic canola oil) and 35.6% PHCO. The authors used 27% polar compounds as a regulatory parameter for frying oils which resulted in a stability ranking of the oils as: PHCO > low-linolenic canola oil > HOSO > PO > medium-linolenic canola oil > high-linolenic canola oil. However, the authors concluded from the small differences between PO and high-oleic canola oil that only PHCO could have been used for a longer time.

The amount of free fatty acids increased in all oils during frying, but the highest increase was found for PO, HOSO and PHCO. The three high-oleic canola oils had significantly lower rates, but the differences between these oils were not significant.

The fried products were tasted with a large group consisting of 36 tasters with 10 trained oil tasters. The results showed that chips from canola oil with low and medium linolenic acid were significantly better than chips from the other oils. Chips from PHCO had a very different taste with a higher intensity of unpleasant aroma components, typically for hydrogenated oils.

In summary, the result of this investigation was that PO had a similar frying performance as high-oleic, low-linolenic (HOLL) canola oil, while it was better than the other oils.

In a later paper, Xu et al. (2000) found slightly different results. PO was compared with HOLL canola oil as well as two blends of canola oil and PO (70:30 and 30:70, respectively), in two 80 h frying trials. In all oils, the amount of free fatty acids and total polar compounds increased significantly during the processing. HOLL canola oil and blended canola oil (70:30) had higher oxidative stability, less free fatty acids and polar compounds with continually frying time. Concerning the sensory scores for taste and overall quality, HOLL canola oil was evaluated better than the blended oils and PO. Gertz (2006) presented a comprehensive investigation comparing several commercial fats and oils. In this work, the increase of polar compounds was comparable for PO and HOSO, while HOLL canola oil showed a significant faster formation of polar compounds during the 16 h frying trial at 180°C.

From the results, it can be concluded that HOLL canola oil is a good alternative to other commonly used oils for deep frying, with some advantages regarding nutritional aspects as well as the sensory quality of the oil and products. The low level of saturated fatty acids, no *trans*-fatty acids and the high content of oleic acid comparable to olive oil makes HOLL canola oil an attractive recommendation for the use in the preparation of deep-fried food. In addition, the results show that the use of HOLL canola oil during frying results in high quality products with a long shelf life. Therefore, this oil seems to be an interesting alternative for applications using higher temperature during the preparation of food.

11.5 INFLUENCE OF THE FRYING MEDIUM ON THE STORAGE STABILITY OF THE FRIED PRODUCT

The high thermal stability of the frying medium must be taken into consideration as the sensory quality of products produced with oils high in linolenic acid becomes rancid very fast during storage. It is known that potato crisps fried in conventional canola oil had the best flavour directly after frying in comparison to other oils. However, product quality greatly diminished during storage while product quality remained stable for products fried in palm and peanut oil over a period of 16 weeks (Weber and Putz, 2004). This means that frying with conventional canola oil results in tasty food which consists of healthy oil, but during storage, the product becomes inedible in a very short period of time. Consequently, oils low in linolenic acid and high in oleic acid could dramatically improve the storage stability of the products.

In a storage experiment, the behaviour of Berlin doughnuts and potato crisps fried in HOLL canola oil at 170°C or 180°C and 175°C, respectively, was compared over a storage period of 12– 24 weeks, respectively, with products fried in HOSO, PO and different types of partially hydrogenated fats (PHF), high-oleic, low-*trans* (HOLT), high-palmitic, low-*trans* (HPLT) and high-*trans* (HT). Berlin doughnuts were stored at –18°C in plastic bags, while potato crisps were stored at room temperature under nitrogen and normal atmosphere, respectively. During storage, the quality of products fried in HOLL canola oil was comparable with products fried in the other commonly used oils with regard to parameters characterizing the oxidative state of the products.

Often the peroxide value is useful to follow the oxidative deterioration of fats and oils. In the case of deep-fat frying, the use of this parameter is problematical because peroxides are destroyed by high temperature and during cooling new peroxides are formed (Augustin and Berry, 1983). Therefore, Fritsch (1981) concluded that the determination of the peroxide value is not suitable for the assessment of used frying oils. In contrast to the peroxide value, the anisidine value does not measure primary products of the oxidation process, but secondary decomposition products such as carbonyl compounds (aldehydes and ketones). The totox value is calculated as twofold the peroxide value plus the anisidine value. Therefore, the totox value describes the development of the primary and secondary degradation products during oxidation giving sufficient information about the oxidative state of a product.

A totox value of 30 has been suggested by the industry and official authorities as a maximum limit. All samples of potato crisps stored under nitrogen came out below this value after 24 weeks of storage (Figure 11.3). Samples stored under normal atmosphere had totox values that exceeded the limit during storage. For all samples stored under nitrogen, the totox value was comparable in the range between 26 (HOSO) and 30 (PO). Only the totox value of potato crisps fried in HOSO was significantly lower than the totox values of the other samples ($P = 0.01$). The differences between the different oils were a little higher for storage under normal atmosphere. These differences were statistically significant ($P = 0.01$) and were found in the range between

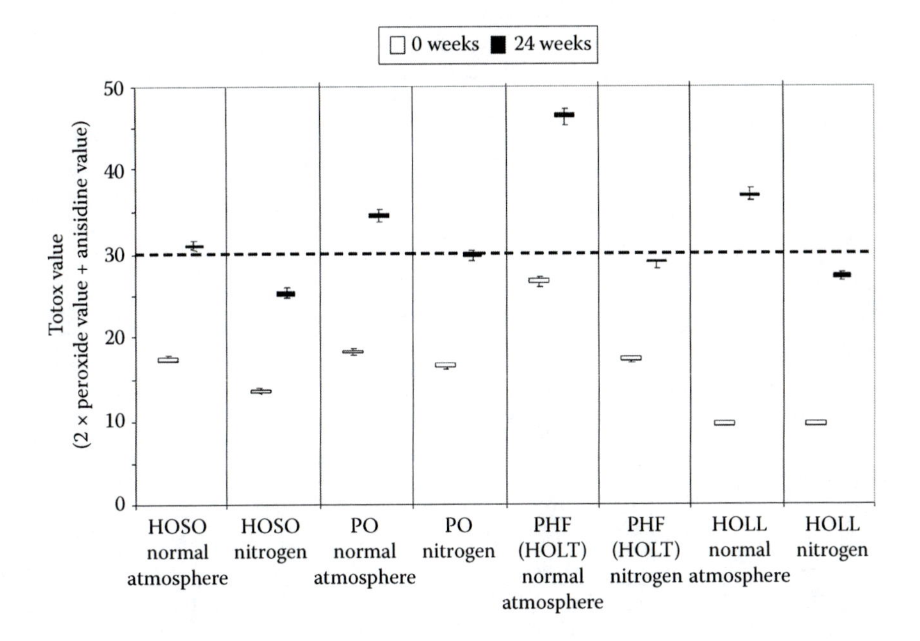

FIGURE 11.3 Totox value in potato crisps during storage.

31 (HOSO) and 47 (PHF (HOLT). The totox value for potato crisps fried in HOLL canola oil was the lowest just after preparation. The situation was different for the storage of Berlin doughnuts. During storage for 12 weeks, only products fried in PHF (HT) at 170 and 180°C, respectively and HOLL canola oil at 170°C were below a limit of 30 for the totox value (Figure 11.4). All other oils reached the limit in a very short period of time. In the case of PHF (HPLT) and PO used at 180°C, the limit was already exceeded directly after preparation of Berlin doughnuts. The result also showed the negative effect of a high frying temperature. While the increase of the totox value was moderate when using a temperature of 170°C, the increase was more pronounced at 180°C, because of a higher initial formation of oxidation products during processing.

In contrast to the oligomer triacylglycerols, the totox value is more suitable as an indicator for the deterioration of the products during storage. After heating the oil, the formation of deterioration products goes further on in the fried food depending on the storage conditions and the nature of food fried.

Tocopherols/tocotrienols are characterized by a high susceptibility against autoxidation at high temperatures. The highest amount of tocopherols/tocotrienols was in the potato crisps fried in PO, while the concentration in the products fried in other oils was significantly lower ($P = 0.01$), but quite similar to each other. After 24 weeks of storage of potato crisps, the highest degradation of tocopherols/tocotrienols was found for products fried in PO. The reduction came to about 50%, while the rate of degradation in products fried in the other oils came to about 25% (Figure 11.5).

One reason for the faster degradation of tocopherols/tocotrienols in PO could be that this oil contained mainly tocotrienols. They have a higher antioxidant activity

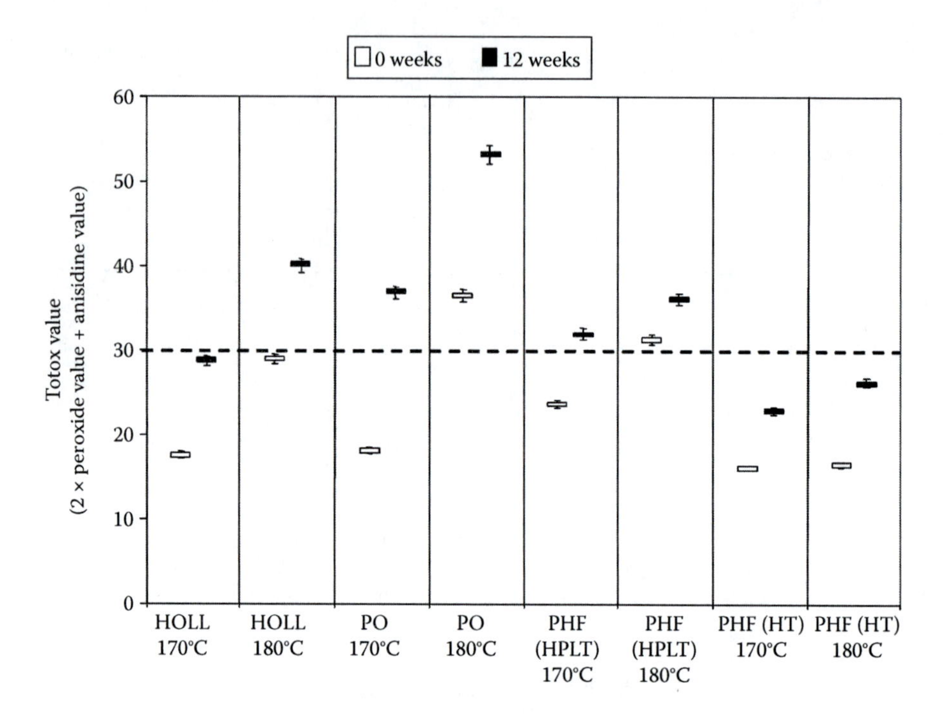

FIGURE 11.4 Totox value in Berlin doughnuts during storage.

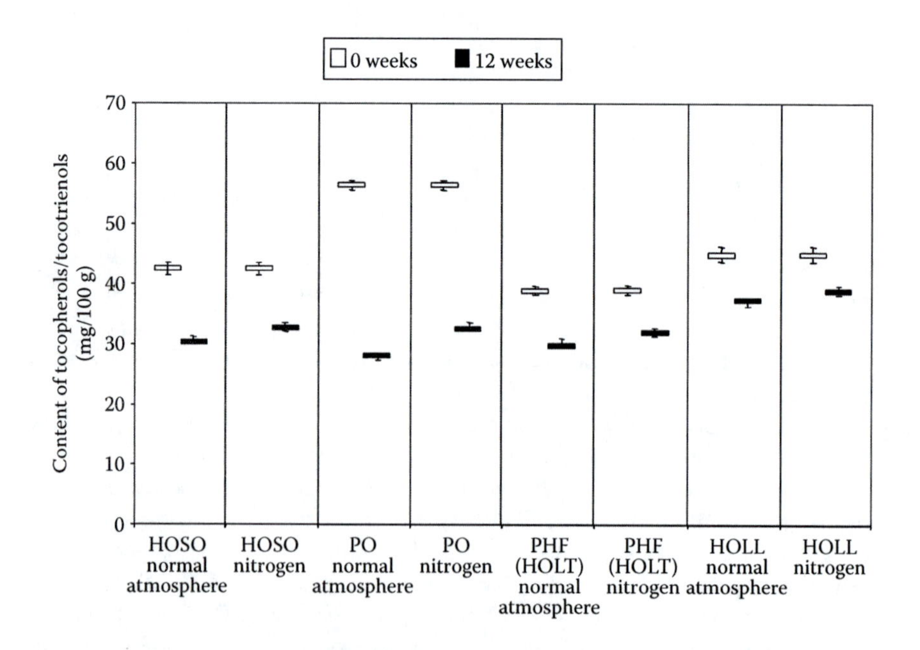

FIGURE 11.5 Content of tocopherols/tocotrienols in potato crisps during storage.

than tocopherols, resulting in a faster degradation during oxidation reactions (Packer et al., 2001).

Products stored over a period of 24 weeks, after being fried in HOLL canola oil, still contained the highest amount of tocopherols/tocotrienols. Again, a positive effect of a nitrogen atmosphere was found. All samples stored under nitrogen contained slightly higher concentrations of tocopherols/tocotrienols, although, the difference was only statistically significant ($P = 0.01$) for PO stored under normal atmosphere and nitrogen.

Depending on the composition, a certain degradation of tocopherols/tocotrienols was found during storage of potato crisps. But after 24 weeks of storage, about 30 mg/100 g tocopherols/tocotrienols were detectable in all the products. No degradation of tocopherols/tocotrienols took place (results not shown) in Berlin doughnuts stored over 12 weeks at −18°C.

The sensory evaluation of the potato crisps, appearance, consistency and smell and taste were tested by a trained sensory panel with the results combined to a weighted quality score in the range from 0 to 5. The results showed the sensory quality of potato crisps fried in HOLL canola oil was comparable with potato crisps fried in PO and PHF (HOLT) with no significant difference between the different oils ($P = 0.01$) when the samples were stored under normal atmosphere (Figure 11.6a).

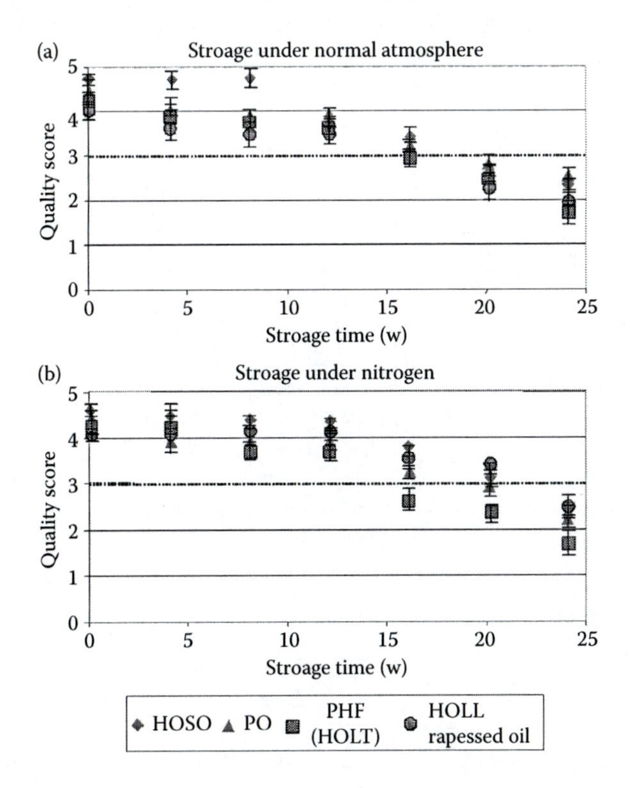

FIGURE 11.6 Result of the sensory evaluation of potato crisps stored under (a) normal and (b) nitrogen atmospheres.

Under normal atmosphere, the samples were storable for 16 weeks before the quality score fell below 3, which is the limit for product acceptability. The quality score of potato crisps fried in HOSO was significantly better than for products fried in the other oils in the first 8 weeks of storage. After 8 weeks of storage, there was no significant difference between the quality score of all the samples ($P = 0.01$). The storage time was extended up to 20 weeks for HOSO, HOLL canola oil and PO, for samples stored under nitrogen (Figure 11.6b). However, sensory scores of samples fried in PHF (HOLT) fell below a score of 3 at the 16-week test. Again, no significant difference was found between samples fried in HOSO, HOLL canola oil and PO after 20 weeks of storage ($P = 0.01$).

At the beginning of the storage experiment, the taste and smell of all fresh Berlin doughnuts was agreeable, independent of the oil used for frying and the frying temperature (Table 11.2). Only frying in HOLL canola oil at 180°C resulted in a slight abnormal smell, which was different from high quality Berlin doughnuts. At 170°C, this negative smell was not noticeable. During storage over a period of 12 weeks, the taste and smell of nearly all products changed significantly. While products fried in PHF (HPLT) showed an abnormal taste and smell after 12 weeks of storage, products fried in PHF (HT) only had a slight strange taste. The best results were obtained with PO. After 12 weeks of storage, no deterioration of the sensory characteristics was detected. HOLL canola oil had a slight abnormal smell after 12 weeks for products fried at 170°C. The products were inedible after 12 weeks when 180°C was used to fry the product.

TABLE 11.2
Result of the Sensory Evaluation of Berlin Doughnuts

	Taste		Smell	
	Fresh	3 Months	Fresh	3 Months
Frying Medium	**Frying Temperature: 170°C**			
High-oleic, low-linolenic rapeseed oil	Perfect	Slight oily, abnormal taste	Normal	Slight abnormal smell
Palm olein	Perfect	Slight oily	Neutral	Normal
Partially hydrogenated fat (HPLT)	Perfect	Abnormal taste	Neutral	Abnormal smell
Partially hydrogenated fat (HT)	Perfect	Slight abnormal taste	Neutral	Slight abnormal smell
Frying Medium	**Frying Temperature: 180°C**			
High-oleic, low-linolenic rapeseed oil	Perfect	Abnormal taste	Slight abnormal smell	Abnormal smell
Palm olein	Perfect	Normal	Neutral	Normal
Partially hydrogenated fat (HPLT)	Perfect	Abnormal taste	Neutral	Abnormal smell
Partially hydrogenated fat (HT)	Perfect	Slight abnormal taste	Neutral	Slight abnormal smell

11.6 CONCLUSION

The search for healthier fats and oils as frying media is an ongoing process. HOLL canola oil can be an alternative to commonly used frying media. The oil showed comparable oxidative and thermal stability during frying similar to commonly used frying media and produced tasty food of good quality. During storage, products fried in HOLL canola oil varied depending on the product. While the change in quality of potato crisps is comparable to other oils, Berlin doughnuts were significantly less acceptable than Berlin doughnuts fried in PO.

REFERENCES

Anonymous. 2005. *U.S. Department of Health and Human Services and U.S. Department of Agriculture. Dietary Guidelines for Americans.* 6th Edition, Washington, DC: U.S. Government Printing Office.

Anonymous. 2000. Referenzwerte für die Nährstoffzufuhr. Deutsche Gesellschaft für Ernährung, Österreichische Gesellschaft für Ernährung, Schweizerische Gesellschaft für Ernährungsforschung, Schweizerische Vereinigung für Ernährung, 1. Auflage, Umschau Braus GmbH, Verlagsgesellschaft, Frankfurt am Main.

Augustin, M.A. and Berry, S.K. 1983. Efficacy of the antioxidants BHA and BHT in palm olein during heating and frying. *J. Am. Oil Chem. Soc.* 60: 1520–1522.

Carré, P., Dartenuc, C., Evrard, J., Judde, A., Labalette, F., Renard, R. and Raoux, M. 2003. Frying stability of rapeseed oils with modified fatty acid compositions. In: *Proceedings of the 11th International Rapeseed Congress.* Sorensen, H., Sorensen, J.C., Sorensen, S., Muguerza, N.B. and Bjergegaard, C. eds. Narayana Press. pp. 540–543.

Gertz, Ch. 2006. What happens in the fryer? *Workshop 'Frittieren, Backen, Braten'*, pp. 29–30. Wien, Austria.

Chang, S.S., Peterson, R.J. and Ho, C. 1978. Chemical reactions involved in the deep-fat frying of foods. *J. Am. Oil Chem. Soc.* 55: 718–727.

Eskin, N.A.M., Vaisey-Genser, M., Durance-Todd, S. and Przybylski, R. 1989. Stability of low linolenic acid canola oil to frying temperatures. *J. Amer. Oil Chem. Soc.* 66: 1081–1084.

Fritsch, C.W. 1981. Measurements of frying fat deterioration. *J. Amer. Oil Chem. Soc.* 55: 718–727.

Hahn, A., Ströhle, A., Wolters, M., Siekmann, D. and Lechler, T. 2005. Atherosklerose und Dyslipoproteinämien: *Trans*-Fettsäuren. In: *Ernährung—Physiologische Grundlagen, Prävention, Therapie*, pp. 371–372. Wissenschaftliche Verlagsgesellschaft mbH, 70191 Stuttgart.

Jutteland, A. 2004. *Trans* fats: Status and solutions. *Food Technol.* 58: 20–22.

Mounts, T.L., Warner, K., List, G.R., Neff, W.E. and Wilson, R.F. 1994. Low linolenic acid soybean oils: Alternatives to frying oils. *J. Am. Oil Chem. Soc.* 71: 495–499.

Kratz, M., Cullen, P., Kannenberg, F., Kassner, A., Fobker, M., Abuja P.M., Asmann, G. and Wahrburg, U. 2002. Effects of dietary fatty acids on the composition and oxidizability of low-density lipoprotein. *Eur. J. Clin. Nutr.* 56: 72–81.

Packer, L., Weber, S.U. and Rimbach, G. 2001. Molecular aspects of alpha-tocotrienol antioxidant action and cell signalling. *J. Nutr.* 131: 369–373.

Precht, D. and Molkentin, J. 1995. *Trans* fatty acids: Implications for health, analytical methods, incidence in edible fats and intake. *Die Nahrung.* 39: 343–374.

Sanchez- Muniz, F., Viejo, M. and Medina, R. 1992. Deep frying of sardines in different culinary fats. Change in the fatty acid composition of sardines and frying fats. *J. Agric. Food Chem.* 40: 2252–2256.

Stender, S., Dyerberg, J., Holmer, G., Ovesen, L. and Sandström, B. 1995. The influence of trans fatty acids on health: A report from The Danish Nutrition Council. *Clin. Sci.* 88: 375–392.

Stender, S., Dyerberg, J. and Astrup, A. 2006. High levels of industrially produced trans fat in popular fast foods. *N. Engl. J. Med.* 354: 1650–1652

Stevenson, S., Vaisey, M. and Eskin, N.A.M. 1984. Quality control in the use of deep fat frying oils. *J. Am. Oil Chem. Soc.* 61: 1102–1108.

Trautwein, E.A., Rieckhoff, D., Kunath-Rau, A. and Erbersdobler, H.F. 1999. Replacing saturated fat with PUFA-rich (sunflower oil) or MUFA-rich (rapeseed, olive and high-oleic sunflower oil) fats resulted in comparable hypocholesterolemic effects in cholesterol-fed hamsters. *Ann. Nutr. Metabo.* 43: 159–172.

Warner, K. and Mounts, T.L. 1993. Frying stability of soybean and canola oils with modified fatty acid compositions. *J. Am. Oil Chem. Soc.* 70: 983–988.

Warner, K., Orr, P., Parrott, L. and Glynn, M. 1994. Effects of frying oil composition on potato chip stability. *J. Am. Oil Chem. Soc.* 71: 1117–1121.

Warner, K., Orr, P. and Glynn, M. 1997. Effect of fatty acid composition of oils on flavor and stability of fried foods. *J. Am. Oil Chem. Soc.* 74: 347–356.

Weber, L. and Putz, B. 2004. Einfluss des Herstellungsprozesses auf die Haltbarkeit von Chips. *Kartoffelbau.* 7: 274–276.

Xu, X.-Q., Tran, V.H., Palmer, M., White, K. and Salisury, P. 1999. Chemical and physical analyses and sensory evaluation of six deep-frying oils. *J. Am. Oil Chem. Soc.* 76: 1091–1099.

Xu, X.-Q., Tran, V.H., Palmer, M.V., White, K. and Salisbury, P. 2000. Chemical, physical and sensory properties of Monola oil, palm olein, and their blends in deep frying trails. *Food Aust.* 52: 77–82.

12 Biodiesel from Mustard Oil

Titipong Issariyakul and Ajay K. Dalai

CONTENTS

12.1 Introduction 217
12.2 Mustard Oil as Feedstock for Biodiesel Production 220
12.3 Biodiesel Quality 222
12.4 Biodiesel Production from Mustard Oil 229
12.5 Reaction Kinetics 230
12.6 Lubricity Property of Biodiesel 233
12.7 Biodiesel Production in Canada 237
Acknowledgement 239
References 239

12.1 INTRODUCTION

Biodiesel is composed of monoalkyl esters of long-chain fatty acids derived from renewable sources such as vegetable oils or animal fats (Ma and Hanna, 1999; Fukuda et al., 2001; Knothe, 2005; Knothe and Dunn, 2005; Moser, 2011). It can be used as an alternative fuel to petroleum diesel fuel. The advantages of the use of biodiesel over petroleum diesel fuel include lower overall exhaust emissions (Knothe and Dunn, 2005; Reaney et al., 2005; Knothe, 2010), superior lubricity and flash point (Reaney et al., 2005), renewability, low toxicity and biodegradability (Knothe, 2010). In addition, it is miscible in petroleum diesel fuel in all proportion and can be used in diesel engine with no engine modification required as pure or blended with petroleum diesel fuel (Knothe, 2005). The disadvantages of biodiesel include high feedstock cost, lower heating values, inferior low-temperature operatability and oxidative stability, and in some cases, higher NO_x exhaust emissions (Knothe, 2010; Moser, 2011).

Biodiesel is commonly produced from a chemical reaction called 'transesterification' of lipid sources such as vegetable oils and animal fats. Fats and oils are composed mainly of triacylglyceride (TAG), which is three fatty acid chains attached to a glycerol backbone. Each vegetable oil and animal fat is differentiated by the type of fatty acid chain attached to the glycerol backbone. Figure 12.1 shows the transesterification scheme where TAG reacts with 3 mol of a short-chain monohydric alcohol such as methanol usually in the presence of a catalyst to form 3 mol of fatty acid acyl ester (FAAE) and glycerol. The reaction mechanism consists of three

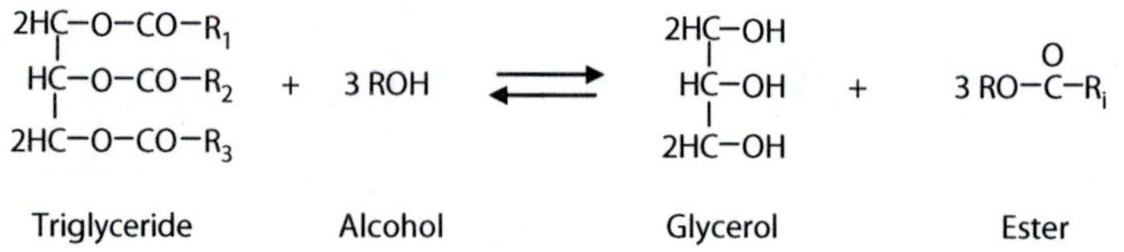

$$
\begin{array}{l} 2HC\text{–}O\text{–}CO\text{–}R_1 \\ \;\;HC\text{–}O\text{–}CO\text{–}R_2 \\ 2HC\text{–}O\text{–}CO\text{–}R_3 \end{array} + 3\,ROH \rightleftharpoons \begin{array}{l} 2HC\text{–}OH \\ \;\;HC\text{–}OH \\ 2HC\text{–}OH \end{array} + 3\,RO\text{–}\overset{O}{\overset{\|}{C}}\text{–}R_i
$$

Triglyceride Alcohol Glycerol Ester

FIGURE 12.1 Scheme for transesterification.

consecutive reaction steps starting from triacylglyceride (TAG) to diacylglyceride (DAG) to mono-acyl-glyceride (MAG) to glycerol (GL), respectively as shown in Figure 12.2 (Ma and Hanna, 1999; Moser, 2011). In each step, the reaction consumes 1 mol of alcohol and produces 1 mol of ester. Stoichiometrically, each mole of TAG requires 3 mol of alcohol to yield 3 mol of FAAE as shown in Figure 12.1; however, due to the reversible nature of the reaction steps, excess alcohol is usually required to shift the reaction equilibrium to the product.

The alcohol used in transesterification is usually methanol due to its beneficial economics (Ma and Hanna, 1999) and superior reactivity (Sridharan and Mathai, 1974). The disadvantages of using methanol are dependency on petroleum sources and low solubility of TAG in methanol. It is reported that a minimum mixing time of 3 min is required to sustain methanolysis of soyabean oil (Zhou and Boocock, 2006). The lag time of 2–3 min during methanolysis of soyabean oil and sunflower oil is also reported (Freedman et al., 1986; Mittelbach and Trathnigg, 1990). These reports illustrate the immiscible behaviour of TAG in methanol. This immiscibility behaviour is often referred to as mass transfer resistance or mass transfer limitation which can be overcome by several methods, including the use of rigorous mechanical stirring (Lifka and Ondruschka, 2004; Vicente et al., 2005; Meher et al., 2006a,

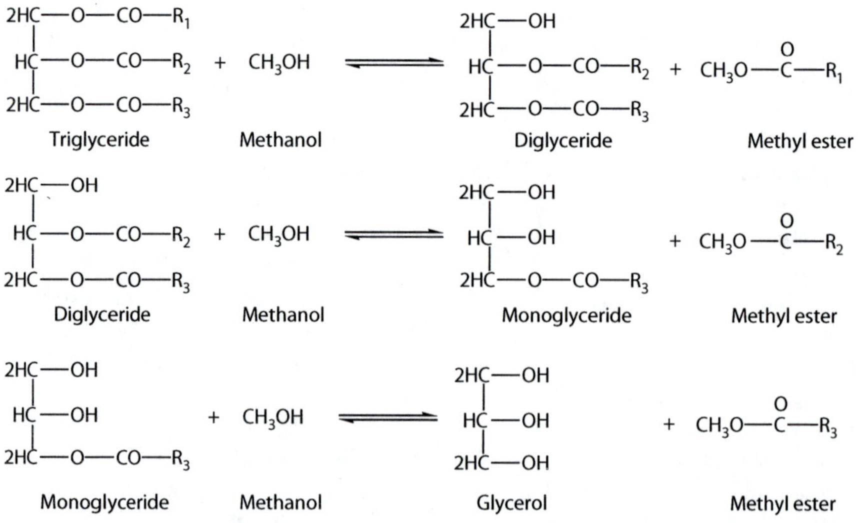

$$
\begin{array}{l} 2HC\text{—}O\text{—}CO\text{—}R_1 \\ \;\;HC\text{—}O\text{—}CO\text{—}R_2 \\ 2HC\text{—}O\text{—}CO\text{—}R_3 \end{array} + CH_3OH \rightleftharpoons \begin{array}{l} 2HC\text{—}OH \\ \;\;HC\text{—}O\text{—}CO\text{—}R_2 \\ 2HC\text{—}O\text{—}CO\text{—}R_3 \end{array} + CH_3O\text{—}\overset{O}{\overset{\|}{C}}\text{—}R_1
$$

Triglyceride Methanol Diglyceride Methyl ester

$$
\begin{array}{l} 2HC\text{—}OH \\ \;\;HC\text{—}O\text{—}CO\text{—}R_2 \\ 2HC\text{—}O\text{—}CO\text{—}R_3 \end{array} + CH_3OH \rightleftharpoons \begin{array}{l} 2HC\text{—}OH \\ \;\;HC\text{—}OH \\ 2HC\text{—}O\text{—}CO\text{—}R_3 \end{array} + CH_3O\text{—}\overset{O}{\overset{\|}{C}}\text{—}R_2
$$

Diglyceride Methanol Monoglyceride Methyl ester

$$
\begin{array}{l} 2HC\text{—}OH \\ \;\;HC\text{—}OH \\ 2HC\text{—}O\text{—}CO\text{—}R_3 \end{array} + CH_3OH \rightleftharpoons \begin{array}{l} 2HC\text{—}OH \\ \;\;HC\text{—}OH \\ 2HC\text{—}OH \end{array} + CH_3O\text{—}\overset{O}{\overset{\|}{C}}\text{—}R_3
$$

Monoglyceride Methanol Glycerol Methyl ester

FIGURE 12.2 Scheme for stepwise transesterification mechanism.

2006), an aid of co-solvent (Boocock et al., 1996), the use of supercritical conditions (Kusdiana and Saka, 2004; Saka et al., 2010) and the use of other techniques such as microwave (El Sherbiny et al., 2010; Kumar et al., 2011) and ultrasonic (Colucci et al., 2005; Singh et al., 2007). Once the initial mass transfer is overcome, the reaction is initiated; DAG and MAG are formed as the reaction intermediates and act as surfactants to enhance the mass transfer of TAG into methanol. Attempts to improve the mass transfer of TAG have been made by using other alcohols such as ethanol, propanol and butanol (Lang et al., 2001a; Meneghetti et al., 2006; Kucek et al., 2007). Biodiesel produced using bioethanol is completely renewable. The main disadvantage of ethanolysis is the lower reactivity of ethoxide. When alcohol reacts with homogeneous base catalysts, alkoxides, which are the actual catalysts, are formed. If ethanol is used instead of methanol, the carbon chain length is increased which leads to a decrease in nucleophilicity and consequently a reduction in reactivity of ethoxide as compared to methoxide (Sridharan and Mathai, 1974). It was found that when waste fryer grease is transesterified with a mixture of methanol and ethanol at equal molar ratio, the resulting biodiesel contains 50% more FAME than FAEE (Issariyakul et al., 2007), which illustrates the higher reactivity of methoxide as compared to ethoxide. The lower polarity of ethanol has advantage and disadvantage on transesterification process. On the one hand, the lower polarity of ethanol alleviates the initial mass transfer resistance encountered in the case of methanolysis, hence increasing the initial rate of the reaction. On the other hand, it improves mutual miscibility of ester and glycerol in which the catalyst resides and therefore promotes saponification. In the case of ethanolysis, saponification occurs faster and soap concentration in biodiesel phase is higher than methanolysis (Mendow et al., 2011). Saponification if occurred would result in a reduction in ester yield as well as consumption of the catalyst. It was found that during ethanolysis of sunflower oil, 95% of sodium hydroxide initially loaded in the reactor is converted into sodium soap within 5 min. The soap formation not only lowers the ester yield, but also complicates the glycerol separation step in biodiesel purification process. In order for phase separation to occur, an additional step such as ethanol evaporation (Bouaid et al., 2009) or glycerol addition (Issariyakul et al., 2008) is necessary. An alternative solution is to use mixtures of methanol and ethanol (Kulkarni et al., 2007; Issariyakul et al., 2007; Issariyakul and Dalai, 2010).

The most common catalysts used commercially in transesterification are homogeneous bases such as KOH, NaOH, $KOCH_3$ or $NaOCH_3$ due to fast reaction rate, less corrosion, ambient temperature operatibility and economical advantages (Lang et al., 2001a; Colucci et al., 2005; Meneghetti et al., 2006; Issariyakul et al., 2007; Kucek et al., 2007; Kulkarni et al., 2007; Singh et al., 2007; Bouaid et al., 2009; Issariyakul and Dalai, 2010; Mendow et al., 2011). The disadvantage of using hydroxides of potassium and sodium over their methoxide form is that the water produced during the alkoxide-generation step favours saponification. When the feedstock contains higher amounts of free fatty acids (FFA), homogeneous acid catalysts such as H_2SO_4 is preferred to avoid saponification (Ramadhas et al., 2005; Meneghetti et al., 2006; Veljković et al., 2006; Zheng et al., 2006; Issariyakul et al., 2007; Zhang and Jiang, 2008). Recently, heterogeneous base catalysts such as alkaline earth metal oxides (i.e., MgO, CaO, SrO and BaO) and K_2CO_3/Al_2O_3 have been focussed in numerous research works due to the simplicity of biodiesel purification process and the reusability of the catalysts (Kulkarni et al., 2006; Meher et al., 2006b; D'Cruz et al., 2007; Babu et al., 2008; Kawashima et al., 2008; Liu et al., 2008; Lee et al., 2009). In addition, heterogeneous acid catalysts offer simultaneous esterification and transesterification catalysis (Furuta et al., 2004; Yadav and Murkute, 2004; Jacobson et al., 2008; Peng et al., 2008; Suwannakarn et al., 2009). However, further research is required to improve the catalyst activity and the reaction rate. Alternatively, transesterification can be enzymatically catalyzed (Dizge et al., 2008; Chen et al., 2009; Raita et al., 2010; Wang et al., 2011; Zhang et al., 2011). The process neither produces soap nor waste water but it has expensive operating cost and stricted reaction conditions. On the other hand, there have been interests to carry out non-catalytic transesterification reaction under supercritical conditions (Saka and Kusdiana, 2001; Kusdiana and Saka, 2004; Saka et al., 2010; Tan et al., 2011). The process does not require catalysts and has short reaction time. However, it requires extreme reaction temperatures and pressures; therefore, the process is susceptible to polymerization (D'Ippolito et al., 2007). Consequently, the purification step becomes difficult due to the increase in viscosity.

12.2 MUSTARD OIL AS FEEDSTOCK FOR BIODIESEL PRODUCTION

Mustards are plants in *Brassica* and *Sinapis* species whose seeds can be turned into a condiment known as mustard (by grinding the seed and mixing with water, vinegar and other liquid) and can be pressed to yield mustard oil. In addition to mustard, the genus *Brassica* also includes turnips, rapeseed, cabbage, cauliflower, rutabagas, broccoli and Brussels sprouts (Sauer and Kramer, 1983). Mustards have several varieties including *Brassica nigra* (black mustard), *Brassica carinata* (Abyssinian mustard), *Brassica juncea* (brown, oriental and leaf mustard), *Sinapis arvensis* (wild mustard) and *Sinapis alba* (white mustard). The unique fatty acid compositions of mustard oil are due to the substantial amounts of the erucic acid (C22:1) contained in this oil as shown in Table 12.1 (Basu et al., 1973; Ali and McKay, 1982; Sauer and Kramer, 1983; Cardone et al., 2003; Matthaus et al., 2003; Jham et al., 2009; Issariyakul et al., 2011). The erucic acid results from pathways of fatty acid biosynthesis, including the addition of a two-carbon fragment to oleic acid to form eicosenoic acid (C20:1), followed by the addition of another two-carbon fragment to eicosenoic acid to form erucic acid (Downey, 1983). Erucic acid is distinguished by its high melting point (33°C), which is very high for a *cis*-monounsaturated fatty acid while oleic acid melts at 16°C.

Many researchers report that cardiac fat infiltration in experimental animals is caused by erucic acid and thus conclude erucic acid as toxic compound. This compound if fed in large quantities would result in heart lesions (Sauer and Kramer, 1983). Since there are fewer experiments done on the effects of erucic acid on people compared to the number of experiments on animals, the effects of erucic acid on human health are not fully understood. Historically, the use of high-erucic-acid oil as edible oil has been objected by many organizations. The Canadian regulations state that in cooking oil, margarine, salad oil, simulated dairy product, shortening or food that resembles margarine or shortening, the erucic and cetoleic acid may not exceed 5% of the total fatty acid (Government of Canada, 1978).

TABLE 12.1
Fatty Acid Compositions of Various Mustard Oils

Vegetable Oils		Fatty Acid Composition (wt.%)										
Common Name	**Species**	**14:0**	**16:0**	**16:1**	**18:0**	**18:1**	**18:2**	**18:3**	**20:0**	**22:0**	**22:1**	**Reference**
Black mustard	*Brassica nigra*	1.5	5.3	0.2	1.3	11.7	16.9	2.5	9.2	0.4	41.0	Basu et al. (1973)
Oriental mustard	*Brassica juncea*	—	2.3	0.2	1.0	8.9	16.0	11.8	0.8	5.7	43.3	Matthaus et al. (2003)
Brown mustard	*Brassica juncea*	—	2.2	0.2	1.2	17.4	20.5	14.1	0.7	0.5	28.1	Ali and McKay (1982)
Wild Brazilian mustard	*Brassica juncea*	0.1	2.6	0.2	0.9	7.8	14.2	13.0	0.8	1.5	45.7	Jham et al. (2009)
White mustard	*Sinapis alba*	—	3.1	0.2	0.7	9.1	11.7	12.5	0.7	—	46.5	Ali and McKay (1982)
White mustard	*Sinapis alba*	0.1	2.8	0.2	1.1	25.0	11.6	8.6	0.7	0.6	32.8	Issariyakul et al. (2011)
Abyssinian mustard	*Brassica carinata*	—	3.1	—	1.0	9.7	16.8	16.6	0.7	—	42.5	Cardone et al. (2003)

Canadian mustard seed production has been ranging from 105,000 t in 2001–2002 to 306,000 t in 2004–2005. In 2006, the total world mustard exports were 315,000 t, 55% of which were Canadian mustard. In 2006–2007, Saskatchewan dominated Canadian mustard seed production, with 78% of total production. The area seeded for mustard in 2006 in Saskatchewan was 280,000 acres, which yielded 776 pounds per acre (Agriculture and Agri-Food Canada, 2007). These data show that mustard seeds are available in large quantity in Canada. Because it contains a high level of erucic acid, mustard oil does not meet Canadian specifications for edible purpose, but it could be utilized for other purposes such as feedstock for biodiesel production.

12.3 BIODIESEL QUALITY

The use of low-quality biodiesel due to incomplete reaction or contaminants in a diesel engine could result in several engine problems (Ma and Hanna, 1999). In order to protect consumers from unknowingly purchasing substandard fuel, several fuel standards have been adopted for quality control. Among these standards, ASTM D6751 (the American Society for Testing and Materials) (ASTM Standard specification for biodiesel fuel, 2008) and EN 14214 (European Committee for Standardization, 2003) are the most referred standards for pure biodiesel and are presented in Table 12.2. In addition, AOCS (American Oil Chemists' Society, 1998) has established official test methods for biodiesel quality and these methods are also listed in Table 12.2 (ASTM Standard specification for diesel fuel oil, biodiesel blend, 2008). It is reported that FAAE can be added at a low ratio to petroleum diesel fuel without substantially changing fuel properties (Reaney et al., 2005). The low-temperature flow property of the blended fuel with lower than 30% FAAE is not significantly changed from its parent petroleum diesel fuel. When FAAE that meets standard specifications is properly blended into petroleum diesel fuel and is handled according to standard techniques, the resulting fuel is of high quality and should perform well in a diesel engine. In the United States, ASTM D7467 is adopted for quality control of blended fuel containing 6–20% FAAE and is shown in Table 12.3 (ASTM Standard specification for diesel fuel oil, biodiesel blend, 2008). It is imperative that FAAE must meet standards for pure biodiesel prior to blending. Blends up to 5% are allowable in ASTM D957 for diesel fuel and ASTM D396 for heating oil provided that FAAE meets standards for pure biodiesel. In Canada, the Canadian General Standard Board has issued standard CAN/CGSB-3.520 for biodiesel–petroleum diesel blends up to 5% in 2005 and is shown in Table 12.3 (Canadian General Standard Board, 2005). The Canadian standard is intended for quality control of Type A-LS blends used in urban transit buses and passenger automobiles and Type B-LS blends used in engines in services involving relatively high loads as found in industrial and heavy mobile equipment, and the ASTM methods are adopted for testing the blended fuels.

The heating value of biodiesel and its parent oils is approximately 10% less than those of petroleum base diesel fuel on a mass basis (Lang et al., 2001b; Issariyakul et al., 2007, 2008). However, the higher viscosity of biodiesel reduces the amount of fuel that leaks past the plungers in the diesel fuel injection pump. In addition to heat of combustion, ignition delay time is also an important fuel burning characteristics. The ignition delay time is the time that passes between injection of fuel into the

TABLE 12.2
Fuel Standards and Test Methods for Pure Biodiesel

Property	AOCS Method	ASTM Method	EN Method	ASTM Limits	EN Limits
Acid value	Cd 3d-63	ASTM D664	EN14104	0.5 max[a] (mg KOH/g)[b]	0.5 max (mg KOH/g)
Water and sediment	Ca 2e-84	ASTM D2709	EN ISO 12937	0.05 max (% vol.)	500 max (mg/kg)
Ester content	—	—	EN 14103	—	96.5 min (% mol)
MAG content	Cd 11b-91 Cd 11d-96	—	EN 14105	—	0.8 max (% mol)
DAG content	Cd 11b-91 Cd 11d-96	—	EN 14105	—	0.2 max (% mol)
TAG content	Ce 5-86 Ce 5b-89	—	EN 14105	—	0.2 max (% mol)
Free glycerol	Ca 14-56 Ca 14b-96	ASTM	EN 14105 EN 14106	0.02 (% mass)	0.02 max (% mol)
Total glycerol	Ca 14-56	ASTM	EN 14105	0.24 (% mass)	0.25 max (% mol)
Methanol	—	—	EN 14110	0.2 max (% vol.)	0.2 max (% mol)
Ash content	Ca 11-55	ASTM D874	ISO 3987	0.02 max (% mass)	0.02 max (% mol)
Sulphur	Ca 8a-35	ASTM D5453	EN ISO 20846	0.0015 max (% mass)	10.0 max (mg/kg)
S15 grade	Ca 8b-35		EN ISO 20884	0.05 max (% mass)	
S500 grade					
Copper strip corrosion	—	ASTM D130	EN ISO 2160	No. 3 max	1.0 (degree of corrosion)
Phosphorus content	Ca 12-55 Ca 12b-92	ASTM D4951	EN 14107	0.001 max (% mass)	10.0 max (mg/kg)
Sodium and potassium, combined	Ca 15b-87	—	EN 14108 EN 14109	5.0 max (ppm)	5.0 max (mg/kg)
Calcium and magnesium, combined	Ca 15b-87	—	EN 14538	5.0 max (ppm)	5.0 mix (mg/kg)
Cetane number	—	ASTM D613	EN ISO 5165	47.0 min[a]	51.0 min
Iodine value	Cd 1-25	—	EN 14111	—	120 max (g I_2/100 g)

continued

TABLE 12.2 (continued)
Fuel Standards and Test Methods for Pure Biodiesel

Property	AOCS Method	ASTM Method	EN Method	ASTM Limits	EN Limits
Linolenic acid content	—	—	EN 14103	—	12.0 max (% mol)
Polyunsaturated (≥4 double bonds) FAME	—	—	EN 14103	—	1.0 max (% mol)
Cloud point	Cc 6-25	ASTM D2500	—	—	—
Cold soak filterability	—	ASTM D7501	—	360 max (s)	—
Carbon residue	—	ASTM D4530	EN ISO 10370	0.05 max (% mass)	0.3 max; 10% distillation residue (% mol)
Oxidation stability	Cd 12b-92	—	EN 14112	3.0 min (h)	6.0 min (h)
Flash point	Cc 9b-55	ASTM D93	EN ISO 3679	93 min (°C)	120 min (°C)
Density, 15°C	Cc 10a-25	—	EN ISO 3675 EN ISO 12185	—	860 – 900 (kg/m^3)
Kinematic viscosity, 40°C	—	ASTM D445	EN ISO 3104 ISO 3105	1.9–6.0 (mm^2/s)	3.5–5.0 (mm^2/s)
Distillation temperature, atmospheric equivalent, 90% recovered	—	ASTM D1160	—	360 max (°C)	—
Total contamination		—	EN 12662	—	24.0 max (mg/kg)

[a] Max, maximum; min, minimum.
[b] Units of the corresponding limits are displayed in parentheses.

TABLE 12.3
Fuel Standards ASTM D7467 for B6 to B20 and CAN/CGSB-3.520 for B1 to B5 Blended Biodiesel-Petroleum Diesel Fuel

Property	ASTM Method	ASTM Limits	CGSB Limits	
			Type A-LS[a]	Type B-LS[b]
Acid value	ASTM D664	0.3 max[c] (mg KOH/g)	0.1 max (mg KOH/g)	0.1 max (mg KOH/g)
Water and sediment	ASTM D2709	0.05 max (% vol.)	0.05 max (% vol.)	0.05 max (% vol.)
Ash content	ASTM D482	0.01 max (% mass)	0.01 max (% mass)	0.01 max (% mass)
Sulphur			500 max (mg/kg)	500 max (mg/kg)
S15 grade	ASTM D5453	15 max (μg/g)		
S500 grade	ASTM D2622	0.05 max (% mass)		
Copper corrosion, 3 h 50°C	ASTM D130	No. 3 max	No. 1 max	No. 1 max
Cetane number	ASTM D613	40.0 min[c]	40.0 min	40.0 min
One of the following must be met				
1. Cetane index	ASTM D976	40.0 min	—	—
2. Aromaticity	ASTM D1319	35.0 max (% vol.)	—	—
Cloud point	ASTM D2500 ASTM D4539 ASTM D6371	—	—	—
Electrical conductivity at point, time and temperature of delivery to purchaser	ASTM D2624	—	25.0 min (pS/m)	25.0 min (pS/m)
Carbon residue, 10% bottoms	ASTM D524	0.35 max (% mass)	0.10 max (% mass)	0.16 max (% mass)
Oxidation stability	—	6.0 min (h)	—	—
Flash point	ASTM D93	52 min (°C)	40 min (°C)	40 min (°C)
Kinematic viscosity, 40°C	ASTM D445	1.9–4.1 (mm²/s)	1.3–3.6 (mm²/s)	1.7–4.1 (mm²/s)
Distillation temperature, atmospheric equivalent, 90% recovered	ASTM D86	343 max (°C)	290 max (°C)	360 max (°C)
Lubricity, HFRR 60°C	ASTM D6079	520.0 max (μm)	—	—
Biodiesel content	ASTM D7371	6–20 (% vol.)	—	—

[a] Type A-LS is intended for use in urban transit buses and passenger automobiles or when ambient temperatures require better low-temperature properties than Type B-LS.
[b] Type B-LS is intended for use in engines in services involving relatively high loads as found in industrial and heavy mobile equipment, such as intercity trucks and construction equipment, and when ambient temperatures and fuel storage conditions allow use of such fuel.
[c] Max, maximum; min, minimum.

cylinder and onset of ignition and is characterized by cetane number (CN) (Knothe and Dunn, 2005). The higher CN represents a shorter ignition delay time and vice versa. Cetane (hexadecane; $C_{16}H_{34}$) is a long straight-chain hydrocarbon and has been assigned a CN of 100. Most biodiesel from vegetable oils have CN higher than 51 and CN of specific ester such as that of stearic can be as high as 87 while the CN of petroleum base diesel is usually ranged at 40–52 (Graboski and McCormick, 1998; Azam et al., 2005). The higher CN of biodiesel stems from the fact that biodiesel is composed of linear-chain molecules similar to that of cetane itself while petroleum base diesel is a mixture of hydrocarbons that typically contains 8–12 carbon atoms per molecule which is composed of 75% saturated hydrocarbon, including stretch, branched chains and cycloalkanes and 25% aromatics. The branched chains, cycloalkanes and aromatics are responsible to the lower CN in petroleum base diesel. CN is usually characterized by ASTM D613. Alternatively, since the CN of biodiesel increases with chain length and decreases with number of double bonds, the CN of FAME can be estimated with reasonable accuracy using its saponification value and iodine value (Krisnangkura, 1986). It is worthy to note that although CN of biodiesel increases with chain length, the use of longer-chain alcohols such as ethanol or butanol as reacting alcohols in transesterification yields an insignificant effect on CN of the resulting biodiesel (Azam et al., 2005).

Fuel flow property is an important characteristic as it determines the performance of the fuel flow system and can be evaluated by viscosity which measures the fluid's resistance to flow. A highly viscous fuel could lower the performance of the fuel flow system. One of the main reasons that the use of neat vegetable oil as diesel fuel has been considered to be unsatisfactory and impractical is because of its high viscosity (Ma and Hanna, 1999). In order to reduce its viscosity, the glycerol backbone of TAG is required to be stripped off usually by the transesterification reaction. The resulting FAAE has shown a significant reduction in viscosity compared to its parent oils. Due to the reduction of viscosity during transesterification, viscosity can also be used as means to monitor transesterification progress (Ellis et al., 2008). Since the viscosity of diesel fuels is a strong function of temperature and usually increases at lower temperatures, operating engines at cold climate regions are often challenging and therefore the low-temperature flow properties of the fuel should be monitored closely. These properties can be examined by cloud point (CP), pour point (PP) and cold filter plugging point (CFPP). Cloud point is the temperature at which a cloud of wax crystals first appears in the oil when it is cooled and a cloudy fuel is visible to the naked eye. At temperatures below CP, crystals grow larger and agglomerate together to the point that they prevent the fluid to flow. The lowest temperature at which the fluid will pour is defined as pour point. The CFPP is defined as the lowest temperature at which biodiesel will flow under vacuum condition through a wire mesh filter screen within 60 s. In addition to CP, PP and CFPP, differential scanning calorimeter (DSC) has been used to evaluate low-temperature properties of biodiesel (Lang et al., 2001b; Issariyakul and Dalai, 2010; Issariyakul et al., 2011). At an adequately low temperature, crystal is formed and the heat associated with crystallization is released and measured by DSC, and the temperature is recorded as onset crystallization temperature (OCT) which is the temperature at which the first crystal is formed. In addition to OCT, DSC is used to measure the melting temperature, polymorphic transition temperature (temperature at which crystal changes its form) and the corresponding endothermic and exothermic heats. The low temperature property of biodiesel is dependent mainly on its compositions. It is well known that unsaturated FAAE crystallized at lower temperature than saturated FAAE due to their different three-dimensional conformations. Saturated molecules are in its minimum energy when fully extended and are well stacked, thereby strengthening the intermolecular attraction force (Norris, 2007). Unlike saturated ester, especially *cis*-formation, unsaturated FAAE molecules have weaker intermolecular interactions and therefore crystallize at a lower temperature. The *trans*-formation fatty acids that usually occur unnaturally have similar a molecular arrangement to those saturated fatty acids and therefore would crystallize at temperature higher than that of the corresponding *cis*-formation fatty acids. Branched molecules also have weak intermolecular force and therefore crystallize at low temperatures. Based on this knowledge, there have been attempts to improve low-temperature flow property of biodiesel by introducing branched structure to the originally straight-chain FAAE either by means of transesterification with branched alcohols (Lee et al., 1995) or by isomerization reaction (Reaume and Ellis, 2011). Alternatively, low-temperature additives such as glyceryl ethers produced from etherification of glycerol with isobutylene or *tert*-butanol in the presence of solid acid catalysts such as sulphonated carbon and amberlyst-15 have been used to improve CP biodiesel (Noureddini, 2001; Klepáčová et al., 2007; Janaun and Ellis, 2010). In addition to fatty acid compositions, transesterification intermediates such as DAG and MAG if present in FAAE can greatly deteriorate low-temperature flow properties of biodiesel. The transesterification intermediates, especially saturated MAG, induce stronger intermolecular force mainly due to molecular stacking and hydroxyl moiety in their molecules and therefore raise the biodiesel's low-temperature properties such as CP, PP, CPFF and OCT. In addition, it was found that the presence of saturated MAG in biodiesel induces precipitation even at temperatures higher than CP, which cause problems with fuel filterability (Chupka et al., 2011; Lin et al., 2011).

Biodiesel is susceptible to oxidation which leads to fuel degradation; therefore, the oxidation stability of biodiesel is crucially important as it determines the resistance to chemical changes brought about by oxidation reaction. The oxidation of biodiesel is similar to those of lipid oxidations in that the initial step involves an abstraction of hydrogen from unsaturated fatty acid to form free radical (R·) followed by an attack of molecular oxygen to these locations to form peroxide radicals (ROO·). The propagation phase involves intermolecular interactions, whereby the peroxide radical abstracts hydrogen from an adjacent molecule, which gives rise to hydroperoxides (ROOH) and a new free radical. Carbon–hydrogen bond dissociation energies of fatty acid are lowest at biallylic followed by allylic positions (see Figure 12.3). It is reported that lower bond energies for bisallylic and allylic hydrogens are 75 and 88 kcal/mol, respectively, while those of methylene hydrogens are 100 kcal/mol (Erickson, 2002). As a result, hydrogens at bisallyic and allylic locations are favoured sites for abstraction by peroxide radical. Once formed, hydroperoxides tend to proceed towards further oxidation degradation leading to secondary oxidation derivatives such as aldehydes, acids and other oxygenates (Nawar, 1984). In addition, polymerization occurs due to the presence of double bonds to form higher-molecular-weight products, which, in turn, raises

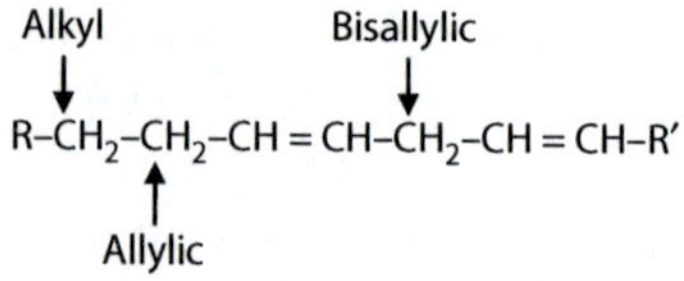

Alkyl Bisallylic

$R{-}CH_2{-}CH_2{-}CH = CH{-}CH_2{-}CH = CH{-}R'$

Allylic

FIGURE 12.3 Carbon–hydrogen bond positions in fatty acids. (Reaney, M.J.T., Hertz, P.B. and McCalley, W.W.: Vegetable oils as biodiesel. In *Bailey's Industrial Oil & Fat Products.* Vol. 6. Shahidi F. ed. Copyright Wiley-VCH Verlag GmbH & Co. KGaA. Reproduced with permission.)

the biodiesel's viscosity. The oxidation stability of biodiesel depends greatly on the fatty acid compositions and the degree of unsaturation. Saturated FAAE is more stable than unsaturated FAAE, while polyunsaturated FAAE is at least two times more reactive to autoxidation than monounsaturated FAAE (Gunstone, 1967; Neff et al., 1997). For the same number of double bond per molecule, FAAE with longer chain or higher molecular weight would be less prone to autoxidation due to the lower molar concentration of double bond (Knothe and Dunn, 2003). As an example of this phenomenon, ethyl ester has shown higher oxidation stability compared to that of methyl ester (Issariyakul et al., 2007; Issariyakul and Dalai, 2010). In addition to the degree of unsaturation, the position at which double bonds are located in an unsaturated molecule is also an important parameter to determine oxidation stability of biodiesel. It is reported that η-3 fatty acids autoxidize faster than η-6 fatty acids (Adachi et al., 1995). Some metals can accelerate the oxidation of biodiesel. It has been shown in the literature that elemental copper has strong catalytic effects on biodiesel oxidation (Knothe and Dunn, 2003) and the peroxide value of biodiesel increases more rapidly when a copper strip is immersed in a glass container of biodiesel when compared to that when a steel strip is used (Canakci et al., 1999). In addition, biodiesel is prone to hydrolytic degradation in the presence of water. The hydrolytic reaction is strongly influenced by the initial acid value of biodiesel due to the catalytic effects of free fatty acid on the reaction (Bondioli et al., 1995). Biodiesel with high concentration of transesterification intermediates, that is, DAG and MAG, has a high tendency to absorb water, therefore promoting hydrolytic reaction. Most vegetable oils contain natural anti-oxidant reagents, that is, tocopherol or vitamin E, which hinder the oxidation reaction. Once the amount of anti-oxidants is depleted, the rate of oxidation increases rapidly. The addition of synthesis anti-oxidants such as *tert*-butyl hydroquinone (TBHQ), 3-*tert*-butyl-4-hydroxyanisole (BHA), pyrogallol (PY) and *n*-propyl gallate (PG) up to 1000 mg/kg may be required as these compounds have been shown to improve the oxidation stability of biodiesel. The effects of another widely used anti-oxidant 2,6-di-*tert*-butyl-4-methyl-phenol (BHT) in the food industry are controversial when it is used to improve biodiesel stability (Mittelbach and Schober, 2003; Dunn, 2005). Most biodiesel properties such as viscosity, density, CFPP and carbon residue are not affected by the addition of anti-oxidants. However, the addition of high amounts of anti-oxidants can alter the acid value of biodiesel (Schober and Mittelbach, 2004). The oxidation stability of biodiesel is preferably determined by the rancimat method as per EN 14112 or AOCS Cd 12b-92. During the rancimat test, the biodiesel sample is heated to 110°C and the oxygen is supplied. In the presence of oxygen at high temperature, the oxidation reaction takes place and the oxidation derivatives are transferred to the measuring chamber containing Millipore water. The increase in conductivity of the water is detected as the oxidation derivatives are transferred into the water. The induction time is defined as the time required for the conductivity of the water to be increased rapidly and is used as an indication of biodiesel oxidation stability. Alternatively, oxidation stability of biodiesel can be evaluated by peroxide value (PV) and iodine value (IV). The PV of biodiesel increases when FAAE oxidation is initiated and propagates to form peroxides and hydroperoxides. However, PV is not a very suitable parameter for determining oxidation stability because its value drops during further degradation of hydroperoxides to form secondary oxidation derivatives (Canakci et al., 1999; Dunn, 2002). IV indicates the degree of unsaturation in terms of mg iodine per 100 g sample and is often used to correlate with the oxidation stability of the test sample. The major flaw of this method as an oxidation stability indicator is that it does not take into account the positions at which double bonds are located in a molecule, which is proved to be a contributing factor for autoxidation of fatty acids (Adachi et al., 1995). Pressurized differential scanning calorimeter (PDSC) has also been used to determine the oxidation stability of biodiesel. Since oxidation is an exothermic reaction, the reaction heat makes it possible to use DSC to monitor the biodiesel oxidation process. Operating DSC at high pressure helps to increase the number of moles of oxygen available for the reaction, thereby accelerating oxidation to take place at lower temperature (Dunn, 2006). The results from the DSC method are in line with those obtained from the rancimat method and it requires lesser amounts of sample and shorter analysing time (Gouveia et al., 2006). DSC was concluded to be a reliable alternative method to determine the oxidation stability of biodiesel.

12.4 BIODIESEL PRODUCTION FROM MUSTARD OIL

Biodiesel was produced from mustard oil (*Sinapis alba*) via transesterification using 6:1 alcohol to oil molar ratio at 60°C for 1.5 h with potassium hydroxide as a catalyst (Issariyakul et al., 2011). The alcohols chosen in this study include methanol, ethanol, propanol and butanol. After the reaction, the glycerol was separated from the ester phase by gravity in a separatory funnel. Heated-distilled water was used to remove KOH, soap and alcohol that remained in the ester phase. BÜCHI rotavapor was then used to remove the remaining alcohol and water in ester phase, followed by passing biodiesel through anhydrous sodium sulphate to remove traces of moisture. In addition, further purification was performed in a spinning band distillation to eliminate residual glycerides. Biodiesel was then extensively characterized for its fuel and lubricant properties (see Table 12.4).

The resulting biodiesel from this process is very high in purity as no residual glycerides and glycerol can be detected in HPLC. Acid value (AV) represents the mass percentage of free fatty acids contained in the biodiesel sample. High AV could cause corrosion problems to the engine and oxidation problems to the fuel while diesel fuel containing excessive water could cause irreversible damages to the fuel injection system in a very short time. This is because many parts of the fuel injection system are made of high-carbon steels which are subjected to corrosion when in contact with water. Damages caused by water corrosion lead to premature failure of the fuel injection system. The water content of biodiesel should be controlled during the

TABLE 12.4
Properties of Mustard Oil (*S. alba*) and Biodiesel Produced from Mustard Oil

Property	MO[a]	MME[b]	MEE[c]	MPE[d]	MBE[e]
AV (mg KOH/g)	0.9	0.4	0.5	0.6	4.0
Triglyceride (mass%)	96.9	0	0	0	0
Diglyceride (mass%)	2.5	0	0	0	0
Monoglyceride (mass%)	0	0	0	0	0
Free glycerol (mass%)	0	0	0	0	0
Ester (mass%)	0	99.8	99.7	99.7	98.0
Water (ppm)	241	231	62	187	345
Kinematic viscosity at 40°C (cSt)	37.5	4.2	4.5	5.0	5.5
Wear reduction, HFRR, 1% ester (%)	n/a	43.7	23.2	30.7	30.6
Onset crystallization temperature (°C)	n/a				
Saturated compounds		−16.4	−16.5	−12.3	−16.6
Monounsaturated compounds		−42.5	−51.0	−51.9	−58.2
Polyunsaturated compounds		−65.4	−93.5	n/a	n/a

Source: Adapted from Issariyakul, T., Dalai, A.K. and Desai, P. 2011. *J. Amer. Oil Chem. Soc.* 88: 391–402.

[a] MO = mustard oil.
[b] MME = mustard methyl ester.
[c] MEE = mustard ethyl ester.
[d] MPE = mustard propyl ester.
[e] MBE = mustard butyl ester.

production process to meet standards. The acid value and water content of biodiesel prepared from mustard oil are sufficiently low so that it meets the ASTM D6751 specifications (see Table 12.4). The viscosity of esters is reduced significantly from their parent oil (viscosity of mustard oil = 37.5 cSt) and ranged from 4.2 to 5.5 cSt due to transesterification and distillation. The crystallization temperature of biodiesel is measured using differential scanning calorimetry (DSC) and tends to decrease when a higher alcohol is used in transesterification. For unsaturated compounds, if the number of double bonds is the same, a molecule with a higher carbon chain length would have poorer molecular stacking and therefore poorer intermolecular interactions leading to a lower crystallization temperature. The low-temperature property of biodiesel can be improved by using higher alcohols, that is, the cloud point and pour point of ethyl ester were reported to be lower than those of methyl ester (Lang et al., 2001b; Issariyakul and Dalai, 2010). The lubricating property of biodiesel derived from mustard oil will be discussed in Section 12.6.

12.5 REACTION KINETICS

The kinetics of transesterification is studied using conditions mentioned in Section 12.4. The reaction temperature ranged from 40°C to 60°C and the samples were taken during the first 30 min of the reaction. Each sample was taken at 5 mL and was immediately mixed with 5 mL of 0.01 N HCl aqueous solutions in order to stop the reaction. The mixtures were centrifuged and the aqueous layer was removed. Dichloromethane was used to extract organic compounds and dried sodium sulphate anhydrous was used to adsorb the trace moisture. The samples were then centrifuged and evaporated.

In order to measure the triglyceride, diglyceride, monoglyceride and methyl ester content, the organic phase was analysed by a GC model agilent 7890A using J&W 123-5711 DB-5HT column (15 m × 320 μm × 0.1 μm; 400°C max temperature), cool on-column inlet with track oven temperature mode, 7.6 psi, 1 μL injection volume, and FID detector, at 380°C, 40 mL/min H_2 flow rate, and 400 mL/min air flow rate. The program was set to start at 50°C, ramp from 50°C to 230°C at 5°C/min, and ramp from 230°C to 380°C at 30°C/min and hold for 18 min with a total runtime of 1 h. Methanol concentrations were calculated based on a concept of number of moles of methanol consumed equals to number of moles of methyl ester formed. Based on the concept of number of moles of glycerol group in the reaction mixture is constant, glycerol concentrations were calculated.

The sequential reaction scheme shown in Figure 12.2 can be divided into six irreversible reactions:

$$\text{TAG} + \text{MeOH} \xrightarrow{k_1} \text{DAG} + \text{ME} \quad \text{(r1)}$$

$$\text{DAG} + \text{ME} \xrightarrow{k_2} \text{TAG} + \text{MeOH} \quad \text{(r2)}$$

$$\text{DAG} + \text{MeOH} \xrightarrow{k_3} \text{MAG} + \text{ME} \quad \text{(r3)}$$

$$\text{MAG} + \text{ME} \xrightarrow{k_4} \text{DAG} + \text{MeOH} \quad \text{(r4)}$$

$$\text{MAG} + \text{MeOH} \xrightarrow{k_5} \text{GL} + \text{ME} \quad \text{(r5)}$$

$$\text{GL} + \text{ME} \xrightarrow{k_6} \text{MAG} + \text{MeOH} \quad \text{(r6)}$$

Upon applying rate law to these reactions, the six differential equations can be written as

$$\frac{\text{dTAG}}{\text{d}t} = -k_1[\text{TAG}][\text{MeOH}] + k_2[\text{DAG}][\text{ME}] \quad (12.1)$$

$$\frac{\text{dDAG}}{\text{d}t} = k_1[\text{TAG}][\text{MeOH}] - k_2[\text{DAG}][\text{ME}] - k_3[\text{DAG}][\text{MeOH}] + k_4[\text{MAG}][\text{ME}] \quad (12.2)$$

$$\frac{\text{dMAG}}{\text{d}t} = k_3[\text{DAG}][\text{MeOH}] - k_4[\text{MAG}][\text{ME}] - k_5[\text{MAG}][\text{MeOH}] + k_6[\text{ME}][\text{GL}] \quad (12.3)$$

$$\frac{dME}{dt} = k_1[TAG][MeOH] - k_2[DAG][ME] + k_3[DAG][MeOH] - k_4[MAG][ME] + k_5[MAG][MeOH] - k_6[ME][GL] \quad (12.4)$$

$$\frac{dGL}{dt} = k_5[MAG][MeOH] - k_6[ME][GL] \quad (12.5)$$

$$\frac{dMeOH}{dt} = -k_1[TAG][MeOH] + k_2[DAG][ME] - k_3[DAG][MeOH] + k_4[MAG][ME] - k_5[MAG][MeOH] + k_6[ME][GL] \quad (12.6)$$

MATLAB® program was used to estimate the rate constants and the Arrhenius equation was used to calculate the activation energy (Fogler, 1999).

Figure 12.4 shows the experimental versus simulated data obtained from the MATLAB program during reaction at 50°C. It is observed that the simulated curves adequately fit with the experimental data. An increasing trend in the rate of methyl ester formation with reaction temperature found in Figure 12.5 confirms that the reaction is favoured at higher temperatures, in line with those reported in the literature (Noureddini and Zhu, 1997; Kusdiana and Saka, 2001; Zhou et al., 2003; Schumacher, 2005; Vicente et al., 2005, 2006; Issariyakul and Dalai, 2010).

Table 12.5 shows the rate constants calculated using the MATLAB program. It is observed that the values of reverse rate constants k_2 are not zero, which indicates that the reaction step of TAG to DAG is reversible. The exceptionally low values of k_6 indicate that the reaction step of MAG to GL is less reversible. This observation is due to phase separation of glycerol from oil phase; however, the reverse reaction can still take place at the GL–ME interface rendering a small positive value of k_6. The reverse rate constants k_4 are unnoticeable due to the low value of k_5. This is because MAG has a better chance to proceed with the forward reaction step by reacting with methanol to form glycerol rather than to reverse the reaction step by reacting with ME to form DAG. In addition, it is found that the rate constant k_1 is the lowest among forward rate constants indicating that the reaction step involving TAG to DAG is the rate-determining step (RDS) that controls the kinetic of overall transesterification of mustard oil. Moreover, when the reaction temperature is increased, the rate constant of RDS is also increased. This finding indicates that the reaction is favoured at higher reaction temperatures.

Activation energy (E_a) of the rate-determining step was calculated from Arrhenius plots (Figure 12.6) and is presented in Table 12.6. The activation energy is a minimum energy required for a reaction to take place. The activation energy of RDS of mustard oil (*Sinapis alba*) transesterification is found to be 26.8 kJ/mol, which is less than that using *Brassica carinata* as feedstock (104.8 kJ/mol). This finding indicates that mustard oil with different species can greatly affect the kinetics of the reaction.

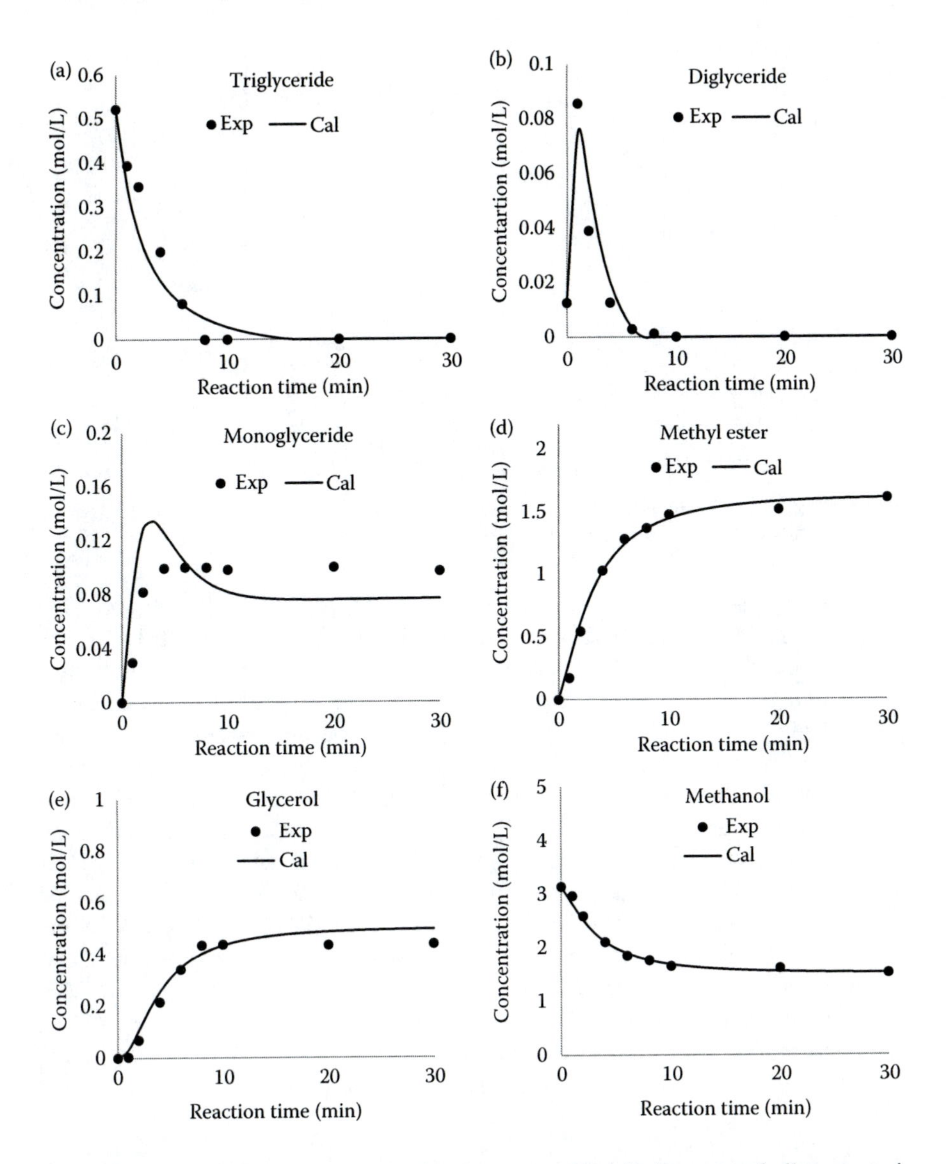

FIGURE 12.4 Experimental and simulated concentrations during mustard oil transesterification at 60°C: (a) triglyceride concentration; (b) diglyceride concentration; (c) monoglyceride concentration; (d) methyl ester concentration; (e) glycerol concentration; (f) methanol concentration.

12.6 LUBRICITY PROPERTY OF BIODIESEL

The lubricating property of fuel is defined as the quality that prevents wear when two moving metal parts come into contact with each other (Schumacher, 2005). Oxygen- and nitrogen-containing compounds are responsible for the natural lubricating property of diesel fuel (Mirchell, 2001). In petroleum refineries, processes such as

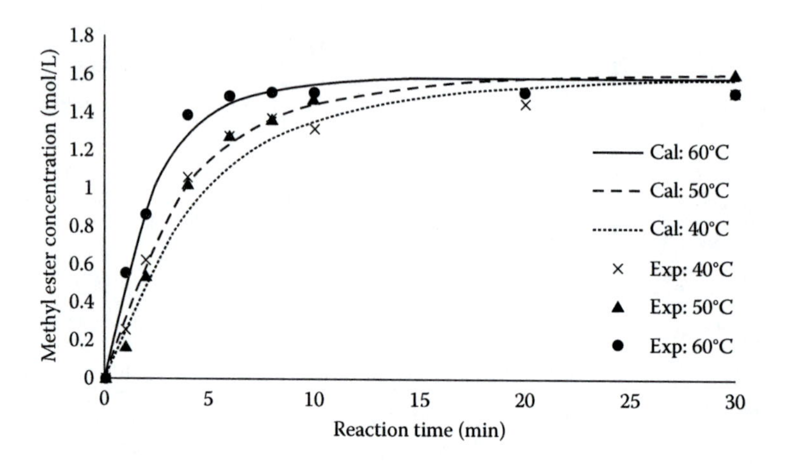

FIGURE 12.5 Experimental and simulated methyl ester concentrations during mustard oil transesterification.

hydrotreating usually used to remove sulphur also destroy heterocyclic oxygen- and nitrogen-containing compounds which are responsible for providing lubricity to the fuel (Barbour et al., 2000). Consequently, this typically ultra-low sulphur diesel fuel exhibits poor lubricity. ASTM D6079 is typically used to evaluate the lubricating property of biodiesel and diesel fuel by the high-frequency reciprocating rig (HFRR). In this method, the ball and disc are submerged in the test fluid and rubbed against each other for 75 min at 50 Hz to generate a wear. At the end of the test, the wear diameter was measured on the ball and the high wear diameter indicates poor lubricating property of the test fluid and vice versa. In order to evaluate the mustard biodiesel as lubricant, the biodiesel sample is added to the reference diesel fuel as specified in ASTM D6079 at different ratio. In addition, commercial diesel is purchased and compared with biodiesel-blended samples. Mustard biodiesel shows great potential as a lubricity additive (see Table 12.7). At 0.1% and 1%, mustard methyl ester (DMME) blended with diesel fuel, the wear scar diameter was reduced by 11.1% and 43.7%, respectively. The blends of biodiesel–petrodiesel beyond 1% biodiesel level do not show a significant improvement. Therefore, an addition of biodiesel to petrodiesel at

TABLE 12.5
Rate Constants of Each Reaction Step during Transesterification of Mustard Oil

Reaction	Direction	Rate Constant	40°C	50°C	60°C
TG ↔ DG	Forward	k_1	0.11	0.14	0.21
	Reverse	k_2	0.10	0.11	0.02
DG ↔ MG	Forward	k_3	0.55	0.63	1.04
	Reverse	k_4	0	0	0
MG ↔ GL	Forward	k_5	0.19	0.26	0.64
	Reverse	k_6	0	0.04	0.01

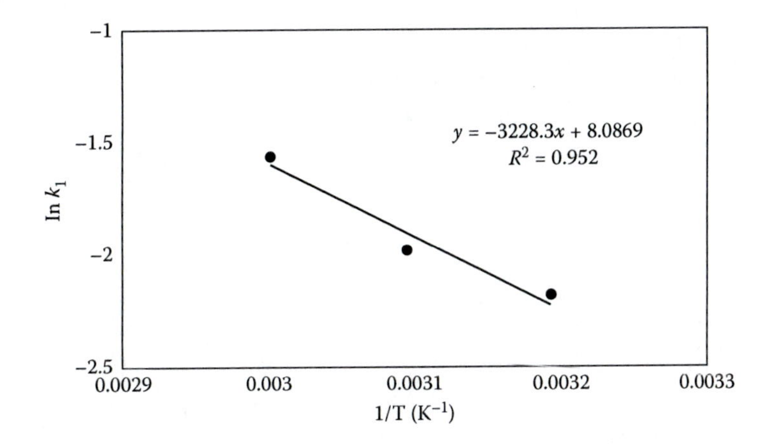

FIGURE 12.6 Arrhenius plot of the rate-determining step during mustard oil transesterification.

1% is sufficient to improve the fuel lubricity. Methyl ester shows superior performance as a lubricity additive when compared to other esters prepared from higher alcohols such as ethanol, propanol and butanol (see Table 12.4). This is explained by the presence of $COOCH_3$ moeity in methyl ester while the lower lubricating performance of esters prepared from higher alcohols is explained by an absence of $COOCH_3$ moeity. It was reported that the order of oxygenated moiety that provides lubricity is COOH > OH > $COOCH_3$ > C=O > C–O–C (Knothe and Steidley, 2005). In addition, four commercial diesel samples were purchased from different gas stations (Esso, Shell, Petro-Canada and Co-op) and tested for their lubricity (see Table 12.7). The blended mustard biodiesel–petrodiesel samples showed superior lubricating property compared to those of commercial diesel fuels. In addition, the lubricity of these commercial diesel fuels can be improved by the addition of mustard biodiesel.

Although the biodiesel lubricating property is tested, compared with petroleum-based diesel, and reported widely in the literature, the tribological mechanism of biodiesel is still not available. Nevertheless, the tribological mechanism of other model compounds such as zinc dialkyl-dithiophosphate (ZDDP) (Hsu, 2004) may be useful in explaining the lubricity behaviour of biodiesel. Initially, lubrication fluids are used to generate hydrostatic and hydrodynamic pressures to support the load. This condition is referred to as the elastohydrodynamic lubrication (EHL) regime where the fluid pressure is used to provide lubrication. Further increase in contact pressure causes the thickness of the fluid film to decrease. When the average

TABLE 12.6
Activation Energy of the Rate-Determining Step of Transesterification of Mustard Oil

Feedstock	Activation Energy (kJ/mol)
Sinapis alba	26.8
Brassica carinata [69]	104.8

TABLE 12.7
Wear Scar Diameter of Mustard Biodiesel Blends and Petro Diesel Using ASTM D6079 Method (HFRR)

Sample	Wear Scar Diameter (μm)
RDF[a]	608
B0.1[b]	541
B0.5[b]	451
B1[b]	368
B2[b]	362
B5[b]	356
Esso[c]	568
Shell[c]	516
Petro-Canada[c]	475
Co-op[c]	669
B1 Esso[d]	487
B1 Shell[d]	379
B1 Petro-Canada[d]	403
B1 Shell[d]	327

[a] RDF = Reference diesel fuel.
[b] Bx = Blend of biodiesel—petrodiesel with x% of biodiesel.
[c] These samples are petrodiesel purchased from corresponding gas stations.
[d] These samples are mustard biodiesel–petrodiesel blends at 1% biodiesel.

thickness of the fluid film falls below the average surface roughness, the boundary lubrication (BL) regime is applied. Under BL regime, the temperature is usually high enough to cause chemical reactions between the lubricant and the solid surface to take place, resulting in a chemical film that protects the surface. The reaction yields metallic-organo compounds which polymerize to form higher-molecular-weight products. These polymers (MW = 3000–5000) are critical in providing lubrication to the contacting surfaces. Petroleum diesel is a mixture of hydrocarbons that typically contains 8–12 carbon atoms per molecule with 75% saturated hydrocarbon and 25% aromatics. The reaction rate between petroleum diesel and the contacting surfaces in diesel engine is insufficient to form a film quickly enough. Unlike petroleum diesel, biodiesel contains a polar functional group such as $-COOCH_3$ in case of FAME in its molecule. This functional group promotes reactivity between biodiesel and metal surfaces forming a chemical film quickly enough to protect the surfaces. However, if the reaction rate is too rapid, chemical corrosion can occur causing an increase in wear. The proposed chemical solution model of biodiesel blends in petroleum-based diesel involves aggregation of biodiesel molecules in reverse micelle formation (polar group in the inside and hydrocarbon tail on the outside) if biodiesel concentration is high enough (see Figure 12.7). The outside reverse micelle of FAAE lays a free molecular region in which each molecular species compete freely for

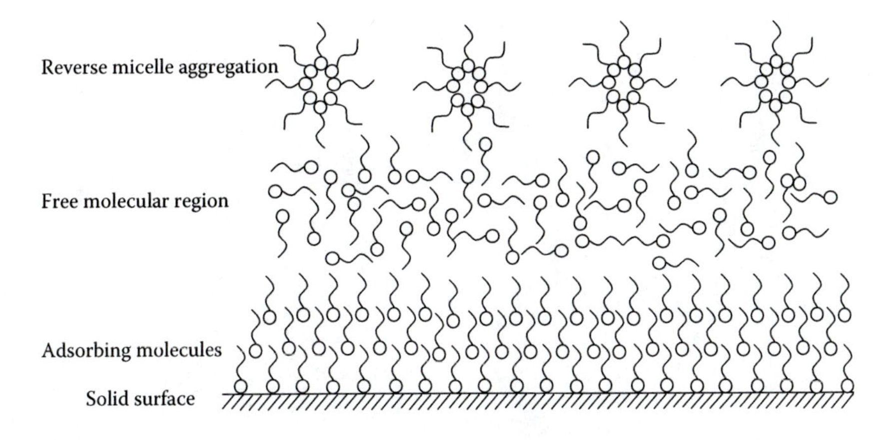

FIGURE 12.7 Chemical solution model for biodiesel blends.

adsorption on the solid surface. When these free molecules are depleted, the reverse micelle dissociates to release more free species. This model is used to explain how lubricant maintains its functionality throughout its lubricating life. In addition to the polar head, the hydrocarbon chain has great impacts on biodiesel lubricating properties. Hydrocarbon chain length, degree of branching and the presence of double bond influence how the lubricants pack themselves on the solid surface, resulting in the packing density. Low-packing-density film allows lubricating molecules to move about, hence providing flexibility and longevity of the lubricant. On the other hand, high-packing-density film has mechanical strength necessary for load-bearing ability. Increase in hydrocarbon chain length results in lower-packing-density film which improves lubricating longevity but the load-bearing ability is decreased. In addition, an increase in alkyl chain length leads to reduction in the molar concentration of the functional group resulting in a slower rate of the reaction between lubricant and the solid surface. However, if the chain length is insufficient, FAAE would lose its durability as a lubricant. A good lubricating biodiesel should be composes of varieties of FAAE to provide molecular mobility as well as solid adhesion strength.

12.7 BIODIESEL PRODUCTION IN CANADA

Biodiesel production in Canada was below 50 million litres per year in 2005. In December 2006, the federal government had announced an intention to mandate 2% renewable content in diesel fuel, which would create approximately 500 million litres per year of biodiesel demand across the country. This announcement has served as a major driving force for tremendous growth in Canadian biodiesel industry. The Canadian biodiesel production capacity has been increased to ~150 million litres per year in 2008 and ~200 million litres per year in 2010 (Canadian Renewable Fuels Association, 2010). The implementation date of the 2% federal mandate for biodiesel was later set on July 1, 2011 (CRFA, 2011). Prior to the federal mandate, there are a number of provincial renewable fuel mandates such as 2% in Alberta and Manitoba and 3% in British Columbia. The current major Canadian biodiesel plants using various feedstocks are listed in Table 12.8 indicating that the current total Canadian

TABLE 12.8
Biodiesel Plants in Canada

Plant	Status	Feedstock	Capacity (million litres per year)	City	Province
BioStreet Canada	Proposed plant	Oilseed	22	Vegreville	Alberta
Canadian Bioenergy Corporation–Northern Biodiesel Limited Partnership	Proposed plant	Canola	265	Lloyminster	Alberta
FAME Biorefinery	Demonstration facility	Canola, camelina and mustard	1	Airdire	Alberta
Kyoto Fuels Corporation	Under construction	Multi-feedstock	66	Lethbridge	Alberta
Western Biodiesel Inc.	Operational	Multi-feedstock	19	Calgary	Alberta
City-Farm Biofuel Ltd.	Operational	Recycled oil/tallow	10	Delta	British Columbia
Consolidated Biofuels Ltd.	Operational	Yellow grease	10.9	Delta	British Columbia
Bifrost Bio-Blends Ltd.	Operational	Canola	3	Arborg	Manitoba
Eastman Bio-Fuels Ltd.	Operational	Canola	5	Beausejour	Manitoba
Speedway International Inc.	Operational	Canola	20	Winnipeg	Manitoba
Bioversel Sarnia	Proposed plant	Multi-feedstock	170	Sarnia	Ontario
BIOX Corporation	Operational	Multi-feedstock	66	Hamilton	Ontario
BIOX Corporation (Plant 2)	Proposed plant	Multi-feedstock	67	Hamilton	Ontario
Methes Energies Canada	Operational	Yellow grease	5	Mississauga	Ontario
Methes Energies Canada	Under construction	Multi-feedstock	50	Sombra	Ontario
Noroxel Energy Ltd.	Operational	Yellow grease	5	Springfield	Ontario
Biocardel Quebec Inc.	Proposed plant	Multi-feedstock	40	Richmond	Quebec
Bio-Lub Canada.com	Operational	Yellow grease	10	St-Alexis-des-Monts	Quebec
QFI Biodiesel Inc.	Operational	Multi-feedstock	5	St-Jean-d'Iberville	Quebec
Rothsay Biodiesel, a member of Maple Leaf Foods Inc.	Operational	Multi-feedstock	45	Sainte-Catherine	Quebec
TRT-ETGO	Proposed plant	Vegetable oil	100	Bécancour	Quebec
Milligan Bio-Tech Inc.	Operational	Canola	1	Foam Lake	Saskatchewan

Source: Adapted from Zhou, W. and Boocock, D.G.B. 2006. *J. Amer. Oil Chem. Soc.* 83(12): 1041–1045.

biodiesel production is 205.9 million litres per year (Canadian Renewable Fuels Association, 2010). The feedstock for biodiesel production includes animal fats and waste vegetable oils (yellow grease) and only a small quantity of canola oil is used to produce biodiesel. A fraction of Canadian canola oil has been shipped to the United States for the production of biodiesel, which is then shipped back to Canada to meet the mandate. In addition, Germany has been importing canola oil from Canada for their biodiesel production process and biodiesel usage. The Canadian biodiesel production industry is relatively new compared to that in the United States and many European countries since the first provincially mandated market was established in 2009. The new Canadian 2% renewable fuel standard (RFS) requirement is anticipated to drive biodiesel production and market growth for a sustainable future.

ACKNOWLEDGEMENT

The authors acknowledge financial supports from Natural Sciences and Engineering Research Council of Canada (NSERC), the Agricultural Biorefinery Innovation Network (ABIN), Canada Research Chair program (CRC), the Saskatchewan Canola Development Commission (SCDC), the Saskatchewan Mustard Development Commission (SMDC) and Mustard 21.

REFERENCES

Adachi, S., Ishiguro, T. and Matsuno, R. 1995. Autoxidation kinetics for fatty acids and their esters. *J. Amer. Oil Chem. Soc.* 72(5): 547–551.

Agriculture and Agri-Food Canada. 2007. Mustard seed: Situation and outlook. *Bi-Weekly Bulletin* 20(11). Winnipeg, MN, Canada: Market Analysis Division. Available at http://www.agr.gc.ca/mad-dam/index_e.php?s1=pubs&s2=bi#v20

Ali, A. and McKay, J.E. 1982. The chemical and physical characteristics and fatty acid composition of seed oils extracted from cruciferous species cultivated in Pakistan. *Food Chem.* 8: 225–231.

AOCS. 1998. *Official Methods and Recommended Practices of the AOCS.* 5th edition. Champaign, IL: American Oil Chemists' Society.

ASTM Standard specification for diesel fuel oil, biodiesel blend (B6 to B20). 2008. In *Annual Book of ASTM Standards*, ASTM International, West Conshohocken, Method D7467-08a.

ASTM Standard specification for biodiesel fuel (B100) blend stock for distillate fuels. 2008. In *Annual Book of ASTM Standards*, ASTM International, West Conshohocken, Method D6751-08.

Azam, M.M., Waris, A. and Nahar, N.M. 2005. Prospects and potential of fatty acid methyl esters of some non-traditional seed oils for use as biodiesel in India. *Biomass Bioenergy.* 29: 293–302.

Babu, N.S., Sree, R., Prasad, P.S.S. and Lingaiah, N. 2008. Room-temperature transesterification of edible and non-edible oils using a heterogeneous strong basic Mg/La catalyst. *Energy Fuels.* 22: 1965–1971.

Barbour, R.H., Rickeard, D.J. and Elliot, N.G. 2000. Understanding diesel lubricity. SAE Technical Paper Series. 2000- 01-1918.

Basu, A.K., Ghosh, A. and Dutta S. 1973. Fatty acid composition of mustard (*Brassica nigra*) seed oil by gas-liquid chromatography. *J. Chromatog*. 86: 232–233.

Bondioli, P., Gasparoli, A., Lanzani, A., Fedeli, E., Veronese, S. and Sala, M. 1995. Storage stability of biodiesel. *J. Amer. Oil Chem. Soc.* 72(6): 699–702.

Boocock, D.G.B., Konar, S.K., Mao, V. and Sidi, H. 1996. Fast one-phase oil-rich processes for the preparation of vegetable oil methyl esters. *Biomass Bioenergy*. 11(1): 43–50.

Bouaid, A., Martinez, M. and Aracil, J. 2009. Production of biodiesel from bioethanol and *Brassica carinata* oil: Oxidation stability study. *Biores. Technol.* 100: 2234–2239.

Canadian Renewable Fuels Association. 2010. Growing beyond oil delivering our energy future: A report card on the Canadian renewable fuels industry. www.greenfuels.org. November.

Canadian General Standard Board. 2005. Automotive low-sulphur diesel fuel containing low levels of biodiesel esters (B1-B5). National Standard of Canada, CAN/CGSB-3.520-2005, Gatineau, Canada.

Canakci, M., Monyem, A. and Van Gerpen, J. 1999. Accelerated oxidation processes in biodiesel. *Trans. ASAE.* 42: 1565–1572.

Cardone, M., Mazzoncini, M., Menini, S., Rocco, V., Senatore, A., Seggiani, M. and Vitolo, S. 2003. *Brassica carinata* as an alternative oil crop for the production of biodiesel in Italy: Agronomic evalution, fuel production by transesterification and characterization. *Biomass Bioenergy.* 25: 623–636.

Chen, Y., Xiao, B., Chang, J., Fu, Y., Lv Pa. and Wang X. 2009. Synthesis of biodiesel from waste cooking oil using immobilized lipase in fixed bed reactor. *Energy Conversion Manage.* 50(3): 668–673..

Chupka, G.M., Yanowitz, J., Chiu, G., Alleman, T.L. and McCormick, R.L. 2011. Effect of saturated monoglyceride polymorphism on low-temperature performance of biodiesel. *Energy Fuels*. 25(1): 398–405.

Colucci, J.A., Borrero, E.E. and Alape, F. 2005. Biodiesel from an alkaline transesterification reaction of soybean oil using ultrasonic mixing. *J. Amer. Oil Chem. Soc.* 82(7): 525–530.

Committee for Standardization Automotive fuels—Fatty acid (FAME) for diesel engines—Requirements and test methods. 2003. European Committee for Standardization, Brussels; Method EN 14214.

CRFA. 2011. The benefits of biodiesel and the new 2% RFS. Posted April 8, 2011 on the biofuels journal website: http://www.biofuelsjournal.com/info/bf_articles.html?ID=107419.

D'Cruz, A., Kulkarni, M.G., Meher, L.C. and Dalai, A.K. 2007. Synthesis of biodiesel from canola oil using heterogeneous base catalyst. *J. Amer. Oil Chem. Soc*. 84(10): 937–943.

D'Ippolito, S.A., Yori, J.C., Iturria, M.E., Pieck, C.L. and Vera, C.R. 2007. Analysis of a two-step, noncatalytic, supercritical biodiesel production process with heat recovery. *Energy Fuels.* 21: 339–346.

Dizge, N., Aydiner, C., Imer, D.Y., Bayramoglu, M., Tanriseven, A. and Keskinler, B. 2008. Biodiesel production from sunflower, soybean, and waste cooking oils by transesterification using lipase immobilized onto a novel microporous polymer. *Biores. Technol.* 100(6): 1983–1991.

Downey, R.K. 1983. The origin and description of the *Brassica* oilseed crops. In *High and Low Erucic Acid Rapeseed Oils*. Kramer, J.K.G., Sauer, F.D. and Pigden, W.J. eds., Ontario, Canada: Academic Press.

Dunn, R.O. 2002. Effect of oxidation under accelerated conditions on fuel properties of methyl soyate (biodiesel). *J. Amer. Oil Chem.* 79(9): 915–920.

Dunn, R.O. 2005. Effect of antioxidants on the oxidative stability of methyl soyate (biodiesel). *Fuel Proc. Technol*. 86: 1071–1085.

Dunn, R.O. 2006. Oxidative stability of biodiesel by dynamic mode pressurized—differential scanning calorimetry (P–DSC). *Trans. ASABE.* 49(5): 1633–1641.

Ellis, N., Guan, F., Chen, T. and Poon C. 2008. Monitoring biodiesel production (transesterification) using *in situ* viscometer. *Chem. Eng. J.* 138(1–3): 200–206.

El Sherbiny, S.A., Refaat, A.A. and El Sheltawy, S.T. 2010. Production of biodiesel using the microwave technique. *J. Adv. Res.* 1(4): 309–314.

Erickson, M. 2002. Lipid oxidation of muscle foods. In *Food Lipids*. Akoh, C.C. and Min, D.B., eds. 2nd edition. New York: Marcel Dekker, Inc.

Fogler, H.S. 1999. *Elements of Chemical Reaction Engineering*. 3rd edition. New Jersey, USA: Prentice Hall PTR.

Freedman, B., Butterfield, R.O. and Pryde, E.H. 1986. Transesterification kinetics of soybean oil. *J. Amer. Oil Chem. Soc.* 63(10): 1375–1380.

Fukuda, H., Kondo, A. and Noda, H. 2001. Review: Biodiesel fuel production by transesterification of oils. *J. Biosci. Bioeng.* 92(5): 405–416.

Furuta, S., Matsuhashi, H. and Arata, K. 2004. Biodiesel fuel production with solid superacid catalysis in fixed bed reactor under atmospheric pressure. *Catalysis Commun.* 5: 721–723.

Graboski, M.S. and McCormick, R.L. 1998. Combustion of fat and vegetable oil derived fuels in diesel engines. *Prog. Energy Combust. Sci.* 24(2): 125–164.

Gouveia, A.F., Duarte, C., Beirão da Costa, M.L., Bernardo-Gil, M.G. and Moldão-Martins, M. 2006. Oxidative stability of olive oil flavoured by *Capsicum frutescens* supercritical fluid extracts. *Eur. J. Lipid Sci. Technol.* 108: 421–428.

Government of Canada. 1978. Consolidated Regulations of Canada, c.870, Food and Drugs Regulations. B.09.022. (revised 2009).

Gunstone, F.D. 1967. *An introduction to the Chemistry and Biochemistry of Fatty Acids and Their Glycerides*. 2nd edition. London: Chapman & Hall, pp. 105–114.

Hsu, S.M. 2004. Molecular basis of lubrication. *Tribol. Int.* 37: 553–559.

Issariyakul, T. and Dalai, A.K. 2010. Biodiesel production from greenseed canola oil. *Energy Fuels*. 24(9): 4652–4658.

Issariyakul, T., Dalai, A.K. and Desai, P. 2011. Evaluating esters derived from mustard oil (*Sinapis alba*) as potential diesel additives. *J. Amer. Oil Chem. Soc.* 88: 391–402.

Issariyakul, T., Kulkarni, M.G., Dalai, A.K. and Bakhshi, N.N. 2007. Production of biodiesel from waste fryer grease using mixed methanol/ethanol system. *Fuel Proc. Technol.* 88: 429–436.

Issariyakul, T., Kulkarni, M.G., Meher, L.C., Dalai, A.K. and Bakhshi, N.N. 2008. Biodiesel production from mixtures of canola oil and used cooking oil. *Chem. Eng. J.* 140: 77–85.

Jacobson, K., Gopinath, R., Meher, L.C. and Dalai, A.K. 2008. Solid acid catalyzed biodiesel production from waste cooking oil. *Appl. Catal. B: Environ.* 85: 86–91.

Janaun, J. and Ellis, N. 2010. Glycerol etherification by *tert*-butanol catalyzed by sulfonated carbon catalyst. *J. Appl. Sci.* 10(21): 2633–2637.

Jham, G.N., Moser, B.R., Shah, S.N., Holser, R.A., Dhingra, O.D., Vaughn, S.F., Berhow, M.A. et al. 2009. Wild Brazilian mustard (*Brassica juncea L.*) seed oil methyl esters as biodiesel fuel. *J. Amer. Oil Chem. Soc.* 86: 917–926.

Kawashima, A., Matsubara, K. and Honda K. 2008. Development of heterogeneous base catalysts for biodiesel production. *Biores. Technol.* 99: 3439–3443.

Klepáčová, K., Mravec, D., Kaszonyi, A. and Bajus M. 2007. Etherification of glycerol and ethylene glycol by isobutylene. *Appl. Catal. A: General.* 328(1): 1–13.

Knothe, G. 2005. Introduction. In *The Biodiesel Handbook*. Knothe, G., Gerpen, J.V. and Krahl, J. eds. Champaign, IL: AOCS Press.

Knothe, G. 2010. Biodiesel and renewable diesel: A comparison. *Prog. Energy Combustion Sci.* 36: 364–373.

Knothe, G. and Dunn, R.O. 2003. Dependence of oil stability index of fatty compounds on their structure and concentration and presence of metals. *J. Amer. Oil Chem. Soc.* 80(10): 1021–1026.

Knothe, G. and Dunn, R.O. 2005. Biodiesel: An alternative diesel fuel from vegetable oils or animal fats. In *Industrial Uses of Vegetable Oils*. Erhan, S.Z., ed. Champaign, IL: AOCS Press.

Knothe, G. and Steidley, K.R. 2005. Lubricity of components of biodiesel and petrodiesel: The origin of biodiesel lubricity. *Energy Fuels.* 19: 1192–1200.

Krisnangkura, K. 1986. Simple method for estimation of cetane index of vegetable oil methyl esters. *J. Amer. Oil Chem. Soc.* 63(4): 552–553.

Kucek, K.T., César-Oliveira, M.A.F., Wilhelm, H.M. and Ramos, L.P. 2007. Ethanolysis of refined soybean oil assisted by sodium and potassium hydroxides. *J. Amer. Oil Chem. Soc.* 84: 385–392.

Kulkarni, M.G., Dalai, A.K. and Bakhshi, N.N. 2007. Transesterification of canola oil in mixed methanol/ethanol system and use of esters as lubricity additive. *Biores. Technol.* 98: 2027–2033.

Kulkarni, M.G., Gopinath, R., Meher L.C. and Dalai, A.K. 2006. Solid acid catalyzed biodiesel production by simultaneous esterification and transesterification. *Green Chem.* 8: 1056–1062.

Kumar, R., Kumar, G.R. and Chandrashekar, N. 2011. Microwave assisted alkali-catalyzed transesterification of *Pongamia pinnata* seed oil for biodiesel production. *Biores. Technol.* 102(11): 6617–6620.

Kusdiana, D. and Saka, S. 2001. Kinetics of transesterification in rapeseed oil to biodiesel fuel as treated in supercritical methanol. *Fuel.* 80: 693–698.

Kusdiana, D. and Saka, S. 2004. Two-step preparation for catalyst-free biodiesel fuel production. *Appl. Biochem. Biotechnol.* 115: 781–791.

Lang, X., Dalai, A.K., Bakhshi, N.N., Reaney, M.J. and Hertz, P.B. 2001a. Preparation and characterization of bio-diesels from various bio-oils. *Biores. Technol.* 80: 53–62.

Lang, X., Dalai, A.K., Reaney, M.J. and Hertz, P.B. 2001b. Biodiesel esters as lubricity additives: Effects of process variables and evaluation of low-temperature properties. *Fuels Int.* 1–3: 207–227.

Lee, I., Johnson, L.A. and Hammond, E.G. 1995. Use of branched-chain esters to reduce the crystallization temperature of biodiesel. *J. Amer. Oil Chem. Soc.* 72: 1155–1160.

Lee, D.W., Park, Y.M. and Lee, K.Y. 2009. Heterogeneous base catalysts for transesterification in biodiesel synthesis. *Catal. Surveys Asia.* 13: 63–77.

Lifka, J. and Ondruschka, B. 2004. Influence of mass transfer on the production of biodiesel. *Chem. Eng. Technol.* 27(11): 1156–1159.

Lin, H., Haagenson, D.M., Wiesenborn, D.P. and Pryor, S.W. 2011. Effect of trace contaminants on cold soak filterability of canola biodiesel. *Fuel.* 90(5): 1771–1777.

Liu X., He, H., Wang, Y., Zhu, S. and Piao, X. 2008. Transesterification of soyabean oil to biodiesel using CaO as a solid base catalyst. *Fuel.* 87: 216–221.

Ma, F. and Hanna, M.A. 1999. Biodiesel production: A review. *Biores. Technol.* 70: 1–15.

Matthaus, B., Vosmann, K., Pham, L.Q. and Aitzetmüller, K. 2003. FA and tocopherol composition of Vietnamese oilseeds. *J. Amer. Oil Chem. Soc.* 80: 1013–1020.

Meher, L.C., Dharmagadda, V.S.S. and Naik, S.N. 2006a. Optimization of alkali-catalyzed transesterification of *Pongamia pinnata* oil for production of biodiesel. *Biores. Technol.* 97: 1392–1397.

Meher, L.C., Kulkarni, M.G., Dalai, A.K., Naik, S.N. 2006b. Transesterification of karanja (*Pongamia pinnata*) oil by solid basic catalysts. *Eur. J. Lipid Sci. Technol.* 108: 389–397.

Meneghetti, S.M.P., Meneghetti, M.R., Wolf, C.R., Silva, E.C., Lima, G.E.S., Silva, L.L., Serra, T.M., Cauduro, F. and de Oliveira, L.G. 2006. Biodiesel from caster oil: A comparison of ethanolysis versus methanolysis. *Energy Fuels.* 20(5): 2262–2265.

Mendow, G., Veizaga, N.S. and Querini, C.A. 2011. Ethyl ester production by homogeneous alkaline transesterification: Influence of the catalyst. *Biores. Technol.* 102: 6385–6391.

Mirchell, K. 2001. Diesel Fuel Lubricity—Base Fuel Effects. SAE Technical Paper Series 2001-01-1928 (2001).

Mittelbach, M. and Schober, S. 2003. The influence of antioxidants on the oxidation stability of biodiesel. *J. Amer. Oil Chem. Soc.* 80(8): 817–823.

Mittelbach, M. and Trathnigg, B. 1990. Kinetics of alkaline catalyzed methanolysis of sunflower oil. *Fat Sci. Technol.* 4: 145–148.

Moser, B.R. 2011. Biodiesel production, properties, and feedstocks. In *Biofuels. Global Impact on Renewable Energy, Production Agriculture, and Technological Advancements.* Tomes D, Lakshmanan, P. and Songstad, D., eds. New York, NY: Springer.

Nawar, W.W. 1984. Chemical changes in lipids produced by thermal processing. *J. Chem. Educ.* 61(4): 299–302.

Neff, W.E., Mounts, T.L. and Rinsch, W.M. 1997. Oxidative stability as affected by triacylglycerol composition and structure of purified canola oil triacylglycerols from genetically modified normal and high stearic and lauric acid canola varieties. *LWT-Food Sci. Technol.* 30: 793–799.

Norris, S. 2007. Trans Fats: The Health Burden, Parliamentary Information and Research Service from Library of Parliament, Retrieved February 7, 2007, from the parliament of Canada Web site: http://www.parl.gc.ca/information/library/PRBpubs/prb0521-e.pdf.

Noureddini, H. 2001. System and process for producing biodiesel fuel with reduced viscosity and a cloud-point below thirty two (32) degree Fahrenheit. United States of America Patent. 6,174,501

Noureddini, H. and Zhu, D. 1997. Kinetics of transesterification of soybean oil. *J. Amer. Oil Chem. Soc.* 74(11): 1457–1462.

Peng, B.X., Shu, J.F.Q., Wang, G.R., Wang, D.Z. and Haan, M.H. 2008. Biodiesel production from waste oil feedstocks by solid acid catalysis. *Process Safety Environ. Protect.* 86: 441–47.

Raita, M., Champreda, V. and Laosiripojana, N. 2010. Biocatalytic ethanolysis of palm oil for biodiesel production using microcrystalline lipase in *tert*-butanol system. *Process Biochem.* 45(6): 829–834.

Ramadhas, A.S., Jayaraj, S. and Muraleedharan, C. 2005. Biodiesel production from high FFA rubber seed oil. *Fuel.* 84: 335–340.

Reaney, M.J.T., Hertz, P.B. and McCalley, W.W. 2005. Vegetable oils as biodiesel. In *Bailey's Industrial Oil & Fat Products.* Vol. 6. Shahidi F. ed. Hoboken, NJ: John Wiley & Sons, Inc.

Reaume, S.J. and Ellis, N. 2011. Optimizing reaction conditions for the isomerization of fatty acids and fatty acid methyl esters to their branch chain products. *J. Amer. Oil Chem. Soc.* 88: 661–671.

Saka, S., Isayama, Y., Ilham, Z. and Jiayu X. 2010. New process for catalyst-free biodiesel production using subcritical acetic acid and supercritical methanol. *Fuel.* 89(7): 1442–1446.

Saka, S. and Kusdiana, D. 2001. Biodiesel fuel from rapeseed oil as prepared in supercritical methanol. *Fuel.* 80(2): 225–231.

Sauer, F.D. and Kramer, J.K.G. 1983. The problems associated with the feeding of high erucic acid rapeseed oils and some fish oils to experimental animals. In *High and Low Erucic Acid Rapeseed Oils.* Kramer, J.K.G., Sauer, F.D., Pigden, W.J. eds. New York: Academic Press.

Schober, S. and Mittelbach, M. 2004. The impact of antioxidants on biodiesel oxidation stability. *Eur. J. Lipid Sci. Technol.* 106: 382–389.

Schumacher, L. 2005. Biodiesel lubricity. In *The Biodiesel Handbook.* Knothe, G., Krahl, J. and Gerpan, J.V. eds., Champaign, IL: AOCS Press (2005).

Singh, A.K., Fernando, S.D. and Hernandez, R. 2007. Base-catalyzed fast transesterification of soybean oil using ultrasonic. *Energy Fuels.* 21: 1161–1164.

Sridharan, R. and Mathai, I.M. 1974. Transesterification reaction. *J. Sci. Ind. Res.* 33: 178–186.

Suwannakarn, K., Loreto, E., Ngaosuwan, K. and Goodwin Jr., J.G. 2009. Simultaneous free fatty acid esterification and triglyceride transesterification using a solid acid catalyst with *in situ* removal of water and unreacted methanol. *Ind. Eng. Chem. Res.* 48: 2810–2818.

Tan, K.T., Lee, K.T. and Mohamed, A.R. 2011. Potential of waste palm cooking oil for catalyst-free biodiesel production. *Energy.* 36(4): 2085–2088.

Veljković, V.B., Lakićević, S.H., Stamenković, O.S., Todorović, Z.B. and Lazic, M.L. 2006. Biodiesel production from tobacco (*Nicotiana tabacum L.*) seed oil with a high content of free fatty acids. *Fuel.* 85: 2671–2675.

Vicente, G., Martinez, M., Aracil, J. and Esteban, A. 2005. Kinetics of sunflower oil methanolysis. *Ind. Eng. Chem. Res.* 44: 5447–5454.

Vicente, G., Martinez, M. and Aracil, J. 2006. Kinetics of *Brassica carinata* oil methanolysis. *Energy Fuels.* 20: 1722–1726.

Wang, X., Liu, X., Zhao, C., Ding, Y. and Xu, P. 2011. Biodiesel production in packed-bed reactors using lipase–nanoparticle biocomposite. *Bioresource Technol.* 102(10): 6352–6355.

Yadav, G.D. and Murkute, A.D. 2004. Preparation of a novel catalyst UDCaT-5: Enhancement in activity of acid-treated zirconia-effect of treatment with chlorosulfonic acid vis-à-vis sulphuric acid. *J. Catal.* 224: 218–223.

Zhang, J. and Jiang, L. 2008. Acid-catalyzed esterification of *Zanthoxylum bungeanum* seed oil with high free fatty acids for biodiesel production. *Biores. Technol.* 99: 8995–8998.

Zhang, K.P., Lai, J.Q., Huang, Z.L. and Yang, Z. 2011. *Penicillium expansum* lipase-catalyzed production of biodiesel in ionic liquids. *Bioresource Technol.* 102(3): 2767–2772.

Zheng, S., Kates, M., Dubé, M.A. and McLean, D.D. 2006. Acid-catalyzed production of biodiesel from waste frying oil. *Biomass Bioenergy.* 30: 267–272.

Zhou, W. and Boocock, D.G.B. 2006. Phase behavior of the base-catalyzed transesterification of soybean oil. *J. Amer. Oil Chem. Soc.* 83(12): 1041–1045.

Zhou, W., Konar, S.K. and Boocock, D.G.B. 2003. Ethyl ester from the single-phase base-catalyzed ethanolusis of vegetable oils. *J. Amer. Oil Chem. Soc.* 80: 367–371.

13 Canola Oil and Heart Health

A Historical Perspective

Bruce E. McDonald

CONTENTS

13.1 Introduction 245
13.2 Canola Oil and CVD 246
13.2.1 Unique Characteristic of Canola Oil 246
13.2.2 Response of Serum Lipids to Diets Containing Canola Oil 246
13.2.2.1 Normolipidemic Subjects 246
13.2.2.2 Hyperlipidemic Subjects 247
13.3 Response of Serum Lipids to Diets Containing High-Oleic Acid Canola Oil 247
13.4 Effect of Canola Oil on Lipid Oxidation 247
13.5 Conversion of LNA into Long-Chain Omega-3 Homologs 248
13.6 Beyond Serum Cholesterol and Lipoproteins 248
References 249

13.1 INTRODUCTION

An association between dietary fat and cardiovascular disease (CVD) has been widely accepted for half a century. Much of the research over the first half of this period concentrated on type of fat, in particular the adverse effect of amount of fat, especially the amount of saturated fat. The rationale for this position came from the famous Seven Countries Study by Ancel Keys and associates (Keys et al., 1965). The one region in their study that did not fit their conclusion was the Mediterranean. People on the Island of Crete had a high-fat intake, an intake equivalent to that of populations living in North America and Northern Europe, but they had a significantly lower incidence of CVD. The diet of the inhabitants of this region was characterized by a relatively high intake of olive oil. However, the dogma of the day held that saturated fatty acids (SFA) increased the risk of CVD, polyunsaturated fatty acids (PUFA) decreased the risk, and monounsaturated fatty acids (MUFA), such as oleic acid (OA) in olive oil, had no effect on CVD risk; MUFA neither increased nor decreased blood cholesterol level. Elevated serum cholesterol level was believed the primary cause of CVD; a view still prominent in clinical practice. The concept has been refined over the past 30 years, from an emphasis on serum total cholesterol (TC) to an emphasis on the level of serum low-density lipoprotein cholesterol

(LDL-C) and over the past decade a concern with low serum levels of high-density lipoprotein cholesterol (HDL-C).

13.2 CANOLA OIL AND CVD

13.2.1 Unique Characteristic of Canola Oil

The importance of the work by Stefansson and Downey* is universally recognized, but it is unlikely, on the basis of the dogma of the day, that they would have set out to develop an oilseed with the unique fatty acid composition of canola oil. Canola oil is characterized by a very low level of SFA but only an intermediate level of PUFA. However, the PUFA content is unique in that one-third is contributed by α [alpha] linolenic acid (LNA); linoleic acid (LA) makes up the other two-thirds. In fact, Stefansson and Downey probably would have preferred a much lower level of LNA in the new cultivar. LNA was not only considered physiologically unimportant 50 years ago, it was but also regarded as the primary reason for the instability of soyabean and rapeseed oils. Fortuitously, Stefansson and Downey's objective was to eliminate or, at least, markedly reduce the level of long-chain monoenoic fatty acids in rapeseed oil, in particular erucic acid. The new cultivar, however, was not adopted by farmers because it was not as well adapted agronomically as its progenitor rape. Furthermore, there was no convincing evidence that erucic acid had any obvious adverse physiological effects. However, when it was announced in 1972 that high erucic acid rapeseed oil had deleterious effects on the hearts of weanling rats, Canada changed the entire rapeseed crop to canola.†

Canola oil is a rich source of OA. In fact, it is second only, among common vegetable oils, to olive oil in OA content. In addition, canola oil contains a relatively high level of phytosterols; it is second only to corn oil among common edible oils in phytosterol content.

13.2.2 Response of Serum Lipids to Diets Containing Canola Oil

13.2.2.1 Normolipidemic Subjects

Our laboratory immediately embarked on human metabolic studies with canola oil following the announcement that Canada would change from rape to canola production. To our surprise, canola oil resulted in a significant decrease in the serum TC level of healthy, young male subjects (McDonald et al., 1974). Although canola oil contains a low level of SFA, OA is the main fatty acid in canola oil and the dogma of the day maintained that MUFA were neutral with respect to their effect on serum cholesterol level. However, the report by Mattson and Grundy (1985), a decade later, that high-oleic safflower oil was equally as effective as regular safflower oil (high in LA) in lowering plasma lipid and lipoprotein levels, explained our earlier results

* Dr. Baldur Stefansson and Dr. Keith Downey are credited with the development of canola; a low erucic acid cultivar of rapeseed (Stefansson et al., 1961).

† The new cultivar was not canola but rather a low erucic acid progenitor of canola. The name canola was adopted later to describe the rapeseed cultivar with a very low erucic acid content oil and much lower glucosinolate (goitrogen) level in the meal (oil-free residue portion of the seed).

with canola oil. Studies at the University of Manitoba (McDonald et al., 1989; Chan et al., 1991), in the United States (Wardlaw et al., 1991) and in Finland (Valsta et al., 1992), showed canola oil equally as effective as sunflower oil, soyabean oil and safflower oil in lowering serum total and LDL cholesterol levels. Serum TC decreased 12–20% and LDL-C 17–23% from baseline levels on the canola and PUFA diets. These results are consistent with the current view that MUFA, namely OA, are equally as effective as PUFA in lowering serum TC and LDL-C levels. Studies also found that LNA, like OA and LA, produced lower serum TC and LDL-C levels when it replaced SFA in the diet (Chan et al., 1991). The positive effect of LNA on serum TC and LDL-C contrast with the effect of the long-chain omega-3 fatty acids in fish oils (namely, eicosapentaenoic acid [EPA] and docosahexaenoic acid [DHA]), which have little effect on serum TC and LDL-C levels.

13.2.2.2 Hyperlipidemic Subjects

Canola oil also was found to be equally as effective as corn oil and sunflower oil in lowering serum TC and LDL-C of subjects with elevated serum lipid levels (Lichtenstein et al., 1993; Gustafsson et al., 1994). All three dietary fats produced similar decreases in TC and LDL-C (−12% to −17% from baseline). Lichtenstein et al. (1993) and Gustafsson et al. (1994) reported a decrease in HDL-C on the canola and corn oil diets which coincided with the decrease in HDL-C reported by Mattson and Grundy (1985) when hyperlipidemic subjects were fed a high PUFA diet. Consistent with the results with normolipidemic subjects, a study by Södergren et al. (2001) with hyperlipidemic subjects found canola oil resulted in a decrease in TC and LDL-C from baseline values whereas there was no change in the blood lipid levels on an SFA diet.

13.3 RESPONSE OF SERUM LIPIDS TO DIETS CONTAINING HIGH-OLEIC ACID CANOLA OIL

High-oleic acid (Hi-OA) canola oil, which was developed for use in deep frying, was found equally as effective as canola oil and sunflower oil in lowering serum TC and LDL-C of normolipidemic subjects (McDonald et al., 1995). However, this observation does not mean that they are nutritional equivalent. Nonetheless, the stability of Hi-OA canola oil in deep frying and its replacement of partially hydrogenated vegetable oil (PHVO) in this application has made a significant contribution to the lowering of CVD risk; PHVO with its high trans fatty acid content not only results in an increase in serum LDL level, but also a decrease in serum HDL level.

13.4 EFFECT OF CANOLA OIL ON LIPID OXIDATION

Although canola oil contains a high level of OA, it also contains a relatively high level of LNA and thus the potential to increase oxidative stress *in vivo*. Oxidized LDL (ox-LDL) plays a fundamental role in the development of atherosclerosis. High PUFA intakes were found to promote the formation of ox-LDL whereas LDL enriched with OA were stabler to oxidation. *In vitro*-conjugated diene formation (a measure of lipid oxidation) of the LDL fraction of subjects fed diets, where canola oil or high oleic (Hi-OA) canola oils replaced SFA was significantly lower than when sunflower oil was substituted for SFA (McDonald et al., 1995). Turpeinen et al. (1995) and Kratz et al. (2002) also reported significantly greater formation of conjugated dienes on a sunflower oil diet than on a canola oil diet. In addition, Turpeinen et al. (1998) found no change in urinary 8-iso-prostaglandin $F_{2\alpha}$ (8-iso-$PGF_{2\alpha}$, a biomarker of *in vivo* lipid peroxidation), from baseline values on a canola diet whereas there was a significant increase on a sunflower oil diet while Södergren et al. (2001) found that the baseline levels of plasma and urinary 8-iso-$PGF_{2\alpha}$, did not change when subjects were changed to either a canola oil or an SFA diet.

13.5 CONVERSION OF LNA INTO LONG-CHAIN OMEGA-3 HOMOLOGS

Interest in long-chain omega-3 PUFA (n-3 LC-PUFA) in fish oils (namely, EPA, 20:5n-3; and DHA, 22:6n-3) arose with the report of a much lower incidence of CVD among Greenland Eskimos than among Danes (Dyerberg, 1986) This observation led to an interest in the effect of n-3 LC-PUFA, in particular EPA, on clot formation. Clot formation and blockage of blood flow in a major vessel to the heart or brain manifests as a heart attack or a stroke. Interest in the antithrombotic effect of n-3 LC PUFA raised the question of the possible role of LNA on clot formation. Although there is some data suggesting dietary LNA increases clotting time, the results are highly variable. Some of the variance may relate to a failure to account for the effect of the n-6–n-3 ratio of the dietary fat. Chan et al. (1993) found that the level of EPA in serum phospholipids was higher when subjects were on a canola oil diet than when they were on a soyabean oil diet. Although the level of LNA was only slightly higher on the canola oil diet, the ratio of LA to LNA was appreciably lower than on the soyabean oil diet (2:1 vs 7:1). Lieu et al. (2007), who used flax oil and safflower oil to vary the LA to LNA ratio, also found the ratio important in the conversion of LNA to EPA. Most literature reviews, however, discount the ratio as a factor in this conversion. In addition, there is little evidence to suggest that the level of LNA in the diet is an overriding factor in the conversion of LNA into EPA. Nevertheless, there is general acceptance that LNA can be converted into EPA by humans but the common consensus maintains that the conversion is relatively slow.

13.6 BEYOND SERUM CHOLESTEROL AND LIPOPROTEINS

In spite of a continued emphasis on serum lipid levels in clinical practice, in particular LDL level, there is an increasing awareness of the need to move beyond serum cholesterol and lipoproteins in the study of dietary fat and heart disease. Even within the realm of serum lipids and lipoproteins, there is evidence that the total-to-HDL cholesterol (T/HDL-C) ratio is a better indicator of CVD risk than serum LDL level and that T/HDL-C ratio together with elevated C-reactive protein level (a biomarker of systemic inflammation) is an even better indicator of CVD risk (Blake and Ridker, 2002).

There is appreciable evidence that the unique composition of canola oil accounts for its favourable effect on CVD risk factors. The fact that canola oil is equivalent to high-PUFA content vegetable oils (e.g., corn, soyabean, sunflower and safflower) in lowering serum total and LDL cholesterol levels and that it may have additional nutritional benefits to high LA oils, such as lower risk of *in vivo* lipid peroxidation, suggests that the virtual collapse of nutrition research on canola oil over the last 15 years needs to be addressed. There is a need to compare the effect of canola oil and its relatively high LNA content and relatively narrow LA-to-LNA ratio (namely, 2:1) with the effects of high LA oils (e.g., sunflower oil, soyabean oil) and Hi-OA canola oil on markers of: inflammation (e.g., C-reactive protein); artery endothelial function (e.g., flow-mediated dialatation [FMD]); and endothelial cell activity (e.g., vascular and intercellular cell adhesion molecules [VCAM-1 and ICAM-1]). In addition, there is a need to assess the extent of the conversion of the LNA in canola oil into n-3 LC PUFA by humans and to assess the effect of LA level on this conversion and the significance of this conversion into the nutritional properties of canola oil.

REFERENCES

Blake, G.J. and Ridker, P.M. 2002. Inflammatory biomarkers and cardiovascular risk prediction. *J. Intern. Med.* **252**: 283–294.

Chan, J.K., Bruce, V.M. and McDonald, B.E. 1991. Dietary α [alpha] linolenic acid is as effective as oleic acid and linoleic acid in lowering blood cholesterol in normolipidemic men. *Am. J. Clin. Nutr.* **53**: 1230–1234.

Chan, J.K., McDonald, B.E., Gerrard, J.M., Bruce, V.M., Weaver, B.J. and Holub, B.J. 1993. Effect of dietary α[alpha] linolenic acid its ratio to linoleic acid platelet and plasma fatty acids and thrombogenesis. *Lipids* **28**: 811–817.

Dyerberg, J. 1986. Linolenate-derived polyunsaturated fatty acids and prevention of atherosclerosis. *Nutr. Rev.* **44**: 125–133.

Gustafsson, I.-B., Vessby, B., Ohrvall, M. and Nydahl, M. 1994. A diet rich in monounsaturated rapeseed oil reduces the lipoprotein cholesterol concentration and increases the relative level of n-3 fatty acids in hyperlipidemic subjects. *Am. J. Clin. Nutr.* **59**: 667–674.

Keys, A., Anderson, J.T. and Grande, F. 1965. Serum cholesterol response to changes in the diet. IV. Particular saturated fatty acids in the diet. *Metabolism* **14**: 776–787.

Kratz, M., Cullen, P., Kannenberg, F., Kassner, A., Fobker, M., Abuja, P.M., Assman, G. and Wahrburg, U. 2002. Effects of dietary fatty acids on the composition and oxidizability of low-density lipoproteins. *Eur. J. Clin. Nutr.* **56**: 72–81.

Lichtenstein, A.H., Ausman, L.M., Currasco, W., Jenner, J.I., Gualatieri, I.J., Goldin, B.R, Ordovas, J.M. and Schaefer, E.J. 1993. Effect of canola, corn and olive oils on fasting and postprandial lipoproteins in humans as part of the National Education Program Step 2 Diet. *Arterioscler. Thromb.* **13**: 1533–1542.

Lieu, Y.A., King, J.H., Zibrik, D. and Innis, S.M. 2007. Decreasing linoleic acid with constant alpha-linolenic acid in dietary fat increases (n-3) eicosapentaenoic acid in plasma phospholipids in healthy men. *J. Nutr.* **137**: 945–952.

Mattson, F.H. and Grundy, S.M. 1985. Comparison of the effect of saturated, monounsaturated and polyunsaturated fatty acids on plasma lipids and lipoproteins in man. *J. Lipid Res.* **26**: 575–581.

McDonald, B.E., Bruce, V.M., LeBlanc, E.I. and King, D.J. 1974. Effect of rapeseed oil on serum lipid patterns and blood hematology of young men. *Proceedings 4 Internationaler Rapskongress*, Geissen, Germany, pp. 693–700.

McDonald, B.E., Bruce, V.M., Murthy, V.G. and Latta, M. 1995. Assessment of the nutritional properties of low-linolenic acid (LL) canola oil with human subjects. *Proceedings of the Ninth International Rapeseed Congress*, Cambridge, UK, pp. 849–851.

McDonald, B.E., Gerrard, J.M., Bruce, V.M. and Corner, E.J. 1989. Comparison of the effect of canola oil and sunflower oil on plasma lipids and lipoproteins and on *in vivo* thromboxane A_2 and prostacyclin production in young men. *Am. J. Clin. Nutr.* **50**: 1382–1388.

Södergren, E., Gustafsson, I.-B., Basu, S., Nourooz-Zadek, J., Nälsen, C., Turpeinen, A., Berglund, L. and Vessby, B. 2001. A diet containing rapeseed oil-based fats does not increase lipid peroxidation in humans when compared to a diet rich in saturated fatty acids. *Eur. J. Clin. Nutr.* **55**: 922–931.

Stefansson, B.R., Hougen, F.W. and Downey, R.K. 1961. The isolation of rape plants with seed oil free from erucic acid. *Can. J. Plant Sci.* **41**: 218–219.

Turpeinen, A.M., Alfthan, G., Valsta, I., Hietanen, E., Salonen, J.T., Schunk, H., Nyyssönen, K. and Mutanen, M. 1995. Plasma and lipoprotein lipid peroxidation in humans on sunflower and rapeseed oil diets. *Lipids* **30**: 485–490.

Turpeinen, A.M., Basa, S. and Mutanen, M. 1998. A high linoleic acid diet increases oxidative stress *in vivo* and affects nitric oxide metabolism in humans. *Pros. Leuk. Ess. Fatty Acids* **59**: 229–233.

Valsta, L.M., Jauhianinen, A., Aro, M.B., Katan, M.B. and Mutanen, M. 1992. Effects of monounsaturated rapeseed oil and a polyunsaturated sunflower oil diet on lipoprotein levels in humans. *Arterioscler. Thromb.* **12**: 50–57.

Wardlaw, G.M., Snook, J.T., Lin, L.-C., Puangco, M. and Kwon, J.S. 1991. Serum lipid and apolipoprotein concentration in healthy men on diets containing either canola oil or safflower oil. *Am. J. Clin. Nutr.* **54**: 104–110.

14 Canola Oil
Evolving Research in Obesity and Insulin Resistance

Danielle Hanke, Karin Love, Amy Noto, Peter Zahradka and Carla Taylor

CONTENTS

14.1 Canola Oil 252
14.2 Obesity and Insulin Resistance 252
  14.2.1 Methods to Assess Obesity and IR 253
  14.2.2 The Metabolic Syndrome 254
14.3 Canola Oil Fatty Acids as Modulators of Obesity and IR 255
  14.3.1 Monounsaturated Fatty Acids versus Saturated Fatty Acids 256
  14.3.2 Polyunsaturated Fatty Acids 257
  14.3.3 MUFA versus Carbohydrate 260
  14.3.4 Possible Synergistic Effects of Canola Oil Fatty Acids 260
14.4 Hypotheses for Metabolic Effects of Canola Oil 261
  14.4.1 Regulation of Transcription Factors 261
    14.4.1.1 Peroxisome Proliferator-Activated Receptors and PUFAs 262
    14.4.1.2 Sterol Regulatory Element-Binding Proteins and PUFA 263
    14.4.1.3 Relationship of MUFA to PPARs and SREBPs 264
  14.4.2 Tissue Lipid Accumulation and Fatty Acid Composition 264
    14.4.2.1 Liver Fatty Acid Metabolism 265
    14.4.2.2 Adipose Function and Inflammatory Markers 266
    14.4.2.3 Fatty Acids and Insulin Signalling 267
  14.4.3 Fatty Acid-Independent Mechanisms 268
14.5 Summary and Conclusions 269
14.6 Limitations and Implications for Future Research 269
References 269

14.1 CANOLA OIL

Canola was developed in the 1970s by breeding a novel variety of rapeseed with reduced erucic acid content (Shahidi, 1990). It is now abundantly grown in Canada since it is well suited to the Canadian climate. It has become an economically important crop, for example, adding 13.8 billion dollars in economic activity annually and bringing back 2.8 billion dollars in revenue to the Canadian economy (Canola Council of Canada, 2008). According to the United States Department of Agriculture (USDA, 2007), canola oil was the third most consumed vegetable oil in the United States in 2007. Although canola meal, which is normally used in animal feed, is an excellent source of protein, canola oil is the most valuable part of the canola seed and is considered to be a 'healthy' fat compared to other popular vegetable oils on the market (Canola Council of Canada, 2008).

In the United States, the Food and Drug Administration (FDA, 2006) has approved a health claim for conventional canola oil that states 'canola is high in unsaturated fats and consuming 1.5 tablespoons of canola oil per day may reduce the risk of coronary heart disease'. Potential health benefits of conventional canola oil are largely due to its relatively low levels of saturated fatty acids (SFA; 7% of total fatty acids) and high amounts of the monounsaturated fatty acid (MUFA), oleic acid (OA; 61% of total fatty acids; Canola Council of Canada, 2008). Conventional canola oil is also a good source of two essential polyunsaturated fatty acids (PUFA), linoleic acid (LA; 21% of total fatty acids), an n-6 PUFA, and alpha-linolenic acid (ALA; 11% of total fatty acids), an n-3 PUFA. This composition of LA and ALA results in a low, 2:1 ratio of n-6:n-3.

High oleic canola oil is the type of canola oil that is most commonly used in commercial food production and service (Canola Council of Canada, 2008). High oleic canola oil is more heat stable and has a longer shelf life than conventional canola oil because it contains less PUFA, mainly ALA. In addition, as its name implies, high oleic canola oil contains more OA than conventional canola oil. High oleic canola oil has a fatty acid profile that consists of 7% SFA, 70% MUFA and 23% PUFA; n-3 PUFAs make up only 3% of total fatty acids, whereas n-6 PUFAs compose 20% (Canola Council of Canada, 2008). High oleic canola oil contains 8% less ALA and only 1% less LA than conventional canola oil, resulting in a higher n-6 to n-3 ratio of about 7:1.

Diet modelling has demonstrated that the recommended intakes of SFA, MUFA and ALA for prevention of heart disease can be achieved with conventional canola oil as the primary dietary fat source (Johnson et al., 2007). However, there is a gap in knowledge regarding the canola oil itself, as well as the synergistic effects of the fatty acids found in canola oil, on obesity and insulin resistance (IR). The unique fatty acid profile of canola oil may be beneficial in this regard and related data and possible mechanisms of action are described in the following sections.

14.2 OBESITY AND INSULIN RESISTANCE

Obesity occurs at epidemic rates in both youth and adults around the globe and this rate continues to increase with time (WHO, 2012). Obesity does not occur without consequence in the body. Obesity increases an individual's risk of developing various diseases such as cardiovascular disease, type 2 diabetes mellitus (DM2), certain types of cancer and osteoarthritis (WHO, 2012). In most instances, obesity is caused by an imbalance between calories consumed and calories expended thus resulting in a positive energy balance. A positive energy balance is often obtained when energy dense or empty calorie foods, such as fats and sugars, are over-consumed and when physical activity is lacking (WHO, 2012).

The prevalence of DM2 has increased dramatically in North America over the past 20 years due to a number of factors, such as escalating obesity rates, the ageing population and increasingly sedentary lifestyles. DM2 is characterized by IR and hyperglycaemia and is strongly associated with obesity, hypertension and the metabolic syndrome (discussed below). IR is defined as a normal to high production of insulin, which produces a less than normal biological response leading to hyperglycaemia (De Vries et al., 1989). IR occurs in skeletal muscle, adipose tissue and the liver. It is widely accepted that diet and exercise can effectively prevent or postpone the onset of IR and DM2 largely by decreasing visceral obesity and improving membrane fluidity and insulin sensitivity (McCarty, 2000). Realistically, however, such lifestyle changes often require more discipline than many people are willing to give (McCarty, 2000). This has led to the search for new compounds to improve glucose uptake and metabolism, even when diet and exercise habits remain suboptimal.

It is critical to prevent and treat obesity and IR to improve the health of the global population. The dietary strategies recommended by the World Health Organization (2006) to battle obesity include eating more fruit and vegetables, as well as nuts and whole grains; cutting the amount of fatty, sugary foods in the diet; and moving from saturated animal-based fats to unsaturated vegetable-oil-based fats. Nutritional guidelines for pre-diabetes and DM2 management, conditions where IR is present, suggest that SFA and PUFA should be limited to <7% and 10% of energy intake, respectively, and intake of *trans* fatty acids minimized. Additionally, fat intake should favour MUFA and n-3 PUFA from fatty fish and plant oils (CDA, 2008).

These recommendations suggest that there is utility in MUFA from nuts and plant oils including canola oil to combat obesity, however, dietary guidelines for diabetes and general health are largely based on the research specific to heart disease. There is a lack of knowledge and agreement regarding the optimal fatty acid profile of the diet with regard to obesity or IR. The following sections will discuss the possible role of canola oil or its specific fatty acid components for prevention or management of obesity, IR and related components of the metabolic syndrome as defined below.

14.2.1 Methods to Assess Obesity and IR

Obesity can be measured in two main ways: body mass index (BMI), and waist circumference (WC; Douketis et al., 2005). BMI is a measure of weight (in kilograms) divided by height (in metres) squared and a BMI > 30 kg/m^2 is classified as obese. Furthermore, BMI levels are associated with high (BMI 30–34.9 kg/m^2), very high (BMI 35–39.9 kg/m^2) and extremely high (BMI ≥40 kg/m^2) risks of developing health problems such as DM2. BMI is a relatively easy measurement to obtain, but it may not be fully accurate since it does not take body composition into account.

For example, BMI can misclassify people with large muscle mass as obese even though their body fat percentage is low. Therefore, WC should also be measured when determining obesity. A WC ≥102 cm in men, and ≥88 cm in women, is associated with increased risk of health problems including DM2. In animal models, BMI and WC do not apply, but measuring weight gain and adipose tissue mass, as well as adipocyte size, can provide insights into the development of obesity in these models.

Both genetic and environmental factors, such as obesity, influence the development of IR and its progression to DM2. The ability to measure IR is therefore important both for diagnosis of the disease and for testing potential therapeutic interventions. A number of well-established tests are available to estimate glucose homeostasis and insulin sensitivity, including model assessments, glucose/insulin infusion sensitivity tests and clamps (Heikkinen et al., 2007; Muniyappa et al., 2009; Matsuda 2010). Homeostatic model assessment (HOMA) is a mathematical calculation using fasting plasma glucose and fasting insulin levels to determine IR. The application to rodents can be of concern since the underlying parameters used for the basis of the assessment are based on human data. In contrast, the oral glucose tolerance test (OGTT) measures the clearance of glucose from the blood. The test is based on the consumption, while in the fasted state, of a standardized glucose amount after which blood glucose levels are monitored for 3 h. The data are plotted (glucose versus time) and the area under the curve is calculated. Higher values are indicative of IR. Similar but less frequently used tests are the intraperitoneal glucose tolerance test, intraperitoneal insulin sensitivity test and the meal tolerance test. The gold standard, however, remains the hyperinsulinaemic–euglycaemic clamp. In this procedure, insulin is infused to lower blood glucose levels, and glucose is infused to balance the effect of insulin thus maintaining euglycaemia. The amount of glucose that is infused determines the degree of insulin sensitivity, with higher values representative of good sensitivity. One advantage of this method is the fact that there is no need to measure insulin levels. On the other hand, this procedure is technically more difficult. For the latter reason, the clamp is not often used. At the same time, it is more sensitive and accurate than the OGTT.

Conclusions drawn from available data can often depend on assessment methods and diagnostic criteria at the time of study. Components of obesity (WC) and IR are central to the metabolic syndrome, as defined next.

14.2.2 The Metabolic Syndrome

The Adult Treatment Panel (ATP III) diagnostic criteria for the metabolic syndrome include at least three of: elevated WC (≥102 cm in men; ≥88 cm in women), elevated plasma triacyglycerols (TAG; ≥1.7 mmol/L), reduced plasma high-density lipoprotein cholesterol (HDL-C; <1.03 mmol/L in men; <1.3 mmol/L in women), elevated blood pressure (≥130 mmHg systolic or ≥85 mmHg diastolic or drug treatment for hypertension) or elevated fasting plasma glucose (≥5.5 mmol/L or drug treatment for hyperglycaemia). Each diagnostic parameter can be related to IR (Grundy et al., 2005).

Dyslipidaemia is simply excess lipids in the blood including TAG, phospholipids (PL), free fatty acids (FFA) and cholesterol, and can lead to cardiovascular disease and hepatic steatosis. Insulin acts to promote free fatty acid uptake into muscle cells and adipocytes by lipoprotein lipase (LPL), resulting in TAG storage (Nugent, 2004).

However, in a state of IR, there is less stimulation of LPL for breakdown of TAG to FFA for uptake by the cells leading to hyperlipidaemia. The lipid profile that is characteristic of the metabolic syndrome consists of reduced high-density lipoprotein (HDL) and elevated apolipoprotein B (apoB), TAG and intermediate density lipoprotein levels in plasma (Nugent, 2004). Apolipoprotein Bs (apoB; subtypes apoB48 and apoB100) are structural components of the atherogenic lipoproteins LDL, intermediate density lipoprotein (IDL) and very-low-density lipoprotein (VLDL; Grundy, 2002) and thus indicate circulating levels of the various apoB containing lipoproteins.

Hypertension refers to chronically elevated blood pressure in the arteries and is a major risk factor for cardiovascular disease, including heart attack, heart failure and stroke, as well as kidney disease (Chobanian et al., 2003). Hypertension is diagnosed when systolic blood pressure and/or diastolic blood pressure are above 140 mmHg and/or 90 mmHg, respectively. The metabolic syndrome criteria for hypertension, as noted above, are blood pressure above 130 mmHg systolic and/or 85 mmHg diastolic. The presence of diabetes and high serum cholesterol increase the risk of developing hypertension, thus, an individual who has the metabolic syndrome commonly has hypertension as one of the components.

Additionally, it has been suggested that non-alcoholic fatty liver disease (NAFLD) should be added to the classical components of the metabolic syndrome given its close association to IR as a central feature (Marchesini et al., 2001). NAFLD is defined as a broad spectrum of liver pathology, ranging from fatty liver (hepatic steatosis) without inflammation, to severe inflammatory activity with significant fibrosis or even cirrhosis (Marchesini et al., 2001). The release of inflammatory mediators, including C-reactive protein (CRP), tumour necrosis factor (TNF)-α, interleukin (IL)-6 and IL-8, from the liver and adipose tissue are also characteristic of NAFLD (Hijona et al., 2010).

The prevalence of the metabolic syndrome is on the rise, in conjunction with rapidly increasing obesity rates (Haffner, 2006). A sample of 1276 multi-ethnic Canadians revealed that the prevalence of the metabolic syndrome in Canada was 25.8% (Anand et al., 2003). The prevalence of the metabolic syndrome was highest in Native Americans (42%), followed by South Asians (26%), Europeans (22%) and Chinese (11%). The implications of having the metabolic syndrome are severe as it increases the risk of coronary heart disease and stroke by threefold compared with individuals with normal glucose tolerance (reviewed by Nugent, 2004).

In summary, obesity and IR are central features of the metabolic syndrome and related to abdominal obesity/WC, dyslipidaemia, hypertension, NAFLD and inflammation. Each of these components will be discussed within the context of how fatty acids, particularly those found in canola oil, may play a beneficial role in the prevention or treatment of obesity and IR.

14.3 CANOLA OIL FATTY ACIDS AS MODULATORS OF OBESITY AND IR

In the past, dietary fats were merely seen as a source of calories, whereas today, it is known that dietary fats and oils have an important role in health. MUFAs are considered to have less of a negative impact on health than SFA and may even be beneficial to people with DM2 (CDA, 2008; ADA, 2009). PUFAs are considered to be the most 'healthy' types of fatty acids, however, over the past 50 years dietary consumption of n-6 PUFAs has greatly increased whereas consumption of n-3 PUFAs has decreased. The imbalance between n-6 and n-3 PUFAs may negatively affect health. In light of what is currently known about the various types of fatty acids, vegetable oils and fats that are low in SFA, have moderate amounts of MUFA and have adequate n-3 PUFA may be especially important for the prevention and treatment of many diseases.

Most of the clinical and experimental research that has investigated the effects of dietary fatty acids specifically on obesity and IR has focused on total fat or the effects of the fatty acid classes: SFA, MUFA and PUFA. Some study has also been devoted to the very long-chain marine n-3 PUFA [eicosapentanoic acid (EPA) and docosapentanoic acid (DHA)] but less is known about the plant-based n-3 PUFA, ALA. The study designs (controls, population, total amount of fat) and results vary but overall some consistent patterns with regard to fatty acid type can be extracted.

14.3.1 Monounsaturated Fatty Acids versus Saturated Fatty Acids

MUFAs refer to a family of fatty acids that are characterized as having one double bond. MUFAs in food have the double bond located either at 7 (n-7) or 9 (n-9) carbon atoms from the methyl end. The MUFAs in the diet include myristoleic acid (C14:1n-7), palmitoleic acid (C16:1n-7), vaccenic acid (C18:1n-7), OA (C18:1n-9), eicosenoic acid (C20:1n-9) and erucic acid (C22:1n-9; National Academy of Sciences et al., 2005). The body uses MUFAs to generate energy and as an important lipid in structural membranes, particularly nervous tissue myelin (National Academy of Sciences et al., 2005). MUFAs are not essential in the diet as they can be biosynthesized from other fuel sources. No adequate intake (AI), estimated average requirement (EAR) or recommended dietary allowance (RDA), has been set for MUFAs.

Dietary SFAs are abundantly present in animal products, but can also be found in plant products. The major SFAs in the diet include caprylic acid (C8:0), caproic acid (C10:0), lauric acid (C12:0), myristic acid (C14:0), palmitic acid (C16:0) and stearic acid (C18:0; National Academy of Sciences et al., 2005). SFAs have two primary functions in the body; they serve as a source of energy and are structural components of cell membranes (National Academy of Sciences et al., 2005). SFAs are not essential in the diet as they can be synthesized as needed from other fuel sources. In addition, SFAs are not associated with a beneficial role in the prevention of chronic disease, and neither an AI, EAR nor RDA has been set for SFA intake (National Academy of Sciences et al., 2005).

In general, a high SFA-diet negatively affects obesity and IR (reviewed in Funaki, 2009; Melansun et al., 2009; Risérus, 2008). Epidemiological data have shown that a relatively high saturated fatty acid plasma status is related to IR (Vessby et al., 1994, 2002; Laaksonen et al., 2002).

Important to the current discussion on canola oil, a few clinical trials have shown that diets high in SFA exacerbate IR compared to high MUFA diets. The KANWU study compared a high SFA diet (17% energy) to a high MUFA diet (21% energy) in which participants received butter and high SFA margarine or high-oleic sunflower oil margarine, respectively. The high-SFA diet reduced insulin sensitivity by 12.5%, while the high MUFA diet did not affect insulin sensitivity in randomly selected, healthy individuals. Insulin sensitivity was assessed by the intravenous glucose tolerance test (Vessby et al., 2001). Additional supplementation with 2.4 g/day of EPA and DHA did not further affect insulin sensitivity or insulin secretion in this study. Similarly, studies by Pérez-Jiménez et al. (2001) and Paniagua et al. (2007) showed that high SFA diets impaired insulin sensitivity compared to high MUFA diets. First, in a crossover design, healthy men and women were randomized to receive a high fat (38% energy)/SFA-enriched diet (20% energy) or a high carbohydrate/moderate fat (28% energy)/MUFA-enriched diet (22% energy). Those in the latter group had improved insulin sensitivity according to a modified insulin suppression test and steady-state plasma glucose levels, however, the lower fat content of the treatment diet may have been a confounding factor (Pérez-Jiménez et al., 2001). Secondly, insulin-resistant men and women (aged 62 ± 9.4 years) fed a high-SFA diet (38% total fat, 23% SFA) had lower insulin sensitivity compared to those fed a high-MUFA diet (38% total fat, 23% MUFA), as assessed by the frequently sampled insulin-assisted intravenous glucose tolerance test, in conjunction with reduced central body fat distribution (Paniagua et al., 2007).

In a diet-induced obesity (DIO) rat model, Buettner et al. (2006) examined the effect of standard chow versus various high-fat diets (42% energy) of lard, olive oil, coconut oil or fish oil on insulin sensitivity in Wistar rats. The high-fat olive oil diet (MUFA) and lard diets lead to the most pronounced worsening of IR, when assessed by the insulin tolerance test (but not by HOMA), and the most weight gain compared to the standard chow and high-fat fish oil diets. On the other hand, Rocca et al. (2001) showed that lean Zucker rats fed olive oil (5% energy) had improved area under the curve during a glucose tolerance test compared to a similar amount of coconut oil despite no differences in feed intake or body weight. These discrepancies may be attributed to the different genetic models (Wistar versus lean Zucker rats) and diets (high versus low fat).

Overall, the data suggest that SFAs are detrimental to obesity and IR, while MUFA appear at the very least neutral on these parameters based on limited clinical data. The recommendations to reduce SFA intake are therefore important, however, whether MUFA is superior to PUFA for the prevention or treatment of obesity and IR requires further investigation.

14.3.2 Polyunsaturated Fatty Acids

PUFAs consist of a group of fatty acids that have two or more double bonds. The first double bond can begin either six carbons from the methyl end (n-6) or three carbons from the methyl end (n-3).

Dietary n-6 PUFAs include the fatty acids, LA (C18:2n-6), γ-linolenic acid (C18:3n-6), dihomo-γ-linolenic acid (C20:3n-6), arachidonic acid (AA; C20:4n-6), adrenic acid (C22:4n-6) and docosapentaenoic acid (C22:5n-6; National Academy of Sciences et al., 2005). LA is an essential fatty acid because humans cannot synthesize it. Without dietary LA, deficiency occurs, producing adverse clinical symptoms, including reduced growth and a scaly rash (National Academy of Sciences et al., 2005). In the body, n-6 PUFAs function as a component of structural cell membranes and are involved in cell-signalling pathways. LA is also desaturated and elongated to AA and dihomo-γ-linolenic acid, which are substrates for eicosanoid production (National Academy of Sciences et al., 2005). Eicosanoids, such as prostaglandins, thromboxanes and leukotrienes, are signalling molecules and are important to human health because they exert complex control over many bodily systems (Simopoulos, 1999). A diet rich in n-6 PUFAs increases n-6 eicosanoid production, which is thought to shift the physiological state to one that is more pro-thrombotic, pro-constrictive and pro-inflammatory (reviewed by Simopoulos, 2002). It has been shown that the eicosanoids produced from AA contribute to the formation of thrombus, atheroma, allergic and inflammatory disorders as well as the proliferation of cells (reviewed by Simopoulos, 2002). The AI of LA for men aged between 19 and 50 years is 17 g/day and for men more than 50 years is 14 g/day. The AI of LA for women aged between 19 and 50 years is 12 g/day and for women over the age of 50, 11 g of LA/day is recommended (National Academy of Sciences et al., 2005). However, although n-6 PUFAs are essential to the diet, the typical North American population consumes excessive amounts of n-6 PUFAs (Simopoulos, 2002).

N-3 PUFAs include ALA which is an essential fatty acid that cannot be synthesized by humans. A deficiency in ALA leads to adverse clinical symptoms including neurological abnormalities and reduced growth (National Academy of Sciences et al., 2005). Common n-3 PUFAs in the diet include ALA (C18:3n-3), EPA (C20:5n-3), docosapentaenoic acid (DPA; C22:5n-3) and DHA (C22:6n-3; National Academy of Sciences et al., 2005). ALA is the parent compound of the n-3 series; the body uses ALA mainly as a source of energy and carbon, but also as a precursor for all n-3 very-long-chain PUFA derivatives including EPA and DHA (Thomas, 2002). The amount of conversion of dietary ALA into EPA and DHA by humans is not conclusive but is estimated to be up to 15% for EPA and 0.05%–5% for DHA, and strongly depends on the concentration of n-6 PUFAs in the diet (Thomas, 2002). However, Legrand et al. (2010) have recently demonstrated that plasma EPA and DHA levels can be maintained in humans without fish oils if adequate sources of ALA are consumed. EPA, which is desaturated and elongated from ALA, is a precursor for n-3 eicosanoids. In contrast to n-6 eicosanoids, eicosanoids produced by n-3 PUFAs are considered anti-inflammatory, anti-thrombotic, anti-arrhythmic, hypolipidemic and vasodilatory (reviewed by Simopoulos, 2002). They may play an important role in the prevention and treatment of coronary heart disease, hypertension, diabetes, cancer, arthritis and other inflammatory and autoimmune disorders (reviewed by Simopoulos, 1999). The AI of ALA for male and female adults is 1.6 g/day and 1.1 g/day, respectively (National Academy of Sciences et al., 2005).

There is much controversy around the optimal dietary ratio of n-6 to n-3 PUFAs. Increased dietary consumption of n-6 PUFAs has been shown to decrease the production of n-3 eicosanoids, and vice versa (reviewed by Simopoulos, 2002). This is due to competition *in vivo* of ALA and LA for the elongation and desaturation enzymes that are involved in the synthesis of long-chain PUFAs (Thomas, 2002). Humans evolved on a diet in which the n-6 to n-3 ratio was about 1, however, over the past 50–100 years there has been rapid changes in the human diet (Simopoulos, 2002). Currently, the typical North American diet is rich in n-6 PUFAs, which has resulted in an n-6 to n-3 ratio of ~16:1 (Simopoulos, 2006). Intakes of n-3 PUFAs are much lower and intakes of n-6 PUFAs are much higher than in the past because of the decrease in fish consumption and the increase in consumption of both oils that are rich in n-6, such as soyabean and safflower oil, and cereal grains that have a high n-6/n-3 ratio (Simopoulos, 1999). Also, the industrial production of animal feed rich in grains containing n-6 PUFAs has led to the production of meat with a high n-6 PUFA content, further offsetting the ratio of n-6 to n-3 (Simopoulos, 1999). Based on limited studies that have been done on animals, children and adults, the Food and Agriculture Organization/World Health Organization (1995) recommends that adults consume a LA:ALA ratio of 5–10:1 to maintain health. However, many researchers recommend a ratio of 5:1, or less, to reduce the risk of many chronic diseases (Simopoulos, 2002). Others point out that it is not the ratio, but rather the absolute intake of the different n-6 and n-3 fatty acids that is important for health (reviewed in Harris, 2006). For example, Harris et al. (2007) demonstrates that in heart disease LA, ALA, EPA and DHA all appear to reduce coronary heart disease risk. The determining factor for health, possibly also in relation to obesity and IR, may be consuming adequate amounts of both select n-6 and n-3 fatty acids, regardless of the ratio.

The notion that fatty acid type and specifically, n-3 fatty acids, could influence insulin action was first demonstrated under conditions of euglycaemic hyperinsulinaemic clamp in Wistar rats (standard healthy rat strain) fed a high-fat diet. Compared to rats fed a high-fat diet (59% energy) containing safflower oil that is primarily LA, replacing 20% of the fat with tuna oil led to a marked improvement in insulin sensitivity and, in particular, increased skeletal muscle glucose disposal during the euglycaemic hyperinsulinaemic clamp (Storlien et al., 1987). In this study, there was replacement of just 6% of the LA with long-chain n-3 EPA and DHA, however, plant-based ALA sources were not investigated. Several other studies using animal models of obesity have shown that EPA- and DHA-containing diets can protect against weight gain and IR compared to both high n-6 PUFA diets and high SFA diets via mechanisms that include improved skeletal muscle glucose disposal and reduced adipocyte size (Storlien et al., 1987, 1991; Baillie et al., 1999; Takahashi and Ide, 2000; Lombardo et al., 2007; Pérez-Echarri et al., 2008).

Human studies using n-3 fatty acids from fish oil have shown either a beneficial effect (Rasic-Milutinovic et al., 2007; Lombardo et al., 2007; Tsitouras et al., 2008) or no effect (Vessby et al., 2001; Browning et al., 2007) on overall insulin sensitivity, although there has been considerable variation in the experimental design (e.g., model, dose, duration, procedures for evaluation of insulin sensitivity). There is one report of fish oil supplementation in people with diabetes having negative effects on insulin sensitivity (assessed by isoglycaemic clamp) compared to controls consuming corn-oil (Mostad et al., 2006). In the OPTILIP study, insulin sensitivity and glycaemic control (evaluated by the homeostasis model assessment (HOMA) and quantitative insulin sensitivity check (QUICKI)) in 45–70-year-old people were not altered when the dietary n-6 to n-3 ratio was lowered from 10:1 to 3:1 (Griffin et al., 2006), but this was not a hyperglycaemic or hyperinsulinaemic population and thus changes in these measures may have been difficult to detect.

Research with ALA as the n-3 source and effects on insulin sensitivity has been limited, and the question remains whether the type of unsaturation or n-3 position/chain length is important for insulin sensitivity. In a study by Storlien et al. (1991), adult male Wistar rats were fed high-fat diets (34% energy) containing primarily SFA (tallow and safflower oil), MUFA (olive oil), PUFA (safflower oil), PUFA + fish oil (~10% energy), PUFA + flaxseed oil (~7% energy) or SFA + flaxseed oil for 30 days. Flaxseed oil is a rich source of ALA (55% of fatty acids). When substituted for SFA, but not when substituted for PUFA, the flaxeed oil (ALA) containing diet prevented IR as assessed by euglycaemic clamp. The PUFA + fish oil diet also prevented IR in these rats. Takahashi and Ide (2000) demonstrated that ALA-containing perilla oil and EPA/DHA-containing fish oil similarly normalized fasting serum glucose levels and reduced fat pad weights compared to safflower oil-fed DIO rats. In this study, rats were fed a high-fat diet (30% energy) for 3 weeks.

When comparing PUFA to MUFA on a population level ($n = 538$), the Pizarra study from Spain showed less IR, measured by HOMA, in individuals who reported consuming a high MUFA (olive oil) or mixed oil diet compared to those who consumed a diet rich in sunflower oil (high n-6 PUFA; Soriguer et al., 2006). The subjects with higher OA levels in plasma phospholipids had the lowest odds ratio for IR. Similarly, when comparing the fatty acid composition of serum phospholipids to the beta-cell function index of HOMA, and adjusted for age, BMI and an IR index, Rojo-Martínez et al. (2006) documented that of the fatty acid classes, only MUFA accounted for the variation in this index. The authors speculated that MUFA consumption is favourable for beta-cell insulin secretion.

Clinically, in overweight people with DM2, Brynes et al. (2000) did not find an association with dietary fatty acid manipulations (MUFA, 20.3 ± 3.5% energy versus PUFA, 13.4 ± 1.3% energy) on insulin sensitivity, assessed by the short-insulin tolerance test. This study was limited by a small sample size ($n = 9$).

In summary, both long- (ALA) and very-long-chain (EPA, DHA) n-3 fatty acids as well as MUFA (OA) may be beneficial for insulin sensitivity, however, this is based on very limited animal or population data.

14.3.3 MUFA versus Carbohydrate

Diets of <35% fat, favouring MUFA, and 45–60% carbohydrate are recommended by the Canadian Diabetes Association for people with diabetes (CDA, 2008). In a meta-analysis by Garg (1998) that focused on patients with DM2, a high MUFA diet was shown to significantly reduce the fasting plasma glucose concentrations compared to a high carbohydrate diet (−0.23 mmol/L), however, no improvement was seen in fasting serum insulin or insulin sensitivity when the euglycaemic hyperinsulinaemic glucose clamp technique was used. The author postulated that improved glycaemia in this case may have been attributed to a reduction in the carbohydrate load rather than improved insulin sensitivity. The studies reported in this meta-analysis provided higher total fat (37–50% energy) and lower carbohydrate intakes (35–40% energy) than are currently recommended.

14.3.4 Possible Synergistic Effects of Canola Oil Fatty Acids

The unique combination of MUFA and ALA in canola oil may provide synergistic benefits for obesity and/or IR. Louheranta et al. (2002) documented that in 31 subjects, a high MUFA diet containing canola oil, canola-oil-based margarines and high-OA sunflower oil (40% fat, 11% SFA, 19% MUFA, 8% PUFA) compared to a high SFA diet containing butter and a small amount of canola oil (37% fat, 18% SFA, 11% MUFA, 5% PUFA) increased the proportions of both OA and ALA in plasma phospholipids, and both of these fatty acids were found to be associated with lower fasting plasma glucose concentrations in people with impaired glucose tolerance. The high MUFA diet resulted in lower fasting plasma glucose concentrations and a better glucose effectiveness index, when assessed by the frequently sampled intravenous-glucose-tolerance test.

In mice fed high-fat diets (41% energy), those fed the canola oil diet had less weight gain and lower fat pad weights compared to those fed the beef fat diet (Bell et al., 1997). In fact, the mice fed the high-fat canola-based diets did not differ in body or fat pad weights compared to mice fed a low-fat control diet. IR was not assessed in this study.

In a model of genetic obesity, Mustad et al. (2006) investigated the effects of high-fat diets (43–45% energy) rich in MUFA (85% high-oleic safflower oil, 10% canola oil, 5% lecithin), or MUFA plus ALA, EPA or DHA (11–14% energy) on IR in *ob/ob* mice. After 29 days, only animals consuming the MUFA control and ALA/MUFA blend diets showed a trend to lower non-fasting glucose concentrations. Additionally, fasting plasma glucose values were significantly elevated in the animals consuming the MUFA + EPA and MUFA + DHA blends. When insulin sensitivity was assessed with the insulin tolerance test, only the MUFA + ALA diet proved beneficial.

Although the data are extremely limited, the ALA content of canola oil may not only provide benefits for IR, and the combination of MUFA and ALA may prove particularly beneficial for obesity and IR.

14.4 HYPOTHESES FOR METABOLIC EFFECTS OF CANOLA OIL

There is currently next to no data to support mechanisms of action for positive effects of canola oil on obesity, IR and the metabolic syndrome. Some hypotheses can be summarized based on the literature surrounding other fatty acids, particularly very long chain n-3 and other PUFAs.

14.4.1 Regulation of Transcription Factors

It is well documented that, independent of whole body obesity, inappropriate lipid storage in the muscle, heart and liver is closely related to whole body insulin action (reviewed by Storlien et al., 1996). A mechanism by which n-3 PUFAs are suggested to improve IR is by their ability to inhibit lipid accumulation in non-adipose tissues by directing fatty acids away from intracellular storage and towards fatty acid oxidation (reviewed by Clarke, 2000). The ability of n-3 PUFAs to improve IR by altering lipid metabolism has mainly been documented with marine n-3 PUFAs. Peroxisome proliferator-activated receptors (PPARs) and sterol regulatory element-binding proteins (SREBPs) are two important transcription factors that may explain the actions of certain fatty acids on obesity and IR, although more research is required to determine if the fatty acids in canola oil are biologically significant ligands for these transcription factors.

14.4.1.1 Peroxisome Proliferator-Activated Receptors and PUFAs

PPARs are ligand-activated nuclear transcription factors that belong to the steroid hormone nuclear receptor family (Sampath and Ntambi, 2005). In general, PPARs act to increase fatty acid elongation, transport and oxidation. There are three PPAR isoforms: PPARα, PPARβ and PPARγ. PPARα is the major isoform found in hepatocytes and has an important function in lipid homeostasis by regulating genes encoding lipid metabolism enzymes, lipid transporters, apolipoproteins, and Δ5, Δ6 and Δ9 desaturases (Costet et al., 1998; Jump 2002; Sampath and Ntambi, 2005). PPARs regulate genes involved in long-chain fatty acid oxidation including fatty acyl-CoA synthase (FACS), acyl-CoA oxidase (ACO), 2-enoyl-CoA hydratase and 3-hydroxy acyl-CoA dehydrogenase (reviewed by Clarke, 2000). ACO is the most widely used marker of peroxisome proliferator action and its activity increases during peroxisomal proliferation (Tugwood et al., 1992).

PUFAs are naturally occurring PPARα ligands, which are hypothesized to activate fatty acid oxidation. Although n-6 PUFAs can activate PPARα, n-3 PUFAs are more potent PPARα activators *in vivo* (reviewed by Schmitz and Ecker, 2008). Among n-3 PUFAs, EPA is the strongest PPARα activator while ALA and DHA are weak activators but can be converted *in vivo* into EPA (Jump, 2008). Interestingly, eicosanoids are even stronger activators of PPARα than EPA (reviewed by Schmitz and Ecker, 2008).

A study by Neschen et al. (2007) demonstrated that n-3 PUFAs from fish oil protect against high-fat diet-induced hepatic IR in mice by acting in a PPARα-dependent manner. In this study, both wild type and PPARα null mice that were fed high-fat diets (59% energy) based on safflower oil developed IR as assessed by the euglycaemic clamp method. However, IR was prevented in wild-type mice but not in PPARα null mice when both groups were fed a high-fat safflower oil diet where 8% of the safflower oil had been replaced with fish oil. In another study by Neschen et al. (2002), the mechanism by which fish oil protects against fat-induced IR was determined by examining the effects of high-fat (59% energy) fish oil and safflower oil diets on markers of peroxisomal fatty acid oxidation. Fish oil-fed rats had a 150% increase in the peroxisomal enzymes ACO and 3-ketoacyl-CoA thiolase in the liver and an almost 2-fold increase in hepatic peroxisome content compared to rats fed the high-fat safflower oil and control diet containing soyabean oil (17% energy). Additionally, these changes in the fish oil-fed rats were associated with significantly lower hepatic TAG content. Despite the massive peroxisome proliferation in the fish oil-fed rats, there was no associated increase in hepatic PPAR gene expression. To further support n-3/PPAR regulation of fatty acid oxidation, Baillie et al. (1999) studied Fisher rats fed a high-fat diet (40% energy) containing either fish oil or corn oil. After 6 weeks, the fish oil group had a nearly three fold higher gene expression of ACO in the liver. When comparing the effects of different high fat diets (42% energy) in Wistar rats, Buettner et al. (2006) found that high-fat-fed fish oil rats had upregulation of key lipid oxidation genes compared to rats fed high-fat lard, olive oil, or coconut oil diets. Carnitine palmitoyl transferase and enoyl-CoA, major enzymes of fatty acid oxidation, were downregulated in all high-fat-fed diet groups except for the high-fat-fed fish oil group. PPARα was only upregulated in the high-fat fish oil group and, in particular, 8 out of 10 PPAR-dependent genes were upregulated in the high-fat fish oil group, whereas only minor changes were seen in the mRNA levels of PPAR-dependent genes of the other high-fat-fed groups, including the group fed OA-containing olive oil group.

Taken together, these data suggest that n-3 PUFAs from fish oil act as naturally occurring PPAR ligands which bind and activate PPAR receptors and lead to peroxisome proliferation, increased hepatic fat oxidation and less hepatic fat storage. All of these studies strongly support the hypothesized mechanism that n-3 PUFAs protect against fat-induced IR by enhancing lipid oxidation by acting as a PPAR ligand. It is possible that the relatively high ALA content in canola oil as opposed to olive oil can affect PPAR metabolism, either directly as ALA or indirectly through metabolism to EPA and DHA.

14.4.1.2 Sterol Regulatory Element-Binding Proteins and PUFA

It seems as though dietary PUFAs also favourably alter lipid metabolism by suppressing lipogenic genes and reducing fat synthesis. SREBP-1c is a nuclear transcription factor in the liver that is required for the insulin-mediated induction of hepatic fatty acid and TAG synthesis. The expression and nuclear localization of SREBP-1c is suppressed by dietary PUFAs (Worgall et al., 1998; Xu et al., 1999). There are three isoforms of SREBP: SREBP-1a, SREBP-1c and SREBP-2. The SREBP-1c isoform is the most prominent in rodent and human liver and is the key regulator of fatty acid synthesis (reviewed by Price et al., 2000). Acetyl-CoA carboxylase (ACC) and fatty acid synthase (FAS) are two important enzymes that are regulated by SREBP-1c; ACC is the rate-limiting enzyme in long-chain fatty acid synthesis (Hardie, 1989; Horton, 2002). Other genes that are regulated by SREBP include stearoyl-CoA carboxylase and glycerol 3-phosphate acyltransferase, an enzyme involved in TAG production (Horton, 2002).

Both n-3 and n-6 PUFAs have been shown to decrease the expression of genes that are regulated by SREBP. Wilson et al. (1990) demonstrated that PUFAs can decrease the hepatic production of malonyl-CoA, suggesting that hepatic ACC transcription is suppressed by dietary PUFAs. Malonyl-CoA is an indicator of acetyl-CoA carboxylation, as acetyl-CoA is converted into malonyl-CoA by ACC (Wilson et al., 1990).

Buettner et al. (2006) demonstrated the ability of n-3 PUFAs from fish oil to suppress hepatic FAS. In this study, rats that were fed high-fat (42% energy) lard, olive oil or coconut oil diets for 12 weeks had increased hepatic FAS and stearoyl-CoA desaturase, which are major enzymes of fatty acid synthesis, however, in high-fat fish oil-fed rats, there was no upregulation of these genes compared to standard chow fed rats.

Further studies have demonstrated that, of the n-3 PUFAs, DHA is the most potent fatty acid regulator of SREBP (reviewed by Jump, 2008). The mechanism by which DHA seems to work is by lowering SREBP-1 nuclear content (reviewed by Jump, 2008). Other n-3 and n-6 PUFAs seem to suppress SREBP-1 by regulating SREBP-1c gene transcription and by decreasing the stability of SREBP-1 mRNA (reviewed by Jump, 2008; Xu et al., 1999). More research specific to MUFA and ALA is needed in the future.

14.4.1.3 Relationship of MUFA to PPARs and SREBPs

Although most of the attention for the fatty acid regulation of PPARs has focused on very-long-chain n-3 fatty acids, there are some suggestions that MUFA may also play a role in PPAR metabolism. As part of the Pizarra study, Soriguer et al. (2006) have shown that people with the Pro12Ala polymorphism had a substantially reduced odds ratio for impaired fasting glucose, impaired glucose tolerance and DM2. Those with this genetic variation were found to have higher HOMA values when MUFA intake was low. It is possible that MUFAs may also improve insulin sensitivity by activating PPARα and fatty acid oxidation. However, although OA can efficiently bind PPARα *in vitro*, OA has not actually been shown to activate PPARα in hepatocytes in rats (Kliewer et al., 1997; Jump, 2002).

Another possible role of dietary MUFA with regard to obesity and IR may be related to the regulation of stearoyl coA desaturase (SCD). SCD is the enzyme responsible for converting SFA into MUFA (e.g., C18:0 to C18:1) by introducing a *cis* double bond between carbons 9 and 10 from the carboxyl end of the fatty acid chain. SCD contains promoter sites for both SREBP-1 and PPARs in mice and humans (Zhang et al., 1999, 2001, 2005; Bene et al., 2001). Of four SCD isoforms (SCD-1 to -4; of which SCD-1 and -2 have been identified in humans; Zhang et al., 1999, 2005), SCD-1 has received considerable attention because its inhibition protects against obesity, IR and other components of the metabolic syndrome in mice (Cohen et al., 2003; Dobrzyn and Ntambi, 2005). SCD is also thought to stimulate fat storage rather than oxidation and as such, SCD-1-deficient mice are protected from diet- and genetically induced obesity (Ntambi et al., 2002; Chu et al., 2006; Macdonald et al., 2008). Insulin sensitivity is improved within the liver, muscle and adipose of the SCD-1-deficient mice (Rahman et al., 2003, 2005; Gutierrez-Juárez et al., 2006). However, there are some contradictions in the literature to suggest that upregulating, rather than inhibiting, SCD-1 is beneficial (reviewed in Popeijus et al., 2008). This may be due to the differences in mouse and human lipid metabolism and, although the data are limited, it appears that upregulation may be beneficial in humans. Risérus et al. (2005) showed that treatment with the diabetes drug rosiglitazone, a known PPARγ agonist, reduces IR coincidently with increased SCD activity (based on the SCD index). Mauvoisin et al. (2007, 2010) have shown that in HepG2 cells insulin upregulates SCD-1 expression via SREBP-1, while leptin downregulates SCD-1 expression. The extent by which dietary MUFAs such as OA may inhibit SCD in humans in relation to obesity and IR is unclear. What is known is that SCD-1 is expressed predominantly in liver and adipose in humans, making it an interesting potential target.

14.4.2 Tissue Lipid Accumulation and Fatty Acid Composition

The mechanism that is most frequently used to describe the effect of n-3 PUFAs on IR is the ability of n-3 PUFAs to increase the unsaturation and the fluidity of structural membrane lipids (reviewed by Storlien et al., 1996; Glatz et al., 2010). Although more rigid cell membranes are able to bind as much or more insulin as fluid membranes, the unsaturation induced by n-3 PUFAs may enhance events following insulin binding such as the movement of the glucose transporter to the cell membrane (Storlien et al., 1987). Although n-6 PUFAs are also highly unsaturated, and should also be able to increase membrane fluidity, n-3 PUFAs are elongated and desaturated to a greater extent than is true for the PUFAs in the n-6 pathway where AA is the normal end point.

However, it is also suggested that the degree of membrane unsaturation may not be as important as the overall changes in the membrane fatty acid composition. For example, Mustad et al. (2006) found that insulin sensitivity was improved in *ob/ob* mice that were fed a high-fat diet rich in MUFA and ALA, but not MUFA plus EPA or DHA. The rats fed the MUFA plus ALA diet had a smaller reduction in total MUFAs and a more modest increase in total n-3 PUFAs in liver and muscle PL compared to animals fed diets rich in MUFA plus EPA or DHA. It may be possible that it is the combination of MUFA plus ALA in PL that allows for more insulin sensitivity and uptake of glucose.

14.4.2.1 Liver Fatty Acid Metabolism

The primary cause of excess lipid accumulation in the liver, or hepatic steatosis, is hyperlipidaemia induced by IR. In the insulin resistant state, TAG that are normally stored in adipocytes are also stored in the liver leading to hepatic steatosis. In addition, more fat storage in the liver increases hepatic VLDL production, resulting in elevated serum TAG concentrations. However, TAG also continues to accumulate in the liver because there are limits to VLDL production (e.g., limits on apoB-100; reviewed by Neuschwander-Tetri and Caldwell, 2003).

The n-3 PUFAs and MUFA can help prevent hepatic steatosis in a number of different ways. It has been proposed that n-3 PUFAs alter the hepatic fatty acid composition of TAG and PL and this may reduce hepatic steatosis. Studies that have investigated the hepatic lipid composition of patients with NAFLD reveal a depletion of n-3 and n-6 PUFAs in hepatic TAG, decreased n-3 PUFAs in hepatic PL, and an increase in the n-6 to n-3 ratio in hepatic tissue (Allard et al., 2008).

The liver is responsible for the conversion of ALA into EPA and DHA via a series of elongation and desaturation steps. The Δ5 and Δ6 desaturases are important enzymes in the biosynthesis of 20 carbon PUFAs. However, very little is known about the ability of the body to convert large amounts of ALA to its long-chain derivatives (Morise et al., 2004). Impairment in the Δ5 and Δ6 desaturase index is associated with NAFLD (Burdge et al., 2002; Allard et al., 2008). A reduction in Δ5 desaturase activity is also associated with IR (reviewed by Vessby, 2000) and obesity (Pan et al., 1994). It is important to determine if dietary ALA can elevate EPA and DHA in hepatic TAG and PL by increasing Δ5 and Δ6 desaturase activity. This suggests a possible mechanism for improved hepatic steatosis, IR and obesity.

Additionally, an increase in long-chain n-3 PUFAs in hepatic TAG and PL may also reduce inflammation associated with hepatic steatosis by increasing the biosynthesis of anti-inflammatory eicosanoids. In general, dietary PUFAs have been suggested to suppress Δ5 and Δ6 desaturase activity (Sekiya et al., 2003); however, the effects of dietary ALA on the regulation of these enzymes are controversial. A study by Morise et al. (2004) found no increase in the Δ5 or Δ6 desaturase index in hamsters when they were fed ALA in various amounts (the LA/ALA ratio varied from

22.5 to 0.6). However, in this study, circulating EPA concentration was strictly linear and proportional to dietary ALA, even though the Δ5 and Δ6 desaturase indexes were identical among groups, suggesting that ALA even in very large amounts does not regulate its own desaturation, at least in the hamster. It is the amount of substrate (versus desaturase levels) that appears to be important.

Along with the liver, adipose tissue is also important for whole body insulin-sensitivity and possible adipose-related mechanisms are explained next.

14.4.2.2 Adipose Function and Inflammatory Markers

When adipocytes become enlarged, namely due to obesity, their endocrine and metabolic functions are altered, resulting in adipocyte dysfunction (reviewed by Weisberg et al., 2003; reviewed by DeClercq et al., 2008). White adipose tissue and/or infiltrated macrophages not only secrete adipokine hormones such as pro-inflammatory leptin and anti-inflammatory adiponectin, but also pro-inflammatory cytokines such as TNF-α and IL-6, and acute-phase proteins such as haptoglobin and CRP (reviewed by DeClercq et al., 2008; Pérez-Echarri et al., 2008; Ahima 2000). The synthesis and secretion of these pro- and anti-inflammatory markers are altered by changes in adipocyte size and number (Guerre-Millo, 2003). Larger adipocytes are more insulin resistant and produce more pro-inflammatory and less anti-inflammatory mediators (reviewed by Weisberg et al., 2003).

There is limited research available on the effects of MUFAs on adipose function and inflammatory markers. A cross-sectional study evaluated the effects of various components of the Mediterranean diet on inflammatory markers in 339 men and 433 women with diabetes. This study showed that subjects with the highest consumption of nuts and olive oil (rich in MUFAs) had the lowest circulating concentrations of IL-6 and CRP (Salas-Salvadó et al., 2008). In a clinical trial, insulin-resistant patients who consumed MUFA-rich diet, containing 47% (energy) carbohydrate and 38% fat (9% SFA; 23% MUFA of which 75% was provided as extra virgin olive oil; and 6% PUFA) had elevated adiponectin mRNA expression in adipose tissue along with improved insulin sensitivity (assessed by euglycaemic clamp) compared to subjects who consumed carbohydrate-rich diets (Paniagua et al., 2007). Elevated levels of adiponectin are beneficial given its anti-inflammatory and cardio-protective properties (DeClercq et al., 2008). Further studies on the effects of OA, ALA and other components of canola oil on inflammatory markers and adipose function are warranted.

Numerous mechanisms have been suggested for how n-3 PUFAs may improve inflammation and adipocyte function. N-3 PUFAs may decrease adiposity, adipocyte size and macrophage infiltration, enhance the production of anti-inflammatory adipokines and cytokines, and reduce the production of pro-inflammatory adipokines and cytokines (Calder et al., 2009). Research suggests that the ability of n-3 PUFAs to normalize the concentrations of the adipokines leptin and adiponectin may be related to the role of n-3 PUFAs in adiposity and insulin sensitivity. Lombardo et al. (2007) used 2-month-old male Wistar rats to investigate the effects of FAs on adipokines. The diets consisted of a starch-rich control diet and two sucrose-rich diets (to induce obesity) where corn oil or fish oil were the fat sources (8% by weight); the intervention period lasted for 2 months. Plasma leptin and adiponectin levels in rats fed the fish oil diet were comparable to those on the control diet, while the corn oil diet produced a decrease in both adipokines. Furthermore, leptin and adiponectin mRNA levels in WAT were unchanged by diet.

An epidemiological study from Tuscany, Italy, revealed that there is a negative association between dietary intake of ALA, EPA and DHA, as well as the n-6 fatty acid, AA, and pro-inflammatory markers such CRP and IL-1ra (Ferrucci et al., 2006). In another study, 24 obese subjects with elevated inflammatory markers were involved in a prospective, double-blind crossover study and randomized into two groups, a flaxseed flour group, receiving 5 g ALA/day, and a placebo group. After 2 weeks, the flaxseed group had a significant reduction in the inflammatory markers CRP, serum amyloid A and fibronectin, whereas there was no change in these inflammatory markers in the placebo group (Faintuch et al., 2007).

Smaller, more insulin-sensitive adipocytes have a direct, positive effect on insulin sensitivity and it remains to be seen if the combination of fatty acids found in canola oil may reduce adipocyte size and improve adipocyte function.

14.4.2.3 Fatty Acids and Insulin Signalling

An effect on insulin signalling may further define the relationship between fatty acids and IR. The insulin signalling cascade can be viewed as a complex series of phosphorylation events that begin with insulin binding to a transmembrane receptor and ends with a number of different outcomes including gene regulation, growth, differentiation, glycogen and protein synthesis and glucose uptake into the cell (Glund and Zierath, 2005). Increases in FFA in the blood, such as what occurs in obesity, are associated with impairment of these parameters (Belfort et al., 2005). Dysfunction of the insulin signalling cascade is the basis for IR.

The first step in the insulin signalling pathway involves insulin binding to its receptor in the cell membrane; this receptor is a tyrosine kinase that spans the phospholipid bilayer and insulin binding induces autophosphorylation of the receptor (Glund and Zierath, 2005). Normal insulin binding with a 40% reduction in insulin receptor tyrosine kinase activity has been observed in human muscle in obesity with and without DM2 (Arner et al., 1987). Further investigation into this observation has shown a direct role for TNF-α in inhibiting insulin receptor tyrosine kinase activity in muscle tissue (Hotamisligil et al., 1994; Hotamisligil, 1999); since TNF-α is increased in obesity due to increased leptin (Loffreda et al., 1998), the resultant inhibition of the insulin receptor tyrosine kinase increases IR.

Autophosphorylation of the insulin receptor leads to phosphorylation of insulin receptor substrate (IRS). IRS comes in four different forms (IRS-1, IRS-2, IRS-3 and IRS-4). In muscle tissue, IRS-1 is the most important form for mediating insulin-signal transduction and IRS-1 impairment has been observed in muscle tissue of humans with DM-2 (Glund and Zierath, 2005). IRS-1 has many tyrosine phosphorylation sites. When these sites are phosphorylated by the insulin receptor, multiple insulin signals are enabled (Sun et al., 1993). IRS-1 also has several serine phosphorylation sites; phosphorylation of serine residue 1101 results in inhibition of insulin signalling and provides a possible mechanism for IR (Li et al., 2004). After IRS is phosphorylated, it recruits and activates phosphatidylinositol 3-kinase (PI3-kinase). PI3-kinase phosphorylates phosphatidylinositol-4,5-bisphosphate (PIP_2) to form phosphatidylinositol-3,4,5-triphosphate (PIP_3). PIP_3 then serves as an activator of various serine–threonine kinases including Akt.

Taouis et al. (2002) investigated the effects of dietary fatty acids on insulin signalling in muscle tissue. For their study, 5-week-old male Wistar rats were fed one of three diets for 4 weeks: control (high carbohydrate), n-6 PUFA (58% energy from safflower oil), or n-3 PUFA (39% energy from safflower oil and 19% energy from fish oil). To determine effects of insulin stimulation, the rats were injected with insulin 7 min before termination. The results of this study showed that insulin-induced tyrosine phosphorylation of IR and IRS was similar in the muscle of the animals fed control and n-3 PUFA diets, but depressed in the animals fed the n-6 PUFA diet.

Like IRS, Akt also has many phosphorylation sites; in order for Akt to become activated, serine residue 473 and threonine residue 308 must be phosphorylated (Persad et al., 2001). Akt activation is reduced in muscle tissue of people with DM-2 (Glund and Zierath, 2005). Chavez and Summers (2003) treated C_2C_{12} myotubes with 0.75 mM FFA for 16 h, 4 days after differentiation and found that 16:0, but not OA-inhibited Akt activation. Additionally, in Wistar rats, Le Foll et al. (2007) found that a diet containing fish oil (9.7% energy from peanut/rapeseed and 4.9% energy from fish oil) resulted in non-significant reductions in Akt phosphorylation compared to the control diet (14.6% energy as a peanut/rapeseed oil mix), which coincidentally was a treatment providing MUFA and ALA.

Ultimately, dietary fatty acids seem to influence insulin sensitivity not only by altering cell membrane lipid composition, but also by affecting fatty acid oxidation and synthesis. The transcription factors involved with the ability of n-3 PUFAs to improve adiposity and insulin sensitivity, namely by PPARα and SREBP-1, may also work to improve adipocyte function, inflammation and insulin signalling. However, more research is needed to determine if OA and ALA can have the same effect on membrane PL composition and the transcription of genes involved in fatty acid synthesis and oxidation as the longer chain marine n-3 PUFAs.

14.4.3 Fatty Acid-Independent Mechanisms

Minor components of canola oil include tocopherols (700–1200 ppm of mainly α and γ tocopherols) and chlorophylls (5–35 ppm). The α-tocopherol (vitamin E) content of canola oil is 2.44 mg/tablespoon (USDA, 2010). This is higher than most vegetable oils except sunflower and safflower oils (USDA, 2010). The γ-tocopherol content is not readily reported, but in canola oil is typically about 1.5 times that of the α-tocopherol content (Przybylski, 2010). The RDA for Vitamin E for adults is 15 mg/day. Most of the trace elements found in the canola plant such as phosphorus, iron, calcium, sulphur, zinc and lead are removed or minimzed during processing (Przybylski, 2010).

Some of the minor components that remain in the refined oil may act as antioxidants within the body and thus may be beneficial for chronic disease prevention, including metabolic syndrome, however, there are no data as to the levels of these compounds present in canola oil and their effects on health. For example, Siger et al. (2008) have documented a relatively high amount of phenolic compounds (256.6 ± 0.73 μg/100 g) and antioxidant activities in cold-pressed canola oil compared to other cold-pressed oils. The potential health effects as related to obesity and IR are as yet unknown.

14.5 SUMMARY AND CONCLUSIONS

Obesity and IR are affecting human health worldwide. Canola oil is thought to have a favourable fatty acid profile for health, however, very few studies have examined canola oil itself and the synergistic effects of its fatty acid profile on obesity and IR directly. On a population level, high MUFA intake appears to be favourable for reducing IR. However, the effects in experimental and clinical trials are varied, and study of the unique fatty acid profile of canola oil itself is relatively scarce, although there is emerging data of a beneficial, synergistic effect of ALA and OA. There are several potential mechanisms including effects on transcription factors such as PPARs and SREBPs. Alterations in tissue lipid accumulation, fatty acid composition and adipocyte size, as affected by these transcription factors or by independent mechanisms, may explain how canola oil fatty acids could be beneficial, although much more data are required.

14.6 LIMITATIONS AND IMPLICATIONS FOR FUTURE RESEARCH

Very few of the studies cited in this chapter have tested the effects of canola oil itself, which is high in MUFA and ALA, and low in SFA, on obesity and IR. Many of the studies cited that offer mechanisms to explain the beneficial actions of fats/oils on health have used the marine fatty acids EPA and DHA as the n-3 PUFAs in their diet formulations and not ALA. Additionally, there is a lack of comprehensive comparison of various fats and oils that represent different SFA/MUFA/PUFA and n-6/n-3 compositions. Genetically or pharmacologically induced obesity in animal models have been used to study obesity and IR but may not be representative of human obesity. High-fat fed, DIO models may be more useful when studying gene–environment interactions. Research on the metabolic syndrome and DM2 has focused on how dietary lipids affect hyperlipidaemia, insulin signalling in the muscle tissue, or muscle fatty acid composition. However, hepatic steatosis, inflammation and adipose function are important parts of the pathogenesis of obesity, IR and the metabolic syndrome. Future research needs to include hepatic and adipose tissue to get a better overall picture of how different dietary interventions and fatty acid compositions influence all components of the metabolic syndrome.

REFERENCES

Ahima, R.S. Adipose tissue as an endocrine organ. *Trends Endocrinol Metab* 2000, 11, 327–332.

Allard, J.P.; Aghdassi, E.; Mohammed, S.; Ramn, M.; Avand, G.; Arendt, B.M.; Jalali, P. et al. Nutritional assessment and hepatic fatty acid composition in non-alcoholic fatty liver disease (NAFLD): A cross-sectional study. *J Hepatol* 2008, 48, 300–307.

American Diabetes Association (ADA). Fats and diabetes. http://www.diabetes.org/food-nutrition-lifestyle/nutrition/meal planning/fatand-diabetes.jsp (April 2, 2009).

Anand, S.S.; Yi, Q.; Gerstein, H.; Lonn, E.; Jacobs, R.; Vuksan, V.; Teo, K.; Davis, B.; Montague, P.; Phil, S.Y. Relationship of metabolic syndrome and fibrinolytic dysfunction to cardiovascular disease. *Circulation* 2003, 108, 420–425.

Arner, P.; Pollare, T.; Lithell, H.; Livingston, J.N. Defective insulin receptor tyrosine kinase in human skeletal muscle in obesity and type 2 (non-insulin-dependent) diabetes mellitus. *Diabetologia* 1987, 30, 437–440.

Baillie, R.A.; Takada, R.; Nakamura, M.; Clarke, S.D. Coordinate induction of peroxisomal acyl-CoA oxidase and UCP-3 by dietary fish oil a mechanism for decreased body fat deposition. *Prostaglandins, Leukotrienes and Essential Fatty Acids* 1999, 60, 351–356.

Belfort, R.; Mandarino, L.; Kashyap, S.; Wirfel, K.; Pratipanawatr, T.; Berria, R.; DeFronzo, R.A.; Cusi, K. Dose–response effect of elevated plasma free fatty acid on insulin signaling. *Diabetes* 2005, 54, 1640–1648.

Bell, R.R.; Spencer, M.J.; Sherriff, J.L. Voluntary exercise and monounsaturated canola oil reduce fat gain in mice fed diets high in fat. *J Nutr* 1997, 127, 2006–2010.

Bene, H.; Lasky, D.; Ntambi, J.M. Cloning and characterization of the human stearoyl-CoA desaturase gene promoter: Transcriptional activation by sterol regulatory element binding protein and repression by polyunsaturated fatty acids and cholesterol. *Biochem Biophys Res Commun* 2001, 284, 1194–1198.

Browning, L.M.; Krebs, J.D.; Moore, C.S.; Mishra, G.D.; O'Connell, M.A.; Jebb, S.A. The impact of long chain n-3 polyunsaturated fatty acid supplementation on inflammation, insulin sensitivity and CVD risk in a group of overweight women with an inflammatory phenotype. *Diabetes Obes Metab* 2007, 9, 70–80.

Brynes, A.E.; Edwards, C.M.; Jadhav, A.; Ghatei, M.A.; Bloom, S.R.; Frost, G.S. Diet-induced change in fatty acid composition of plasma triacylglycerols is not associated with change in glucagon-like peptide 1 or insulin sensitivity in people with type 2 diabetes. *Am J Clin Nutr* 2000, 72, 1111–1118.

Buettner, R.; Parhofer, K.G.; Woenckhaus, M.; Wrede, C.E.; Kunz-Schughart, L.A.; Scholmerich, J.; Bollheimer, L.C. Defining high-fat diet rat models: Metabolic and molecular effects of different fat types. *J Mol Endocrinol* 2006, 36, 485–501.

Burdge, G.C.; Jones, A.E.; Wootton, S.A. Eicosapentaenoic and docosapentaenoic acids are the principal products of alpha-linolenic acid metabolism in young men. *Br J Nutr* 2002, 88, 355–363.

Calder, P.S.; Albers, R.; Antoine, J-M.; Blum, S.; Broudet-Sicard, R.; Ferns, G.A.; Folkerts, G. et al. Inflammatory disease processes and interaction with nutrition. *Br J Nutr* 2009, 101, S1–S45.

Canadian Diabetes Association (CDA). Clinical practice guidelines for the prevention and management of diabetes in Canada. *Can J Diabetes* 2008, 32, S1–S201.

Canola Council of Canada. Canola oil. http://www.canola-council.org (December 16, 2008).

Chavez, J.A.; Summers, S.A. Characterizing the effects of saturated fatty acids on insulin signaling and ceramide and diacylglycerol accumulation in 3T3-L1 adipocytes and C2C12 myotubes. *Arch Biochem Biophys* 2003, 419, 101–109.

Chobanian, A.V.; Bakris, G.L.; Black, H.R.; Cushman, W.C.; Green, L.A.; Izzo, J.L. Jr.; Jones, D.W. et al. Seventh report of the joint national committee on prevention, detection, evaluation, and treatment of high blood pressure. *Hypertension* 2003, 42, 1206–1252.

Chu, K.; Miyazaki, M.; Man, W.C.; Ntambi, J.M. Stearoyl-coenzyme A desaturase 1 deficiency protects against hypertriglyceridemia and increases plasma high-density lipoprotein cholesterol induced by liver X receptor activation. *Mol Cell Biol* 2006, 26, 6786–6798.

Clarke, S.D. Polyunsaturated fatty acid regulation of gene transcription: A mechanism to improved energy balance and insulin resistance. *British J Nutr* 2000, 83, 59–66.

Cohen, P.; Ntambi, J.M.; Friedman, J.M. Stearoyl-CoA desaturase-1 and the metabolic syndrome. *Curr Drug Targets Immune Endocr Metabol Disord* 2003, 3, 271–280.

Costet, P.; Legendre, C.; Moré, J.; Edgar, A.; Galtier, P.; Pineau, T. Peroxisome proliferator-activated receptor α-isoform deficiency leads to progressive dyslipidemia with sexually dimorphic obesity and steatosis. *J Biol Chem* 1998, 273, 29577–29585.

DeClercq, V.; Taylor, C.; Zahradka, P. Adipose tissue: The link between obesity and cardiovascular disease. *Cardiovasc Haematolog Disord-Drug Targets* 2008, 8, 228–237.

De Vries, C.P.; Van Haeften, T.W.; Wieringa, T.J.; Van der Veen, E.A. The insulin receptor. *Diabetes Res* 1989, 11, 155–165.

Dobrzyn, A.; Ntambi, J.M. Stearoyl-CoA desaturase as a new drug target for obesity treatment. *Obes Rev* 2005, 6, 169–174.

Douketis, J.D.; Paradis, G.; Keller, H.; Martineau, C. Canadian guidelines for body weight classification in adults: Application in clinical practice to screen for overweight and obesity and to assess disease risk. *CMAJ* 2005, 172, 995–998.

Faintuch, J.; Horie, L.M.; Barbeiro, H.V.; Barbeiro, D.F.; Soriano, F.G.; Ishida, R.K.; Cecconello, I. Systemic inflammation in morbidly obese subjects: Response to oral supplementation with alpha-linolenic acid. *Obesity Surgery* 2007, 17, 341–347.

Ferrucci, L.; Cherubini, A.; Bandinelli, S.; Bartali, B.; Corsi, A.; Lauretani, F.; Martin, A.; Andres-Lacueva, C.; Senin, U.; Guralnik, J.M. Relationship of plasma polyunsaturated fatty acids to circulating inflammatory markers. *J Clin Endocrin Metab* 2006, 91, 439–436.

Food and Agricultural Organization/World Health Organization. WHO and FAO joint consultation: Fats and oils in human nutrition. *Nutr Rev* 1995, 53, 202–205.

Food and Drug Administration. Unsaturated Fatty Acids from Canola Oil and Reduced Risk of Coronary Heart Disease. http://www.fda.gov/Food/LabelingNutrition/LabelClaims/QualifiedHealthClaimsucm073992.htm#canola (December 16, 2006).

Funaki, M. Saturated fatty acids and insulin resistance. *J Med Invest* 2009, 56, 88–92.

Garg, A. High-monounsaturated-fat diets for patients with diabetes mellitus: A meta-analysis. *Am J Clin Nutr* 1998, 67, 577–582.

Glatz, J.F.; Luiken, J.J.; Bonen, A. Membrane fatty acid transporters as regulators of lipid metabolism: Implications for metabolic disease. *Physiol Rev* 2010, 90, 367–417.

Glund, S.; Zierath, J.R. Tackling the insulin-signalling cascade. *Can J Diabetes* 2005, 29, 239–245.

Griffin, M.D.; Sanders, T.A.; Davies, I.G.; Morgan, L.M.; Millward, D.J.; Lewis, F.; Slaughter, S., Cooper, J.A.; Miller, G.J.; Griffin, B.A. Effects of altering the ratio of dietary n-6 on 3 fatty acids on insulin sensitivity, lipoprotein size, and postprandial lipemia in men and post menopausal women aged 45–70 y: The OPTILIP study. *Am J Clin Nutr* 2006, 84, 1290–1298.

Grundy, S.M. Low-density lipoprotein, non-high-density lipoprotein, and apolipoprotein B as targets of lipid-lowering therapy. *Circulation* 2002, 106, 2526–2529.

Grundy, S.M.; Cleeman, J.I.; Daniels, S.R.; Donato, K.A.; Eckel, R.H.; Franklin, B.A.; Gordon, D.J. et al. Diagnosis and management of the metablic syndrome. An American Heart Association/National Heart, Lung and Blood Institute scientific statement: Executive summary. *Circulation* 2005, 112, e285–e290.

Guerre-Millo, M. Extending the glucose/fatty acid cycle: A glucose/adipose tissue cycle. *Biochem Soc Transact* 2003, 31, 1161–1164.

Gutierrez-Juárez, R.; Pocai, A.; Mulas, C.; Ono, H.; Bhanot, S.; Monia, B.P.; Rossetti, L. Critical role of stearoyl-CoA desaturase-1 (SCD1) in the onset of diet-induced hepatic insulin resistance. *J Clin Invest* 2006, 116, 1686–1695.

Haffner, S.M. The metabolic syndrome: Inflammation, diabetes mellitus, and cardiovascular disease. *Am J Cardiol* 2006, 97, 3A–11A.

Hardie, D.G. Regulation of fatty acid synthesis via phosphorylation of acetyl CoA carboxylase. *Prog Lipid Res* 1989, 28, 117–146.

Harris, W.S. The omega-6/omega-3 ratio and cardiovascular disease risk: Uses and abuses. *Curr Cardio Risk Rep* 2006, 1, 39–45.

Harris, W.S.; Poston, W.C.; Haddock, C.K. Tissue n-3 and n-6 fatty acids and risk for coronary heart disease events. *Arteriosclerosis* 2007, 193, 1–10.

Heikkinen, S.; Argmann, C.A.; Champy, M.F.; Auwerx, J. Evaluation of glucose homeostasis. *Curr Protoc Mol Biol* 2007, Chapter 29: Unit 29B.3.

Hijona, E.; Hijona, L.; Arenas, J.I.; Bujanda, L. Inflammatory mediators of hepatic steatosis. *Mediators of Inflammation* 2010, 2010, 837419–837428.

Horton, J.D. Sterol regulatory element-binding proteins: Transcriptional activators of lipid synthesis. *Biochem Soc Transact* 2002, 30, 1091–1095.

Hotamisligil, G.S. The role of TNF alpha and TNF receptors in obesity and insulin resistance. *J Int Med* 1999, 245, 621–625.

Hotamisligil, G.S.; Budavari, A.; Murray, D.; Spiegelman, B.M. Reduced tyrosine kinase activity of the insulin receptor in obesity-diabetes. Central role of tumor necrosis factor-alpha. *J Clin Invest* 1994, 94, 1543–1549.

Johnson, G.H.; Keast, D.R.; Kris-Etherton, P.M. Dietary modeling shows that the substitution of canola oil for fats commonly used in the United States would increase compliance with dietary recommendations for fatty acids. *J Am Diet Assoc* 2007, 107, 1726–1734.

Jump, D.B. The biochemistry of n-3 polyunsaturated fatty acids. *J Biochem Chem* 2002, 277, 8755–8758.

Jump, D.B. N-3 polyunsaturated fatty acid regulation of hepatic gene transcription. *Curr Opin Lipidol* 2008, 19, 242–247.

Kliewer, S.A.; Sundseth, S.S.; Jones, S.A.; Brown, P.J.; Wisel, G.B.; Kobles, C.S.; Devchand, P. et al. Fatty acids and eicosanoids regulate gene expression through direct interactions with peroxisome proliferator-activated receptors α and γ. *Proc Nat Acad Sci* 1997, 94, 4318–4323.

Laaksonen, D.E.; Lakka, T.A.; Lakka, H.M.; Nyyssönen, K.; Rissanen, T.; Niskanen, L.K.; Salonen, J.T. Serum fatty acid composition predicts development of impaired fasting glycaemia and diabetes in middle-aged men. *Diabet Med* 2002, 19, 456–464.

Le Foll, C.; Corporeau, C.; Le Guen, V.; Gouygou, J.P.; Berge, J.P.; Delarue, J. Long-chain n-3 polyunsaturated fatty acids dissociate phosphorylation of Akt from phosphatidylinositol 3′-kinase activity in rats. *Am J Physiol Endocrinol Metab* 2007, 292, E1223–E1230.

Legrand, P.; Schmitt, B.; Mourot, J.; Catheline, D.; Chesneau, G.; Mireaux, M.; Kerhoas, N.; Weill, P. The consumption of food products from linseed-fed animals maintains erythrocyte omega-3 fatty acids in obese humans. *Lipids* 2010, 45, 11–19.

Li, Y.; Soos, T.J.; Li, X.; Wu, J.; Degennaro, M.; Sun, X.; Littman, D.R.; Birnaum, J.; Polakiewicz, R.D. Protein kinase C theta inhibits insulin signaling by phosphorylating IRS1 at ser(1101). *J Biol Chem* 2004, 279, 45304–45307.

Loffreda, S.; Yang, S.Q.; Lin, H.Z.; Karp, C.L.; Brengman, M.L.; Wang, D.J.; Klein, A.S. et al. Diehl, A.M. Leptin regulates proinflammatory immune responses. *FASEB J* 1998, 12, 57–65.

Lombardo, Y.B.; Hein, G.; Chicco, A. Metabolic syndrome: Effects of n-3 PUFAs on a model of dyslipidemia, insulin resistance and adiposity. *Lipids* 2007, 42, 427–437.

Louheranta, A.M.; Sarkkinen, E.S.; Vidgren, H.M.; Schwab, U.S.; Uusitupa, M.I.J. Association of the fatty acid profile of serum lipids with glucose and insulin metabolism during 2 fat-modified diets in subjects with impaired glucose tolerance. *Am J Clin Nutr* 2002, 76, 331–337.

Macdonald, M.L.; Singaraja, R.R.; Bissada, N.; Ruddle, P.; Watts, R.; Karasinska, J.M.; Gibson, W.T. et al. Absence of stearoyl-CoA desaturase-1 ameloriates features of the metabolic syndrome in LDLR-deficient mice. *J Lipid Res* 2008, 49, 217–229.

Marchesini, G.; Brizi, M.; Bianchi, G.; Tomassetti, S.; Bugianesi, E.; Lenzi, M.; McCullough, A.J.; Natale, S.; Forlani, G.; Melchionda, N. Nonalcoholic fatty liver disease: A feature of the metabolic syndrome. *Diabetes* 2001, 50, 1844–1850.

Matsuda, M. Measuring and estimating insulin resistance in clinical and research settings. *Nutr Metab Cardiovasc Dis* 2010, 20, 79–86.

Mauvoisin, D.; Rocque, G.; Arfa, O.; Radenne, A.; Boissier, P.; Mounier, C. Role of the PI3-kinase/mTor pathway in the regulation of the stearoyl CoA desaturase (SCD1) gene expression by insulin in liver. *J Cell Commun Signal* 2007, 1, 113–125.

Mauvoisin, D.; Prévost, M.; Ducheix, S.; Arnaud, M.P.; Mounier, C. Key role of the ERK1/2 MAPK pathway in the transcriptional regulation of the Stearoyl-CoA Desaturase (SCD1) gene expression in response to leptin. *Mol Cell Endocrinol* 2010, 319, 116–128.

McCarty, M.F. Towards practical prevention of type two diabetes. *Medical Hypotheses* 2000, 54, 786–793.

Morise, A.; Combe, N.; Boué, C.; Legrand, P.; Catheline, D.; Delplanque, B.; Fenart, E.;Weill, P.; Hermier, D. Dose effect of α-linolenic acid on PUFA conversion, bioavailability, and storage in the hamster. *Lipids* 2004, 39, 325–334.

Mostad, I.L.; Bjerve, K.S.; Bjorgaas, M.R.; Lydersen, S.; Grill, V. Effects of n-3 fatty acids in subjects with type 2 diabetes: Reduction of insulin sensitivity and time-dependent alteration from carbohydrate to fat oxidation. *Am J Clin Nutr* 2006, 84, 540–550.

Muniyappa, R.; Chen, H.; Muzumdar, R.; Einstein, F.H.; Yan, X.; Yue, L.Q.; Barzilai, N.; Quon, M.J. Comparison between surrogate indexes of insulin sensitivity/resistance and hyperinsulinemic euglycemic clamp estimates in rats. *Am J Physio Endocrinol Metab* 2009, 297, 1023–1029.

Mustad, V.A.; DeMichele, S.; Huang, Y-S.; Mika, A.; Lubbers, N.; Berthiaume, N.; Polakowski, J.; Zinker, B. Differential effects of n-3 polyunsaturated fatty acids on metabolic control and vascular reactivity in the type 2 diabetic ob/ob mouse. *Metab Clin Exp* 2006, 55, 1365–1374.

National Academy of Sciences. Institute of Medicine. Food and Nutrition Board. Dietary reference intakes for energy, carbohydrate, fiber, fat, fatty acids, cholesterol, protein, and amino acids (macronutrients). http://www.nal.usda.gov/fnic/DRI//DRI_Energy/422–541.pdf (February 9, 2009).

Neschen, S.; Moore, I.; Regittnig, W.; Yu, C.L.; Wang, Y.; Pypaert, M.; Petersen, K.F.; Shulman, G.I. Contrasting effects of fish oil and safflower oil on hepatic peroxisomal and tissue lipid content. *Am J Physiol, Endocrinol Metab* 2002, 282, 395–401.

Neschen, S.; Morino, K.; Dong, J.; Wang-Fischer, Y.; Cline, G.W.; Romanelli, A.J.; Rossbacher, J.C. et al. N-3 fatty acids preserve insulin sensitivity *in vivo* in a peroxisome proliferator-activated receptor-α-dependent manner. *Diabetes* 2007, 56, 1034–1041.

Neuschwander-Tetri, B.A.; Caldwell, S.H. Nonalcoholic steatohepatitis: Summary of an ASLD single topic conference. *Hepatology* 2003, 37, 1202–1219.

Ntambi, J.M.; Miyazaki, M.; Stoehr, J.P.; Lan, H.; Kendziorski, C.M.; Yandell, B.S.; Song, Y.; Cohen, P.; Friedman, J.M.; Attie, A.D. Loss of stearoyl-CoA desaturase-1 function protects mice against adiposity. *Proc Natl Acad Sci USA* 2002, 99, 11482–11486.

Nugent, A.P. The metabolic syndrome. *Br Nutr Found Nutr Bull* 2004, 29, 36–43.

Pan, D.A.; Hulbert, A.J.; Storlien, L.H. Dietary fats, membrane phospholipids and obesity. *J Nutr* 1994, 124, 1555–1565.

Paniagua, J.A.; Gallego De La Sacristana, A.; Romero, I.; Vidal-Puig, A.; Sanchez, E.; Perez-Martinez, P.; Lopez-Miranda, J.; Pérez-Jiménez, F. Monounsaturated fat-rich diet prevents central body fat distribution and decreases postprandial adiponectin expression induced by a carbohydrate-rich diet in insulin resistance subjects. *Diabetes Care* 2007, 30, 1717–1723.

Pérez-Echarri, N.; Pérez Matute, P.; Marcos-Gómez, B.; Baena, M.J.; Marti, A.; Martinez, J.A.; Moreno-Aliaga, M.J. Differential inflammatory status in rats susceptible or resistant to diet-induced obesity: Effects of EPA ethyl ester treatment. *Eur J Nutr* 2008, 47, 380–386.

Pérez-Jiménez, F.; López-Miranda, J.; Pinillos, M.D.; Gómez, P.; Paz-Rojas, E.; Montilla, P.; Marín, C. et al. A Mediterranean and a high-carbohydrate diet improve glucose metabolism in healthy young persons. *Diabetologia* 2001, 44, 2038–2043.

Persad, S.; Attwell, S.; Gray, V.; Mawji, N.; Deng, J. T.; Leung, D.; Yan, J.; Sanghera, J.; Walsh, M. P.; Dedhar, S. Regulation of protein kinase B/Akt-serine 473 phosphorylation by integrin-linked kinase: Critical roles for kinase activity and amino acids arginine 211 and serine 343. *J Biol Chem* 2001, 276, 27462–27469.

Popeijus, H.E.; Saris, W.H.; Mensink, R.P. Role of stearoyl-CoA desaturases in obesity and the metabolic syndrome. *Int J Obes (Lond)* 2008, 32, 1076–1082.

Price, P.T.; Nelson, C.M.; Clarke, S.D. Omega-3 polyunsaturated fatty acid regulation of gene expression. *Curr Opin Lipidol* 2000, 11, 3–7.

Przybylski, R. Canola oil: Physical and chemical properties. http://www.canolacouncil.org/uploads/Chemical1–6.pdf. Accessed August 16th, 2010.

Rahman, S.M.; Dobrzyn, A.; Dobrzyn, P.; Lee, S.H.; Miyazaki, M.; Ntambi, J.M. Stearoyl-CoA desaturase 1 deficiency elevates insulin-signaling components and down-regulates protein-tyrosine phosphate 1B in muscle. *Proc Natl Acad Sci USA* 2003, 100, 11110–11115.

Rahman, S.M.; Dobrzyn, A.; Lee, S.H.; Dobrzyn, P.; Miyazaki, M.; Ntambi, J.M. Stearoyl-CoA desaturase 1 deficiency increases insulin signaling and glycogen accumulation in brown adipose tissue. *Am J Physiol Endocrinol Metab* 2005, 288, E381–E387.

Rasic-Milutinovic, Z.; Perunicic, G.; Pljesa, S.; Gluvic, Z.; Sobajic, S.; Djuric, I.; Ristic, D. Effects of n-3 PUFAs supplementation on insulin resistance and inflammatory biomarkers in hemodialysis patients. *Renal Failure* 2007, 29, 321–329.

Risérus, U. Fatty acids and insulin sensitivity. *Curr Opin Clin Nutr Metab Care* 2008, 11, 100–105.

Risérus, U.; Tan, G.D.; Fielding, B.A.; Neville, M.J.; Currie, J.; Savage, D.B.; Chatterjee, V.K.; Frayn, K.N.; O'Rahilly, S.; Karpe, F. Rosiglitazone increases indexes of stearoyl-CoA desaturase activity in humans: Link to insulin sensitization and the role of dominant-negative mutation in peroxisome proliferator-activated receptor-gamma. *Diabetes* 2005, 54, 1379–1384.

Rocca, A.S.; LaGreca, J.; Kalitsky, J.; Brubaker. P.L. Monounsaturated fatty acid diets improve glycemic tolerance through increased secretion of glucagon-like peptide-1. *Endocrinology* 2001, 142, 1148–1155.

Rojo-Martínez, G.; Esteva, I.; Ruiz de Adana, M.S.; García-Almeida, J.M.; Tinahones, F.; Cardona, F.; Morcillo, S.; García-Escobar, E.; García-Fuentes, E.; Soriguer, F. Dietary fatty acids and insulin secretion: A population-based study. *Eur J Clin Nutr* 2006, 60, 1195–1200.

Salas-Salvado, J.; Garcia-Arellano, A.; Estruch, R.; Marquez-Sandoval, F.; Corella, D.; Fiol, M.; Gómez-Gracia, E. et al. Components of the Mediterranean-type food pattern and serum inflammatory markers among patients at high risk for cardiovascular disease. *Eur J Clin Nutr* 2008, 62, 651–659.

Sampath, H.; Ntambi, J.M. Polyunsaturated fatty acid regulation of genes in lipid metabolism. *Ann Rev Nutr* 2005, 25, 317–340.

Schmitz, G.; Ecker, J. The opposing effects of n-3 and n-6 fatty acids. *Prog Clin Res* 2008, 47, 147–155.

Sekiya, M.; Yahagi, N.; Matsuzaka, T.; Najima, Y.; Nakakuki, M.; Nagai, R.; Ishibashi, S.; Osuga, J.; Yamada, N.; Shiman, H. Polyunsaturated fatty acids ameliorate hepatic steatosis in obese mice by SREBP-1 Suppression. *Hepatology* 2003, 38, 1529–1539.

Shahidi, F. *Canola and Rapeseed: Production, Chemistry, Nutrition, and Processing Technology*. New York, NY: Springer, 1990.

Siger, A.; Nogala-Kalucka, M.; Lampart-Szczapa, E. The content and antioxidant activity of phenolic compounds in cold-pressed plant oils. *J Food Lip* 2008, 15, 137–149.

Simopoulos, A.P. Essential fatty acids in health and chronic disease. *Am J Clin Nutr* 1999, 70, 560–569.

Simopoulos, A.P. The importance of the ratio of omega-6/omega-3 fatty acids. *Biomed Pharmacother* 2002, 56, 365–379.

Simopoulos, A.P. Evolutionary aspects of diet, the omega-6/omega-3 ratio and genetic variation: Nutritional implications for chronic disease. *Biomed Pharmacother* 2006, 60, 502–507.

Soriguer, F.; Morcillo, S.; Cardona, F.; Rojo-Martínez, G.; Almaraz, M.C.; Adana, M.S.R.; Olveira, G.; Tinahones, F.; Esteva, I. Pro12Ala polymorphism of the PPARG2 gene is associated with type 2 diabetes mellitus and peripheral insulin sensitivity in a population with a high intake of oleic acid. *J Nutr* 2006, 136, 2325–2330.

Storlien, L.H.; Jenkins, A.B.; Chisholm, D.J.; Pascoe, W.S.; Khouri, S.; Kraegen, E.W. Influence of dietary fat on development of insulin resistance in rats: Relationship to muscle triglyceride and n-3 fatty acids in muscle phospholipid. *Diabetes* 1991, 40, 280–289.

Storlien, L.H.; Kraegen, E.W.; Chisholm, D.J.; Ford, G.L.; Bruce, D.G.; Pascoe, W.S. Fish oil prevents insulin resistance induced by high-fat feeding in rats. *Science* 1987, 237, 885–888.

Storlien, L.H.; Pan, D.A.; Kriketos, A.D.; O'Connor, J.; Caterson, I.D.; Cooney, G.J.; Jenkins, A.B.; Baur, L.A. Skeletal muscle membrane lipids and insulin resistance. *Lipids* 1996, 31, 261–265.

Sun, X.J.; Crimmins, D.L.; Myers, M.G., Jr.; Miralpeix, M.; White, M.F. Pleiotropic insulin signals are engaged by multisite phosphorylation of IRS-1. *Mol Cell Biol* 1993, 13, 7418–7428.

Takahashi, Y.; Ide, T. Dietary n-3 fatty acids affect mRNA level of brown adipose tissue uncoupling protein 1, and white adipose tissue leptin and glucose transporter 4 in the rat. *Br J Nutr* 2000, 84, 175–184.

Taouis, M.; Dagou, C.; Ster, C.; Durand, G.; Pinault, M.; Delarue, J. N-3 polyunsaturated fatty acids prevent the defect of insulin receptor signaling in muscle. *Am J Physiol Endocrin Metab* 2002, 282(3), E664–E671.

Thomas, B.J. Efficiency of conversion of [alpha]-linolenic acid to long chain n-3 fatty acids in man. *Lipid Metab Therapy* 2002, 5, 127–132.

Tsitouras, P.D.; Gucciardo, F.; Salbe, A.D.; Heward, C.; Harman, S.M. High omega-3 fat intake improves insulin sensitivity and reduces CRP and IL6, but does not affect other endocrine axes in healthy older adults. *Horm Metab Res* 2008, 40, 199–205.

Tugwood, J.D.; Issemann, I.; Anderson, R.G.; Bundel, K.R.; McPheat, W.L.; Green, S. The mouse peroxisome proliferator activated receptor recognizes a response element in the 5′ flanking sequence of the rat acyl CoA oxidase gene. *EMBO J* 1992, 11, 433–439.

United States Department of Agriculture (USDA). World statistics: World vegetable oil consumption 2007. http://www.soystats.com/2008/page_35.htm (April 1, 2009).

United States Department of Agriculture (USDA). National nutrient database for standard reference, release 22. http://www.ars.usda.gov/SP2UserFiles/Place/12354500/Data/SR22/nutrlist/sr22w323.pdf. Accessed August 16th, 2010.

Vessby, B.; Tengblad, S.; Lithell, H. Insulin sensitivity is related to the fatty acid composition of serum lipids and skeletal muscle phospholipids in 70-year-old men. *Diabetologia* 1994, 37, 1044–1050.

Vessby, B. Dietary fat and insulin action in humans. *Br J Nutr* 2000, 83, S91–S96.

Vessby, B.; Uusitupa, M.; Hermansen, K.; Riccardi, G.; Rivellese, A.A.; Tapsell, L.C.; Nälsén, C. et al. Substituting dietary saturated for monounsaturated fat impairs insulin sensitivity in healthy men and women: TheKANWUStudy. *Diabetologia* 2001, 44, 312–319.

Vessby, B.; Gustafsson, I.B.; Tengblad, S.; Boberg, M.; Andersson, A. Desaturation and elongation of fatty acids and insulin action. *Ann N Y Acad Sci* 2002, 967, 183–195.

Weisberg, S.P.; McCann, D.; Desai, M.; Rosenbaum, M.; Leibel, R.L.; Ferrante, A.W. Obesity is associated with macrophage accumulation in adipose tissue. *J Clin Invest* 2003, 111, 1796–1808.

Wilson, M.D.; Blake, W.L.; Salati, L.M.; Clarke, S.D. Potency of polyunsaturated and saturated fats as short-term inhibitors of hepatic lipogenesis in rats. *J Nutr* 1990, 120, 544–552.

World Health Organization. *Obesity and Overweight.* http://www.who.int/mediacentre/factsheets/fs311/en/index.html (May, 2012).

Worgall, T.S.; Sturley, S.L.; Seo, T.; Osborne, T.F.; Deckelbaum, R.J. Polyunsaturated fatty acids decrease expression of promoters with sterol regulatory elements by decreasing levels of mature sterol regulatory element binding protein. *J Biol Chem* 1998, 273, 25537–25540.

Xu, J.; Nakamura, M.T.; Cho, H.P.; Clarke, S.D. Sterol regulatory element binding protein-1 expression is suppressed by dietary polyunsaturated fatty acids. *J Biol Chem* 1999, 274, 23577–23583.

Zhang, L.; Ge, L.; Parimoo, S.; Stenn, K.; Prouty, S.M. Human stearoyl-CoA desaturase: Alternative transcripts generated from a single gene by usage of tandem polyadenylation sites. *Biochem J* 1999, 340, 255–264.

Zhang, L.; Ge, L.; Tran, T.; Stenn, K.; Prouty, S.M. Isolation and characterization of the human stearoyl-CoA desaturase gene promoter: Requirement of a conserved CCAAT *cis*-element. *Biochem J* 2001, 357, 183–193.

Zhang, S.; Yang, Y.; Shi, Y. Characterization of human SCD2, an oligomeric desaturase with improved stability and enzyme activity by cross-linking in intact cells. *Biochem J* 2005, 388, 135–142.

15 Rapeseed and Canola Phenolics

Antioxidant Attributes and Efficacy

Usha Thiyam-Holländer and Karin Schwarz

CONTENTS

15.1 Introduction 278
15.1.1 Oxidative Stability of Commercial Rapeseed and Canola Oils 278
15.1.2 Antioxidants and Auto-Oxidation 279
15.1.3 Application of Phenolic Ingredients in Rapeseed and Canola Oil 279
15.1.4 Phenolic Compounds of Rapeseed and Canola 281
15.2 Fractionation of 70% Methanolic Extract 282
15.3 Quantification and Characterization of Main Phenolics in Rapeseed Meal Extract 282
15.4 Free Radical Scavenging Activity 285
15.4.1 DPPH Free Radical Scavenging Activity 285
15.4.2 Free Radical Scavenging Activity of Sinapoyl Glucose, Sinapine and Sinapic Acid 286
15.4.3 Free Radical Scavenging Activity of Sinapic Acid as Compared to Other Standard Antioxidants 286
15.4.4 Free Radical Scavenging Activity of Rapeseed Extracts and Their Fractions 288
15.5 Antioxidative Activity of Rapeseed Meal Extracts 291
15.6 Antioxidative Activity of Major Phenolic Compounds during Lipid Oxidation 292
15.6.1 Effect of Rapeseed Meal Extracts as Compared with Sinapic Acid in Purified Rapeseed Oil Emulsion 293
15.6.2 Formation of Primary Oxidation Products 294
15.6.3 Secondary Oxidation Products-Pattern 294
15.7 Conclusion and Future Perspectives 296
References 297

15.1 INTRODUCTION

Rapeseed, known in different countries by different names, ranks as the one of three most plentiful oilseed crops. In North America and some countries such as Canada and Japan, it is generally recognized by the name of canola. In the EU, where it is known as rapeseed, it continues to be the major oilseed crop of the region. Mustard also belongs to the same *Brassicaceae* family, and remains an important oilseed crop in Asian countries such as India. Rapeseed has been used as a source of oil since ancient times. The high content of erucic acid in rapeseed oil, however, limited its use as an edible oil. Positive developments in breeding changed the fatty acid composition of rapeseed oil making it a preferred vegetable oil for human nutrition. The historical development of rapeseed and canola is discussed in Chapters 1 and 4. Compared to other vegetable fats and oils, rapeseed oil has a distinct fatty acid composition. It is extremely low in saturated fatty acids and is an important source of the monounsaturated oleic acid which is with ~58–60% the most abundant fatty acid. In addition, rapeseed oil is a good source of the essential fatty acids linoleic acid, and in particular the omega-3-fatty acid, alpha-linolenic acid. Thus, rapeseed oil remains attractive to consumers as high-quality oil. To guarantee the high quality of the oil, the use of suitable antioxidants is needed to prevent oxidative degradation of the oil. However, the retention of antioxidants in the pressed and extracted oils is low except for tocopherols. This is also true for the widely occurring endogenous antioxidants, sinapic acid and derivatives. Therefore, it is of interest to investigate the by-products of oil processing as a source of antioxidants, especially sinapic acid derivatives. The effect of endogenous naturally occurring phenolic compounds from rapeseed to impart free radical scavenging activity and prevent oxidative deterioration could further stabilize oils such as rapeseed oil. This chapter will discuss work on the investigation of endogenous phenolic compounds in rapeseed meal, and their ability to stabilize an oil-in-water (o/w) emulsion (oil-enriched model emulsion) rapeseed oil-containing system as a model food system. The chapter includes material taken from published work of Thiyam et al. (2006a) and Usha Thiyam (2005) (PhD thesis) with the permission of Shaker Verlag and Wiley.

15.1.1 Oxidative Stability of Commercial Rapeseed and Canola Oils

Foods without natural or synthetic antioxidants become spoiled when oxidation takes place. An antioxidant can be defined as a substance that prevents the reaction of various food constituents with oxygen and prevents oxidative damage (Pszczola, 2001). Common oxidative stability tests monitor the formation of hydroperoxides (indicating primary oxidation products) using different standardized tests.

Currently, refined and cold-pressed rapeseed oils are readily available in the edible oil markets of European countries like Germany. In Canada and the United States, the predominant frying oil is high oleic canola oil which has replaced hydrogenated fats because of its suitability for frying foods (see Chapter 11). Other canola oils that are emerging include high oleic and/or low linolenic canola oil, in addition to value-added virgin oils (see Chapters 5 and 9). Studies comparing some rapeseed and olive oils highlighted the fact that rapeseed oils have low initial peroxide values (PVs).

However, the hydrophilic phenol content in rapeseed oils is low (3–4 μg/g compared to olive oils which contain 40–100 times more hydrophilic phenols) (Koski et al., 2003). When comparing the oxidative stability and minor constituents of cold-pressed low erucic acid rapeseed oils and virgin olive oils, rapeseed oils oxidized more rapidly due to their higher levels of polyunsaturated fatty acids and lower phenol content even though the initial PVs of fresh olive oils were much higher.

15.1.2 Antioxidants and Auto-Oxidation

In light of rapid technological changes and customer preferences, the inherent antioxidant properties of all the plant-based naturally occurring phenolic compounds offer natural options to food manufacturers for potential antioxidants. These natural extracts also satisfy two basic conditions required for an antioxidant. Firstly, when present in low concentration they can delay, retard or prevent the auto-oxidation or free radical-mediated oxidation. Secondly, the resulting radical formed after scavenging must be stable through intra-molecular hydrogen bonding to prevent further oxidation. In addition, many *in vitro* studies have defined the antioxidant potential of these polyphenols as direct radical scavengers and in some systems they show greater efficiency. The main purpose of adding antioxidants to food systems is to delay the accumulation of free radicals and thus, enhance their oxidative stability. However, factors affecting antioxidative efficiency must be carefully studied as antioxidant efficiency is system- and method-dependent (Frankel, 1998).

Phenolic antioxidants act to inhibit lipid oxidation by trapping the peroxy radical. This can be accomplished in one of the two ways:

$$LOO^{\circ} + ArOH = LOOH + ArO^{\circ} \tag{15.1}$$

$$LO^{\circ} + ArO^{\circ} = LOOAr \tag{15.2}$$

In the first mechanism (Equation 15.1), the peroxy radical (LOO°) abstracts a proton from the antioxidants (ArOH) to yield an antioxidant radical (ArO°) and the hydroperoxide (LOOH). In the second mechanism (Equation 15.2), a peroxy and an antioxidant radical react by radical–radical coupling to form a non-radical product (Chimi et al., 1999).

15.1.3 Application of Phenolic Ingredients in Rapeseed and Canola Oil

There is great interest in using extracts with antioxidative properties from natural sources to replace the now banned commercial antioxidants BHT and butylated hydroxylanisole (BHA). In addition to tocopherols, sage and rosmarin extracts are the most commercially produced natural antioxidants used today (Cuvelier et al., 1996). The structure (Figure 15.1) and range of tocopherol content in rapeseed oil is shown in Table 15.1.

During the extraction and processing of rapeseed oil, many phenolic compounds (Figure 15.2), including sinapic acid derivatives (Figure 15.3), are removed. The amount of phenolics was highest in the post-expelled crude rapeseed oil but decreased

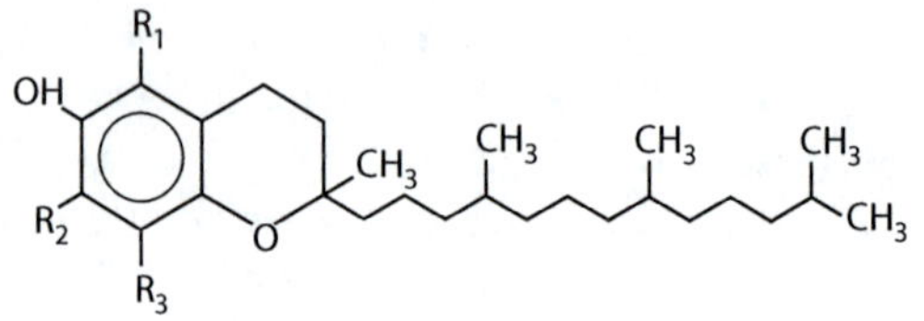

Tocopherol	R_1	R_2	R_3
Alpha	CH_3	CH_3	CH_3
Beta	CH_3	H	H
Gamma	H	CH_3	CH_3
Delta	H	H	CH_3

FIGURE 15.1 Structure of tocopherols.

TABLE 15.1
Ranges (Means) of Tocopherol Levels in Rapeseed Oil (mg/kg)

Tocopherol	High-Erucic Rapeseed	Low-Erucic Rapeseed
Alpha-tocopherol	39–305	100–320 (202)
Beta-tocopherol	24–158 (27)	16–140 (65)
Gamma-tocopherol	230–500	287–753 (490)
Delta-tocopherol	5–14	4–22 (9)
Total (mean)	312–928	424–1,054 (766)

Source: Adapted from King, B.J., Turrel, J.A. and Zilka, S.A. 1986. Analysis of minor fatty acid components by capillary column GLC and of triglycerides by HPLC. Research Report no. 563. Leatherhead Food Research association. Leatherhead, Surrey, United Kingdom.

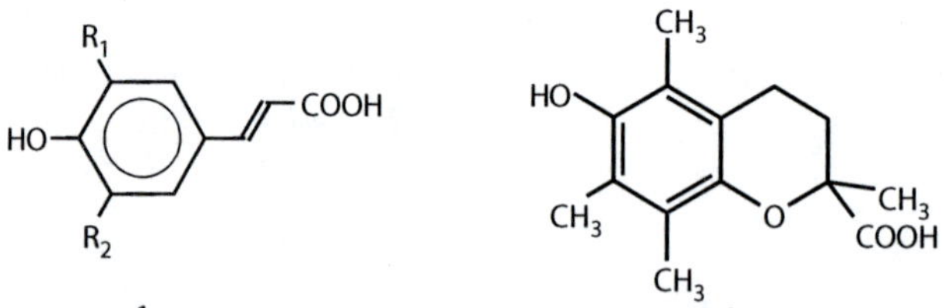

1a

2a

R_1	R_2	
H	H	*p*-Coumaric acid
H	OH	Caffeic acid
CH_3O	H	Ferulic acid

FIGURE 15.2 Chemical structures of cinnamic acids derivatives (1a) and Trolox (2a).

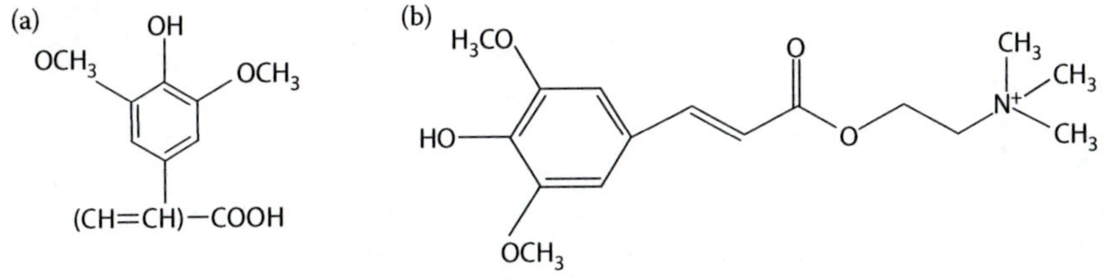

FIGURE 15.3 (a) Sinapic acid. (b) Sinapine.

with an increasing degree of refining (Koski et al., 2003). However, cold-pressed rapeseed oil was still more susceptible to oxidation than refined rapeseed oil (Pekkarinen et al., 1998). The lower stability of cold-pressed rapeseed was attributed to the higher degree of oxidation prior to the incubation experiment. Sinapic acid, the main phenolic constituent of rapeseed and mustard, is known to cause inhibition of peroxides in bulk lipid systems as well as in emulsions (Pekkarinen et al., 1999). This implies that the natural phenolic extracts from the rapeseed meal could be used commercially for stabilizing different food formulations apart from oils, for example, salad dressings, mayonnaise and meat systems. 4-vinyl-2,6-dimethoxyphenol (vinylsyringol or canolol), a compound with natural antioxidative potential, and its dimer were subsequently identified in rapeseed oil (Kuwahara et al., 2004; Harbaum-Piayda et al., 2010).

15.1.4 Phenolic Compounds of Rapeseed and Canola

Once oil is extracted or pressed from oilseeds for edible applications, the fat-free residues of different oilseeds contain considerable amounts of phenolic compounds in the meal press-cake or the by-products of oil processing. Rapeseed meal is known to have a much higher phenolic content of over 50 mg/100 g flour compared to ~23.4 mg/100 g for soyabean flour.

Over the past decade, the negative qualities of the phenolic compounds have dominated the positive attributes. In general, they are associated with a darker colour, bitter taste and astringency of rapeseed, canola or mustard feed. They are further known to affect the nutritional quality of the meal for animal feed (Shahidi, 1990; Shahidi and Naczk, 1992, 1995). The main phenolic compound, sinapine, is also responsible for fishy odours in brown-shelled eggs when incorporated in poultry rations. At dietary levels higher than 5%, rapeseed meal may result in enlarged thyroids, kidneys and livers in young and growing swine as shown by feed trails.

Despite these negative attributes, there are opportunities for these phenolic compounds to be extracted using pure or aqueous solvents like ethanol to be further utilized as natural antioxidants. Studies showed that the extracts obtained from the oilseed residues displayed remarkable antioxidant activity, the extent of which depends on the type of residue and the solvent used for the extraction (Amarowicz et al., 2000). Wanasundara et al. (1994) reported that the best antioxidant activity was exhibited by a fraction of canola meal phenolics that contained only 34 mg of phenolic compounds/g of sample. On the other hand, Amarowicz et al. (1996) observed that the antioxidant activity of ethanolic extracts of mustard correlated well with the total content of phenolic compounds in its isolated fractions. The high antioxidant activity of rapeseed/canola fractions, low in total phenolic content, may be dictated by the molecular structure of phenolic compounds involved. According to Zadernowski et al. (1991), the molecular structure of rapeseed phenolic compounds plays an important role in their antioxidant activity. Furthermore, Wanasundara et al. (1994) proposed that synergism of phenolic compounds with one another and/or other components present in each fraction may contribute to the higher antioxidant activity of rapeseed/canola fractions lower in phenolic compounds. Plant extracts may attribute their different mode of antioxidative nature to the system used to prove the antioxidative power (Schwarz et al., 2001).

15.2 FRACTIONATION OF 70% METHANOLIC EXTRACT

The main phenolic compounds of rapeseed meal are commonly sinapic acid (Figure 15.3a) and its derivatives—sinapine the choline ester of sinapic acid (Figure 15.3b), or as the glucosidic ester, glucopyranosyl sinapate. About 80–90% of all the phenolics in the meal are sinapic acid esters (SAEs) as discussed earlier. Thus, 70% methanolic rapeseed meal extracts of the meal have been classified into free-phenolics, esterified phenolics and released-phenolics according to Krygier et al. (1982). Krygier et al. (1982) extracted free and esterified phenolics, which were methanol soluble and demonstrated that only a small fraction of the total phenolic compounds of rapeseed occurs as free sinapic acid (Koski et al., 2002; Vuorela et al., 2003).

These results concurred with the findings of Thiyam et al. (2006a) that rapeseed meal extracts contained free sinapic acid, which was equivalent to just one-tenth of the content of sinapine. This was further illustrated by the free-phenolic fractions of the meal extracts that could recover the free sinapic acid satisfactorily. Usually in analysis, the phenolic extracts are hydrolysed with NaOH and the released-phenolics are extracted with diethyl ether, ethyl acetate or both. Comparisons between the aqueous fraction (rich in sinapine) before and after hydrolysis producing the released fraction (rich in sinapic acid) showed reasonable results with minimum hydrolysis losses affecting the accuracy of the process. Additionally, fractionation of the 70% methanolic extract showed comparable extraction efficiency to the original extract before fractionation.

Rapeseed meal extract was fractionated following the procedure of Krygier as described in Figure 15.4. Thus, 70% methanolic extract of rapeseed meal was fractionated to obtain fractions that were rich in free, esterified and released-phenolic compounds (Table 15.2). The fractionation of the 70% methanolic extract with an initial content of free sinapic acid: 1.15–1.38 mg/g fat-free meal and sinapine: 13.85 mg/g fat-free meal.

15.3 QUANTIFICATION AND CHARACTERIZATION OF MAIN PHENOLICS IN RAPESEED MEAL EXTRACT

Phenolic constituents of the 70% methanolic extracts, mainly sinapic acid derivatives including free sinapic acid, sinapoyl glucose and sinapine (Figure 15.5), were quantified by high pressure liquid chromatography (HPLC) at 275 and 330 nm. Figure 15.5a and b indicates the HPLC chromatograms of the 70% methanolic extract showing the identified and non-identified peaks. At 275 nm, no significant peaks

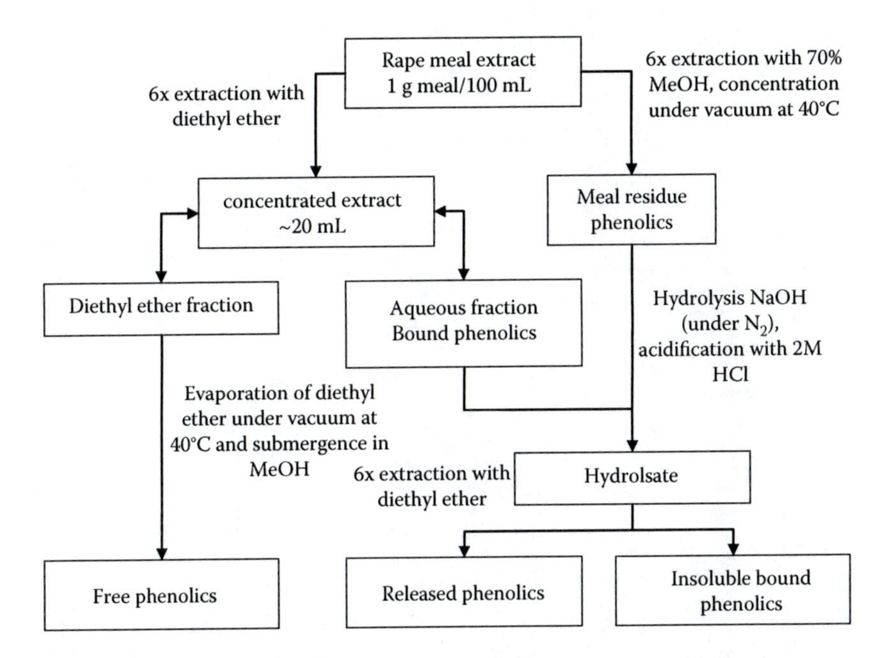

FIGURE 15.4 Fractionation procedure of rapeseed meal extract. (Adapted from Krygier, K., Sosulski, F. and Hogge, L. 1982. *J. Agric. Food Chem.* 30: 330–334.)

TABLE 15.2
Phenolic Content of Different Fractions of 70% Methanolic Extract Estimated Using HPLC (330 nm) and Folin–Ciocalteu Assay (750 nm)

Assay	Sinapine Equivalent (mg/g dm)	Sinapic Acid Equivalent (mg/g dm)	Sinapic Acid Content (mg/g dm)
Phenolic fraction	Folin–Ciocalteu[a] (±SD)	Folin–Ciocalteu[a] (±SD)	HPLC (330 nm)[b] (±SD)
Free fraction (diethyl ether fraction)	3.84 ± 0.06	1.92 ± 0.03	1.13 ± 0.04
Aqueous fraction	36.96 ± 1.10	18.50 ± 0.60	—
Released fraction	27.29 ± 0.10	13.65 ± 0.05	12.07 ± 0.08

Note: Free fraction (diethyl ether fraction with free-phenolic compounds), aqueous fraction (bound-phenolic acid fraction) and released fraction (diethyl ether fraction containing released-phenolic compounds).

[a] Principal analysis of phenolic compounds of the extracts was carried out according to the method of Singleton and Rossi (1965) using Folin–Ciocalteu reagent and denoted as total content of phenolic compounds (Folin–Ciocalteu method).

[b] HPLC method with detection at 330 nm.

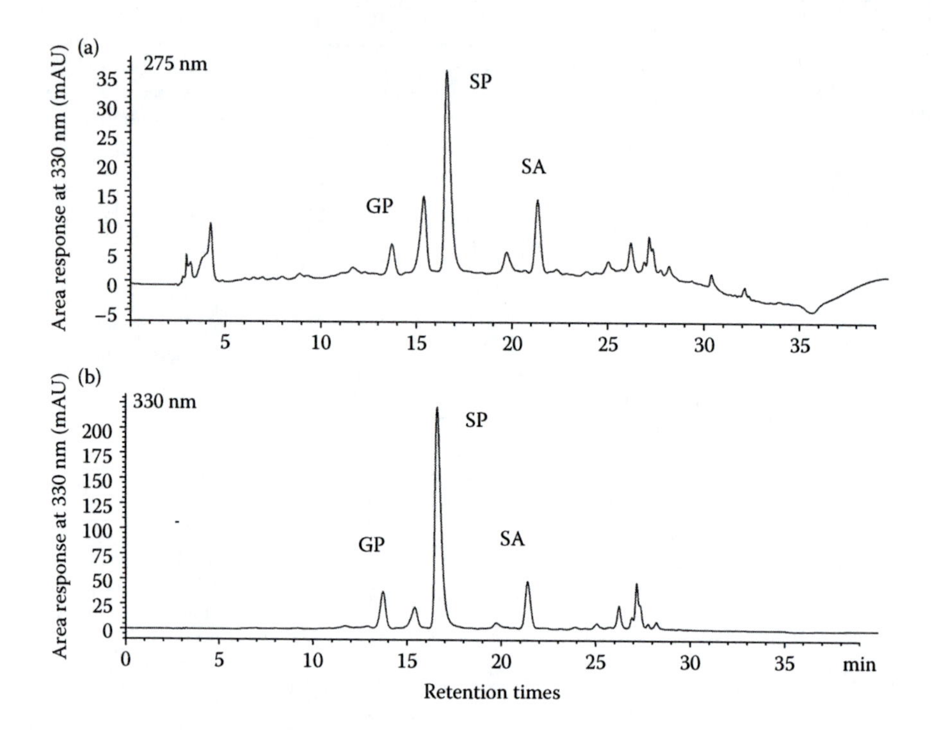

FIGURE 15.5 HPLC chromatograms of 70% methanolic extract of rapeseed meal indicating benzoic acid derivatives (a) at 275 nm and sinapic acid derivatives (b) at 330 nm. Chromatographic conditions: elution using water/methanol (90:10) with 1.25% *O*-phosphoric acid as solvent A and methanol (100%) with 0.1% *O*-phosphoric acid solvent B in a C-8 Chrospher column (Knauer). Sinapoyl glucose (GP), sinapine (SP), sinapic acid (SA), others non-identified phenolic constituents.

were obtained indicating negligible of benzoic acid derivatives and vinylsyringol for the 70% methanolic extract.

Figure 15.6 indicates the ranges of the phenolic constituents of the sinapic acid derivatives detected at 330 nm using HPLC for the commercial rapeseed meal extracts. Commercially available meals of rapeseed and mustard procured from Germany and

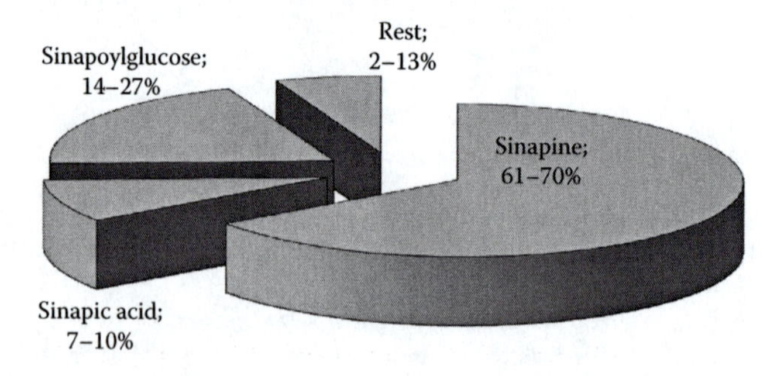

FIGURE 15.6 Percent distribution (ranges) of sinapic acid derivatives of the rapeseed meal extracts.

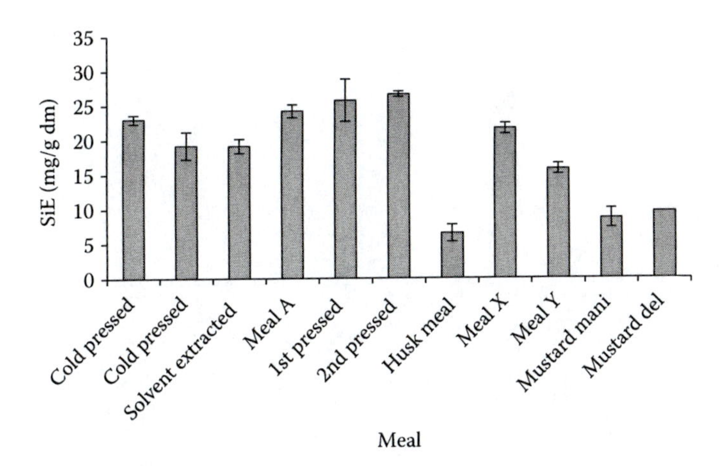

FIGURE 15.7 Total phenolic compounds (750 nm) of 70% methanolic extract of commercial meals expressed as sinapine equivalents (SiE mg/g fat-free meal). Right to left: mustard Delhi, mustard Manipur, meals X, Y, A* (non-specified), husk meal*, second-pressed*, first-pressed*, solvent-extracted and cold-pressed meals. *From the same company. Each error bar represents the mean of two measurements ($p < 0.05$).

India were extracted with 70% methanol and then analysed for the range of content of total phenolic compounds and total cinnamic acids using standardized procedures.

Figure 15.7 indicates the broad range of contents of total phenolic compounds from extracts of the commercial rapeseed cakes between 15 and 27 mg/g fat-free meal. Cold-pressed meal extract showed values of ~22–19 mg/g fat-free meal, which was slightly more but not significantly different from the extract of solvent extracted meal showing a range of ~17–19 mg/g fat-free meal. The highest value for total phenols was found in extracts from second-pressed meal with a value of ~27 mg/g fat-free meal, while extracts from first-pressed meal showed a slightly lower value of ~25 mg/g fat-free meal. Husk meal extracts showed more or less three to four times lower total phenolic compounds content to the first- and second-pressed meals. Mustard cake extracts were low in phenolic compound with 8–9 mg/g fat-free meal, which was two to three times lower compared to extracts of cold-pressed commercial rapeseed cake.

15.4 FREE RADICAL SCAVENGING ACTIVITY

15.4.1 DPPH Free Radical Scavenging Activity

1,1-Diphenyl-2-picrylhydrazyl (DPPH) assay is widely adopted for evaluating the ability to scavenge the DPPH free radical activity of numerous plant extracts. The scavenging reactions involve electron/H-atom transfer from antioxidant to DPPH. As the odd electron of DPPH, a stable radical becomes paired off, the absorption vanishes. The deep-purple colour then is reduced to light-purple colour. This decolourization is stoichiometric with respect to the number of electrons taken up (Blois, 1958).

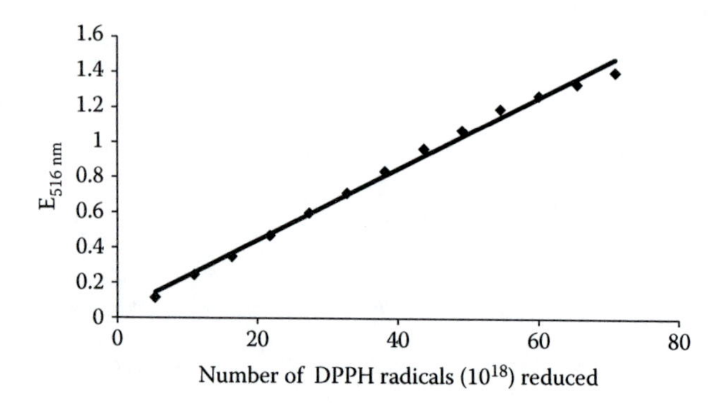

FIGURE 15.8 Calibration curve for DPPH radicals at 516 nm ($R^2 = 0.994$). The calibration curve used for this assay in the current study is shown in Figure 15.1.

The calibration curve used for this assay in the current study is shown in Figure 15.8. The absorbance at 516 nm is related to the radicals of DPPH reduced as shown in Equation 15.3.

$$\text{Extinction}\,(516\,\text{nm}) = 0.0204 \cdot \text{DPPH}_{\text{radicals}} + 0.0358 \tag{15.3}$$

To measure the DPPH radicals scavenged, 50 μL of extracts was dissolved in 0.3 mM DPPH solutions and differences before ($t = 0$ and $t = 10$) and after the sample injection were read. The resulting difference is expressed as the number of radicals scavenged using Equation 15.3. The readings were done in triplicates. For other antioxidants, the same procedure was adopted where the 50 μL of extracts were replaced by the required antioxidant solution. A quantity of 70% methanolic extracts of the commercial meals were extensively investigated for their free radical activity.

15.4.2 Free Radical Scavenging Activity of Sinapoyl Glucose, Sinapine and Sinapic Acid

The antioxidant activities of standards of sinapoyl glucose, sinapine and sinapic acid, the major sinapic acid derivatives, were compared using the free radical scavenging activity. Under the tested concentrations (Figure 15.8), the free radical scavenging activity followed the order:

Sinapic acid > sinapoyl glucose > sinapine cation

To scavenge 25×10^{18} DPPH radicals, the required concentrations (mM) for sinapic acid, sinapoyl glucose and sinapine cation were 30.8, 35.8 and 47.5 mM, respectively, compared to 21.5 mM for Trolox, a water-soluble antioxidant.

15.4.3 Free Radical Scavenging Activity of Sinapic Acid as Compared to Other Standard Antioxidants

Thiyam et al. (2006a) were the first to compare the free radical scavenging activity of test compounds sinapic acid with sinapine and sinapoyl glucose using the DPPH

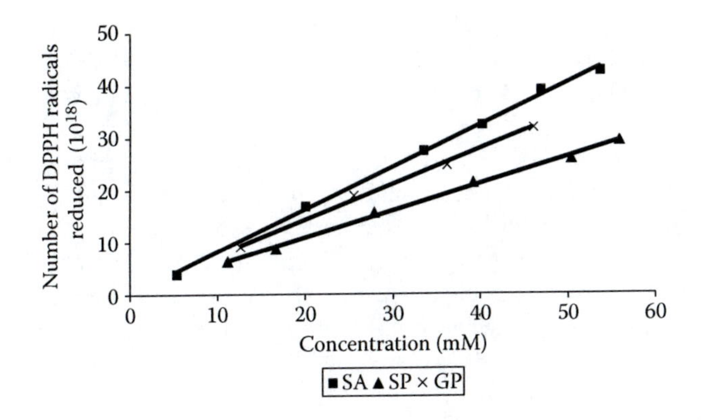

FIGURE 15.9 Free radical scavenging activity of sinapic acid (SA), sinapine (SP) and sinapoyl glucose (GP).

method. This study demonstrated that the free radical scavenging activity of the standards followed the order; sinapic acid > sinapoyl glucose > sinapine based on their molar masses under the tested concentrations (Figure 15.9). This indicated that a glucose moiety attached to the sinapic acid or further esterification of sinapic acid slightly reduced its free radical scavenging activity.

Free radical scavenging activities of different phenolic acids, caffeic acid (CA), ferulic acid (FA) and *p*-coumaric acid (*p* CA) and natural antioxidants alpha tocopherol (alpha-toco) and BHA a synthetic antioxidant were compared with sinapic acid (SA). As indicated in Figure 15.10 under the tested conditions, the radical scavenging activity of the phenolic acids in the DPPH system decreased in the following order:

BHA > alpha-toc > sinapic acid > ferulic acid > caffeic acid

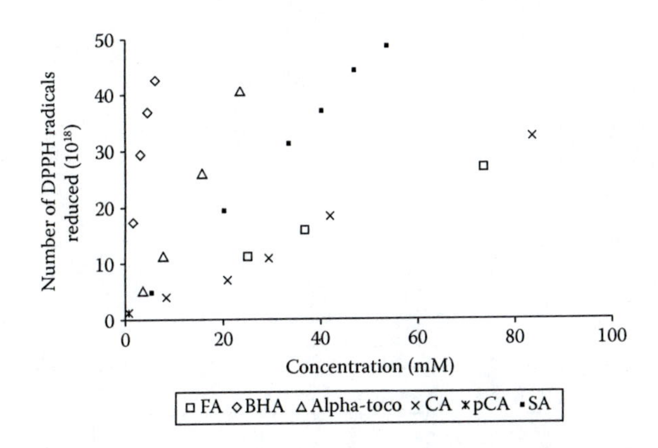

FIGURE 15.10 Radical scavenging activity of sinapic acid as compared with ferulic acid (FEA), butylated hydroxylanisole (BHA), caffeic acid (CA) and *p*-coumaric acid (*p* CA).

To scavenge 25 × 10^{18} DPPH radicals, the required concentrations (mM) for BHA, alpha-toc, sinapic acid, caffeic acid and ferulic acid were 2.5, 15, 30.8, 71.6 and 70.5 mM, respectively. *p* CA showed no significant activity towards the DPPH radical.

Results reported on DPPH radical scavenging activity in literature varies under different test concentrations and systems used. The higher DPPH scavenging activity was higher for caffeic acid compared to sinapic acid was attributed to the presence of two hydroxyl groups in caffeic acid (Kikuzaki et al., 2002). Elsewhere, sinapic acid was cited as a potent free radical scavenger at a concentration of 13.3 μM (Pekkarinen et al., 1998). Bratt et al. (2003) found similar results at a molar ratio 1:1.4 (antioxidant/DPPH) but the results changed for a higher molar ratio (1:5.6).

15.4.4 Free Radical Scavenging Activity of Rapeseed Extracts and Their Fractions

The theoretical contribution of the phenolic constituents, such as free sinapic acid, sinapoyl glucose and sinapine, to the total radical scavenging activity of the extracts is shown in Figure 15.11. The concentration of the phenolic constituents was recorded by HPLC (330 nm). Calibration curves for the RSA were recorded using standard compounds.

The free radical scavenging activity of 70% methanolic extracts of commercial meals was investigated further. Figure 15.12 indicates the variations in the radical scavenging activity of the phenolic extracts for the commercial meals. Extracts from cold-pressed meal showed no differences from that of solvent-extracted meals, which showed the same trend as their phenolic compounds. Similarly, radical scavenging

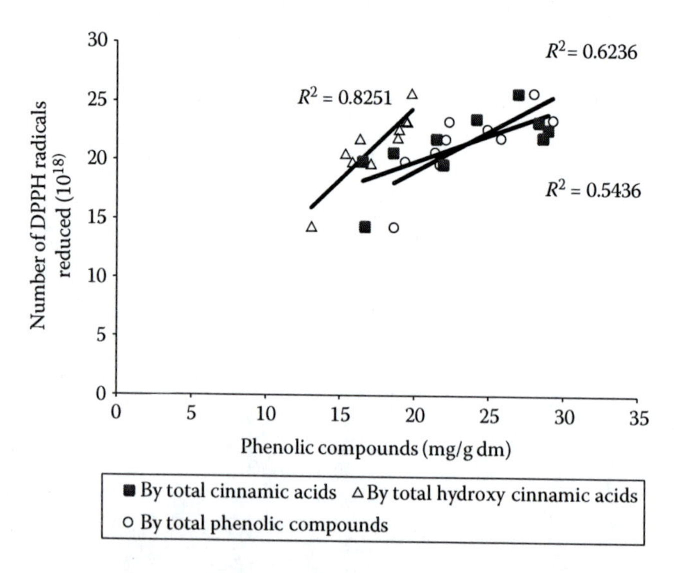

FIGURE 15.11 Correlation between RSA of different extracts and total hydroxycinnamic acids $r = 0.90$, total cinnamic acids, $r = 0.73$, total phenolic compounds $r = 0.79$, $p < 0.05$.

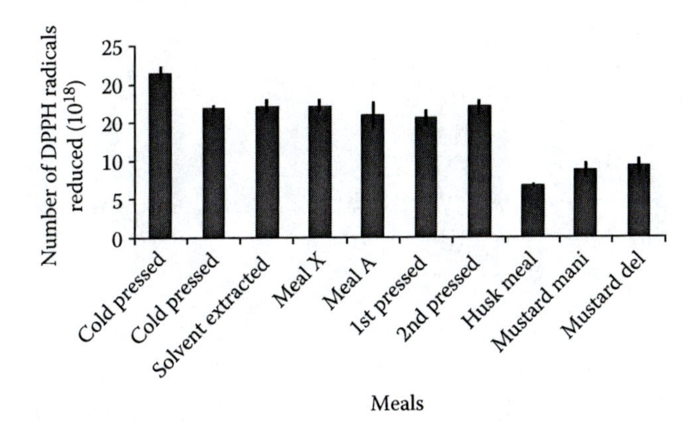

FIGURE 15.12 DPPH radicals scavenged using 70% methanolic extract of commercial meals. Right to left: mustard Delhi, mustard Manipur, meals X, A* (non-specified), husk meal*, second-pressed*, first-pressed*, solvent-extracted and cold-pressed meals. *From the same company.

activity of extracts from second-pressed meal and first-pressed meal did not show any differences exhibiting the pattern of total content of phenolic compounds but slightly deviating from the pattern of total cinnamic acids. Husk meal showed more or less two to three times lower radical scavenging activity than extracts from first- and second-pressed meals corresponding to the pattern of phenolic contents. Mustard cake extracts exhibited two to three times lower activity compared to extracts of cold-pressed rapeseed cake corresponding to the trend of phenolic compounds (total content of phenolic compounds and cinnamic acid content).

Figure 15.12 indicates individual contributions by sinapoyl glucose, sinapine and sinapic acid to the overall radical scavenging activity (100%) theoretically. These three phenolics contributed to a sum of ~50–65% of the overall radical scavenging activity of the cold-pressed and solvent-extracted meal extracts (Figure 15.13). First-pressed meal, second-pressed meal and meal A (procured from the same company) on the other hand contributed over ~70% of its radical scavenging activity to these three sinapic acid derivatives, the highest being by sinapine (40%) followed by sinapic acid and sinapoyl glucose (~10–20% each). For extracts from husk meal and mustard meals, sinapine contributed to ~40% while free sinapic acid and sinapoyl glucose contributed negligibly to the overall radical scavenging activity. The radical scavenging activity correlated positively and strongly, $r = 0.79$ with the total content of phenolic compounds of the commercial meal extracts.

As expected, the content of the principal phenolic compounds, rapeseed meal extracts determined their radical scavenging activity. Thus, the radical scavenging activity was directly related to the major phenolic compound(s) present. For example, the higher radical scavenging activity of sinapic acid alone may account for the high radical scavenging activity of the commercial rapeseed extracts with higher contents of free sinapic acid rather than sinapoyl glucose and sinapine. Furthermore, this could explain the comparatively low radical scavenging activity of the mustard meal extracts as its main phenolic constituent was sinapine, which constituted

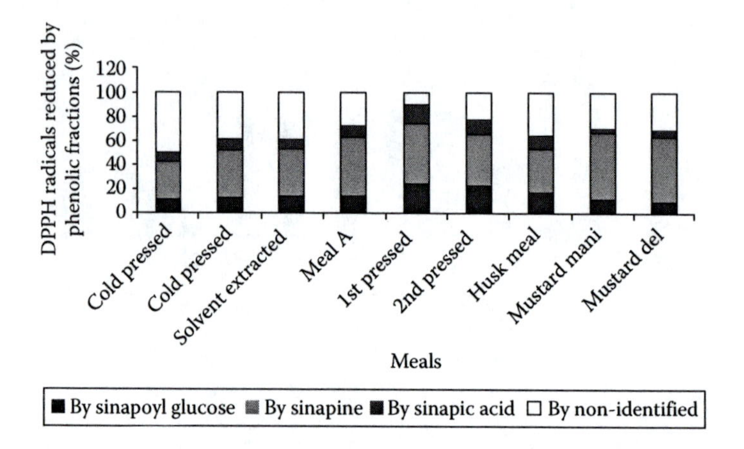

FIGURE 15.13 DPPH radicals scavenged with 70% methanolic extract of commercial meals. Right to left: mustard Delhi, mustard Manipur, meals X, Y, A* (non-specified), husk meal*, second-pressed*, first-pressed*, solvent-extracted and cold-pressed meals. *From the same company. Radicals scavenged by phenolic constituents sinapoyl glucose (SG), sinapine (SP), sinapic acid (SA) and rest from un-identified (non-identified) phenolic constituents.

over 80–90% of the phenolic compounds. This same reason could account for low radical scavenging activity of the hull extracts. Other sinapic acid derivatives with significant antioxidant activity and antimutagenic activity are 4-vinyl-2,6-dimethoxyphenol (vinylsyringol or canolol) isolated from processed rapeseed or canola oil (Kuwahara et al., 2004). However, these compounds have been found only in traces in the commercial meal extracts investigated.

The correlation between total phenolic compounds and radical scavenging activity of the commercial meal extracts measured with Folin–Ciocalteu and DPPH was significant ($r = 0.79$). This means that at least all major phenolic compounds, irrespective of their different structures, may exhibit RSA. This correlation was slightly stronger for total hydroxy cinnamic acids even though hydroxy cinnamic acids were overestimated. The explanation for this may be the non-specificity of the method, as interfering compounds may interfere with the absorbance at 330 nm, but the hydroxy cinnamic acids absorbing at this wavelength possessed RSA. Methodologies for estimating phenolic compounds may be crucial. For example, Kahkonen et al. (1999) found no significant correlation between the total phenolic compound content and the antioxidant activity as measured using a methyl-linoleate system for plant extracts. On the other hand, investigations by Allais et al. (1991) described a strong correlation between the DPPH method and the amount of phenolic compounds; in particular of flavan-3-ols. The reasons cited for the poor correlation between the amount of phenolic compounds and the antioxidant activity was attributed to the methods used to determine the phenolic compounds and individual phenolic compounds may vary, for example, based on sensitivity to Folin–Ciocalteau reagent as discussed in earlier sections.

Additionally, Singleton et al. (1999) described that substances such as sugars or ascorbic acid present in the extracts influence results of various methods intended

TABLE 15.3
DPPH Radical Scavenging Activity of Different Fractions of 70% Methanolic Extract

Assay	Number of DPPH Radicals Reduced (×10[18])	Sinapic Acid Content (SAE mg/g dm)
Phenolic fraction	DPPH assay	Folin–Ciocalteu assay
Free fraction		
(diethyl ether fraction)	2.3 ± 0.1	1.9 ± 0.1
Aqueous fraction	28.8 ± 1.1	18.5 ± 0.6
Released fraction	25.9 ± 0.1	13.6 ± 0.1

Note: Free fraction (diethyl ether fraction with free phenols), aqueous fraction (bound-phenolic fraction) and released fraction. Phenolic contents (Table 15.2).

to register the antioxidant activity. Phenolic compounds are a diverse group of compounds and relating them with their potent antioxidant activity is largely dependent on the methods employed for the determination of the antioxidant activity. Canola and rapeseed hulls are cited to have good antioxidative activity. However, low antioxidative activity was represented by the rapeseed hull extract, as compared with whole rapeseed or dehulled rapeseed extracts. The content of free sinapic acid and sinapoyl glucose, the main antioxidative compounds being present in traces in the hull extracts could be one reason. Secondly, sinapine, the major compound constituting over 80% of the sinapic acid derivatives has less antioxidative activity as reported in this study. This further depicts that total hydroxycinnamic acids that constituted over 70% of the total phenolic compounds contributed significantly to the total radical scavenging activity of all rapeseed extracts.

The phenolic fractions and the DPPH radicals scavenged are shown in Figures 15.12 and 15.13. The results agreed with the phenolic contents in the respective fractions of the 70% methanolic extract. The aqueous fraction when compared with the released fraction showed 1.1 times higher radical scavenging activity corresponding to the 1.36 times higher sinapic acid content (mg/g dm). Free acid fraction when compared with the aqueous fraction showed around 12 times less radical scavenging activity corresponding to the 9.7 times higher total content of phenolic compounds (SAE mg/g dm) (Table 15.3).

15.5 ANTIOXIDATIVE ACTIVITY OF RAPESEED MEAL EXTRACTS

The fractionated and non-fractionated 70% methanolic rapeseed meal extract were also added to 10% o/w emulsion at a concentration of 500 μmol/kg oil. This set of experiments aimed at studying differences in effectiveness of the fractionated rapeseed meal extracts in bulk oils and emulsion using the rate of oxidation as monitored by the formation of hydroperoxides and secondary volatiles. Auto-oxidation was carried out at 40°C in the dark. The oil that was used for preparing the emulsion was purified. Purification of rapeseed oils was done to strip the rapeseed oils of natural antioxidants, trace metals and free fatty acids via adsorption chromatography using the method described by Lampi and Kamal-Eldin (1998).

Peroxide value was measured as an indicator for primary oxidation products using the standardized 'Ferric thiocyanite' method. Peroxide oxidizes ferrous iron to the ferric state, resulting in the formation of a red thiocyanate complex, which was measured at 485 nm. Conjugated dienes were measured according to Stöckmann et al. (2000) and expressed as mmole hydroperoxides per kilogram of oil as described by Frankel et al. (1994). Advanced lipid oxidation products, 'propanal' (specific indicator of the *n*-3 fatty acid) and 'hexanal', were measured as an indicator for secondary oxidation products using static headspace gas chromatography according to Frankel (1993, 1994). Standard solutions (propanal and hexanal) were identified over the retention times (min) with authentic propanal and hexanal standards and calculated by calibration functions of different concentrations. For hexanal, the calibration function (Equation 15.4) was used while that for propanal was calculated using Equation 15.5 as indicated below. These were used for all further analyses irrespective of oil or emulsion.

$$Y_1 = 1.221 \cdot X + 0.242 \quad (R^2 = 0.99) \tag{15.4}$$

$$Y_2 = 1.315 \cdot X - 22.549 \quad (R^2 = 0.99) \tag{15.5}$$

where X: peak area, Y_1 is hexanal concentration [μmol/kg oil] and Y_2 is propanal concentration [μmol/kg oil].

The o/w emulsions were prepared with and without added antioxidants in distilled water containing 1% Emulpur/lecithin (Degussa texturant systems, Germany) and 10% purified rapeseed oil as described by Huang and coworkers (1996). Briefly, Emulpur/lecithin and purified rapeseed oil were homogenized with distilled water, citrate buffer (pH 4.5) and emulsified by sonicating for a total of 5 min. The 20 g emulsions were introduced into standard 50 mL closed flasks and the different antioxidants were added. Samples were stirred manually using glass jars for 1 min for total dispersion of the antioxidants. Antioxidants and extracts were added in ethanol/methanol to the oil. Duplicate samples of purified 10% rapeseed oil-in-water emulsions were oxidised via incubation in an oven at 40°C in the dark and monitored for the formation of oxidation products. In the same manner, rapeseed extracts were added to this emulsified system. Monitoring for the formation of oxidation products was done as described in the following section.

15.6 ANTIOXIDATIVE ACTIVITY OF MAJOR PHENOLIC COMPOUNDS DURING LIPID OXIDATION

As mentioned in Section 15.5 of this chapter, rapeseed meal extracts are potent free radical scavengers. To further investigate the antioxidative power, inhibition of hydroperoxides and propanal/hexanal in o/w emulsion was investigated. During auto-oxidation in the emulsion, different data for oxidation status were determined, such as increases in the primary and secondary oxidation products during the course of incubation, and percent inhibition as compared with the control. It is important to use more than one method to determine the antioxidant activity to evaluate the effect of lipid oxidation at different stages (Frankel, 1993). To get an impression of the overall order of activity of the different antioxidants, cinnamic acids including sinapic acid were compared with reference antioxidants.

15.6.1 Effect of Rapeseed Meal Extracts as Compared with Sinapic Acid in Purified Rapeseed Oil Emulsion

It was further of interest to test the effectiveness and applicability of rapeseed meal extracts and extract fractions as potent antioxidants and determine their effectiveness in inhibiting lipid oxidation in emulsified systems compared to bulk lipid oils. Ethanolic extract fractions of rapeseed (cultivar Jantar) demonstrated antioxidative activity in a beta-carotene-linoleate model system with the free-phenolic fraction showing the highest antioxidative activity while pure sinapic acid and sinapine fractions showed the least activity (Nowak et al., 1992). Ethanolic extracts of canola seeds exhibited antioxidative activity in a meat model system (Shahidi et al., 1993) and in canola oils (Wanasundara et al., 1995) where the effect in canola oil was stronger than that of either BHA or BHT. Aqueous methanolic extracts of low pungency mustard have also exhibited good antioxidative properties in meat model systems (Saleemi et al., 1993).

Evaluation of the fractionated and non-fractionated 70% methanolic rapeseed meal extract added to stripped rapeseed oil at a concentration that was equivalent to 500 μmol/kg oil of total phenolic compounds (as quantified by HPLC, 330 nm) was compared with sinapic acid. The fractionated free-phenolic compounds (free-phenolic fraction), which contain over 85% sinapic acid, showed a similar pattern with the sinapic acid standard with respect to the inhibition of both the hydroperoxides and propanal in the emulsion. This was observed for both the cases, that is, hydroperoxide inhibition and propanal inhibition. The effectiveness of the fractionated free-phenolic compounds (free-phenolic fraction) may be due to the high concentration of sinapic acid in the extracts. These extracts, when added to a 10% o/w system at a concentration of 500 μmol/kg oil exhibited differences in the potencies with respect to inhibition of the primary and secondary products of oxidation.

Results of the present study indicate that the bound and the non-fractionated extract could inhibit the hydroperoxides, propanal and hexanal in a similar manner to sinapine alone when compared with the control sample without any added antioxidant. This was in contrast to the results illustrated in the bulk rapeseed oil system, where these extracts and sinapine functioned as a mild pro-oxidative or ineffective antioxidant. The non-fractionated extract and sinapine represented a comparable manner in inhibiting PV increase, whereas the bound fraction was more effective as compared with sinapine and nonfractionated extract. This means that in this case, the unidentified peaks of the hydrophilic compounds contributed to the enhanced activity of the bound-phenolic fraction. It was also observed that sinapic acid and the free-phenolic fraction functioned in a similar manner until the 18th day of incubation.

With respect to inhibition of propanal and hexanal, sinapine was quite effective in the emulsion in contrast to its activity in the bulk lipid system. The bound-phenolic fraction was also slightly more effective compared to sinapine in the case of propanal and hexanal inhibition. Interestingly, it was observed that the non-fractionated extract acted in a manner similar to sinapic acid and the free-phenolic fraction. The justification as to why fractions rich in sinapine displayed strong antioxidant activities is a difficult task because each fraction is a complex mixture of phenolic compounds; the difference in molecular structure may be in the arrangement of hydroxyl and methoxy groups, in the presence of ester and/or glycosidic bonds, and in the degree of association of the molecules involved. Synergism of phenolic compounds with each other as well as with non-phenolic compounds like the emulsifier may also contribute to the total antioxidative activity of each fraction. Sinapic acid alone, free and the non-fractionated, all behaved as the most effective antioxidant. These high antioxidative activities of sinapic acid could be shown with a 10% oil-in-water emulsion using emulpur as an emulsifier also. In the present study, the lower effectiveness of sinapine in the o/w emulsion could be attributed to the repulsion between the cationic charge of sinapine and the overall cationic charge of the phospholipid system at pH 4.5, while sinapic acid showed a higher activity due to its interaction due to the carboxylic group. In accordance with this study, Barclay and Vinqvist (1994) demonstrated a pH-depended activity for Trolox and the positively charged MDL 73404 ammonium in liposomal models.

15.6.2 Formation of Primary Oxidation Products

The effect of rapeseed extracts has been demonstrated against oxidation using emulsions. Figure 15.13 depicts the formation of hydroperoxides in 10% o/w system treated with the fractionated extracts, namely, free (free-phenolic fraction), bound (bound-phenolic fraction) as compared with the non-fractionated extract (non-fractionated 70% methanolic extract), sinapic acid and sinapine added to stripped rapeseed oil at a concentration of 500 μmol/kg oil.

To reach a hydroperoxide value of ~100 mmol/kg oil, the fractionated extracts, sinapine and sinapic acid conformed to the following order:

Control (no-antioxidant) > sinapine > unfractionated extract > bound fraction > sinapic acid > free fraction.

Unlike in bulk oils (Thiyam et al., 2006b), all the extracts were effective in inhibition of hydroperoxides formation compared to sinapic acid. Thus, unlike in bulk oils, the bound fractions were more effective than the unfractionated 70% methanolic extract and sinapine in the emulsified system. Furthermore, bound fractions were effective in a similar pattern as sinapic acid contrasting its activity in bulk oils. The free fraction of rapeseed extract was slightly more effective than sinapic acid in inhibiting the hydroperoxides. This corresponded to nearly the same activity in bulk oils. The results for hydroperoxides and conjugated dienes formation were in agreement.

15.6.3 Secondary Oxidation Products-Pattern

The patterns of formation of propanal and hexanal (Figures 15.14 and 15.15, respectively) for the above extracts are shown below and decreased in the following order:

Control (no-antioxidant) > sinapine > bound fraction > sinapic acid ≈ free fraction ≈ unfractionated extract.

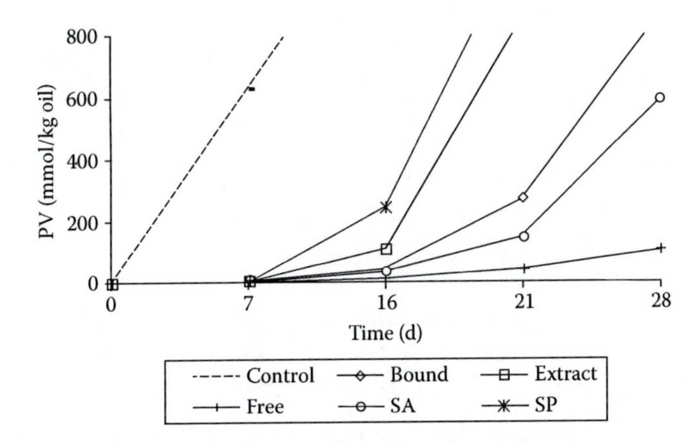

FIGURE 15.14 Effect of fractionated rapeseed meal extracts on the formation of hydroperoxides of rapeseed oil at 40°C in the dark. Control (no antioxidants), sinapic acid (SA), extract (non-fractionated 70% methanolic extract), free (free-phenolic fraction), bound (bound-phenolic fraction), sinapine (SP), all added to stripped rapeseed oil at a concentration of 500 μmol/kg oil.

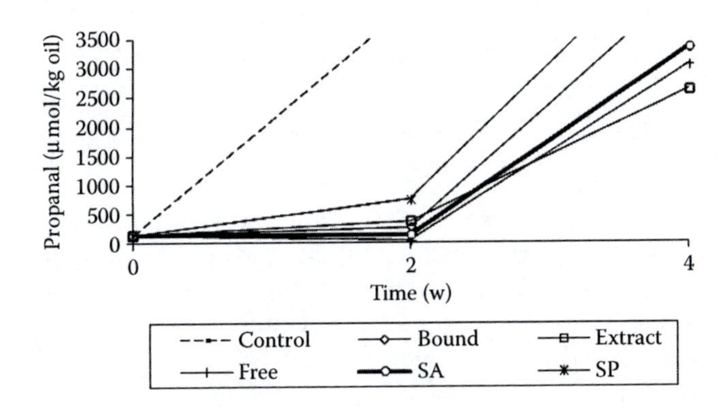

FIGURE 15.15 Effect of fractionated rapeseed meal extracts on the formation of propanal of rapeseed oil at 40°C in the dark. Control (no antioxidants), sinapic acid (SA), extract (non-fractionated 70% methanolic extract), free (free-phenolic fraction), bound (bound-phenolic fraction), sinapine (SP), all added to stripped rapeseed oil at a concentration of 500 μmol/kg oil.

The trend for propanal formation (Figure 15.15) agreed with that for hexanal (Figure 15.16).

This also illustrated that, unlike in bulk oils, all the extracts were effective in inhibiting hydroperoxides as well as secondary volatiles formation compared to sinapic acid. This further suggests that bound fractions were effective in inhibition of propanal and hexanal. However, this inhibition was less than the unfractionated 70% methanolic extract, which was equally effective as sinapic acid and the free fraction of rapeseed extract. This contrasted the effectiveness of the unfractionated 70% methanolic extract compared to sinapic acid in inhibiting hydroperoxide formation.

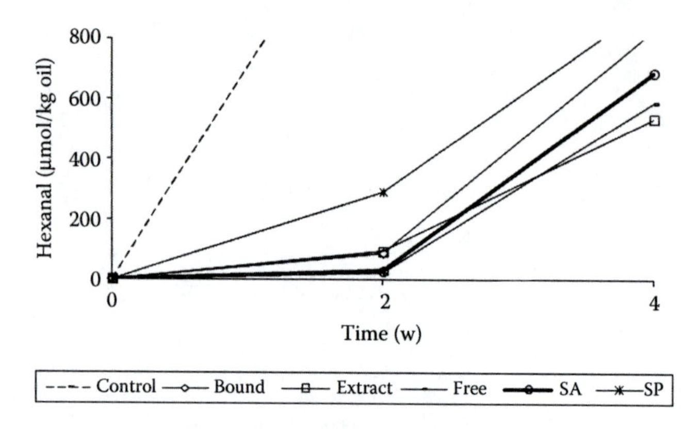

FIGURE 15.16 Effect of fractionated rapeseed meal extracts on the formation of hexanal of rapeseed oil at 40°C in the dark. Control (no antioxidants), sinapic acid (SA), extract (non-fractionated 70% methanolic extract), free (free-phenolic fraction), bound (bound-phenolic fraction), sinapine (SP), all added to stripped rapeseed oil at a concentration of 500 µmol/kg oil.

The overall trends for unfractionated and fractionated extracts were also different for secondary volatiles in the emulsified system compared to that in bulk oil system.

15.7 CONCLUSION AND FUTURE PERSPECTIVES

Vegetable oils and oil-containing food, especially in the context of rapeseed oils and rapeseed-oil-containing systems, are vulnerable to oxidative deterioration. Natural antioxidants are now being widely used to retard oxidation in lipid and lipid-containing systems. The food industry has used emulsification techniques for many years to create a diverse range of food products, such as milk, cream, soft drinks, nutritional beverages, dressings, mayonnaise, sauces, dips, deserts, ice cream, margarine and butter. The majority of these food products are conventional oil-in-water (O/W)- or water-in-oil (W/O)-type emulsions. The rapeseed oil-in-water (o/w) samples incubated at 40°C demonstrated the effectiveness of the sinapic acid and its derivatives as antioxidants by their inhibition of primary oxidation products such as hydroperoxides and conjugated dienes, as well as secondary oxidation products as propanal (headspace-gas chromatography). Furthermore, the free radical scavenging activities of the natural phenolic compounds and rapeseed meal extracts were comparable with standard antioxidants demonstrating the efficacy of rapeseed meal extracts as potential antioxidants. Can we rationally promote rapeseed antioxidants for specific health benefits? A more complete characterization of rapeseed components and their physiological fate may provide mechanistic insights into their potential antioxidant activity observed *in vitro* and *in vivo* studies. The high *in vitro* antioxidant activity of rapeseed meal extract has been largely attributed to its sinapic acid and sinapine, but the antioxidant efficacy of these compounds has to be studied in various food systems before promoting them as potent antioxidants.

REFERENCES

Allais, D.P., Simon, A., Bennini, B., Chulia, A.J. Kaouadji, M. and Delage, C. 1991. Flavone and flavonol glycosides from Calluna vulgaris. *Phytochemistry*. 30: 3099–3101.

Amarowicz, R., Naczk, M. and Shahidi, F. 2000. Antioxidant activity of various fractions of non-tannin phenolics of canola hulls. *J. Agric. Food Chem.* 48: 2755–2759.

Amarowicz, R., Wanasundara, U.N., Karamac, M. and Shahidi F. 1996. Antioxidant activity of ethanolic extract of mustard seed. *Nahrung*. 40: 261–263.

Barclay, L.R.C. and Vinqvist, M.R. 1994. Membrane peroxidation: Inhibiting effects of water-soluble antioxidants on phospholipids of different charge types. *Free Radical Biology and Medicine*. 16: 779–788.

Blois, M.S. 1958. Antioxidant determination by the use of a stable free radical. *Nature*. 181: 1199–1202.

Chimi, H., Cillard, J., Cillard, P. and Rahmani, M. 1991. Peroxyl and hydroxyl radical scavenging activity of some natural phenolic antioxidants. *J. Am. Oil Chem. Soc.* 68: 307–312.

Cuvelier, M.E., Richard, H. and Berset, C. 1996. Antioxidative activity and phenolic composition of pilot-plant and commercial extracts of sage and eosemary. *J. Am. Oil Chem. Soc.* 73: 645–652.

Frankel, E.N. 1993. Formation of headspace volatiles by thermal decomposition of oxidized fish oils vs oxidized vegetable oils. *J. Am. Oil Chem. Soc.* 70: 767–772.

Frankel, E.N. 1994. Methods of evaluating food antioxidants-reply. *Trends Food Sci. Technol.* 5: 55–57.

Frankel, E.N. 1998. *Lipid Oxidation*. The Oily Press LTD, Dundee, Scotland.

Frankel, E.N., Huang S.-W., Kanner J. and German, J.B. 1994. Interfacial phenomena in the evaluation of antioxidants: Bulk oils vs emulsions. *J. Agric. Food Chem.* 42: 1054–1059.

Harbaum-Piayda, B., Oehlke, K., Sönnichsen, F.D., Zacchi, P., Eggers, R. and Schwarz, K. 2010. New polyphenolic compounds in commercial deodestillate and rapeseed oils. *Food Chem*. 123, 607–615.

Kikuzaki, H., Hisamoto, M., Hirose, K., Akiyama, K. and Taniguchi, H. 2002. Antioxidant properties of ferulic acid and its related compounds. *J. Agric. Food Chem.* 50: 2161–2168.

King, B.J., Turrel, J.A. and Zilka, S.A. 1986. Analysis of minor fatty acid components by capillary column GLC and of triglycerides by HPLC. Research Report no. 563. Leatherhead Food Research association. Leatherhead, Surrey, United Kingdom.

Koski, A., Pekkarinen S., Hopia, A., Wähälä K. and Heinonen, M. 2003. Processing of rapeseed oil: Effects on sinapic acid derivative content and oxidative stability. *Eur. Food Res. Technol.* 217: 110–114.

Koski, A., Psomiadou, E., Tsimidou, M., Hopia, A., Kefalas, P., Wähälä, K. and Heinonen, M. 2002. Oxidative stability and minor constituents of virgin olive oil and cold-pressed rapeseed oil. *Eur. Food Res. Technol.* 214: 294–298.

Krygier, K., Sosulski, F. and Hogge, L. 1982. Free, esterified, and insoluble-bound-phenolic acids. 2. Composition of phenolic acids in rapeseed flour and hulls. *J. Agric. Food Chem.* 30: 330–334.

Kuwahara, H., Kanazawa, A., Wakamatu, D., Morimura, S., Kida, K., Akaike, T. and Maeda, H. 2004. Antioxidative and antimutagenic activities of 4-vinyl-2,6-dimethoxyphenol (canolol) isolated from canola oil. *J. Agric. Food Chem.* 52, 4380–4387.

Lampi, A-M. and Kamal-Eldin, A. 1998. Effect of α- and γ-tocopherols on thermal polymerization of purified high-oleic sunflower triacylglycerols. *Journal of the American Oil Chemists' Society*. 75: 1699–170.

Nowak, H., Kujawa, K., Zadernowski, R., Roczniak, B. and KozŁowska, H. 1992. Antioxidative and bactericidal properties of phenolic compounds in rapeseeds. *European Journal of Lipid Science and Technology*. 94: 149–152.

Pekkarinen, S., Hopia, A. and Heinonen, M. 1998. Effect of processing on the oxidative stability of low erucic acid turnip rapeseed oil. *Fett/Lipid*. 100: 69–74.

Pekkarinen, S., Stöckmann, H., Schwarz, K., Heinonen, M., Hopia, A. 1999. Antioxidant activity and partitioning of phenolic acids in bulk and emulsified methyl linoleate. *J. Agric. Food Chem.* 47: 3036–3043.

Pszczola, D.E. 2001. Antioxidants: From preserving food quality to quality of life. *Food Tech.* 55: 51–53.

Saleemi, Z.O., Janitha, P.K., Wanasundara, P.D. and Shahidi, F. 1993. Effects of low-pungency ground mustard seed on oxidative stability, cooking yield, and color characteristics of comminuted pork. *J. Agric. Food Chem.* 41: 641–643.

Schwarz, K., Bertelsen, G., Nissen, L.R., Gardner, P.T., Heinonen, M.I., Hopia, A., Huynh-Ba, T. et al. 2001. Investigation of plant extracts for the protection of processed foods against lipid oxidation. Comparison of antioxidant assays based on radical scavenging, lipid oxidation and analysis of the principal antioxidant compounds. *European Food Research and Technology*. 212: 319–328.

Shahdi, F. and Naczk, M. 1995. *Food Phenolics, Sources Chemistry Effects Applications*. Technomic Publishing Co. Inc. Lancaster, Basel.

Shahidi, F. 1990. *Canola and Rapeseed*. AVI, Van Nostrand Reinhold, New York.

Shahidi, F. and Naczk, M. 1992. An overview of the phenolics of canola and rapeseed: Chemical, sensory and nutritional significance. *J. Am. Oil Chem. Soc.* 69: 917–923.

Shahidi, F., Yang, Z. and Saleemi, Z.O. 1993. Stabilisation of meat lipids with flavonoids and flavomoids and flavonoid-related compounds. *Journal of Food Lipids*. 1: 69–78.

Singleton V.L. and Rossi, J.A. Jr. 1965. Colorimetry of total phenolics with phosphomolybdic-phosphotungstic acid reagents. *Am. J. Enol. Vitic* 16(3): 144–158.

Singleton, V.L., Orthofer, R. and Lamuela-Raventós, R.M. 1999. Analysis of total phenols and other oxidation substrates and antioxidants by means of folin-ciocalteu reagent. *Methods in Enzymology*. 299: 152–178.

Stöckmann, H., Schwarz, K. and Huynh-Ba, T. 2000. The influence of various emulsifiers on the partitioning and antioxidant activity of hydroxybenzoic acids and their derivatives in oil-in-water emulsions. *Journal of the American Oil Chemists' Society*. 77: 535–542.

Thiyam, U. 2005. Antioxidative compounds of rapeeed oil by-products or stabilization of bulk oil and emulsions. PhD Thesis, Shaker Verlag.

Thiyam, U., Stöckmann, H. and Schwarz, K. 2006a. Antioxidative effect of main sinapic acid derivatives from rapeseed and mustard oil by-products. *Eur. J. Lipid Sci. & Tech.* 108: 239–248.

Thiyam, U., Stöckmann, H. and Schwarz, K. 2006b. Antioxidant activity of rapeseed phenolics and their interaction with tocopherols in rapeseed oil triglycerides during lipid oxidation. *J. Am. Oil Chem. Soc.* 83: 523–528.

Vuorela, S., Meyer, A.S. and Heinonen, M. 2003. Quantitative analysis of the main phenolics in rapeseed meal and oils processed differently using enzymatic hydrolysis and HPLC. *Eur. Food Res. Technol.* 217: 517–523.

Wanasundara, U., Amarowicz, R. and Shahidi, F. 1994. Isolation and identification of an antioxidative component in canola meal. *J. Agric. Food Chem.* 42: 1285–1290.

Wanasundara, U., Amarowicz, R. and Shahidi, F. 1995. Partial characterization of natural antioxidants in canola meal. *Food Res. Int.* 28: 525–530.

Zadernowski, R., Nowak, H. and Kozlowska, H. 1991. Natural antioxidants from rapeseed, *Rapeseed in Changing World, Eighth International Rapeseed Congress*, Saskatoon, Canada, July 9–11, pp. 883–887.

16 Nutritional Impact of Fatty Acid Composition of Canola Oil and Its Effect on the Oxidative Deterioration

Kazuo Miyashita

CONTENTS

16.1 Introduction 299
16.2 Nutritional Importance of LN of Canola Oil 300
16.3 Nutritional Impact of OA in Canola Oil 302
16.4 Oxidative Stability of Canola Oil 304
16.5 Formation of CLN in Vegetable Oils and Its Impact on Flavour Deterioration 305
16.6 Conclusion 309
References 310

16.1 INTRODUCTION

Canola oil is rich in oleic acid (18:1n-9, OA; >60%). It also contains a considerable amount of linoleic acid (18:2n-6, LA; ~22%) and α-linolenic acid (18:3n-3, LN; ~10%) (Dolde et al., 1999; Vlahakis and Hazebroek, 2000). The omega-3/omega-6 polyunsaturated fatty acid (PUFA) ratio of canola oil is considered to be favourable for human health (Gunstone et al., 2007). This is based on the fact that people are taking too much LA from the diet in today's society. Simopoulos (2008) found that, in Western societies, the omega-6/omega-3 ratio is about 16/1 due to the high intake of oil soyabean, corn, sunflower and safflower oils, which are high in LA. Indeed, the ratio of omega-6/omega-3 PUFA in the food chain in Europe (Sanders, 2000) and in the United States (Kris-Etherton et al., 2000) is still much higher than that recommended by the Food and Agriculture Organization (FAO) or the World Health Organization (WHO). Although, it is difficult to tell the favourable ratio of omega-6 and omega-3 in the dietary lipids, it is apparent that the adequate intake of LN is higher than that found in Western diet (Russo, 2010). Therefore, canola oil should be regarded as a healthy oil because of its relatively higher level of LN.

The role of monounsaturated fatty acids (MFUA), mainly OA, in human health has also received much attention. Olive oil, the most common OA-rich oil, is a low-risk fat as shown in animal models and through the observation that the incidence of specific diseases is lower in the Mediterranean region, where it is customarily used (Weisburger, 2000). Several clinical and nutritional studies indicated that OA lowers the risk of cardiovascular disease (CVD) (Lusso, 2009), diabetes and obesity (Kien, 2009; Soriguer et al., 2007; Vassiliou et al., 2009), and increases their resistance to oxidation in biological systems (Lusso, 2009), when it substituted for saturated fatty acids (SFA). The lowering effect of OA substitute with SFA on low-density lipoprotein (LDL) oxidation is interesting as SFA are chemically less reactive to oxidation than OA.

The oxidative stability of edible oils is basically dependent on the fatty acid composition. The stability increases with decreasing average number of bis-allylic hydrogens in the molecule (Cosgrove et al., 1987). From many early studies of the oxidative stability of edible oils varying in fatty acid composition, it is now well recognized that the oxidative stability of lipids decreased with increase in their contents of LA and LN, while OA in the lipids increases their resistance to oxidation. Stability is also affected by the position of fatty acid in the glycerol moiety (Miyashita et al., 1990; Neff et al., 1992). Neff et al. (1992) evaluated the effect of the triacylglycerol (TAG) molecular species of soyabean oil on its oxidative stability. They found that OA in the TAG improved its oxidative stability slightly higher than palmitic acid (16:0, PA) did in TAG. Replacing PA in dilinoleoyl-palmitoyl TAG (LLP) with OA improved the oxidative stability by a higher negative correlation in peroxide value and in the formation of selected volatile compounds.

Thus, the fatty acid profile of canola oil, its high level of OA and moderate level of LN will favour both nutritional and product quality. This review will provide a background on the health benefits of canola oil and its oxidative stability. Flavour deterioration is a main problem of food lipid oxidation. Oxidative stability of commercial vegetable oils has been improved by recent progress in oil refining and storage technology. However, there still remains a problem of flavour deterioration noted at unusually low levels of oxidation. This flavour defect is known as 'reversion', a term derived from their flavour characteristic of crude soyabean oil described as 'beany' or 'grassy'. I will discuss in this review the susceptibility of canola oil to this flavour defect.

16.2 NUTRITIONAL IMPORTANCE OF LN OF CANOLA OIL

Lipids play a major role in human nutrition and health, providing a concentrated source of energy, and reduce bulk of the diet. They are indispensable in the diet as major sources of essential fatty acids as well as providing fat-soluble substances, including vitamins and carotenoids. Essential fatty acids play a key role in many metabolic processes and cannot be synthesized by mammals. Because animals lack a Δ-15 or Δ-12 desaturase, they are unable to form omega-3 or omega-6 PUFA *de novo* and they must obtain these essential fatty acids from their diet (Innis, 2003; Jump, 2004; Sampath and Ntambi, 2004). The importance of omega-3 and omega-6 PUFA to human health has been clearly established through research works across the globe. They provide several beneficial health and physiological effects. The functions of each omega-3 or omega-6 PUFA have attracted consumer attention and are often used in functional foods and nutraceuticals.

Traditionally, LA (omega-6) and LN (omega-3) are considered the only essential fatty acids. Sometimes, arachidonic acid (AA; 20:4n-6), eicosapentaenoic acid (EPA; 20:5n-3) and docosahexaenoic acid (DHA; 22:6n-3) are also considered conditional essential fatty acids because their production may be inadequate in certain conditions such as prematurity and periods of growth, thus requiring exogenous supplementation. EPA and DHA are two omega-3 PUFA found in marine lipids. Both long-chain PUFA have been shown to cause significant biochemical and physiological changes in the body (Li et al., 2003; Lands, 2005; Sinclair et al., 2005; Shahidi and Miraliakbari, 2006; Narayan et al., 2006b) that most of the times result in positive influence on human nutrition and health. On the other hand, omega-6 PUFA and their derivatives play an important role in biological systems such as in immune response, thrombosis and in brains (Hoffman et al., 2009; Le et al., 2009).

DHA is the major omega-3 PUFA esterified in the glycerophospholipids that form the structural matrix of brain grey matter and retinal membranes (Belkind-Gerson et al., 2008; Hoffman et al., 2009; Guisto et al., 2002). Humans and other animals can directly intake DHA from marine products or obtain after bioconversion of DHA precursors, LN or intermediate PUFA between LN and DHA. DHA accumulation in the brain and retina, as in other organs, depends on the amount and types of omega-3 PUFA in the diet and on dietary intake of omega-6 PUFA which interact and compete with omega-3 PUFA in the fatty acid metabolic pathway. Thus, the current high intakes of omega-6 PUFA, or low intakes of omega-3 PUFA contribute to poor infant neural development and function, and cause several kinds of biological disorders.

Substantial epidemiological and case–control study data demonstrate that the risk of CVD is lowest among those with the highest fish or long-chain omega-3 PUFA such as EPA and DHA intake (Kris-Etherton et al., 2002; Calder, 2004; Leaf et al., 2008; Wang et al., 2006). The important cardio-protective effect of omega-3 PUFA has also been demonstrated by clinical implications (Russo, 2009) and by genetic and nutrigenetic approaches (Allayee et al., 2009). Thus, American and European heart associations recommend the intake of 1 g/day of EPA and DHA for the prevention of sudden cardiac death and other cardiovascular dysfunctions (De Backer et al., 2003; Smith et al., 2006).

The principal omega-3 PUFAs, LN, EPA and DHA, are believed to each have a constellation of physiological functions. The tissue composition of omega-3 PUFA depends on both dietary intake of these PUFA and metabolism controlled by genetic polymorphisms, resulting that in the same dietary intake of LN, its respective health effects in each tissue may differ due to genetic differences in metabolism (Simopoulos, 2010). Therefore, it is important to understand the extent of their metabolism from LN in the tissue of various mammals. In addition, the metabolism and functions of the omega-3 and omega-6 PUFA interrelate on many levels. High intake of LA inhibits the conversion of LN to DHA. DHA in liver and brain decreased with an intake of LA above 3% energy (Novak et al., 2008; Innis, 2008). Modern human diets contain in excess of 3% energy LA (Innis and Jacobsen, 2007), leading to the argument that omega-6 PUFA intakes are now so high as to flood the fatty acid metabolic pathway and suppress metabolism of the omega-3 PUFA.

Dairy intake of EPA and DHA reduces the risk of CVD. This will be due to the regulation of membrane structure, lipid metabolism, blood clotting, blood pressure and inflammation (Allayee et al., 2009; Givens and Gibbs, 2008; Harris et al., 2008; Leaf et al., 2008; Russo, 2009; Tziomalos et al., 2008). Another important role of DHA is that it is an essential constituent of the mammalian central nervous system, including membrane lipids of brain grey matter and the visual elements of the retina (Belkind-Gerson et al., 2008; Hoffman et al., 2009; Innis, 2008). On the other hand, the nutritional role of their plant-derived omega-3 counterpart, LN, is far less clear, yet it is the principal dietary omega-3 PUFA consumed in the typical Western diet (Barre, 2007; Kris-Etherton et al., 2002).

It may be true that humans have a poor ability to form DHA from LN. Tracer studies have shown that the proportion of the conversion of LN to DHA in infants is very low, <1% (Goyens et al., 2005; Hussein et al., 2005; Carnielli et al., 2007). On the other hand, studies in normal healthy adults consuming Western diets, which are rich in LA, show that supplemental LN raises EPA and DPA status in the blood and in breast milk. Addition of LN to the diets of formula-fed infants does raise DHA, but no level of LN tested raises DHA to levels achievable with preformed DHA at intakes similar to typical human milk DHA supply (Brenna et al., 2009). Males and females differ in their ability to synthesize DHA from LN and this disparity is associated with gender differences in the circulating concentrations of DHA, which is higher in females (Childs et al., 2008).

Though more work is required to identify the differential effects of LN on chronic diseases and to clarify the ability to form DHA from LN in humans, the need for LN is evermore apparent, given that LN is by far the predominant form of omega-3 PUFA consumed while intakes of EPA and DHA are typically very low in the Western diet (Anderson and Ma, 2009). In addition, many studies indicated that the lower intake of LA as compared with LN will be favourable for human health as higher level of LA inhibits conversion of LN to EPA and DHA. Thus, canola oil with relatively higher ratio of LN to LA as compared with other major vegetable oils is a better choice as an edible oil for Western diet.

16.3 NUTRITIONAL IMPACT OF OA IN CANOLA OIL

Several studies have demonstrated the delicate balance in a healthy diet between stearic acid SFA, MUFA and PUFA and their role in LDL/high-density lipoprotein (HDL) composition and oxidation, with MUFA being the most efficacious (Lusso, 2009). OA as the main MUFA has been regarded as a healthy lipid component. Soriguer et al. (2003a,b, 2004) reported that an increase in OA increases adipocyte lipolytic activity and that a diet rich in OA reduces peripheral resistance to the action of insulin. Anti-diabetic and anti-obesity effect of OA has been also reported by others (Vassiliou et al., 2009). The two most common fatty acids in the diet and in tissue stores are PA and OA. Perhaps because in Western diets PA and OA are often derived from the same foods, epidemiologic studies have been done on a differential effect of these two dietary fatty acids on the risk of hyperlipidaemia, insulin resistance, type 2 diabetes and CVD, suggesting that decreasing PA intake or increasing OA intake may be beneficial (Hu et al., 2001; Vessby et al., 2001).

Anti-diabetic and anti-obesity effect of OA intake has been also demonstrated by others (Kien, 2009).

Recent studies in humans and animal models have revealed that modulation of stearoyl-CoA desaturase-1 (SCD1) activity by dietary intervention or genetic manipulation strongly influences several facets of energy metabolism to affect the susceptibility to obesity, insulin resistance, diabetes and hyperlipidaemia (Flowers and Ntambi, 2008, 2009; Paton and Ntambi, 2008). SCD1 catalyzes the D9-*cis* desaturation of a range of fatty acyl-CoA substrates. The preferred substrate is stearoyl-CoA, which produces OA from stearic acid (18:0). The major product of SCD1, OA (18:1n-9), is the key substrate for the formation of complex lipids such as phospholipids, TAG, cholesterol esters, wax esters and alkyl-2,3-diacylglycerols. Reduced OA synthesis is associated with several metabolic changes that elicit protection from obesity, cellular lipid accumulation and insulin resistance (Miyazaki et al., 2000; Ntambi et al., 2002; Sampath et al., 2007).

The importance of SCD1 on the protection against obesity, insulin resistance and hyperlipidaemia is confirmed by studies of mice that have a naturally occurring mutation in the SCD-1 gene isoform (Ntambi et al., 2002). SCD1 is an important metabolic control point (Ntambi and Miyazaki, 2004; Sampath and Ntambi, 2005; Paton and Ntambi, 2008; Flowers and Ntambi, 2008, 2009). SCD1-deficient mice have reduced lipid synthesis and enhanced lipid oxidation, thermogenesis and insulin sensitivity in various tissues, including liver, muscle and adipose tissue due to transcriptional and post-transcriptional effects. Obese people manifest abnormally high activities of this enzyme in skeletal muscle (Hulver et al., 2005). Absent or deficient SCD1 activity causes the down-regulation of acetyl-CoA carboxylase activity, resulting in lower production of malonyl-CoA. This is thought to relieve the inhibitory effects of this compound on carnitine palmitoyltransferase I (CPT-I), a rate-limiting enzyme for catalyzing the inward transport of FA across the inner mitochondrial membrane (permitting β oxidation) (Muoio and Newgard, 2006). Thus, diminished endogenous formation of stearic acid and OA may prevent, respectively, insulin resistance in liver and skeletal muscle. In rats, markedly increasing the OA intake caused an 80% lower hepatic mRNA expression of SCD1 after 3 weeks (Kakuma et al., 2002), suggesting that chronically elevated OA intakes may down-regulate its *de novo* synthesis.

On the contrary, Liu et al. (2010) have shown that OA intake promotes macrophage inflammation and endothelial adhesion response. Although free fatty acids, most notably SFA, such as PA, are important adipocyte-derived mediators in promoting macrophage inflammation (Suganami et al., 2005), the precise contribution of MUFA, mainly OA (18:1n-9) and palmitoleate (16:1n-7), to the cross-talk among adipocytes, macrophages and endothelial cells, has remained largely understudied. Liu et al. (2010) examined the roles of these MUFA in regulating inflammation independent of the effects from SFA and found that OA, but not palmitoleic or LA, contributes to the inflammation in both RAW macrophages and endothelial cells with the doses and time frame of their treatments. In another study (Nguyen et al., 2007), OA was reported to consistently and significantly promote inflammation in RAW264.7 macrophages.

The effect of OA on metabolic disorders has been still unclear and it is only very recently that the importance of OA has been considered. More study will be needed to clarify this point.

16.4 OXIDATIVE STABILITY OF CANOLA OIL

Lipid oxidation proceeds through a free radical chain reaction consisting of chain initiation, propagation and termination processes (Frankel, 1998a; Kamal-Eldin et al., 2003). The rate-limiting step in the reaction is abstraction of hydrogen radical from substrate lipids to form lipid free radicals. Since this hydrogen abstraction occurs at the bis-allylic positions ($CH{=}CH{-}CH_2{-}CH{=}CH$) present in PUFA and the susceptibility of PUFA to oxidation depends on the availability of bis-allylic hydrogens, oxidative stability of each PUFA is inversely proportional to the number of bis-allylic positions in the molecule or the degree of unsaturation of the PUFA. Thus, when the relative oxidative stabilities of typical PUFA are compared, DHA (22:6n-3) is most rapidly oxidized, followed by EPA (20:5n-3), AA (20:4n-6), LN (18:3n-3) and LA (18:2n-6), respectively (Miyashita and Takagi, 1986; Cho et al., 1987; Cosgrove et al., 1987).

The relative rates of autoxidation of different unsaturated fatty acid esters, including OA, were compared on the basis of oxygen absorption measurements (Holman and Elmer, 1947). In neat systems without added initiator, LA was 40 times more reactive than OA, while LN was 2.4 times more reactive than LA. Therefore, it is generally accepted that the oxidative stability of vegetable oils increases with increasing OA content or decreasing LN content. The oxidizability of vegetable oils can be calculated from their fatty acid composition (Fatemi and Hammond, 1980). Though the LN level of canola oil is higher than other major vegetable oils, a little difference has been observed in the oxidative stability of canola oil with soyabean oil (Hung and Slinger, 1981; Liu and White, 1992a,b), with soyabean and corn oils (Frankel and Huang, 1994; Shen et al., 2001), or with soyabean, cottonseed and sunflower oils (Kodali, 2005). In some cases, canola oil showed higher oxidative stability as compared with other vegetable oils. The relative high stability of canola oils will be mainly due to the high OA content.

On the other hand, hydrogen at the allylic carbon-8 or carbon-11 of OA can be abstracted under the presence of free radicals and other initiators to produce two kinds of delocalized three-carbon alkyl radicals (Porter et al., 1995). And then, oxygen attack at the end-carbon positions of these intermediates produces a mixture of four kinds of isomeric OA mono-hydroperoxides (Frankel, 1998a). When the reactivity of OA and SFA such as PA is compared, SFA should be less reactive to oxidation than OA because of no double bond in its molecule. However, results obtained in the comparative study on the oxidative stability of vegetable oil TAG were more complicated.

Neff et al. (1992) oxidized purified soyabean oil TAG at 60°C in the dark and compared the oxidative stability of each molecular species of the TAG by the determination of peroxide value and volatile compounds, and by a high-performance liquid chromatography (HPLC) analysis of the oxidized TAG molecule. They found that an increased rate of peroxide value showed a positive correlation with the average number of double bonds ($r = 0.81$), LA ($r = 0.63$) or LN ($r = 0.85$), but a negative correlation with OA ($r = -0.82$). Resistance of soyabean oil TAG to oxidation decreased with an increase in LN concentration ($r = 0.87$), while that increased with increasing OA level ($r = -0.76$). More interestingly, they found that replacement of PA in dilinoleoyl-palmitoyl TAG (LLP) with OA improved oxidative stability, as shown by a negative correlation coefficient for dilinoleoyl-oleoyl TAG (LLO) ($r = -0.65$ for peroxide value and $r = -0.16$ for total volatiles, respectively) and a positive correlation coefficient for LLP ($r = 0.79$ for peroxide value and $r = 0.62$ for total volatiles, respectively).

Frankel (1998a) demonstrated the difference in kinetic behaviour between TAG and simple esters such as fatty acid methyl esters, and this would be attributed to the tendency of the TAG to form aggregates. The effect on TAG stability of the position of the fatty acids on the glycerol moiety has also been reported (Frankel, 1998a). With synthetic pure and mixed TAG prepared from LA and LN, we have shown (Frankel et al., 1990; Miyashita et al., 1990; Neff et al., 1990) that at oxidation levels pertinent to soyabean oil flavour deterioration, dilinolenoyl-linoleoyl TAG were less stable to oxidation when LN was in the *sn*-1,2 (or *sn*-2,3) (LnLnL) compared to the *sn*-1,3 (LnLLn) glycerol positions. Neff et al. (1992) also reported that the rate of peroxide formation showed a positive correlation with LA ($r = 0.72$) at the *sn*-2-position of the glycerol moiety, showing the higher reactivity of LA in *sn*-2 position to oxidation than those in *sn*-1,3 positions. The distribution of LA in *sn*-2 position in TAG molecule of high-erucic rapeseed oil was 4.56 times higher than those in the *sn*-1,3 positions (Takagi and Ando, 1991), while in low-(canola) erucic rapeseed oil, the ratio was only 1.80 times higher (Ratnayake and Daun, 2004). The decrease in the distribution of LA at *sn*-2 position found in low-(canola) erucic rapeseed oil may be contributing to its higher oxidative stability as compared with traditional high-erucic rapeseed oil.

16.5 FORMATION OF CLN IN VEGETABLE OILS AND ITS IMPACT ON FLAVOUR DETERIORATION

Crude oil is refined by a series of processes to remove impurities that affect taste, smell, appearance and stability of the oil. The refining processes involve degumming, alkali refining, bleaching and deodorization. PUFA—such as LA, LN, EPA and DHA—found in vegetable and marine oils are susceptible to oxidation during storage and refining of crude oils resulting in oxidation products comprising mainly of mono-hydroperoxides. The mono-hydroperoxides may also be formed by enzymatic oxidation of LA and LN by lipoxygenase during storage of oil seeds. Any oxidation is injurious to the flavour and oxidative stability of refined oils as it results in the formation and accumulation of oxidation products. Oxidation products such as mono-hydroperoxides are easily decomposed to produce free radicals, which induce further oxidation. To prevent the oxidation and remove the oxidation products, it is important to select better conditions for storage of oil seeds, extraction of oils, refining processes and packaging.

Yurawecz et al. (1993) found traces (up to 0.2%) of conjugated linolenic acid (CLN) in vegetable oils in their study of 27 oils for CLN content by ultraviolet (UV) measurement. The isomers were identified as α-eleostearic acid (9*cis*(c),11*trans* (t),13t-18:3), β-eleostearic acid (9t,11t,13t-18:3) and 8t,10t,12t-18:3. HPLC analysis of purified soyabean oil methyl esters indicates the presence of small amounts of CLA

TABLE 16.1
Total CLN Content and Fatty Acid Profile of Commercial Vegetable Oils

	Soyabean ($n = 6$)	Corn ($n = 5$)	Sunflower ($n = 4$)	Cottonseed ($n = 4$)	Canola ($n = 6$)	Olive ($n = 6$)
Total CLN (mg/kg oil)	400–1000	300–600	250–500	150–300	80–150	ND[a]
Fatty acid[b] (mg/100 mg oil)						
16:0	11.4	11.3	6.7	23.0	4.1	10.6
18:0	3.9	2.0	4.0	2.0	1.7	3.1
18:1n-9	18.9	29.8	17.9	15.0	59.0	77.0
18:2n-6	53.2	53.7	61.0	55.4	19.1	4.3
18:3n-3	9.5	1.4	1.0	0.2	7.6	0.6

[a] Not detected.
[b] The data is represented as average.

and CLN as shown by UV detection at 233 and 274 nm (Kinami et al., 2007). These conjugated PUFA have been found in commercial vegetable oils such as soyabean, corn, canola, sesame and safflower oils, but little in olive oil (Kinami et al., 2007). The same results were also obtained as shown in Table 16.1 (unpublished data). The highest level of CLN was found in soyabean oil, followed by corn, sunflower, cottonseed and canola oils. On the other hand, little CLN was detected in olive oil. CLN contents in purified soyabean oil vary from 400 to 1000 mg/kg oil, which corresponds to 0.04–0.10% (w/w). Similar values have also been reported by Yurawecz et al. (1993).

Gas chromatography-mass spectrometry (GC-MS) after conversion of methyl esters to 4,4-dimethyloxazoline (DMOX) derivatives and by comparison with authentic CLN isomers on HPLC revealed the formation of 8,10,12- and 9,11,13-18:3 (c,t,t or t,t,c and t,t,t) in the purified soyabean oil. HPLC chromatogram of crude soyabean oil and processed soyabean oil at different stages shows that a significant amount of CLN (8,10,12 or 9,11,13) was found in soyabean oil after bleaching, although it could barely be detected in crude soyabean oil or in the oil after de-gumming and alkali refining (Kinami et al., 2007). The same effect was also found in the refining steps of canola oil (Table 16.2). A slight decrease in CLN after deodorization may be due to the isomerization of the CLN. Combinations of higher percentage of bleaching earth and lower bleaching temperature result in reduced CLN content (Miyashita, 2008). Similar effects of bleaching temperature and earth combinations have been reported by Van Den Bosch (1973a,b).

The possible mechanism for CLN formation is shown in Figure 16.1 (Parr and Swoboda, 1976; Fishwick and Swoboda, 1977). Four kinds of CLN isomers are produced from 9- and 13-LA mono-hydroperoxide isomers, through two chemical reactions, namely, reduction and hydration, occurring in bleaching condition. Figure 16.2 shows the reversed phase HPLC chromatogram of the reaction products of LA mono-hydroperoxides after heating at 100°C for 30 min. LA mono-hydroperoxide (50 mg) was obtained from autoxidized LA methyl ester by thin-layer

TABLE 16.2
CLN Content at Different Stage of Canola Oil Processing

	CLN (mg/kg oil)		
Soyabean Oil	**c,t,t (t,t,c)**	**t,t,t**	**Total**
Crude	ND	ND	ND
De-gumming	ND	ND	ND
Neutralization	ND	ND	ND
Bleaching	84	95	179
Deodorization	79	90	169

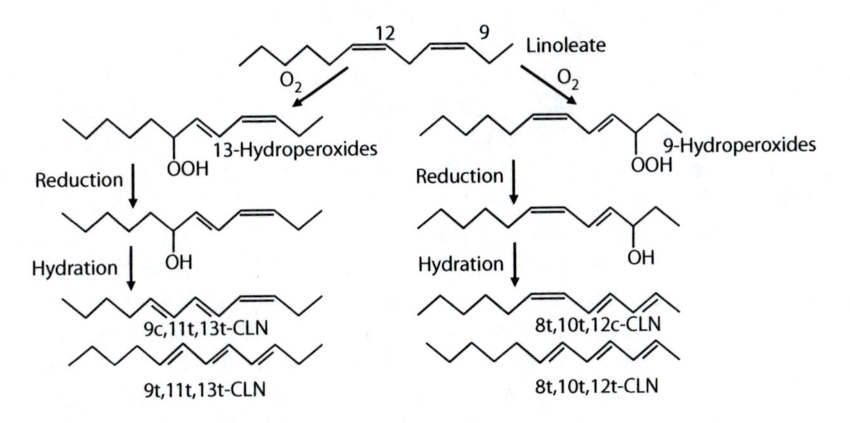

FIGURE 16.1 Possible mechanism for the formation of CLN during bleaching.

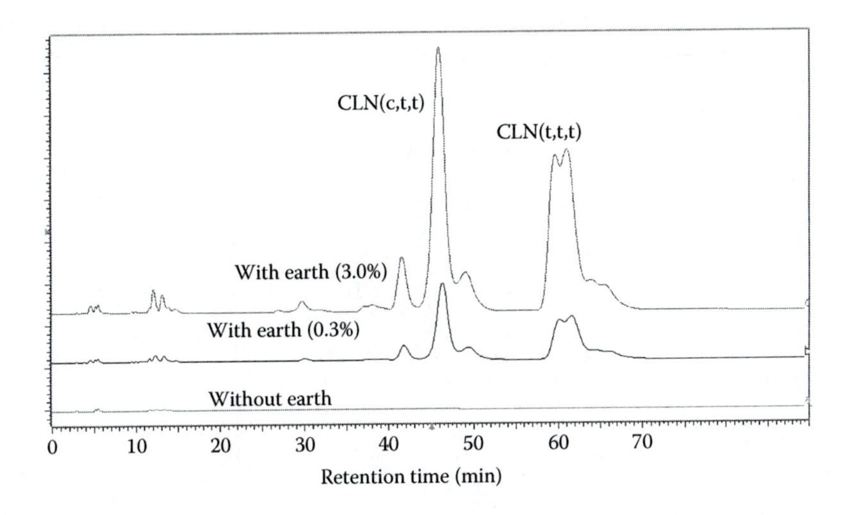

FIGURE 16.2 The formation of CLN after heating LA mono-hydroperoxides under the presence of earth.

chromatography (TLC) and HPLC separation and incubated in a 250 mg middle-chain fatty acid TAG (MCT) with or without activated earth (0.3% or 3.0%). It is apparent that CLN is produced under the presence of activated earth, but not without the earth. Bleaching is usually done under the presence of activated earth at high temperature (around 100°C). Thus, the result in Figure 16.2 confirms the CLN formation from LA mono-hydroperoxides during the bleaching step.

Because CLN is derived from LA mono-hydroperoxides, CLN level found in vegetable oils is basically dependent on LA content in the oils. Table 16.1 shows the relationship between total CLN and fatty acid profile of vegetable oils. The CLN level was strongly associated with LA content in these oils, confirming the possible pathway of CLN formation from LA mono-hydroperoxides (Figure 16.1). Susceptibility of LA to oxidation is another important factor affecting CLN content. TAG containing LA oxidizes more rapidly with increasing LN content of TAG (Frankel, 1998a). LN is easily oxidized to form mono-hydroperoxides during the storage of crude oils even in a low temperature (Figure 16.3). The LN mono-hydroperoxides are susceptible to decomposition to produce free radicals, which initiate LA oxidation to produce LA mono-hydroperoxides. The LA mono-hydroperoxides are relatively stabler than LN mono-hyderoperoxides; therefore, the linoleate hydroperoxides can remain in the oil after de-gumming and neutralization, and produce CLN during bleaching (Figure 16.3). Though there was little difference in the content of LA between soyabean oil and corn oil, CLN level was higher in soyabean oil than in corn oil (Table 16.1). Soyabean oil contained 9.5% LN, while the content of corn oil was <1%. The higher level of CLN found in soyabean oil is attributed to the larger amount of LN in that oil. On the other hand, a little CLN was formed in canola oil, though the LN level of canola oil was relatively high (Table 16.1). This would be due to the lower content of LA of canola oil as CLN precursor and its relatively higher oxidative stability derived from high level of OA.

Soyabean oil tends to develop an undesirable flavour and odour known as reversion when peroxide value is still as low as a few meq/kg. This reversion flavour is characterized as beany and grassy, and is often found in the oil after light

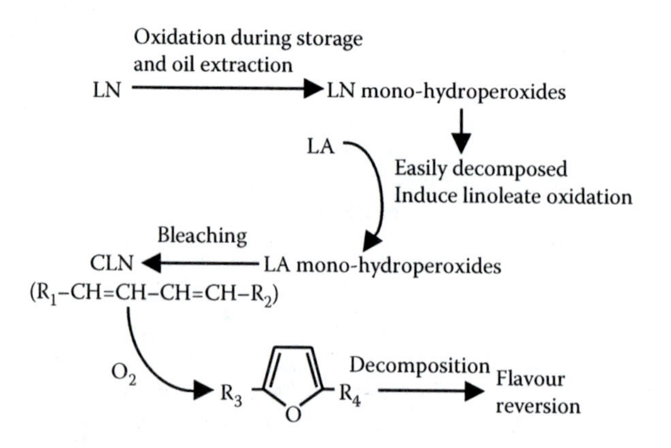

FIGURE 16.3 Possible flavour reversion mechanism from CLN.

irradiation at high temperature even though the peroxide value of the oil is very low. Though the reversion flavour can be detected in other vegetable oils, soyabean oil is the most remarkable oil showing the strong flavour reversion. Guth and Grosch (1991) reported the formation of a potent compound causing this flavour reversion as 3-methyl-2,4-nonanedione. The reversion flavour in soyabean oil is mainly due to furan compound such as 2-pentyl furan (Smouse and Chang, 1967) and 2-pentenyl furan (Ho et al., 1978; Smagula et al., 1979). Min et al. (Min et al., 2003; Cho and Min, 2006) show that these furan compounds are formed from the photooxidation of LA and LN in soyabean oil. The photooxidation is due to singlet oxygen that is produced from triplet oxygen in the presence of chlorophyll under light. On the other hand, conjugated fatty acids have also been considered as a possible source of furan fatty acids (Yurawecz et al., 1995) (Figure 16.3). The furan fatty acids are easily decomposed under the light irradiation to produce the intense flavour compounds (Guth and Grosch, 1991). These compounds such as 3-methyl-2,4-nonanedione shows a similar flavour to that of reversion. Further, a trace amount of CLN plays a vital role in accelerating lipid oxidation. CLN may be one of the important precursors for off-flavour compounds as CLN is easily oxidized in bulk phase (Suzuki et al., 2004).

The intensity of beany and grassy flavour of MCT with or without CLN containing TAG from bitter gourd oil was reported (Miyashita, 2008). Bitter oil TAG contained 9c,11t,13t-CLN (61.6%), 18:0 (25.7%) and OA (6.1%) (Suzuki et al., 2001; Narayan et al., 2006a). Little flavour was detected in MCT without bitter oil TAG after heating at 180°C under light (7000 lux) for 16 h. Beany and grassy flavours were detected in MCT by adding bitter gourd TAG, although the polyvinyl (PV) of the oil was <0.1. This result supports the above hypothesis that CLN will be one of the potent precursors responsible for flavour reversion. The flavour significance of soyabean oil with different amounts of CLN after heating under the light is reported (Miyashita, 2008), showing that flavour reversion was observed in the oil containing CLN, but a little in the oil with low CLN level.

CLN has three double bonds as same as LN. However, CLN is more easily oxidized than LN to produce polymers as the main oxidation products (Suzuki et al., 2004). This oxidation proceeds via free radical chain reaction and the radicals formed initiate the oxidation of PUFA in vegetable oils. Thus, CLN acts as an oxidation inducer as well as flavour reversion precursor. Canola oil contains relatively lower CLN as compared with other vegetable oils (Table 16.1), indicating that canola oil is stabler than oxidative and flavour deterioration.

16.6 CONCLUSION

Breeding developments led to the production of rapeseed low in both erucic acid in the oil and glucosinolates in the meal. There are the so-called double-low varieties. The reduction of erucic acid resulted in the increase in OA, giving a favourable fatty acid composition to canola oil. Canola oil has a good balance of omega-3 to omega-6 ratio and higher OA content. In terms of healthy nutrition, the higher ratio of omega-6/omega-3 PUFA found in Western diet is potentially dangerous. Increase in canola oil in the diet will reduce the risk. OA, the most abundant fatty acid in canola oil, is another contributor to the reduction of the risk of common chronic diseases. The high level of OA in canola oil is also contributing greatly to the improvement of its oxidative stability.

Frankel (1998b) noted the importance of oxidative polymers on the flavour or oxidative deterioration of vegetable oils. The spontaneous decomposition of oxidative polymers has been referred to as 'hidden oxidation' because it cannot be measured by peroxide value analysis. CLN has also no oxygenated functional group in its molecule, although it is formed from LA mono-hydroperoxides. CLN easily decomposes to produce low-molecular compounds which will have strong impact on flavour reversion. CLN cannot be removed from the oil during the refining process because of its similar behaviour to usual fatty acids. CLN content is dependent on LA mono-hydroperoxide level of oil before the bleaching process. CLN content in canola oil is, therefore, relatively low due to the low level of LA. On the other hand, the quality of commercial vegetable oil always depends on the quality of the crude oil used, the processing parameters, temperature and exposure to pro-oxidants such as air, light and heat during storage and processing. More LA mono-hydroperoxides form by inadequate conditions for storage of oil seed and crude oil. This is not exceptional for canola oil even though canola oil has a resistant fatty acid composition against oxidative deterioration and flavour reversion.

REFERENCES

Allayee, H.; Roth, N.; Hodis, H.N. Polyunsaturated fatty acids and cardiovascular disease: Implications for nutrigenetics. *J. Nutrigenet. Nutrigenomics* 2009, 2, 140–148.

Anderson, B.M.; Ma, D.W.L. Are all n-3 polyunsaturated fatty acids created equal? *Lipids Health Dis.* 2009, 8, 33.

Barre, D.E. The role of consumption of alpha-linolenic, eicosapentaenoic and docosahexaenoic acids in human metabolic syndrome and type 2 diabetes: A mini-review. *J. Oleo Sci.* 2007, 56, 319–325.

Belkind-Gerson, J.; Carreón-Rodríguez, A.; Contreras-Ochoa, C.O.; Estrada-Mondaca, S.; Parra-Cabrera M.S. Fatty acids and neurodevelopment. *J. Pediatr. Gastroentrol. Nutr.* 2008, 47, S7–S9.

Brenna, J.T.; Salem Jr., N.; Sinclair, A.J.; Cunnane, S.C. α-Linolenic acid supplementation and conversion to n-3 long-chain polyunsaturated fatty acids in humans. *Prostaglandins Leukot. Essent. Fatty Acids* 2009, 80, 85–91.

Calder, P.C. n-3 Fatty acids and cardiovascular disease: Evidence explained and mechanisms explored. *Clin. Sci.* 2004, 107, 1–11.

Carnielli, V.P.; Simonato, M.; Verlato, G.; Luijendijk, I.; De Curtis, M.; Sauer, P.J.J.; Cogo, P.E. Synthesis of long-chain polyunsaturated fatty acids in preterm newborns fed formula with long-chain polyunsaturated fatty acids. *Am. J. Clin. Nutr.* 2007, 86, 1323–1230.

Childs, C.E.; Romeu-Nadal, M.; Burdge, G.C.; Calder, P.C. Gender differences in the n-3 fatty acid content of tissues. *Proc. Nutr. Soc.* 2008, 67, 19–27.

Cho, E.; Min, D.B. Chemistry and reactions of reactive oxygen species in foods. *Crit. Rev. Food Sci. Nutr.* 2006, 46, 1–22.

Cho, S.-Y.; Miyashita, K.; Miyazawa, T.; Fujimoto, K.; Kaneda, T. Autoxidation of ethyl eicosapentaenoate and docosahexaenoate. *J. Am. Oil Chem. Soc.* 1987, 64, 876–879.

Cosgrove, J.P.; Church, D.F.; Pryor, W.A. The kinetics of the autoxidation of polyunsaturated fatty acids. *Lipids* 1987, 22, 299–304.

De Backer, G.; Ambrosioni, E.; Borch-Johnsen, K.; Brotons, C.; Cifkova, R.; Dallongeville, J.; Ebrahim, S. et al. European guidelines on cardiovascular disease prevention in clinical practice. Third joint task force of European and other societies on cardiovascular disease prevention in clinical practice. *Eur. Heart. J.* 2003, 24, 1601–1610.

Dolde, D.; Vlahakis, C.; Hazebroek, J. Tocopherols in breeding lines and effects of planting location, fatty acid composition, and temperature during development. *J. Am. Oil Chem. Soc.* 1999, 76, 349–355.

Fatemi, S.H.; Hammond, E.G. Analysis of oleate, linoleate, and linolenate hydroperoxides in oxidized ester mixtures. *Lipids* 1980, 15, 379–385.

Fishwick, M.J.; Swoboda, P.A.T. Measurement of oxidation of polyunsaturated fatty acids by spectrophotometric assay of conjugated derivatives. *J. Sci. Food Agric.* 1977, 28, 387–393.

Flowers, M.T.; Ntambi, J.M. Role of stearoyl-coenzyme A desaturase in regulating lipid metabolism. *Curr. Opin. Lipidol.* 2008, 19, 248–256.

Flowers, M.T.; Ntambi, J.M. Stearoyl-CoA desaturase and its relation to high-carbohydrate diets and obesity. *Biochim. Biophys. Acta* 2009, 1791, 85–91.

Frankel, E.N. *Lipid Oxidation*, The Oily Press: Dundee, Scotland, 1998a; pp. 13–77.

Frankel, E.N. *Lipid Oxidation*, The Oily Press: Dundee, Scotland, 1998b; pp. 115–127.

Frankel, E.N.; Huang, S.-W. Improving the oxidative stability of polyunsaturated vegetable oils by blending with high-oleic sunflower oil. *J. Am. Oil Chem. Soc.*, 1994, 71, 255–259.

Frankel, E.N.; Neff, W.E.; Miyashita, K. Autoxidation of polyunsaturated triacylglycerols. II. Trilinolenoylglycerol. *Lipids* 1990, 25:40–47.

Givens, D.I.; Gibbs, R.A. Current intakes of EPA and DHA in European populations and the potential of animal-derived foods to increase them. *Pro. Nutr. Soc.* 2008, 67, 273–280.

Goyens, P.L.; Spilker, M.E.; Zock, P.L.; Katan, M.B.; Mensink, R.P. Compartmental modeling to quantify alpha-linolenic acid conversion after longer term intake of multiple tracer boluses. *J. Lipid. Res.* 2005, 46, 1474–1483.

Guisto, N.M.; Salvador, G.A.; Castagnet, P.I.; Pasquare, S.J.; Ilincheta de Bschero, M.G. Age-associated changes in central nervous system glycerophospholipids composition and metabolism. *Neurochem. Res.* 2002, 27, 1513–1523.

Gunstone, F.D.; Harwood, J.L.; Dijkstra, A.J. *The lipid Handbook*, 3rd edn., CRC Press: New York, 2007; pp. 53–57.

Guth, H.; Grosch, W. Detection of furanoid fatty acids in soya-bean oil—Cause for the light-induced off-flavor. *Fat Sci. Technol.* 1991, 93, 249–255.

Harris, W.S.; Miller, M.; Tighe, A.P.; Davidson, M.H.; Schaefer, E.J. Omega-3 fatty acids and coronary heart disease risk: Clinical and mechanistic perspectives. *Atherosclerosis* 2008, 197, 12–24.

Ho, C.T.; Smagula, M.S.; Chang, S.S. The synthesis of 2-(1-pentenyl) furan and its relationship to the reversion flavor of soybean oil. *J. Am. Oil Chem. Soc.* 1978, 55, 233–237.

Hoffman, D.R.; Boettcher, J.A.; Diersen-Schade, D.A. Toward optimizing vision and cognition in term infants by dietary docosahexaenoic and arachidonic acid supplementation: A review of randomized controlled trials. *Prostaglandins Leukot. Essent. Fatty Acids* 2009, 81, 151–158.

Holman, R.T.; Elmer, O.C. The rates of oxidation of unsaturated fatty acids and esters. *J. Am. Oil Chem. Soc.* 1947, 24, 127–129.

Hu, F.B.; van Dam R.M.; Liu, S. Diet and risk of type 2 diabetes: The role of types of fat and carbohydrate. *Diabetologia* 2001, 44, 805–817.

Hulver, M.W.; Berggren, J.R.; Carper, M.J.; Miyazaki, M.; Ntambi, J.M.; Hoffman, E.P.; Thyfault, J.P. et al. Elevated stearoyl-CoA desaturase-1 expression in skeletal muscle contributes to abnormal fatty acid partitioning in obese humans. *Cell Metab.* 2005, 2, 251–261.

Hung, S.S.O.; Slinger, S.J. Studies of chemical methods for assessing oxidative quality and storage stability of feeding oils. *J. Am. Oil Chem. Soc.* 1981, 58, 785–788.

Hussein, N.; Ah-Sing, E.; Wilkinson, P.; Leach C.; Griffin B.A.; Millward D.J. Long-chain conversion of [13C] linoleic acid and alpha-linolenic acid in response to marked changes in their dietary intake in men. *J. Lipid. Res.* 2005, 46, 269–280.
Innis, S.M. Perinatal biochemistry and physiology of long chain polyunsaturated fatty acids. *J. Pediatr.* 2003, 143, S1–S8.
Innis, S.M. Dietary omega 3 fatty acids and the developing brain. *Brain Res.* 2008, 1237, 35–43.
Innis, S.M.; Jacobson, K. Dietary lipids in early development and intestinal inflammatory disease. *Nutr. Rev.* 2007, 65, 5188–5189.
Jump, D. Fatty acid regulation of gene transcription. *Crit. Rev. Clin. Lab. Sci.* 2004, 41, 41–78.
Kakuma, T.; Lee, Y.; Unger, R.H. Effects of leptin, troglitazone, and dietary fat on stearoyl CoA desaturase. *Biochem. Biophys. Res. Commun.* 2002, 297, 1259–1263.
Kamal-Eldin, A.; Mäkinen, M.; Lampi, A.-M. The challenging contribution of hydroperoxides to the lipid oxidation mechanism. *Lipid Oxidation Pathways*, Kamal-Eldin, A., Ed.; AOCS Press: Champaign, Illinois, USA, 2003; pp. 1–36.
Kien, C.L. Dietary interventions for metabolic syndrome: Role of modifying dietary fats. *Curr. Diab. Rep.* 2009, 9, 43–50.
Kinami, T. Analysis of conjugated fatty acids in edible oils, Master thesis, 2003, Hokkaido University, Hakodate, Japan.
Kinami, T.; Horii, N.; Narayan, B.; Arato, S.; Hosokawa, M.; Miyashita, K.; Negishi, H.; Ikuina, J.; Noda, R.; Shirasawa, S. Occurrence of conjugated linolenic acids in purified soybean oil. *J. Am. Oil Chem. Soc.* 2007, 84, 23–29.
Kodali, D.R. Oxidative stability measurement of high-stability oils by pressure differential scanning calorimeter (PDSC). *J. Agric. Food Chem.* 2005, 53, 7649–7653.
Kris-Etherton, P.M.; Harris, W.S.; Appel, L.J. Fish consumption, fish oil, omega-3 fatty acids and cardiovascular disease. *Circulation* 2002, 106, 2747–2757.
Kris-Etherton, P.M.; Taylor, D.S.; Yu-Poth, S.; Huth, P.; Moriarty, K.; Fishell, V.; Hargrove R.L.; Zhao G.; Etherton T.D. Polyunsaturated fatty acids in the food chain in the United States. *Am. J. Clin. Nutr.* 2000, 71, S179–S188.
Lands, W.E.M. *Fish, Omega-3 and Human Health*, 2nd Edn., AOCS Press: Champaign, IL, 2005; pp. 3–160.
Le, H.D.; Meisel, J.A.; de Meijer, V.E.; Gura, K.M.; Puder, M. The essentiality of arachidonic acid and docosahexaenoic acid. *Prostaglandins Leukot. Essent. Fatty Acids* 2009, 81, 165–170.
Leaf, A.; Kang, J.X.; Xiao, Y.-F. Fish oil fatty acids as cardiovascular drugs. *Curr. Vasc. Pharmacol.* 2008, 6, 1–12.
Li, D.; Bode, O.; Drummond, H.; Sinclair, A.J. Omega-3 (n-3) fatty acids. *Lipids for Functional Foods and Nutraceuticals*, Gunstone, F.D., Ed.; The Oily Press: Bridgwater, England, 2003; pp. 225–262.
Liu, X.; Miyazaki, M.; Flowers, M.T.; Sampath, H.; Zhao, M.; Chu, K.; Paton, C.M.; Joo, D.S.; Ntambi, J.M. Loss of stearoyl-CoA desaturase-1 attenuates adipocyte inflammation effects of adipocyte-derived oleate. *Arterioscler. Thromb. Vasc. Biol.* 2010, 30, 31–38.
Liu, H.R.; White, P.J. Oxidative stability of soybean oils with altered fatty acid compositions. *J. Am. Oil Chem. Soc.* 1992a, 69, 528–532.
Liu, H.R.; White, P.J. Oxidative stability of soybean oils with altered fatty acid compositions. *J. Am. Oil Chem. Soc.*, 1992b, 69, 533–537.
Lusso, G.L. Dietary n-6 and n-3 polyunsaturated fatty acids: From biochemistry to clinical implications in cardiovascular prevention. *Biochem. Pharmacol.* 2009, 77, 937–946.
Min, D.B.; Callison, A.L.; Lee, H.O. Singlet oxygen oxidation for 2-pentylfuran and 2-pentenylfuran formation in soybean oil. *J. Food Sci.* 2003, 68, 1175–1178.
Miyashita, K. Oxidation of long-chain fatty acids. *Lipid Oxidation Pathways*, Kamal-Eldin, A.; Min, D., Eds.; AOCS Press: Champaign, IL, 2008; pp. 54–78.

Miyashita, K.; Frankel, E.N.; Neff, W.E.; Awl, R.A. Autoxidation of polyunsaturated triacylglycerols. III. Synthetic triacylglycerols containing linoleate and linolenate. *Lipids* 1990, 25, 48–53.

Miyashita, K.; Takagi, T. Study on the oxidative rate and prooxidant activity of free fatty acids. *J. Am. Oil Chem. Soc.* 1986, 63, 1380–1384.

Miyazaki, M.; Kim, Y.-C.; Gray-Keller, M.P.; Attie, A.D.; Ntambi, J.M. The biosynthesis of hepatic cholesterol esters and triglycerides is impaired in mice with a disruption of the gene for stearoyl-CoA desaturase 1. *J. Biol. Chem.* 2000, 275, 30132–30138.

Muoio, D.M.; Newgard, C.B. Obesity-related derangements in metabolic regulation. *Annu. Rev. Biochem.* 2006, 75, 367–401.

Narayan, B.; Hosokawa, M.; Miyashita, K. Occurrence of conjugated fatty acids in aquatic and terrestrial plants and their physiological effects. *Nutraceutical and Specialty Lipids and Their Co-Products*, Shahidi, F., Ed.; CRC Taylor & Francis: NY, 2006a; pp. 201–218.

Narayan, B.; Miyashita, K.; Hosokawa, M. Physiological effects of eicosapentaenoic acid (EPA) and docosahexaenoic acid (DHA)—A review. *Food Rev. Inter.* 2006b, 22, 291–307.

Neff, W.E.; Frankel, E.N.; Miyashita, K. Autoxidation of polyunsaturated triacylglycerols. I. Trilinoleoylglycerol. *Lipids* 1990, 25, 33–39.

Neff, W.E.; Selke, E.; Mounts, T.L.; Rinsch, W.; Frankel, E.N.; Zeitoun, M.A.M. Effect of triacylglycerol composition and structures on oxidative stability of oils from selected soybean germplasm. *J. Am. Oil Chem. Soc.* 1992, 69, 111–118.

Ntambi, J.M.; Miyazaki, M.; Stoehr, J.P.; Lan, H.; Kendziorski, C.M.; Yandell, B.S.; Song, Y.; Cohen, P.; Friedman, J.M.; Attie, D. Loss of stearoyl-CoA desaturase-1 function protects mice against adiposity. *Proc. Natl. Acad. Sci. USA* 2002, 99, 11482–11486.

Ntambi, J.M.; Miyazaki, M. Regulation of stearoyl-CoA desaturases and role in metabolism. *Prog. Lipid. Res.* 2004, 43, 91–104.

Nguyen, M.T.A.; Favelyukis, S.; Nguyen, A.-K.; Reichart, D.; Scott, P.A.; Jenn, A.; Liu-Bryan, R.; Glass, C.K.; Neels, J.G.; Olefsky, J.M. A subpopulation of macrophages infiltrates hypertrophic adipose tissue and is activated by free fatty acids via toll-like receptors 2 and 4 and JNK-dependent pathways. *J. Biol. Chem.* 2007, 282, 35279–35292.

Novak, E.; Dyer, R.A.; Innis, S.M. High dietary omega-6 fatty acids contribute to reduced docosahexaenoic acid in the developing brain and inhibit secondary neurite growth. *Brain Res.* 2008, 1237, 136–145.

Parr, L.J.; Swoboda, P.A.T. The assay of conjugable oxidation products applied to lipid deterioration in stored foods. *J. Food Technol.* 1976, 11, 1–12.

Paton, C.M.; Ntambi, J.M. Biochemical and physiological function of stearoyl-CoA desaturase. *Am. J. Physiol. Endocrinol. Metab.* 2008, 297, E28–E37.

Porter, N.A.; Caldwell, S.E.; Mills, K.A. Mechanisms of free radical oxidation of unsaturated lipids. *Lipids* 1995, 30, 277–290.

Ratnayake, W.M.N.; Daun, J.K. Chemical composition of canola and rapeseed oils. *Rapeseed and Canola Oil—Production, Processing, Properties and Uses*, Gunstone, F.D., Ed.; Blackwell Publishing: Oxford, 2004; pp. 37–78.

Russo, G.L. Dietary n-6 and n-3 polyunsaturated fatty acids: From biochemistry to clinical implications in cardiovascularprevention. *Biochem. Pharmacol.* 2009, 77, 937–946.

Russo, G.L. Dietary n-6 and n-3 polyunsaturated fatty acids: From biochemistry to clinical implications in cardiovascularprevention. *Biochem. Pharmacol.* 2010, 235, 785–795.

Sampath, H.; Miyazaki, M.; Dobrzyn, A.; Ntambi, J.M. Stearoyl-CoA desaturase-1 mediates the pro-lipogenic effects of dietary saturated fat. *J. Biol. Chem.* 2007, 282, 2483–2493.

Sampath, H.; Ntambi, J. Polyunsaturated fatty acid regulation of gene expression. *Nutr. Rev.* 2004, 62, 333–339.

Sampath, H.; Ntambi, J.M. Polyunsaturated fatty acid regulation of genes of lipid metabolism. *Annu. Rev. Nutr.* 2005, 25, 317–340.

Sanders, T.A. Polyunsaturated fatty acids in the food chain in Europe. *Am. J. Clin. Nutr.* 2000, 71, 176S–8S.

Shahidi, F.; Miraliakbari, H. Marine oils: Compositional characteristics and health effects. *Nutraceutical and Specialty Lipids and Their Co-Products*, Shahidi, F., Ed.; CRC Press: New York, 2006; pp. 227–250.

Shen, N.; Moizuddin, S.; Wilson, L.; Duvick, S.; White, P.; Pollak, L. Relationship of electronic nose analyses and sensory evaluation of vegetable oils during storage. *J. Am. Oil Chem. Soc.* 2001, 78, 937–940.

Simopoulos, A.P. The importance of the omega-6/omega-3 fatty acid ratio in cardiovascular disease and other chronic diseases. *Exp. Biol. Med.* 2008, 233, 674–688.

Simopoulos, A.P. Genetic variants in the metabolism of omega-6 and omega-3 fatty acids: Their role in the determination of nutritional requirements and chronic disease risk. *Exp. Biol. Med.* 2010, 235, 785–795.

Sinclair, A.; Wallace, J.; Martin, M.; Attar-Bashi, N.; Weisinger, R.; Li, D. The effects of eicosapentaenoic acid in various clinical conditions. *Healthful Lipids*, Akoh, C.C.; Lai, O.-M. Eds.; AOCS Press: Champaign, IL, 2005; pp. 361–394.

Smagula, M.S.; Ho, C.; Chang, S.S. The synthesis of 2-(2-pentenyl) furans and their relationship to the reversion flavor of soybean oil. *J. Am. Oil Chem. Soc.* 1979, 56, 516–519.

Smith, Jr, S.C.; Allen, J.; Blair, S.N.; Bonow, R.O.; Brass, L.M.; Fonarow, G.C.; Grundy, S.M. et al. AHA/ACC guidelines for secondary prevention for patients with coronary and other atherosclerotic vascular disease: 2006 update: Endorsed by the National Heart, Lung and Blood Institute. *Circulation* 2006, 113, 2363–2372.

Smouse, T.H.; Chang, S.S. A systematic characterization of the reversion flavor of soybean oil. *J. Am. Oil Chem. Soc.* 1967, 44, 509–514.

Soriguer, F.; Esteva, I.; Rojo-Martínez, G.; Ruiz de Adana, M.S.; Dobarganes, M.C.; García-Almeida, J.M.; Tinahones, F.; et al. Monounsaturated fatty acids from cooking oils are associated with lower insulin resistance in the general population (Pizarra study). *Eur. J. Endocrinol.* 2004, 150, 33–39.

Soriguer, F.; Moreno, F.; Rojo-Martinez, G.; García-Fuentes, E.; Tinahones, F.; Gómez-Zumaquero, J.M.; Cuesta-Muñoz, A.L.; Cardona, F.; Morcillo, S. Monounsaturated n-9 fatty acids and adipocyte lipolysis in rats. *Br. J. Nutr.* 2003a, 90, 1015–1022.

Soriguer, F.; Moreno, F.; Rojo-Martínez, G.; Cardona, F.; Francisco Tinahones, F.; Gómez-Zumaquero, J.M.; García-Fuentes, E.; Morcillo, S. Redistribution of abdominal fat after a period of food restriction in rats is related to the type of dietary fat. *Br. J. Nutr.* 2003b, 89, 115–122.

Soriguer, F.; Rojo-Martínez, G.; de Fonseca, F.R.; García-Escobar, E.; Fuentes, E.G.; Olveira, G. Obesity and the metabolic syndrome in Mediterranean countries: A hypothesis related to olive oil. *Mol. Nutr. Food Res.* 2007, 51, 1260–1267.

Suganami, T.; Nishida, J.; Ogawa, Y. A paracrine loop between adipocytes and macrophages aggravates inflammatory changes: Role of free fatty acids and tumor necrosis factor α. *Arterioscler. Thromb. Vasc. Biol.* 2005, 25, 2062–2068.

Suzuki, R.; Abe, M.; Miyashita, K. Comparative study of the autoxidation of TAG containing conjugated and nonconnugated C_{18} PUFA. *J. Am. Oil Chem. Soc.* 2004, 81, 563–569.

Suzuki, R.; Noguchi, R.; Ota, T.; Abe, M.; Miyashita, K.; Kawada, T. Cytotoxic effect of conjugated trienoic fatty acids on mouse tumor and human monocytic leukemia cells. *Lipids* 2001, 36, 477–482.

Takagi, T.; Ando, Y. Stereospecific analysis of triscy-*sn*-glycerols by chiral high-performance liquid chromatography. *Lipids* 1991, 26, 542–547.

Tziomalos, K.; Athyros, V.G.; Karagiannis, A.; Mikhailidis, D.P. Omega-3 fatty acids: How can they be used in secondary prevention? *Curr. Atheroscler. Rep.* 2008, 10, 510–517.

Van Den Bosch, G. Bleaching of vegetable oils: I. Conversions in soybean oil, triolein and trilinolein. *J. Am. Oil Chem. Soc.* 1973a, 50, 421–423.

Van Den Bosch, G. Bleaching of vegetable oils: I. Conversions in soybean oil, triolein and trilinolein. *J. Am. Oil Chem. Soc.* 1973b, 50, 487–493.

Vassiliou, E.K.; Gonzalez, A.; Garcia, C.; Tadros, J.H.; Chakraborty, G.; Toney, J.H. Oleic acid and peanut oil high in oleic acid reverse the inhibitory effect of insulin production of the inflammatory cytokine TNF-α both *in vitro* and *in vivo* systems. *Lipids Health Dis.* 2009, 8, 25.

Vessby, B.; Unsitupa, M.; Hermansen, K.; Riccardi, G.; Rivellese, A.A.; Tapsell, L.C.; Nälsén, C. et al. Substituting dietary saturated for monounsaturated fat impairs insulin sensitivity in healthy men and women: The KANWU study. *Diabetologia* 2001, 44, 312–319.

Vlahakis, C.; Hazebroek, J. Phytosterol accumulation in canola, sunflower and soybean oils: Effects of genetics, planting location, and temperature. *J. Am. Oil Chem. Soc.* 2000, 77, 49–53.

Wang, C; Harris, W.S.; Chung, M.; Lichtenstein, A.H.; Balk, E.M.; Kupelnick, B.; Jordan, H.S.; Lau, J. Fatty acids from fish or fish-oil supplements, but not alpha-linolenic acid, benefit cardiovascular disease outcomes in primary- and secondary prevention studies: A systematic review. *Am. J. Clin. Nutr.* 2006, 84, 5–17.

Weisburger, J.H. Eat to live, not live to eat. *Nutrition* 2000, 16, 767–773.

Yurawecz, M.P.; Hood, J.K.; Mossoba, M.M.; Roach, J.A.G.; Ku, Y. Furan fatty acids determined as oxidation products of conjugated octadecadienoic acid. *Lipids* 1995, 30, 595–598.

Yurawecz, M.P.; Molina, A.A.; Mossoba, M.; Ku, Y. Estimation of conjugated octadecatrienes in edible fats and oils. *J. Am. Oil Chem. Soc.* 1993, 70, 1093–1099.

17 Effect of Canolol on Oxidation of Edible Oils

Bertrand Matthäus

CONTENTS

17.1 Introduction 317
17.2 Determination of Canolol 319
17.3 Formation of Canolol during Heating of Canola Seeds 320
17.4 Formation of Canolol during Pressing 321
17.5 Virgin Canola Oils from the Market 322
17.6 Oxidative Stability as a Function of the Canolol Content 323
17.7 Antioxidant Activity of Canolol 324
17.8 Effect of Canolol during Storage of Canola Oil 326
17.9 Conclusions 327
References 327

17.1 INTRODUCTION

Canola oil is one of the most important vegetable oils in the world after palm oil and soyabean oil and is ranked third in world production. The fatty acid composition of the oil is characterized by a high content of oleic acid of about 60% and a moderate content of α-linolenic acid of about 10%. The relative high content of α-linolenic acid and the ratio between ω-6 and ω-3 fatty acids of 2:1 makes canola oil attractive oil nutritionally. In addition to the fatty acids, canola oil is relatively rich in tocopherols and phytosterols, which are important to health, but also improve the oxidative stability of vegetable oils. In comparison with other major oilseeds, canola seeds also contain comparatively high amounts of phenolic compounds (Naczk et al., 1998). However, during oil extraction with a screw press or expeller, in the absence of solvent extraction, only a few of the phenolic compounds go into the oil with the main part remaining in the press cake (Vuorela et al., 2003). Virgin extra olive oil is a particularly important cold-pressed oil. It has a high content of phenolic compounds that significantly improve the oxidative stability of this type of oil (Figure 17.1).

While the main phenolic compounds of olive oil, hydroxytyrosol and oleuropein, give the oil its bitter and pungent taste, the major phenolic compounds in canola seeds are esterified phenolic acids. The main component of the latter is sinapine, the choline-ester of sinapic acid (3,5-dimethoxy-4-hydroxycinnamic acid) (Krygier et al., 1982). Some free phenolic compounds of about 15% are also present with

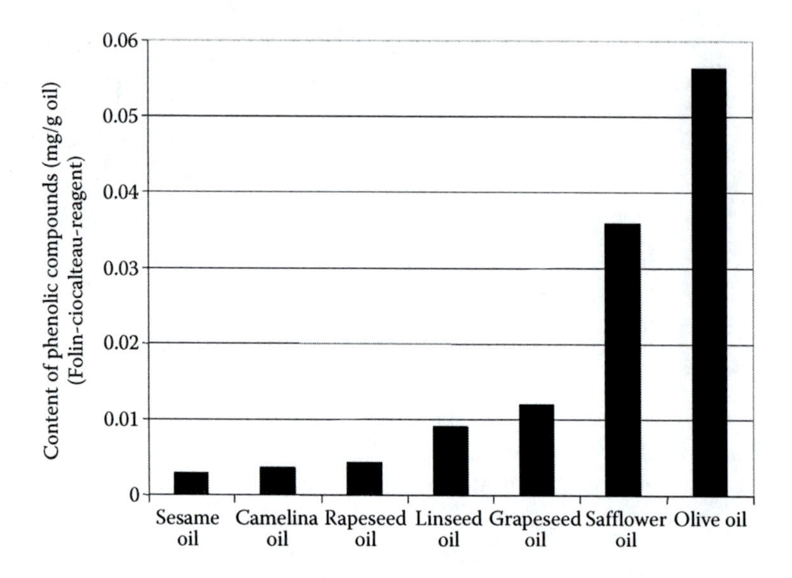

FIGURE 17.1 Content of phenolic compounds in different virgin vegetable oils.

sinapic acid as the major compound of this group (Shahidi and Naczk, 1992; Thiyam et al., 2006). Choline is an important metabolite in the methylation cycle (Byerrum and Wing, 1953), while sinapic acid is necessary for the formation of lignin and flavonoids (Neish, 1960). Artz et al. (1986) showed that phenolic compounds are mainly located in the cotyledons and only trace amounts are found in the seed coats. Similar results were reported by Matthäus (1998) for the distribution of sinapine in canola seeds.

More recently, another derivative of sinapic acid has been identified because of its highly potent antioxidant activity and the antimutagenic and anticarcinogenic properties (Kuwahara et al., 2004; Vuorela et al., 2005; Cao et al., 2008). This derivative, 2,6-dimethoxy-4-vinylphenol (vinylsyringol) or canolol, was first identified in two independent studies by Koski et al. (2003) and Wakamatsu et al. (2005) in crude canola oil. Kuwahara et al. (2004) described the antimutagenic potency of this compound as higher than α-tocopherol, β-carotene, vitamin C

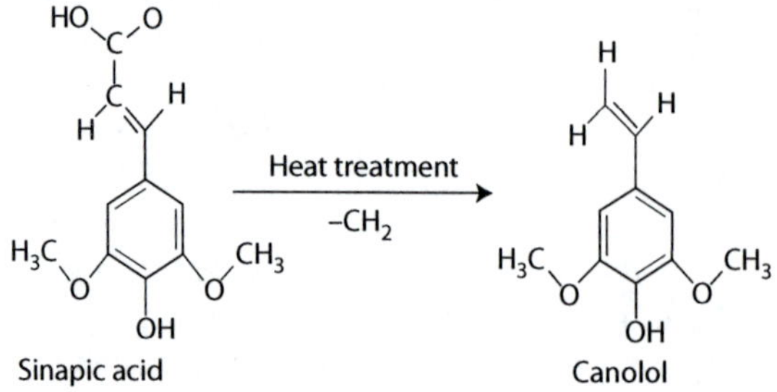

FIGURE 17.2 Formation of canolol.

and different flavonoids such as rutin or quercetin. The compound is formed by decarboxylation of sinapic acid during heating of canola seeds (Figure 17.2). High amounts of canolol can be found in cold-pressed canola oil from roasted seeds or in crude canola oil from big oil processing facilities resulting from the heat treatment during processing (Vuorela et al., 2003; Koski et al., 2003; Wakamatsu et al., 2005).

17.2 DETERMINATION OF CANOLOL

Different methods for the determination of canolol are available (Vuorela et al., 2003; Spielmeyer et al., 2009) based on the extraction of the phenolic compounds by methanol/water and their determination by HPLC with UV-detection. Since canolol shows a good solubility in non-polar solvents like petroleum ether or *n*-hexane, it is possible to determine the compound in canola oil together with the tocopherols according to the method of Balz et al. (1992). 10 mg oil were dissolved in 1 mL *n*-heptane containing 4.85 μg 2,2,5,7,8 pentamethyl-6-chromanol/mL as internal standard. The HPLC analysis was conducted using Merck-Hitachi low-pressure-gradient system, fitted with L-6000 pump, Merck-Hitachi F-1000 Fluorescence Spectrophotometer (detector wavelengths for excitation 295 nm, for emission 330 nm) and Chromgate integration system (Knauer, Berlin, Germany). A volume of 20 μL of the samples was injected by Spark Holland Basic Marathon Autosampler onto a Diol phase HPLC column 25 cm × 4.6 mm ID (Merck, Darmstadt, Germany) at a flow rate of 1.3 mL/min. The mobile phase used was *n*-heptane/tert. butyl methyl ether (99 + 1, v/v). Quantification of canolol was possible using the internal standard with the results expressed as microgram canolol per gram canola seed or canola oil. Figure 17.3 shows a typical HPLC chromatogram of canola oil from unroasted seeds.

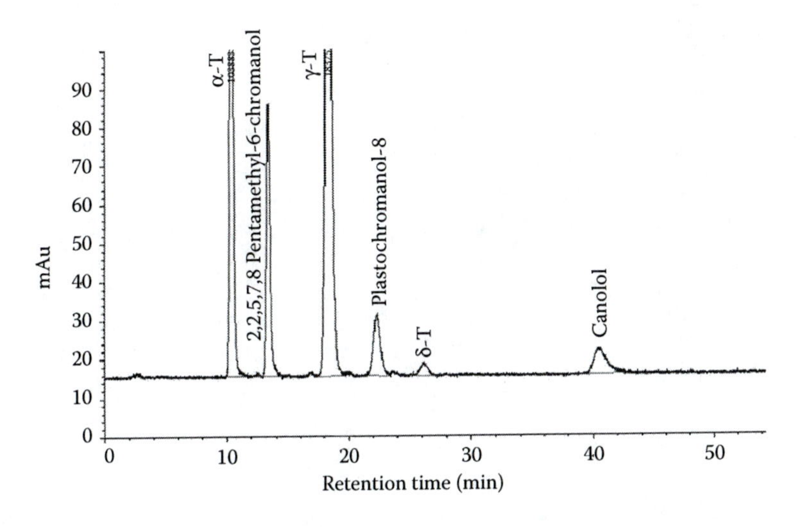

FIGURE 17.3 HPLC chromatogram of virgin canola oil from unroasted seeds.

17.3 FORMATION OF CANOLOL DURING HEATING OF CANOLA SEEDS

While cold-pressed pumpkin seed oil and sesame oil is produced from roasted raw material to form the typical flavour, the production of cold-pressed canola oil from roasted seeds is rather unusual. Koski et al. (2003) and Wakamatsu et al. (2005) both found that canolol is formed during heating of canola seeds by decarboxylation of sinapic acid. This additional production step could be an interesting way to improve the oil quality from a health perspective as well enhance oxidative stability. Figure 17.4 shows the effect of heating on the formation of canolol in the resulting canola oil as a function of the temperature. With increasing temperature, the content of canolol in the oil increases, whereas roasting temperatures between no additional heating and 180°C resulted only in a slow increase of the canolol content in the oil (110–360 µg/g oil). At higher roasting temperature, however, the content of canolol increased and at a temperature of 240°C the canolol content in the oil was about 3230 µg/g oil. This is about 100 times higher than the average content of oil from unroasted canola seeds. The experiment showed that a minimum temperature of 180°C is necessary to form canolol in canola seeds in higher amounts. This observation was consistent with that reported by Spielmeyer et al. (2009), who found a temperature of at least 160°C was required for the fast formation of canolol during roasting. The authors also found a reduction in the content of canolol at higher temperature resulted from the reaction of canolol with other constituents of canola seeds, such as lipid hydroperoxides formed during heating. In addition, degradation of canolol by pyrolysis or thermal decomposition is also possible (Spielmeyer et al., 2009). Similar effects were found for red grape pomace peels which lost antioxidant activity and phenolic compounds by heating at temperatures of 100°C or 140°C (Larrauri et al., 1997). During roasting at higher temperatures, it has to be taken into consideration that in addition to the formation of canolol with roasting time the flavour of

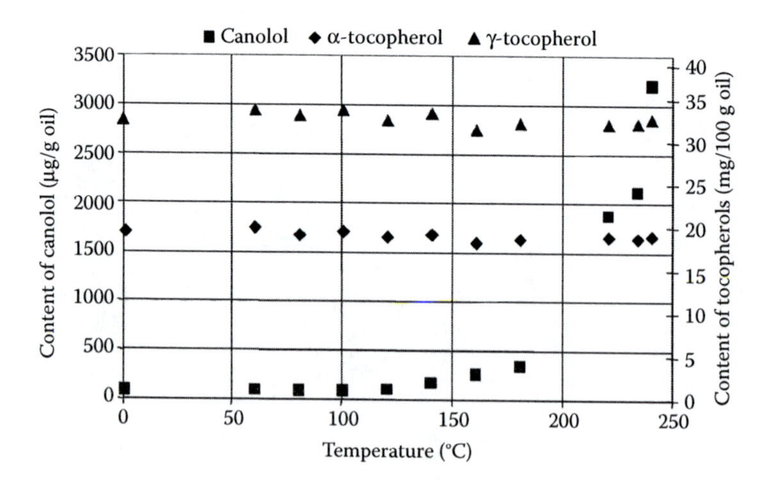

FIGURE 17.4 Influence of temperature during roasting on formation of canolol and content of tocopherols.

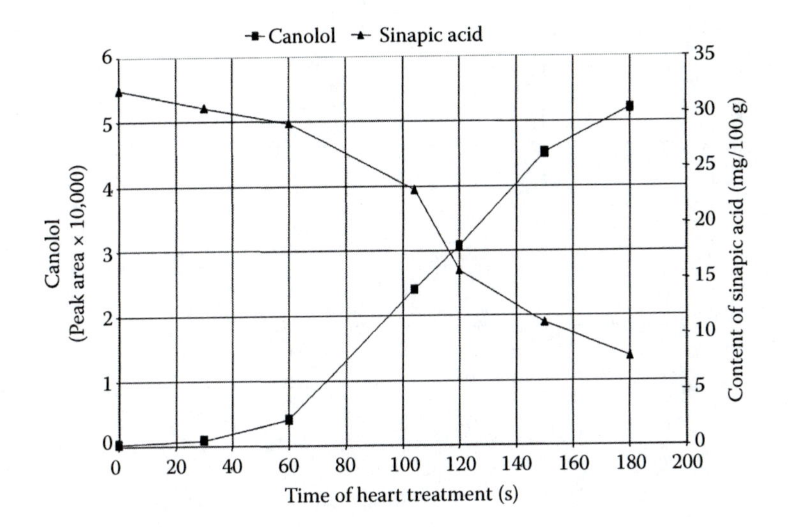

FIGURE 17.5 Influence of heat treatment during roasting on the degradation of sinapic acid and formation of canolol.

the raw material and also of the resulting oil changes remarkably from seed-like and nutty via roasty to burnt and bitter. Under these conditions, the oil was also reported to acquire a darker colour (Thiyam et al., 2001). Therefore, it is necessary to find the critical balance between attaining a high content of canolol and retaining a slightly roasted taste and smell in the resulting canola oil.

Examination of the effect of temperature on the content and composition of tocopherols showed that both were unaffected by the heating process. Irrespective of the temperature used for roasting, the content and the composition of tocopherols in the resulting canola oil remained unchanged. Wakamatsu et al. (2005) and Spielmeyer et al. (2009) both found no significant differences in the tocopherol content of canola oil from unroasted and roasted raw material. It is possible that canolol acts as antioxidant protecting the tocopherols from degradation during the heating process.

The pathway for the formation of canolol is the decarboxylation of sinapic acid during heating of canola seeds. Figure 17.5 shows that heating of canola seeds in a microwave oven at 650 W resulted in the formation of canolol with simultaneous degradation of sinapic acid. While in the first 60 s of heat treatment, only a slight increase of canolol took place, afterwards the formation of canolol increased very rapidly. The reason is that the heat transfer through the hulls of the canola seeds took some time, resulting in a slower increase of the formation of canolol. During the formation of canolol, the content of sinapic acid decreased from about 30 mg/100 g canola seed to about 7 mg/100 g after 200 s of heating.

17.4 FORMATION OF CANOLOL DURING PRESSING

The main part of edible canola oil is produced in big facilities by the screw press, which reduces the oil content to about 20%. This is then followed by solvent

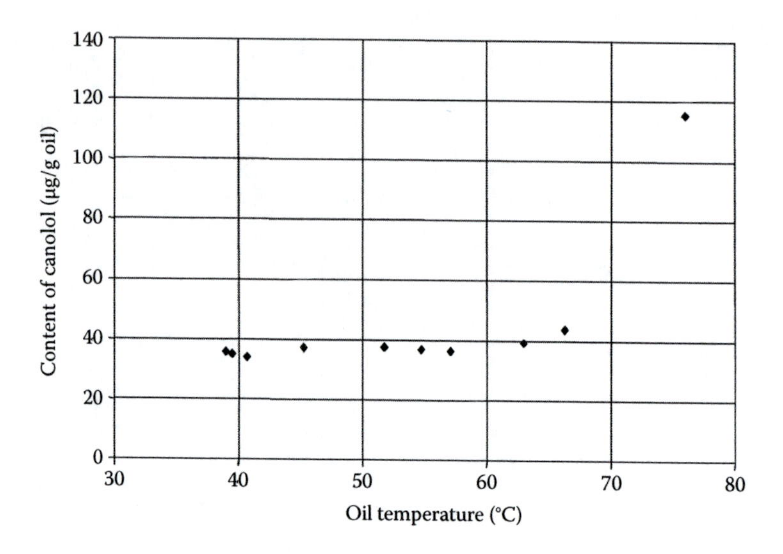

FIGURE 17.6 Correlation between oil temperature during pressing and formation of canolol.

extraction of the press cake. For the production of virgin canola oil, only a screw press is used for the extraction of the oil from the seeds so that between 8% and 15% oil remains in the press cake. The use of high temperature during pressing results in a higher oil yield, which improves the pressing process from an economical point of view.

During cold-press processing, heating of the press head is not allowed. However, the pressing itself causes a rise in temperature so that the raw material within the screw press heats up. Depending on the type of screw press and the residence time of the raw material in the screw press, oil temperatures between 35°C and 60°C can be measured. For higher oil temperatures, an additional external heating source for the press head is necessary. Figure 17.6 shows that during the pressing process, the content of canolol in the resulting oil was not a function of the oil flow temperature over a wide range. The content of canolol in the resulting oil only increases remarkable if the oil temperature reached 75°C or higher by means of an external heating source. This shows that normal pressing conditions during the cold-press process do not result in significant higher contents of canolol in canola oil. Only the use of an external heating source for the press head leads to a sufficient heat transfer from the press head to the raw material which increases the formation of canolol.

17.5 VIRGIN CANOLA OILS FROM THE MARKET

For the production of virgin canola oil, the application of heat during the whole processing chain from the pre-treatment of the raw material to the pressing is not allowed. Thus, the requirements for the formation of canolol in the raw material are not given.

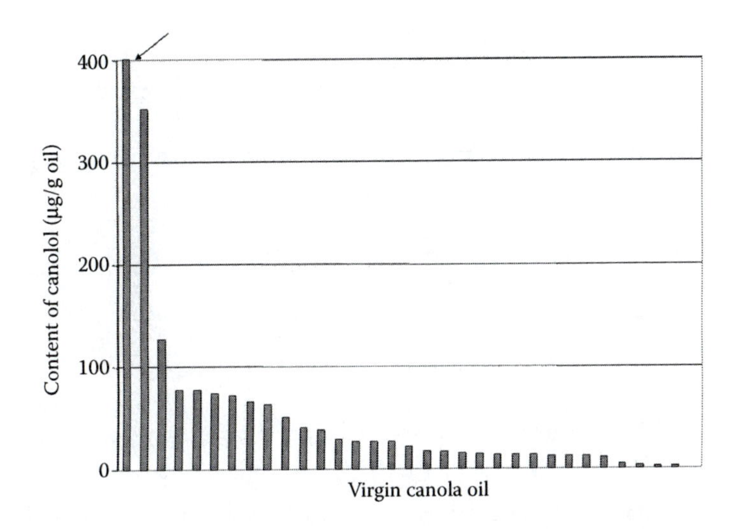

FIGURE 17.7 Canolol content of virgin canola oils from the German market.

Figure 17.7 shows the content of canolol in different canola oils based on a market survey. In most oils, the content of canolol remains clearly below 100 μg/g oil, while some oils showed a remarkable high content of canolol. The mean content of canolol in virgin canola oil was about 30 μg/g. The high contents of canolol in two of the samples raise the question whether these samples were really cold-pressed virgin canola oils. The results of the other experiments showed that higher amounts of canolol in canola oil are always the result of heat-treatment of the raw material. A high content of canolol in canola oil is probably a good indicator for the differentiating between canola oils from heated and unheated raw materials.

In contrast with tocopherols or phytosterols, canolol is completely removed during the refining process (Zacchi and Eggers, 2008; Spielmeyer et al., 2009). Thus, no canolol can be found in refined canola oils, although during processing in big oil mills with conditioning of the raw material by heat and extraction at higher temperatures with the solvent, higher amounts of canolol pass over into the crude oil. Using the Rancimat test at 110°C, Zacchi and Eggers (2008) found crude canola oil with higher amounts of canolol showed remarkably higher oxidative stability compared with completely refined canola oil.

17.6 OXIDATIVE STABILITY AS A FUNCTION OF THE CANOLOL CONTENT

In the literature, canolol is described as an effective antioxidant (Koski et al., 2003; Kuwahara et al., 2004; Vuorela et al., 2005; Wakamatsu et al., 2005). Figure 17.8 shows increased oxidative stability of canola oil accompanied increasing amounts of canolol. Using the Rancimat test at 120°C canolol contents below 200 μg/g in canola oil from roasted seeds resulted in slight decrease of the oxidative stability. In contrast, amounts of canolol higher than 200 μg/g improved oxidative stability of the oil dramatically. Wijesundera et al. (2008) also showed an improvement in

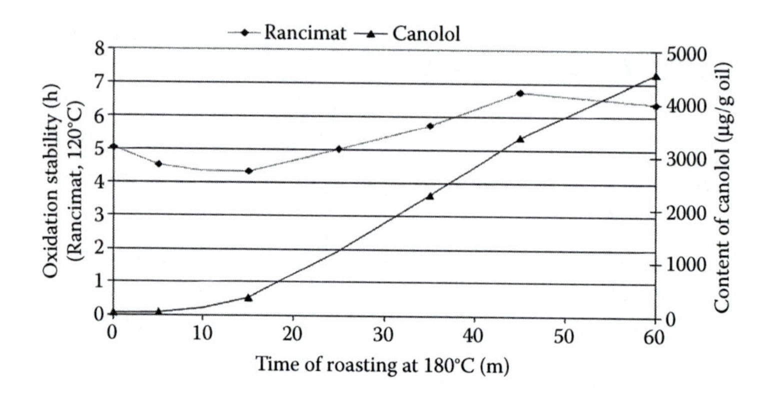

FIGURE 17.8 Formation of canolol during roasting of canola seeds and its effect on the oxidation stability of the resulting oil in the Rancimat test at 120°C.

the oxidative stability of virgin canola oil by roasting the raw material before oil extraction (165°C, 5 min). The roasting process did not change either the fatty acid composition or the content and the composition of tocopherols. They ascribed this effect to the presence of canolol formed during roasting by the decarboxylation of sinapic acid.

At higher contents of canolol in the oil, a good correlation with the oxidation stability using the Rancimat test was found. If the temperature load was <15 min at 180°C, a decrease in the oxidation stability was observed due to the low formation of canolol. With increasing temperature load, the oxidation stability increased from 4 to 7 h, before the oxidation stability decreased again as a result of a temperature load of more than 45 min at 180°C. At a low temperature load, less canolol is formed so that the temperature is sufficient to impair the oxidation stability of the oil. Only when the content of canolol in the oil from roasted seeds increases does oxidative stability improve. If the temperature load is too high, the impairment of the oil is faster, then the formation of canolol can improve the oxidation stability.

17.7 ANTIOXIDANT ACTIVITY OF CANOLOL

To assess the antioxidant activity of canolol, it is necessary to isolate canolol from canola oil by extraction from roasted seeds. For the extraction, about 50 g of oil was diluted with 200 mL mixture composed of ethylacetate/cyclohexane (1:1). From this solution, 7 mL was used for purification by gel permeation chromatography (GPC). The purity of the extract was established by HPLC with recalculation of the used amount of extract. From 1.5 g oil, 3 mg purified extract was obtained.

For the assessment of the antioxidant activity of canolol, the β-carotene–linoleic acid assay as well as the DPPH method was used. Using the β-carotene–linoleic acid assay model system, rapid discolouration was observed in the absence of an antioxidant. The free linoleic acid radical, formed by abstraction of a hydrogen atom from one of its methylene groups, attacks the β-carotene molecules resulting in the loss of double bonds and its characteristic orange colour. The rate of bleaching of the β-carotene solution was determined by measuring the difference between the initial reading in spectral absorbance at 470 nm initially at time 0 min and after 120 min. The determination of the antioxidant activity using a β-carotene/linoleic acid system was carried out according to the method described by Taga et al. (1984). Briefly, 40 mg of linoleic acid and 400 mg Tween 20 were transferred into a flask to which was added 1 mL of a solution of β-carotene (3.34 mg/mL) in chloroform. The chloroform was removed by rotary evaporation at 40°C. Then 100 mL of distilled water was added slowly to the residue and the solution vigorously shaken to form a stable emulsion. To an aliquot of 5 mL of this emulsion, 0.2 mL of an antioxidant solution was added and the absorbance was immediately measured at 470 nm against a blank, consisting of the emulsion without β-carotene. The tubes were placed in a water bath at 50°C and the absorbance was measured every 15 min up to 120 min.

Another method for determining antioxidant activity of canolol is by measuring the decolourization of the purple-coloured stable 1,1-diphenyl-2-picrylhydrazyl (DPPH) (Sigma, Steinheim, Germany) radical. This is a very fast method for determining the antiradical power of an antioxidant by measuring decrease in absorbance of DPPH at 517 nm. As a result of a colour change from purple to yellow, the absorbance decreases, when the DPPH radical is scavenged by an antioxidant through donation of hydrogen to form a stable DPPH-H molecule. In the radical form, this molecule has an absorbance at 515 nm which disappears by acceptance of an electron or hydrogen radical from an antioxidant compound to become a stable diamagnetic molecule.

The method described by Hatano et al. (1988) has a number of modifications. For each extract different concentrations were tested, an aliquot (0.5 mL) of the DPPH solution (50 mg/100 mL) was diluted in 4.5 mL methanol and 0.1 mL of a methanolic solution of the extract added. The mixture was shaken vigorously and allowed to stand for 45 min in the dark. The decrease in absorbance was measured using a spectrophotometer at 515 nm against a blank without added extract. From a calibration curve obtained with different amounts of extract, the ED_{50} was calculated. The ED_{50} is the concentration of an antioxidant sufficient to quench 50% of the initial DPPH radicals under the experimental conditions described. Figure 17.9 compares the effect of canolol and sinapic acid with butylated hydroxytoluene (BHT)

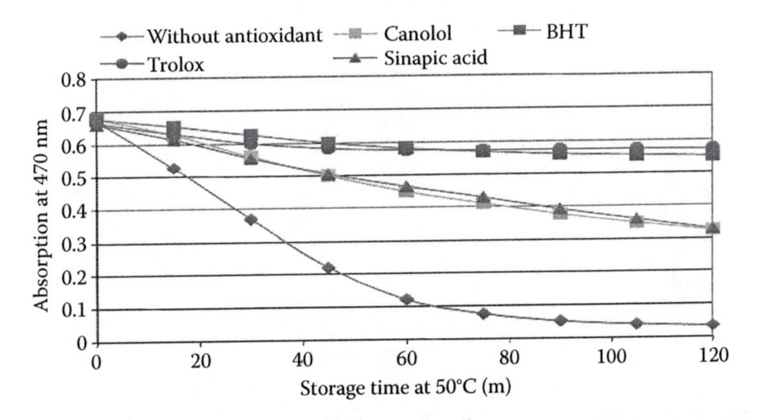

FIGURE 17.9 Purified canolol from oil of roasted canola seeds: β-carotene–linoleic acid assay.

and Trolox in the coupled system of β-carotene and linoleic acid. While the mixture of β-carotene and linoleic acid without addition of an antioxidant results in a very fast decrease of the absorption at 470 nm during storage at 50°C, canolol and sinapic acid improved the stability of β-carotene remarkable by inhibiting the oxidation of linoleic acid and subsequent bleaching of β-carotene. The effect of both compounds was similar. However, in comparison with Trolox and the synthetic antioxidant BHT, the antioxidant activity of canolol was less effective. During 120 min of storage, the absorption of the mixture decreased from 0.7 to 0.3 following addition of canolol or sinapic acid while the addition of BHT or Trolox resulted in an absorption of about 0.5 after the same time of storage.

Also the measurement of the free radical DPPH showed that canolol has an antioxidant activity capable of reducing the concentration of DPPH free radicals in the test tube. However, the antioxidant activity of canolol was only about half of the activity of Trolox or sinapic acid in this test.

17.8 EFFECT OF CANOLOL DURING STORAGE OF CANOLA OIL

The effect of canolol on the storage stability was confirmed by storing canola oil at 60°C over 168 h. The parameters used to monitor the oxidative state of the oil were diene absorption as well as the hexanal content. An increase of absorption at 240 nm was found as a result of a shift of the double bond in unsaturated fatty acids during oxidation. Hexanal, a key compound of the oxidation of fats and oil can be used as an indicator to follow the extent of oxidation.

Canola seeds were roasted at 180°C for different times ranging from 5 to 60 min and the oil extracted and stored at 60°C for 168 h. While the content of tocopherols was similar for all oils, remarkable differences in the content of canolol were found.

Figure 17.10 shows that the diene absorption decreased up to 45 min with increasing roasting time. This indicated a better oxidative state of oils obtained from seeds with

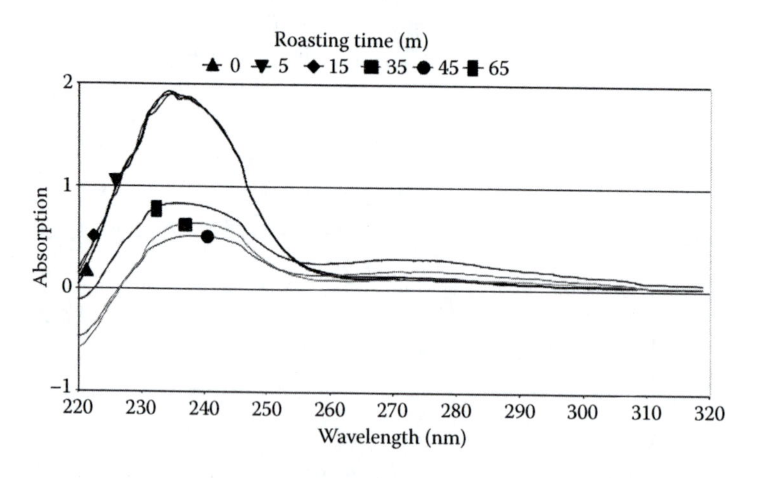

FIGURE 17.10 Diene absorption of canola oils from different roasted seeds after 168 h storage at 60°C.

increasing roasting time. Obviously, more antioxidant active compounds such as canolol are in the oil preventing the formation of conjugated dienes from hydroperoxides. A roasting time longer than 45 min resulted in an increase of the diene absorption. More conjugated dienes are formed from hydroperoxides which are the result of the longer roasting time, but the amount of canolol formed during roasting is not sufficient to prevent this formation. A similar effect was found with respect to the formation of hexanal. While oils from seeds without roasting or only low roasting times showed a higher formation of hexanal, oils from seeds roasted for 35 and 45 min, respectively, had almost no formation of hexanal. Again the high temperature load during roasting for 60 min at 180°C impaired oil quality although the oil showed a higher content of canolol.

17.9 CONCLUSIONS

Canolol is formed during roasting and heating of canola seeds, while simultaneously the content of sinapic acid in the seeds decreases. Virgin canola oil, however, only contains about 30 μg canolol/g canola oil. Substantially higher levels of canolol in virgin canola oil could indicate a heat treatment of the raw material before pressing which is not permitted for virgin cold-pressed canola oils.

Normally, the temperature generated during the cold-pressing process is insufficient to produce high amounts of canolol in the resulting oil. However, temperatures between 140°C and 180°C are required in the raw material, attained during the roasting process, to produce substantial amounts of canolol. Under these conditions, the content and the composition of tocopherols are not affected. Using the Rancimat test, the presence of canolol in canola oil resulted in higher oxidative stability. This was accompanied by changes in the sensory evaluation of the resulting oil if the raw material is roasted.

The results show that roasting of canola seeds before production of cold-pressed canola oil could result in an added-value product with a higher nutritional value and a higher oxidative stability. However, changes in the sensory evaluation of the oil from seed-like and nutty to roasty must be taken into consideration.

REFERENCES

Artz, W. E., Swanson, B. G., Sendzicki J., Rasyid, A. and Birch, R. E. W. 1986. Plant proteins: Applications, biological effects and chemistry. *ACS Symposium Series 312*, R. L. Ory, ed. Washington: American Chemical Society. pp. 126–137.

Balz, M., Schulte, E. and Thier, H.-P. 1992. Trennung von Tocopherolen und Tocotrienolen durch HPLC. *Fat Sci. Technol.* 94: 209–213.

Byerrum, R. U. and Wing, R. E. 1953. The role of choline in some metabolic reactions of *Nicotiana rustica. J. Biol. Chem.* 205: 637–642.

Cao, X., Tsukamoto, T., Seki, T., Tanaka, H., Morimura, S., Cao, L., Mizoshita, T. et al. 2008. 4-Vinyl-2,6-dimethoxyphenol (canolol) suppresses oxidative stress and gastric carcinogenesis in *Helicobacter pylori*-infected carcinogen-treated Mongolian gerbils. *Int. J. Cancer.* 122: 1445–1454.

Hatano, T., Kagaw, H., Yasuhara, T. and Okuda T. 1988. Two new flavonoids and other constituents in licorice root: Their relative astringency and radical scavenging effects. *Chem. Pharm. Bull.* 36: 1090–2097.

Koski, A., Pekkarinen, S., Hopia, A., Wähälä, K. and Heinonen M. 2003. Processing of rapeseed oil: Effects on sinapinic acid derivative content and oxidative stability. *Eur. Food Res. Technol.* 217: 110–114.

Krygier, K., Sosulski, F. and Hogge L. 1982. Free, esterified and insoluble phenolic acids. II. Composition of phenolic acids in rapeseed flour and hulls. *J. Agric. Food Chem.* 30: 334–336.

Kuwahara, H., Kanazanwa, A., Wakamatu, D., Morimura, S., Kida, K., Akaike, T. and Maeda, H. 2004. Antioxidative and antimutagenic activities of 4-vinyl-2,6-dimethoxyphenol (Canolol) isolated from canola oil. *J. Agric. Food Chem.* 52: 4380–4387.

Larrauri, J. A., Rupérez, P. and Saura-Calixto, F. 1997. Effect of drying temperature on the stability of polyphenols and antioxidant activity of red grape pomace peels. *J. Agric. Food Chem.* 45: 1390–1393.

Matthäus, B. 1998. Effect of dehulling on the composition of antinutritive compounds in various cultivars of rapeseed. *Fett/Lipid.* 100: 295–301.

Naczk, M., Amarowicz, R., Sullivan A. and Shahidi F. 1998. Current research developments on polyphenolics of rapeseed/canola: A review. *Food Chem.* 62: 489–502.

Neish, A. C. 1960. Biosynthetic pathways of aromatic compounds. *Ann. Rev. Plant Physiol.* 11: 55–80.

Shahidi, F. and Naczk, M. 1992. An overview of phenolics of canola and rapeseed: Chemical sensory and nutritional significance. *J. Am. Oil Chem. Soc.* 69: 917–924.

Spielmeyer, A., Wagner, A. and Jahreis G. 2009. Influence of thermal treatment of rapeseed on the canolol content. *Food Chem.* 112: 944–948.

Taga, M. S., Miller, E. E. and Pratt D. E. 1984. Chia seeds as a source of natural lipid antioxidants. *J. Am. Oil Chem. Soc.* 61: 928–931.

Thiyam, U., Kuhlmann, A. and Schwarz K. 2001. Extraction of valuable compounds from rape oil side products. *DAAD Bioforum*-Berlin 'Grenzenlos forschen', June 7th–9th, 2001, Berlin. http://www.foodtech.uni-kiel.de/download/rape_oil_Poster.pdf. (accessed 18.06.2012).

Thiyam, U., Stöckmann, H., zum Felde T. and Schwarz K. 2006. Antioxidative effect of the main sinapic acid derivates from rapeseed rapeseed and mustard oil by-products. *Eur. J. Lipid Sci. Technol.* 108: 238–248.

Vuorela, S., Kreander, K., Karonen, M., Nieminen, R., Hämäläinen, M., Galkin, A., Laitinen, L. et al. 2005. Preclinical evaluation of rapeseed, raspberry, and pine bark phenolics for health related effects. *J. Agric. Food Chem.* 53: 5922–5931.

Vuorela, S., Meyer, A. and Heinonen M. 2003. Quantitative analysis of the main phenolics in rapeseed meal and oils processed differently using enzymatic hydrolysis and HPLC. *Eur. Food Res. Technol.* 217: 517–523.

Wakamatsu, D., Morimura, S., Sawa, T., Kida, K., Nakai, C. and Maeda H. 2005. Isolation, identification, and structure of a potent alkyl-peroxyl radical scavenger in crude canola oil, canolol. *Biosci. Biotechnol. Biochem.* 69: 1568–1574.

Wijesundera, C., Ceccato, C., Fagan, P. and Shen Z. 2008. Seed roasting improves the oxidative stability of canola (*B. napus*) and mustard (*B. juncea*) seed oils. *Eur. J. Lipid Sci. Technol.* 110: 360–367.

Zacchi, P. and Eggers, R. 2008. High-temperature pre-conditioning of rapeseed: A polyphenol-enriched oil and the effect of refining. *Eur. J. Lipid Sci. Technol.* 110: 111–119.

18 Canola Oil, Canolol and Cancer

Evolving Research

Pablo Steinberg

CONTENTS

18.1 Introduction 329
18.2 Antimutagenic Activity of Canola Oil and Canolol 329
18.3 Anticarcinogenic Activity of Canola Oil and Canolol 330
18.4 Discussion 333
References 334

18.1 INTRODUCTION

A few years ago 4-vinyl-2,6-dimethoxyphenol, also known as canolol, was identified as a potent antioxidative compound in crude canola oil (Wakamatsu, 2001; Koski et al., 2003; Kuwahara et al., 2004; Wakamatsu et al., 2005), its concentration in crude canola oil being about 200 ppm (Wakamatsu, 2001). Canolol exhibits strong alkyl-peroxyl radical scavenging activity and is even more potent in this respect than antioxidants such as α-tocopherol, ascorbic acid, β-carotene, rutin and quercetin (Wakamatsu et al., 2005). Whereas several papers have described the antioxidative properties of canolol, little is known about its antimutagenic and anticarcinogenic activities. In this chapter, the published evidence regarding the antimutagenic and anticarcinogenic properties of canola oil and canolol are summarized and the remaining open questions in this context highlighted.

18.2 ANTIMUTAGENIC ACTIVITY OF CANOLA OIL AND CANOLOL

In a study by Kuwahara et al. (2004), the effect of canolol on peroxynitrite-mediated mutagenicity in bacteria was analysed. In DNA, purine nucleotides are vulnerable to oxidation and to adduct formation by peroxynitrite, whereby 8-oxoguanine and 8-nitroguanine are two of the major products (Salgo et al., 1995; Szabó and Ohshima, 1997; Burney et al., 1999; Niles et al., 2006). Moreover, peroxynitrite can cause deoxyribose oxidation and DNA strand breaks (Kennedy et al., 1997).

As shown in Table 18.1, canolol was able to significantly inhibit the mutagenic effect of peroxynitrite on the *Salmonella typhimurium* strain TA102, which is

TABLE 18.1
Inhibition of the Peroxynitrite-Mediated Mutation Rate in *Salmonella typhimurium* TA102 by Canolol and Other Compounds

Compound[a]	Inhibition of the Mutation Rate in Bacteria (%)
Canolol (8 μM)	81
Ascorbic acid (100 μM)	13
Ascorbic acid (1 mM)	77
α-Tocopherol (100 μM)	47
α-Tocopherol (1 mM)	93
Caffeine (100 μM)	52
Rutin (10 μM)	56
Protocatechuic acid (1 mM)	55
Sinapinic acid (10 μM)	57
Sinapinic acid (100 μM)	80

Source: Data taken from Kuwahara, H. et al. 2004. *J. Agric. Food Chem.* **52**: 4380–4387.
[a] Concentration of the compounds is given within parentheses.

particularly sensitive to oxidative acting mutagens (Levin et al., 1982), at a concentration of 8 μM (Kuwahara et al., 2004).

Furthermore, if supercoiled plasmid PUC19 DNA is exposed to peroxynitrite, the closed circular form of DNA is converted into the single-nicked open circular form and the double-nicked linear form as a consequence of peroxynitrite-mediated DNA strand breaks. Kuwahara et al. (2004) reported that canolol was also able to prevent the plasmid DNA cleavage induced by peroxynitrite.

Cisplatin is a platinum-based chemotherapeutic agent used to treat various types of cancers, including sarcomas, some carcinomas (e.g., small-cell lung cancer and ovarian cancer), lymphomas and germ cell tumours. The long-term treatment of patients with cisplatin can also lead to a dose-related increase in the frequency of chromosomal damage in non-tumour cells such as peripheral blood lymphocytes (Elsendoorn et al., 2001). Evangelista et al. (2004) treated Wistar rats with a single dose of canola oil (5 mL/kg body weight) by gavage, then administered cisplatin intraperitoneally (5 mg/kg body weight) and sacrificed the animals 24 h after cisplatin injection. The pre-treatment with a single dose of canola oil caused a statistically significant decrease in the total number of chromosomal aberrations and abnormal metaphases induced by cisplatin in bone marrow cells when compared to the experimental group having been treated with cisplatin alone.

18.3 ANTICARCINOGENIC ACTIVITY OF CANOLA OIL AND CANOLOL

Long-chain *n*-3 fatty acids, eicosapentaenoic and/or docosahexaenoic acid, have been shown to suppress the growth of tumour cells. *In vivo*, α-linolenic acid can be converted into eicosapentaenoic or docosahexaenoic. Hardman (2007) hypothesized that substituting canola oil, which contains 10% α-linolenic acid, for corn oil, which includes 1% α-linolenic acid, in the diet of nude mice having been implanted MDA-MB 231 human breast cancer cells subcutaneously would slow down tumour growth by increasing the *n*-3 fatty acid content in the diet. The tumours of mice that consumed the diet supplemented with canola oil contained significantly more eicosapentaenoic and docosahexaenoic, and the mean tumour growth rate as well as the tumour cell proliferation rate was significantly lower than those of mice having been fed with a corn oil containing diet.

Female SV129 mice develop mammary gland tumours due to the expression of the SV40 large T antigen in the mammary gland (Maroulakou et al., 1994). In a recent study by Ion et al. (2010), female SV 129 mice were placed on diets containing either 10% corn oil or 10% canola oil and after 2 weeks on the diets the female mice were bred with homozygous C3(1) TAg transgenic mice. Mother mice consumed the assigned diet throughout gestation and nursing of the offspring. After weaning, all female offspring were maintained on the control diet. Compared to offspring of mothers fed the corn oil diet, offspring of mothers fed the canola oil diet had significantly fewer mammary glands with tumours throughout the experiment. At 130 days of age, the canola oil group had significantly fewer tumours per mouse. Moreover, the tumour incidence and the total tumour weight (per mouse that developed a tumour) was less than one-half that of the corn oil group. At 170 days of age, the total tumour weight per mouse was significantly lower in the canola oil than in the corn oil group and, if a tumour developed, the rate of tumour growth rate was half that of the corn oil group.

Cho et al. (2010) postulated that canola oil reduces breast cancer cell growth by inducing cell death. In a series of *in vitro* experiments, human breast cancer T47D and MCF-7 cells were cultured and treated with canola oil. Cell proliferation and caspase 3 as well as p53 activities were measured (Table 18.2). Reduced cancer cell growth and increased expression of caspase 3 and p53 were seen in T47D and MCF-7

TABLE 18.2
Caspase 3 and p53 Activity Increases as Well Growth Inhibition in Canola Oil-Treated T47D and MCF-7 Cells

Cell Line	Increase in Caspase 3 Activity (%)[a]	Increase in p53 Activity (%)[a]
T47D	16.2	8.4
MCF-7	8.2	14.8
	Growth Inhibition (%)[b]	
T47D	31.4	
MCF-7	21.8	

Source: Data taken from Cho, K. et al. 2010. *Lipids*. **45**: 777–784.

[a] Compared to control caspase 3 and p53 cell activities. Cells were treated for 96 h with 1 mM canola oil.

[b] Compared to control cell growth rates. Cells were treated for 96 h with 1 mM canola oil.

cells treated with canola oil. In a subsequent animal experiment, female Sprague–Dawley rats were randomly assigned to corn oil or canola oil containing diets, and mammary tumours were chemically induced by subcutaneous administration of the carcinogen *N*-nitroso-*N*-methylurea. Rats having been fed with a canola oil-supplemented diet had reduced tumour volumes and showed an increased survival rate as compared to rats having been fed a diet containing corn oil.

In an epidemiological study by Wang et al. (2008), it was reported that breast cancer risk was increased for women cooking with hydrogenated fats (OR = 1.58, 95% CI = 1.20–2.10) or vegetable/corn oil (OR = 1.30, 95% CI = 1.06–1.58) compared to women using olive/canola oil. The authors concluded that a low-fat diet may play a role in breast cancer prevention and speculated that monounsaturated trans fats may have driven the discrepant associations between types of fat and breast cancer risk.

In a very recent study by Akinsete et al. (2012), the influence of a diet rich in ω-3 fatty acids (i.e., containing 5% canola oil and 5% fish concentrate) on prostate cancer development was studied. For this purpose, female SV 129 mice were bred with male mice carrying the SV40 large T antigen with a C3(1) rat prostatic steroid-binding protein promoter (Shibata et al., 1996). The transgenic mice develop prostatic intraepithelial neoplasia that slowly progresses to prostate carcinoma due to the expression of the SV40 large T antigen in the prostate. The male offspring were fed a corn oil containing diet until post puberty and thereafter half of the male mice received the ω-3 fatty acid-rich diet for up to 40 weeks. The other half of the mice received a ω-6 fatty acid-rich (i.e., corn oil containing) diet. Tumour development in the dorsolateral prostate region was slower in the group fed a ω-3 fatty acid-rich diet when compared to the group fed a ω-6 fatty acid-rich diet. This effect on tumour development was accompanied by a significant decrease in the testosterone and estradiol plasma levels as well as in the expression of androgen receptors. Moreover, the ω-3 fatty acid-rich diet led to a decrease in the expression of genes involved in cell proliferation and to an increase in the expression of proapoptotic genes. On the basis of the data obtained, Akinsete et al. (2012) postulated that consumption of a ω-3 fatty acid-rich diet slows down prostate tumourigenesis by lowering estradiol, testosterone and androgen receptor levels, promoting apoptosis and suppressing cell proliferation in C3(1)Tag mice.

In a study by Cao et al. (2008), the effects of canolol on *Helicobacter pylori*-induced gastritis and gastric carcinogenesis using a Mongolian gerbil model were analysed. The animals were exposed to *Helicobacter pylori* or to *Helicobacter pylori* and *N*-methyl-*N*-nitrosourea. After inoculation of *Helicobacter pylori*, they were fed either with or without canolol. *Helicobacter pylori*-induced gastritis, 5′-bromo-2′-deoxyuridine labelling and scores for cyclooxygenase-2 and inducible nitric oxide synthase immunohistochemistry were attenuated in the canolol-treated groups. Expression of interleukin-1β, tumour necrosis factor-α, cyclooxygenase-2 and inducible nitric oxide synthase mRNA in the gastric mucosa as well as serum 8-hydroxy-2′-deoxyguanosine levels were also significantly lower in canolol-treated gerbils. Furthermore, the incidence of gastric adenocarcinomas was markedly reduced in animals treated with *Helicobacter pylori*, *N*-methyl-*N*-nitrosourea and canolol when compared to the corresponding control group. The authors concluded that canolol is able to suppress inflammation, gastric epithelial cell proliferation and gastric carcinogenesis in *Helicobacter pylori*-infected Mongolian gerbils, whereby it should be noted that the viable *Helicobacter pylori* count was not affected by the canolol containing diet. The data suggest that the level of inflammation rather than the existence of the bacteria is the determining factor and in this context the canolol-mediated suppression of mRNAs for inflammatory cytokines is of relevance.

Bhatia et al. (2011) analysed the influence of a control diet (AIN-93), the AIN-93 diet containing 15% corn oil and the AIN-93 diet supplemented with 15% canola oil on the development of colon cancer in Fischer 344 rats treated with the colon carcinogen azoxymethane. Tumour incidence (percentage of rats with a tumour) and tumour multiplicity (number of tumours per animal) were significantly lower in rats having been fed the canola oil diet when compared to the animals receiving the corn oil diet. Moreover, the average tumour size was much higher in the corn oil group than in the canola oil group, but due to the large standard deviation in the corn oil group the difference between the two groups did not reach statistical significance. The α-linolenic acid (i.e., ω-3 fatty acid) levels in colon tissue and plasma samples were significantly higher in the canola oil than in the corn oil group, whereas the cyclooxygenase expression was strongly enhanced in the colon samples of rats fed the corn oil diet if compared to the animals fed the canola oil diet. The authors of the study concluded that canola oil may exert a chemopreventive effect in colon cancer development by increasing ω-3 fatty acid levels and decreasing cyclooxygenase expression.

18.4 DISCUSSION

The limited number of studies demonstrating an anticarcinogenic effect of canola oil and canolol (Hardman, 2007; Cao et al., 2008, 2010; Ion et al., 2010; Akinsete et al., 2012; Bhatia et al., 2011), although promising, do not allow at the present time to definitely conclude that they are potent cancer chemopreventive agents. On the one hand, one important premise when thinking in terms of cancer chemoprevention is that the bioactive compounds are effective when administered p.o., and this was the case in all six above-mentioned studies. On the other hand, the anticarcinogenic effects reported by Hardman (2007), Cho et al. (2010), Ion et al. (2010) and Bhatia et al. (2011) were observed after feeding animals with diets including very high amounts of canola oil (8–15% w/w). Moreover, one should take into account that colon cancer development was inhibited in rats fed a canola oil-rich diet when compared to rats being fed a corn oil-enriched diet, but that the feeding of a canola oil-rich diet did not offer any advantage when compared to the feeding of the standard lab chow (Bhatia et al., 2011). In the study by Akinsete et al. (2012), a diet rich in ω-3 fatty acids suppressed tumour development in C3(1) Tag mice. However, one has to point out that the ω-3 fatty acid-enriched diet included 5% canola oil and 5% fish concentrate, so that the effect cannot alone be ascribed to canola oil as a whole or to one of its constituents.

The fact that Cao et al. (2008) inhibited gastric cancer development with a low dietary concentration of purified canolol (0.1% w/w) strongly suggests that canolol is (one of) the compound(s) responsible for the anticarcinogenic effect of canola oil. In the studies by Hardman (2007), Cho et al. (2010), Ion et al. (2010) and Bhatia et al.

(2011), no purified canolol was administered and no information on the canolol content of the canola oil used was given, so that it is unclear at the present time whether phenolic compounds other than canolol could be responsible for the anticarcinogenic activity of canola oil. Up to now, it has been shown that canola oil can slow down breast (Hardman, 2007; Cho et al., 2010; Ion et al., 2010), prostate (Akinsete et al., 2012), colon (Bhatia et al., 2011) and gastric cancer development (Cao et al., 2008). In the future, it will be important to determine whether the cancer cell growth-inhibiting effects also apply to tumours arising in organs other than the above-mentioned ones and which compound present in canola oil is the 'driving force' underlying the cancer chemopreventive effects discussed in this chapter.

Particularly interesting is the observation made by Cao et al. (2008) that canolol is able to inhibit the inflammatory process in gastric mucosa and the subsequent formation of gastric tumours by repressing the expression of inflammatory cytokines. In this context it should be determined if canolol can also inhibit tumour development in those experimental models of liver and intestinal cancer, in which carcinogenesis is preceded or accompanied by inflammation.

In the study by Ion et al. (2010), maternal consumption of canola oil was associated with the delayed appearance and reduced growth of mammary gland tumours as well as changes in the expression of genes such as those coding for fatty acid synthase and CCAAT/enhancer-binding protein β in the female offspring. From a mechanistic point of view, the following questions remain to be answered: (1) Is the pattern of alterations in gene expression induced by canola oil in the mammary gland tumours also observed in other experimental cancer models and are the changes associated with reduced tumour growth in these experimental cancer models? (2) Which mechanism(s) lead(s) (e.g., altered methylation pattern) to the canola oil-mediated changes in gene expression?

In conclusion, the results obtained up to now show that canola oil possesses a certain anticarcinogenic activity. Future studies addressing the questions posed in this section will demonstrate if canola oil and its phenolic constituents can really be viewed as potent cancer chemopreventive agents.

REFERENCES

Akinsete, J.A., Ion, G., Witte, T.R. and Hardman, W. E. 2012. Consumption of high ω-3 fatty acid diet suppressed prostate tumourigenesis in C3(1) Tag mice. *Carcinogen* **33**: 140–148.

Bhatia, E., Doddivenaka, C., Zhang, X., Bommareddy, A., Krishnan, P., Mathees, D.P. and Dwivedi, C. 2011. Chemopreventive effects of dietary canola oil on colon cancer development. *Nutr. Cancer* **63**: 242–247.

Burney, S., Niles, J.C., Dedon, P.C. and Tannenbaum, S.R. 1999. DNA damage in deoxynucleosides and oligonucleotides treated with peroxynitrite. *Chem. Res. Toxicol.* **12**: 513–520.

Cao, X., Tsukamoto, T., Seki, T., Tanaka, H., Morimura, S., Cao, L., Mizoshita, T. et al. 2008. 4-Vinyl-2,6-dimethoxyphenol (canolol) suppresses oxidative stress and gastric carcinogenesis in *Helicobacter pylori*-infected carcinogen-treated Mongolian gerbils. *Int. J. Cancer* **122**: 1445–1454.

Cho, K., Mabasa, L., Fowler, A.W., Walsh, D.M. and Park, C.S. 2010. Canola oil inhibits breast cancer cell growth in cultures and *in vivo* and acts synergistically with chemotherapeutic drugs. *Lipids* **45**: 777–784.

Elsendoorn, T.J., Weijl, N.I., Mithoe, S., Zwinderman, A.H., Van Dam, F., De Zwart, F.A., Tates, A.D. and Osanto, S. 2001. Chemotherapy-induced chromosomal damage in peripheral blood lymphocytes of cancer patients supplemented with antioxidants or placebo. *Mutat. Res.* **498**: 145–158.

Evangelista, C.M., Antunes, L.M., Francescato, H.D. and Bianchi, M.L. 2004. Effects of the olive, extra virgin olive and canola oils on cisplatin-induced clastogenesis in Wistar rats. *Food Chem. Toxicol.* **42**: 1291–1297.

Hardman, W.E. 2007. Dietary canola oil suppressed growth of implanted MDA-MB 231 human breast tumours in nude mice. *Nutr. Cancer* **57**: 177–183.

Ion, G., Akinsete, J.A. and Hardman, W.E. 2010. Maternal consumption of canola oil suppressed mammary gland tumouri genes is in C3(1) TAg mice off spring. *BMC Cancer* 6: 10–81.

Kennedy, L.J., Moore, K.Jr., Caulfield, J.L., Tannenbaum, S.R. and Dedon, P.C. 1997. Quantitation of 8-oxoguanine and strand breaks produced by four oxidizing agents. *Chem. Res. Toxicol.* **10**: 386–392.

Koski, A., Pekkarinen, S., Hopia, A., Wähälä, K. and Heinonen, M. 2003. Processing of rapeseed oil: Effects on sinapinic acid derivative content and oxidative stability. *Eur. Food Res. Technol.* **217**: 110–114.

Kuwahara, H., Kanazawa, A., Wakamatsu, D., Morimura, S., Kida, K., Akaike, T. and Maeda, H. 2004. Antioxidative and antimutagenic activities of 4-vinyl-2,6-dimethoxyphenol (canolol) isolated from canola oil. *J. Agric. Food Chem.* **52**: 4380–4387.

Levin, D.E., Hollstein, M., Christman, M.F., Schwiers, E.A. and Ames, B.N. 1982. A new *Salmonella* tester strain (TA102) with A T base pairs at the site of mutation detects oxidative mutagens. *Proc. Natl. Acad. Sci. USA* **79**: 7445–7449.

Maroulakou, I.G., Anver, M., Garrett, L. and Green, J.E. 1994. Prostate and mammary adenocarcinoma in transgenic mice carrying a rat C3(1) simian virus 40 large tumour antigen fusion gene. *Proc. Natl. Acad. Sci. USA* **91**: 11236–11240.

Niles, J.C., Wishnok, J.S. and Tannenbaum, S.R. 2006. Peroxynitrite-induced oxidation and nitration products of guanine and 8-oxoguanine: Structures and mechanisms of product formation. *Nitric Oxide* **14**: 109–121.

Salgo, M.G., Bermudez, E., Squadrito, G.L. and Pryor, W.A. 1995. Peroxynitrite causes DNA damage and oxidation of thiols in rat thymocytes. *Arch. Biochem. Biophys* **322**: 500–505.

Shibata, M.A., Ward, J.M., Devor, D.E., Liu, M.L. and Green, J.E. 1996. Progression of prostatic intraepithelial neoplasia to invasive carcinoma in C3(1)/SV40 large T transgenic mice: Histopathological and molecular biological alterations. *Cancer Res.* **56**: 4894–4903.

Szabó, C. and Ohshima, H. 1997. DNA damage induced by peroxynitrite: Subsequent biological effects. *Nitric Oxide* **1**: 373–385.

Wakamatsu, D. 2001. Isolation and identification of radical scavenging compound, canolol, in canola oil. MS Thesis, Graduate School of Natural Science, Kumamoto University, Japan. pp. 1–48.

Wakamatsu, D., Morimura, S., Sawa, T., Kida, K., Nakai, C. and Maeda, H. 2005. Isolation, identification, and structure of a potent alkyl-peroxyl radical scavenger in crude canola oil, canolol. *Biosci. Biotechnol. Biochem.* **69**: 1568–1574.

Wang, J., John, E.M., Horn-Ross, P.L. and Ingles, S.A. 2008. Dietary fat, cooking fat, and breast cancer risk in a multi ethnic population. *Nutr. Cancer* **60**: 492–504.

19 Canolol as a Promising Nutraceutical
Status and Scope

Dayanidhi Huidrom and Usha Thiyam-Holländer

CONTENTS

19.1 Introduction 337
19.2 Status of Canolol: Actual Range in Canola Oil 338
19.3 Review of Functional Properties and Assessment of Efficacy 341
 19.3.1 Radical Scavenging (Antioxidative) 341
 19.3.2 Suppression of Oxidative Stress 342
 19.3.3 Defence of Signalling Molecules 343
 19.3.4 Anti-Mutagenicity 343
 19.3.5 Protection of DNA Breakage 343
 19.3.6 Cytoprotective Effect 343
 19.3.7 Anti-Inflammatory 344
 19.3.8 Inhibition of Chronic Gastritis and Carcinogenesis 344
19.4 Structure–Function Relation 344
19.5 Conclusion 345
Acknowledgements 346
References 346

19.1 INTRODUCTION

Oilseeds contain minor components such as phenolics, which are generally accepted to be potential antioxidants. These antioxidative compounds play a major role in maintaining the genetic integrity of the seeds (Bailly, 2004). Canolol is one of the main phenol compounds derived from canola and rapeseed (seeds and oil) from the precursor sinapic acid. Although sinapic acid is proven to be the parent for its formation, our unpublished recent work seems to indicate that sinapic acid derivatives might have a role in the formation of canolol. Structurally, canolol constitutes a dimethoxy phenol attached with vinyl group at the fourth position of phenol ring (Figure 19.1). Consequently, the chemical name of canolol is 4-vinyl-2,6-dimethoxyphenol. Sinapic acid is regarded as the precursor of canolol on the basis of heat-involved treatments formed by decarboxylation. Discussions on decarboxylation pathways leading to the formation of canolol are mentioned in Chapter 3. Heat treatment such as roasting was found to decarboxylate sinapic acid and as a result, the concentration

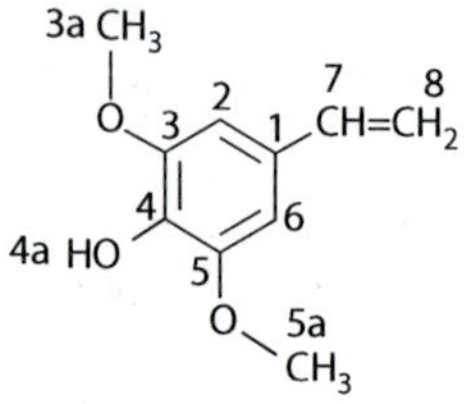

FIGURE 19.1 Structure of canolol. (Numbers denote the possible sites of reactions based on Galano, A., Francisco-Marquez, M. and Alvarez-Idaboy, J. 2011. *J. Phys. Chem. B.* **115**: 8590–8596. With permission.)

of canolol increases with the increase in exposure to heat (Wakamatsu et al., 2005; Spielmeyer et al., 2009). Temperature seems to have a crucial role, in comparison with the form of heat input such as microwave heat or heating block according to Spielmeyer et al. (2009). Most recently, Harbaum-Piayda et al. (2010) also mentions the formation of canolol dimers and trimers in the deodistillates of canola.

Since its discovery in the early 2000 (Wakamatsu, 2001; Tsunehiro et al., 2001; Koski et al., 2003), canolol attracts quite impressively the food scientists, industries and consumers. Thus, a rapidly expanding research on the positive aspects of canolol continued to blossom. The remarkable feature about canolol relates to its potent antioxidative property. It was discovered to possess alkyl-peroxyl radical scavenging capacity, which is much higher than the established antioxidants such as α-tocopherol, vitamin C, β-carotene, rutin and quercetin (Wakamatsu et al., 2005) and the OOH radical scavenger activity of canolol is predicted to be higher than that of allicin and much higher than that of melatonin (Galano et al., 2011). Since the recent positive properties of canolol were proven, it became an intensely studied subject and new functional properties have continued to be revealed. Canolol was also found to possess anticarcinogenic (Cao et al., 2008), antimutagenic and cytoprotective effects (Kuwahara et al., 2004). Chapter 18 provides an overall review of the antimutagenic and anticancer properties of canola oil and canolol. This chapter will focus, in more detail, on the health benefits of canolol as a potential nutraceutical. Additionally, as an update, new data on the occurrence of canolol in various canola oils are given in Section 19.2 as an attempt to reason the existing and probability of higher amounts that can be obtained in commercial or novel processing.

19.2 STATUS OF CANOLOL: ACTUAL RANGE IN CANOLA OIL

Before considering the scope of canolol in canola oils and other oils of value as functional foods, nutraceuticals, cosmetic formulations and other products of pharmacological relevance, it seems logical to correlate the existing content of this phenol. The presence of canolol in seeds, cotyledons or hulls in canola might not seem to be relevant earlier as it is not reported as an important secondary metabolite in canola plants. An overwhelming number of literature suggests the content of various secondary metabolites in plants, especially the well known: cinnamic and benzoic acid derivatives with no mention of canolol in the context of rapeseed and canola, and its close relative mustard. Evolving research in canolol seems to be focused on the pre-treatment of oilseeds or distillation (such as deodistillates) production of this phenol to explore commercial applications. To the best of our knowledge, no data are available on the occurrence of this phenol using non-destructive methods such as near-infrared spectroscopy of the seed substrates indicating that this occurs naturally in raw seeds subjected to no heat or similar treatments. Spielmeyer et al. (2009) mention that there is no report on whether canolol is associated with direct synthesis or the by-product of decarboxylation or other mechanisms in plants. In contrast, canolol seems to present perhaps naturally in very small amounts as low as ~6 μg/g (Wakamatsu et al., 2005; Spielmeyer et al., 2009) in the rapeseed substrates of the unroasted control which is compared with roasted samples. No significant difference was observed concerning the canolol content (2.8 versus 3.2 μg/g respectively) of dried seeds and rapeseed kernels. Vuorela et al. (2003) reported the content of canolol in the range 0–244 μg/g of rapeseed oil associated with pressing of rapeseed. Recent data suggest the occurrence of this valuable phenol only in oils treated with heat (Veldsink et al., 1999), pressing or toasting (with or without steam) as done in our laboratory, or even steam (Zacchi and Eggers, 2008; Harbaum et al., 2010). Thus the question arises, if canolol can be distilled or stripped from canola oils due to its known volatility to find its usage as a nutraceutical. Thus, it is worthwhile to investigate if canola oils can be the substrates for obtaining canolol. If yes, will canola oils obtained from various steps involved in pressing and refining in commercial processing of canola oil be meaningful? Thus, as part of a large project conducted in our laboratory at the University of Manitoba, Winnipeg, Manitoba, we obtained canola oils and seeds from various crushers of canola oil in Canada, the United States and the Canola Council of Canada. Suppliers of these canola oils include Bunge Canada, Richardson Oilseeds Canada, ADM, the United States, Viterra Canola Canada and Dow Agrosciences, the USA. The oils were obtained from 2008 through 2010 and were crude, refined–degummed, expeller–pressed, refined–bleached and refined–bleached–deodorized, refined–washed, acidified in the terminology used by the standards of the canola oil industry. Although, due to issues of confidentiality, we cannot seem to locate or disclose the actual steps of pressing or the steps of refining of these oils or the actual temperature and other relevant conditions that are exposed while refining these oils, it is mutually agreed to share that these oils were either crude oils before refining or oils subjected to the various steps of refining used by each of these commercial crushers. Furthermore, it is well known that due to varying content of the precursor, that is, sinapic acid in the seeds—depending on conventional, genetically modified and affected by other conditions of harvest, canolol content may also be different.

Table 19.1 indicates the content of canolol in various canola oils conducted as a survey recently. Samples that were tested include oils obtained from genetically modified canola, high oleic and conventional canola seeds. Another main aim of this survey was to investigate the content of total phenolic compounds and other minor components such as chlorophyll and other sinapic acid derivatives which are not reported in this chapter. Table 19.1 indicates the most abundant level of canolol which was found in crude canola oils. A wide variation of ranges, that is, negligible to higher but varying amounts, were found in the final steps of the refined oils. Canolol content seems to vary depending on the various degree of refining. This was demonstrated

TABLE 19.1
Quantification of Canolol Was Done as Sinapic Acid Equivalent (SAE) at 270 nm Using the Method of Khattab et al. (2010)

Canola Oil Sample	Canolol Content as SAE (μg/g)
Crude	409.51 ± 24.98
Crude-processed	1067 ± 8.21
Refined–bleached–deodorized	Not detected
Refined–bleached	Not detected
Refined–washed	540.35 ± 2.07
Refined–bleached–deodorized	Not detected
Refined–bleached	Not detected
Refined–bleached–deodorized	Not detected
Crude	1023.09 ± 4.76
Acid–degummed	903 ± 20.79
Crude	129.77 ± 0.69
Refined–bleached	Not detected
Non–GM^{o1}	Not detected
Refined–bleached	Not detected
Conventional oil	47.96 ± 0.71
Non–GM^{o1}	Not detected
Non–GM^{o1+}	34.78 ± 5.75
Refined–neutralized	28.12 ± 0.57
Conventional–refined	16.97 ± 2.79
Crude high oleic oil	80.34 ± 0.44
Non–GM^{o1} refined–degumed	Not detected
Conventional refined–bleached	Not detected

Note: GM^{o1}, Genetically-modified; GM^{o1+}, Genetically-modified but received in a different year/lot. Estimation of canolol was done (270 nm) as SAE by high-performance liquid chromatography (HPLC) conditions reported in Khattab et al. (2010). Spectrum of canolol obtained through this method is indicated in Figure 19.2.

by the oils collected from the various degree of refining such as bleaching, deodorizing, acidification and other washing steps. As indicated in Table 19.1, highest values of canolol were reported in crude oils except in the case of crude high oleic oil. The highest value reported in this survey is 1067 μg/g of canola oil. In refined oils, mostly no canolol is detected. In other oil samples, even if canolol is detected, the values seem to be much less than the 1000 μg range. Thus, it can be concluded that realistically canolol content is the maximum in crude oils and the industrial processes seem to have a negative effect to the high amount. Another important issue is that the different industrial processes, even though, representative of the various processing used commercially might be from various canola seed cultivars. These are also factors that might affect the content of canolol in these oils. Spielmeyer et al. (2009) reported that cold-pressed and rape kernel oils tested contained from 6.7 to 81.4 μg

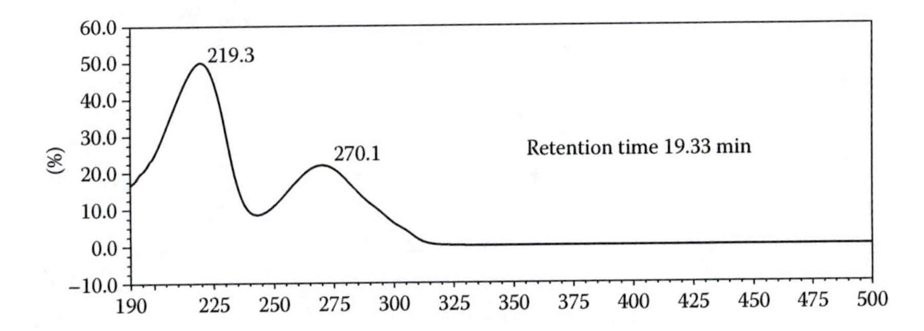

FIGURE 19.2 Spectrum of canolol. Quantification of canolol was done as sinapic acid equivalent (SAE) at 270 nm using Khattab et al. (2010). (From Khattab, R. et al. 2010. *J. Am. Oil Chem. Soc.* **87**(2): 147–155. With permission.)

canolol/g rapeseed oil without distinct differences. Wakamatsu et al. (2005) reported 220–38 μg/g of canolol from degummed and deacidified industrially processed rapeseed oils, respectively. Both these studies reported that after roasting, canolol levels can be elevated to as high as 100–120 times to that of the unroasted samples.

Canolol could also be extracted from the seed and press cake using our novel techniques to as high as 7000 μg (as sinapic acid equivalent), which is a relatively high amount than what is reported in literature. This process was submitted as an intellectual property with the technology transfer office of the University of Manitoba in 2009 and 2010. We are attempting to publish this in future. In general, it is now known that canolol is detected in most industrial crude canola oils, but is often completely lost during refining. However, based on our new process, the potential application of a simplified treatment to produce canolol extracts and canolol-enhanced designer oils for the nutraceutical markets among others is discovered. Canolol can also be extracted from brassica plants and oilseeds containing sinapic acid derivatives. If successful in scaling up to the industrial scale, this innovative approach will enhance the value to both oil and the by-product press cake. New ways to effectively utilize canola and new markets will open up due to these developments on canola phenolics. Natural antioxidant markets remain competitive with products such as rosemary and green tea extracts. Solvent-extracted rosemary products cost an average of $16.2/kg while carbon dioxide extract costs 100% more at $32/kg (Frost and Sullivan, 2007). The price varies according to solubility, concentration and formulation type. The average price of Vitamin E per pound in animal feed was $3.66 in 2005 (Frost and Sullivan, 2006). Let us hope for the best for canolol in the near future.

19.3 REVIEW OF FUNCTIONAL PROPERTIES AND ASSESSMENT OF EFFICACY

19.3.1 Radical Scavenging (Antioxidative)

Lipid radicals can attack and damage a biologically indispensable molecule such as deoxyribose nucleic acid (DNA) and protein and initiate oxidation (Marnett, 2002). Lipid radicals are the potential agents for carcinogenesis (Sawa et al., 1998). One of the widely used assays for testing the effectiveness of antioxidants is the ability to scavenge lipid radicals. Wakamatsu et al. (2005) subjected canolol, separated through a multistep process to alkyl peroxyl radical scavenging assay by chemiluminescence. It was found out that $IPOX_{50}$ was increased to 1050-fold compared with $IPOX_{50}$ of the starting material, that is, degummed crude oil. Interestingly, it was also found out that $IPOX_{50}$ value decreases as the purity of canolol increases. $IPOX_{50}$ is the value at which 50% of the chemiluminescence gets reduced compared with chemiluminescence of control. Lower $IPOX_{50}$ value indicates the higher potency of the antioxidant. The data signify the high antioxidative capacity of canolol. Refining steps used in the edible oil industry is known to minimize several minor components including canolol.

Density functional theory of OOH radical scavenging activity of canolol predicted the overall rate coefficients to be 2.5×10^6 and 6.8×10^5 M^{-1} S^{-1} in aqueous and lipid solutions, respectively. Canolol was predicted to be 'similar to that of carotenes, higher than that of allicin and much higher than that of melatonin in terms of OOH radical scavenging properties' (Galano et al., 2011, P. 8594). Therefore, there exists a high degree of agreement from experimental and theoretical perspectives as far as antioxidant potential is concerned.

19.3.2 Suppression of Oxidative Stress

Reactive oxygen species (ROS) constitutes highly reactive oxygen-bearing molecules such as superoxide anion radicals ($O_2^{\cdot -}$), hydroxyl radicals and so on capable of damaging biomolecules such as DNA. ROS plays an important role in the biological functions such as cell development, growth, ageing, pathogenesis of viral infection and development of cancer (Davies, 1995). t-BH (tertiary-butylated hydroxide) can induce oxidative stress in a human retinal pigment epithelial cell line (ARPE)-19 cells and generate ROS which was cytotoxic and caused cell damage (Giddabasappa et al., 2010). In a study conducted by Dong et al. (2011), the cells' viability was measured by 3-(4,5-dimethylthiazol-2-yl)-2, 5-diphenyl tetrazolium bromide (MTT) assay using t-BH at various ranges (100, 120, 150 and 200 μM) and at 150 μM, 50% of the cells were found to be dead. The effect of canolol at a different concentration was investigated in these oxidative stressed cell lines. Canolol was found to be effective in reducing t-BH-induced cells death upto 100% at 200 μM. Morphology of canolol pretreated cells was also found similar to normal cells. To further confirm that cell death was related to the release of ROS by t-BH-induced oxidative stress, ROS was measured by using a fluorescent ROS indicator, 2′,7′-dichlorodihydrofluorescein diacetate (H_2DCFDA). A 2.3-fold increase in ROS was observed in t-BH-induced cells. Interestingly, canolol pre-treatment appears to have a profound effect in controlling the release of ROS due to oxidative stress. Near-normal ROS production was achieved at a canolol concentration of 200 μm (Dong et al., 2011). This further indicated that canolol in fact helps in the prevention of ROS production during oxidative stress.

Living organisms have an inbuilt system to counteract with the ROS. In fact, ROS should be balanced to avoid damaging situation due to excessive production of ROS. Antioxidative enzymes such as superoxide dimutase (SOD), catalase and glutathione peroxidase allay ROS by allowing them to reduce to non-toxic compounds (Demple and Harrison, 1994). Taking this into consideration, expression levels of antioxidative enzymes such as heme oxygenase (*HO-1*), catalase and glutathione *S*-transferase-pi (GST-pi) were evaluated (Dong et al., 2011). It also helps to understand better the antioxidative mechanisms of canolol against t-BH-induced cell damage in ARPE-19 cells. mRNA level of *HO-1* and catalase were raised up in canolol-treated ARPE-19 cells. Activity of canolol did not limit only upto the enzyme level. mRNA expression of NF-E2-related factor (*Nrf-2*) was also found to be elevated. *Nrf-2* binds to antioxidant response element (ARE) and induces expression of antioxidant genes (Osburn and Kensler, 2008).

19.3.3 Defence of Signalling Molecules

'Extracellular signal-regulated kinase (ERK) cascade is one of the major mitogen-activated protein kinase (MAPK) pathways and its activation is generally thought to mediate cell survival' (Wang et al., 1998). ERK was also responsible in defence signalling against oxidative stressed cells (Glotin et al., 2006). Canolol was found to be capable of playing an active role in the phosphorylation of ERK in ARPE cell lines (Dong et al., 2011). It further relates the role of canolol in cell viability under oxidative stress and ERK phosphorylation. There is a good chance that the property of canolol in combating cell damage is probably due to its active role in ERK phosphorylation.

19.3.4 Anti-Mutagenicity

Salmonella strain TA 102 was shown to have the greatest mutagenic effect of peroxynitrite (ONOO). Mutation frequency was raised to 21% when TA 102 was treated with 8 μM $ONOO^-$ for 20 min. Canolol was found to inhibit the mutation rate to 18% at 8 μM and above (8).

19.3.5 Protection of DNA Breakage

Escherichia coli plasmid phage (pUC 19) DNA when exposed to $ONOO^-$ undergoes structural change by converting the circular DNA into single-nicked open circular form and double-nicked circular form. At higher concentration of $ONOO^-$, the DNA disappeared. As indicated by the fluorescence DNA bands, canolol (>1 μM) could prevent DNA breakage in the presence of 1 μM $ONOO^-$ (Kuwahara et al., 2004). This indicated the DNA protection capacity of canolol.

19.3.6 Cytoprotective Effect

Canolol was shown to possess cytoprotective effect against bactericidal effect of $ONOO^-$. The bactericidal activity of $ONOO^-$ increased considerably with the increasing concentration and exposure time. However, when canolol was applied at various concentration levels, it was shown to protect bacteria, *Samonella typhimurium*, as the survival rate increased upto 100%. This clearly proved the cytoprotective effect of canolol in bacteria. In mammalian cell also (human colon cancer SW 480), canolol showed cytoprotective effect except at high concentration (Kuwahara et al., 2004). This seems to collaborate with the study of Xueyuan Cao et al. (2008), where cell viability of ARPE-19 cells was examined at different concentrations. No cytoxicity was found upto 200 μM. Cytoprotective effect of canolol was also found in human kidney cells (HEK293) and human bronchial cells (HBE140) (Seki et al., 2006).

19.3.7 Anti-Inflammatory

ROS is believed to alter the expression and function of cyclooxygenase (Cox2) and nitric oxide synthase (iNOS) and influence the expression of proteins involved in the regulation of cell cycle progression (Shackelford et al., 2000). Scores of immunoreactivity against Cox-2 and iNOS in the canolol-treated groups were significantly lower than in the canolol-untreated control groups. Further, mRNA expression of IL-1β, TNF- α, COX-2 and iNOS is also indicated to be correlated with *Helicobacter pylori* infection. Upregulation of mRNA expression of IL-12, TNF- α, Cox-2 and iNOS was found in *H. pylori*-infected groups. In a short-term experiment, compared with control (uninfected group), IL-1β was found 16 times more in *H. pylori*-infected groups. Canolol treatment of 0.1% in the diet could attenuate mRNA expression of IL-12 by decreasing upto 50% (Cao et al., 2008). Previous studies have demonstrated that level of TNF-α, IL-12 and IFN-γ was associated with *H. pylori*-infected gastritis (D'Elios et al., 1997; Yamaoka et al., 2005). Expression of IL-12 and TNF-α was also declined in infected rhesus monkeys (Harris et al., 2000). Long-term experiments found higher upregulation of mRNA expression in *H. pylori*-infected groups. IL-1β mRNA expression was upregulated up to 120 times compared with 16 times in short-term experiment. Similar effect of canolol in downregulation was also achieved (Cao et al., 2008).

19.3.8 Inhibition of Chronic Gastritis and Carcinogenesis

H. pylori is an important aetiological agent causing chronic gastritis and ulceration (Parsonnet et al., 1991). Extensive study on the effect of canolol in suppression of the oxidative stress and control of *H. pylori* causing gastric carcinogenesis was carried out by Cao et al. (2008). Effect of canolol was investigated in both short term and long term experiments in gerbils model (Cao et al., 2008). This study concluded that canolol, can prevent *H. pylori*-induced gastritis and carcinogenesis in a gerbil model. Neutrophils and lymphoplasmocytic cell infiltration in antral mucosa of the canolol-treated group were significantly suppressed compared with the *H. pylori*-infected control groups. Besides this, hyperplasia and intestinal metaplasia lesions were found to be decreased in canolol-treated *H. pylori*-infected gerbils. Canolol suppression of gastric carcinogenesis is evident from the low incidence of glandular stomach tumours. Groups which are devoid of canolol showed no difference in tumour development.

19.4 STRUCTURE–FUNCTION RELATION

The antioxidative property of phenolic compounds in general is due to its ease to donate hydrogen atoms to free radicals. Compounds with lower reduction potential can donate hydrogen atoms. Reduction potential of antioxidants is generally below 500 mV (Eunok Choe and Min, 2006).

The mechanism of the antioxidant activity of canolol was critically analysed by Galano et al. (2011). Three possible pathways are

1. Radical adduct formation (RAF)

$$CNL + \bullet OOH \rightarrow (CNL - OOH)\bullet$$

2. Hydrogen atom transfer (HAT), from sites 3a–5a

$$CNL + \bullet OOH \rightarrow CNL(-H)\bullet + H_2O_2$$

3. Single electron transfer (SET)

$$CNL + \bullet OOH \rightarrow CNL\bullet^{+} + OOH^{-}$$

Electron transfer from •OOH to canolol SET was found to be endergonic as shown by Gibbs's free energy values and hence its possibility was ruled out. In both RAF and HAT, the two possible ways of reaction are H transfer from OH moiety from canolol (site 4a) and •OOH addition to site C8. Compared to the other ROS, •OOH has low reactivity. Therefore, it is obvious that canolol can work faster and efficiently in all ROS. It was found out that 99% of all reactions between canolol and •OOH undergo through HAT pathway in all environments. Thus, it can be expected to predominantly form one product. However, it cannot be ruled out that other mechanisms are less important. Reactivity and structure of the radicals are also equally important in deciding the antioxidation mechanisms (Galano et al., 2009).

19.5 CONCLUSION

Crude canola oil seems to be a high source of canolol in industrially processed canola oils. In addition, there are options for the use of pre-treatments such as heating and steaming that can be used to elevate canolol levels in oils. Another way is to use deodistillates as a source of nutraceutical canolol. The results obtained in our laboratory seems to be the only study to the best of our knowledge that seems to be successful in reporting canolol to a very high level that is not reported until now with its scope as a nutraceutical.

Canolol belongs to a new class of naturally derived compounds that show the antioxidant as 'promising' and implicates disease treatment in the near future. The future scope is supported by the current *in vitro* research data and there is no doubt that there is lack of data for *in vivo* research. The accumulated literature of vinyl phenol derivatives including vinyl syringol/canolol indicates the overwhelming role of these compounds in flavour and aroma of beer, wine and coffee (see Chapter 3). It has been already demonstrated to be effective in controlling oxidation in lipid model relevant to food. *In vitro* and *in vivo* studies conducted so far come to an agreement that, besides being a powerful antioxidant, it possesses numerous outstanding properties such as anti-inflammatory, anti-mutagenic, cytoprotective, anti-carcinogenic and so on. Canolol not only represses ROS by antioxidation mechanism, but it also boosts the expression of the enzymes responsible for allaying ROS. Canolol can also work effectively in lipid and aqueous media as well as signifies its capability to exert in physiological conditions.

Given the broad spectrum and the potent which is antioxidative in nature, besides being a good antioxidant in lipids, canolol can effectively be used as a dietary supplement in combating oxidative stress in living organisms. Canolol, as a constituent of canola/rapeseed oil, has already been residual mostly in crude oils. In this context, it can be presumed well that enriching oils with canolol will benefit the value of foods. Nevertheless, to further substantiate its claim, in disease and nutrition, human clinical trials would be necessary. If human trials are in line to the *in vitro* and *in vivo* studies, canolol can be positioned as a new powerful nutraceutical and hit the market in future.

ACKNOWLEDGEMENTS

We acknowledge all the North American Canola Crushers mentioned in this chapter and the Canola Council of Canada for their help in supplying us samples of canola oil and seeds for this research work. Financial support of this project by the Canola Council of Canada, NSERC and Syngenta Crop Protection Inc., Canada is gratefully acknowledged.

REFERENCES

Bailly, C. 2004. Active oxygen species and antioxidants in seed biology. *Seeds Sci. Res.* **14**: 99–107.

Cao, X., Tsukamoto, T., Seki, T., Tanaka, H., Morimura, S., Cao, L., Mizoshita, T. et al. 2008. 4-Vinyl-2,6-dimethoxyphenol (canolol) suppresses oxidative stress and gastric carcinogenesis in *Helicobacter pylori*-infected carcinogen-treated Mongolian gerbils. *Int. J. Cancer* **122**: 1445–1454.

Davies, K.J. 1995. Oxidative stress: The paradox of aerobic life. *Biochem. Soc. Symp.* **61**: 1–31.

D'Elios, M., Manghetti, M., De Carli, M., Costa, F., Baldari, C., Burroni, D., Telford, J., Romagnani, S. and Del Prete, G. 1997. T helper 1 effector cells specific for *Helicobacter pylori* in the gastric antrum of patients with peptic ulcer disease. *J. Immunol.* **158**: 962–967.

Demple, B. and Harrison, L. 1994. Repair of oxidative damage to DNA: Enzymology and biology. *Annu. Rev. Biochem.* **63**: 915–948.

Dong, X., Li, Z., Wang, W., Zhang, W., Liu, S. and Zhang, X. 2011. Protective effect of canolol from oxidative stress-induced cell damage in ARPE-19 cells via an ERK-mediated antioxidative pathway. *Mol. Vis.* **17**: 2040–2048.

Eunok Choe, E. and Min, D. 2006. Mechanisms and factors for edible oil oxidation. *Compr. Rev. Food Sci. Food Saf.* **5**: 169–186.

Frost and Sullivan, 2006. http://www.frost.com/srch/catalog-search.do?queryText=rosemary+solvent+extracts&x=46&y=18&pageSize=12 (access on July 24, 2012)

Frost and Sullivan, 2007. http://www.frost.com/srch/catalog-search.do?queryText=rosemary+solvent+extracts&x=46&y=18&pageSize=12 (Accessed on July 24, 2012)

Galano, A., Francisco-Marquez, M. and Alvarez-Idaboy, J. 2011. Canolol: A promising chemical agent against oxidative stress. *J. Phys. Chem. B.* **115**: 8590–8596.

Galano, A., Alvarez-Diduk, R., Ramirez-Silva, M.T., Alarcon-Angeles, G. and Rojas-Hernandez, A. 2009. Role of the reacting free radicals on the antioxidant mechanism of curcumin. *Chem. Phys.* **363**: 13–23.

Giddabasappa, A., Bauler, M., Yepuru, M., Chaum, E., Dalton, J.T. and Eswaraka, J. 2010. 17-β estradiol protects ARPE-19 cells from oxidative stress through estrogen receptor-β. *Invest. Ophthalmol. Vis. Sci.* **51**: 5278–5287.

Glotin, A.L., Calipel, A., Brossas, J.Y., Faussat, A.M., Tréton, J. and Mascarelli, F. 2006. Sustained versus transient ERK1/2 signaling underlies the anti- and proapoptotic effects of oxidative stress in human RPE cells. *Invest. Ophthalmol. Vis. Sci.* **47**: 4614–4623.

Harbaum-Piayda, B., Oehlke, K., Sönnichsen, F.D., Zacchi, P., Eggers, R. and Schwarz, K. 2010. New polyphenolic compounds in commercial deodistillate and rapeseed oils. *Food Chemistry.* **123**(3): 607–615.

Harris, P., Smythies, L., Smith, P. and Dubois, A. 2000. Inflammatory cytokine mRNA expression during early and persistent *Helicobacter pylori* infection in nonhuman primates. *J. Infect. Dis.* **181**: 783–786.

Khattab, R., Eskin, M., Aliani, M. and Thiyam, U. 2010. Determination of sinapic acid derivatives in canola extracts using high-performance liquid chromatography. *J. Am. Oil Chem. Soc.* **87**(2): 147–155.

Koski, A., Pekkarinen, S., Hopia, A., Wähälä, K. and Heinonen, M. 2003. Processing of rapeseed oil: Effects on sinapinic acid derivative content and oxidative stability. *Eur. Food. Res. Technol.* **217**: 110–114.

Kuwahara, H., Kanazawa, A., Wakamatsu, D., Morimura, S., Kida, K., Akaike, T. and Maeda, H. 2004. Antioxidative and antimutagenic activities of 4-vinyl-2,6-dimethoxyphenol (canolol) isolated from canola oil. *J. Agric. Food Chem.* **52**: 4380–4387.

Marnett, L. 2002. Oxy radicals, lipid peroxidation and DNA damage. *Toxicology* **181**: 219–222.

Osburn, W. and Kensler, T. 2008. Nrf2 signaling: An adaptive response pathway for protection against environmental toxic insults. *Mutat. Res.* **659**: 31–39.

Parsonnet, J., Friedman, G., Vandersteen, D., Chang, Y., Vogelman, J., Orentreich, N. and Sibley, R. 1991. *Helicobacter pylori* infection and the risk of gastric carcinoma. *N. Engl. J. Med.* **325**: 1127–1131.

Sawa, T., Akaike, T., Kida, K., Fukushima, Y., Takagi, K. and Maeda, H. 1998. Lipid peroxyl radicals from oxidised oils and heme iron: Implication of high fat diet in colon carcinogenesis. *Cancer Epidemiol. Biomark. Prev.* **7**: 1007–1012.

Seki, T., Morimura, S., Kida, K., Fang, J. and Maeda, M. 2006. Suppression of inflammatory cytokines including TNF-α, IL-12, antiNOS by a phenolic compound, obtained from crude canola oil. *Nitric Oxide* **14**: A17–A19.

Shackelford, R., Kaufmann, W. and Paules, R. 2000. Oxidative stress and cell cycle checkpoint function. *Free Radic. Biol. Med.* **28**: 1387–1404.

Spielmeyer, A., Wagner, A. and Jahreis, G. 2009. Influence of thermal treatment of rapeseed on the canolol content. *Food Chem.* **112**: 944–948.

Thiyam-Holländer, U. 2012. Unpublished Annual Project Report submitted to NSERC, Canola Council of Canada and Syngenta Inc in 2012.

Tsunehiro, J., Yasuda, F., Wakamatsu, D. and Nakai, C. 2001. Isolation and characterization of lipid-radical scavenging component in crude canola oil. In: *Third International Conference and Exhibition on Nutraceuticals and Functional Foods, from Laboratory to the Real World and the Marketplace*, Nov. 17–20, 2002; San Diego, CA; American Oil Chemists' Society: Champaign, IL.

Veldsink, J.W., Muuse, B.G., Meijer, M.M.T., Cuperus, F.P., v.d. Sande, R.L.K.M. and v. Putte, K.P.A.M. 1999. Heat pretreatment of oilseeds: Effect on oil quality. *Fett. Lipid* **101**: 244–248.

Vuorela, S., Meyer, A.S. and Heinonen, M. 2003. Quantitative analysis of the main phenolics in rapeseed meal and oils processed differently using enzymatic hydrolysis and HPLC. *European Food Research and Technology* **217**: 517–523.

Wakamatsu, D. 2001. Isolation and identification of radical scavenging compound, canolol, in canola oil. MS Thesis, Graduate School of Natural Science, Kumamoto University, pp. 1–48.

Wakamatsu, D., Morimura, S., Sawa, T., Kida, K. and Nakai, C. 2005. Isolation, identification, and structure of a potent Alkyl-Peroxyl radical scavenger in crude canola oil. *Biosci. Biotechnol. Biochem.* **69**: 1568–1574.

Wang, X., Martindale, J., Liu, Y. and Holbrook, N. 1998. The cellular response to oxidative stress: Influences of mitogen-activated protein kinase signaling pathways on cell survival. *Biochem. J.* **333**: 291–300.

Yamaoka, Y., Yamauchi, K., Ota, H., Sugiyama, A., Ishizone, S., Graham, D., Maruta, F., Murakami, M. and Katsuyama, T. 2005. Natural history of gastric mucosal cytokine expression in *Helicobacter pylori* gastritis in Mongolian gerbils. *Infect. Immun.* **73**: 2205–2212.

Zacchi, P. and Eggers, R. 2008. High-temperature pre-conditioning of rapeseed: A polyphenol-enriched oil and the effect of refining. *Eur J Lipid Sci Technol* **110**: 111–119.

Index

A

AACCI, *see* American Association of Cereal Chemists International (AACCI)
ACBP, *see* Acyl-CoA-binding protein (ACBP)
ACCase, *see* Acetyl-CoA carboxylase (ACCase)
ACE-inhibitory peptides, *see* Angiotensin I-converting enzyme-inhibitory peptides (ACE-inhibitory peptides)
Acetyl-CoA carboxylase (ACCase), 103, 104
  cytosolic homomeric, 113
  down-regulation of, 303
  as rate-limiting enzyme, 263
Acid value (AV), 229
  anti-oxidant effect on, 228
  biodiesel, 223, 230, 228
  blended biodiesel-petroleum diesel fuel, 225
  omega-9 oils, 84
  thiobarbituric, 7
ACO, *see* Acyl-CoA oxidase (ACO)
ACP, *see* Acyl carrier protein (ACP)
Activation energy, 232
  of rate-determining step, 232, 235
Acute-phase proteins, 266
Acyl carrier protein (ACP), 104
Acyl-CoA-binding protein (ACBP), 104
Acyl-CoA oxidase (ACO), 262
Acyl-editing reactions, 103, 105
Acyltransferases, 113
  palmitoleic acid into TAG, 107
  in TAG bioassembly pathway, 104
Additives
  food, 52
  low-temperature, 227
  for plastic films, 201
Adequate intake (AI), 256
Adipocyte dysfunction, 266
Adipokine hormones, 266
Adult Treatment Panel diagnostic criteria (ATP III diagnostic criteria), 254
AI, *see* Adequate intake (AI)
AIBN, *see* 2, 2′-Azobisisobutyronitrile (AIBN)
A-IV-S, 62; *see also* Canola protein
ALA, *see* Alpha-linolenic acid (ALA)
Alkaline earth metal oxides, 219
Alpha-linolenic acid (ALA), 104, 246, 252
  measurement, 139–140
  rapeseed oil, 278
Alpha-toco, *see* Tocopherol (Alpha-toco)
AME, *see* Apparent metabolizable energy (AME)
American Association of Cereal Chemists International (AACCI), 130
American Oil Chemists' Society (AOCS
American Society for Testing and Materials (ASTM), 222
America Oil Chemists' Society (AOCS), 126, 222
Angiotensin I-converting enzyme-inhibitory peptides (ACE-inhibitory peptides), 160
Anisidine value, 210; *see also* Peroxide value (PV)
ANN, *see* Artificial neural network (ANN)
Anti-inflammatory agent, 33
Antioxidants, 22, 34, 279
  canolol, 28–29
  dietary, 22
  full paths, 337
  against oxidative deterioration, 296
  phenolic, 22
  reagents, 228
  reduction potential of, 345
  rice bran, 159
  sinapine, 27–28
AOCS, *see* America Oil Chemists' Society (AOCS)
APCI, *see* Atmospheric pressure chemical ionization (APCI)
apoB, *see* Apolipoprotein B (apoB)
Apolipoprotein B (apoB), 255
Apparent metabolizable energy (AME), 31
Aquaculture, 109, 199
  development of, 201
ARA, *see* Arachidonic acid (ARA)
Arachidonic acid (ARA), 110, 111
  conditional essential fatty acids, 301
Aroma compounds, 49, 182; *see also* Phenolic compound
Arrhenius plot, 235
Artificial neural network (ANN), 131
ASTM, *see* American Society for Testing and Materials (ASTM)
Atmospheric pressure chemical ionization (APCI), 27
ATP III diagnostic criteria, *see* Adult Treatment Panel diagnostic criteria (ATP III diagnostic criteria)
Auto-oxidation, 279, 291
AV, *see* Acid value (AV)
2,2′-Azobisisobutyronitrile (AIBN), 46

B

Barton decarboxylation, 46–47
β-Keto-acyl-ACP synthase (KAS), 108
Beta-sitosterol, 153
BHA, *see* Butylated hydroxylanisole (BHA)
BHT, *see* Butylated hydroxytoluene (BHT)
Bioactive extraction, 160
Bioactive phytochemicals, 159
Biodiesel, 217
  advantages of, 217
  anti-oxidants, 228
  CAN/CGS B-3, 520, 225
  chemical solution model, 237
  CN, 226
  consumption, 82
  disadvantages of, 217
  ethanolysis, 219
  fuel flow property, 226
  fuel standards, 225, 223–224
  heating value of, 222
  low temperature property of, 227
  lubricity property of, 233–237
  mustard oil as feedstock, 220–222
  oxidation, 227
  plants in Canada, 238
  production forecast, 81, 229–230, 237–239
  PV of, 229
  quality, 222–229
  rancimat test, 228–229
  reaction kinetics, 230–233
  reaction step rate constant, 234
  soyabean oil and, 82
  transesterification, 217, 218, 228
  vegetable oils, 217
  wear scar diameter of, 236
BioExx Specialty Proteins Ltd., 76
Biorefining model, 162
BL, *see* Boundary lubrication (BL)
Blended biodiesel-petroleum diesel fuel, 225
BMI, *see* Body mass index (BMI)
Body mass index (BMI), 253–254
BOS, *see* *Brassica* oilseed species (BOS)
BOS seed oil content modification, 112
Boundary lubrication (BL), 236
Brassica, 101, 220; *see also* Mustards
  napus L., spp. *oleifera*, *see* Rapeseed
  rapa L. species, *see* Canola oil (Canadian oil, low acid)
  shikimate/phenylpropanoid pathway, 23
  sinapine and related compounds distribution in, 23
Brassica oilseed species (BOS), 101, 115–116
  chain elongation, 104
  erucic acid, 102
  FA modifications, 102
  GE, 102
  high-oleic, low-alpha-linolenic oils, 106–107
  oil production, 109–112
  oil with altered saturated fatty acid content, 107–109
  seed oil composition modification, 106
  seed oil content modification, 112–115
  seed oil formation pathways in, 102–106
Brassicasterol, 153
Burcon NutraScience Corporation, 75
Burcon's process, 75
Butylated hydroxylanisole (BHA), 279, 287
Butylated hydroxytoluene (BHT), 228, 279, 325

C

CA, *see* Caffeic acid (CA)
Caffeic acid (CA), 287
  free radical scavenging activity comparison, 287
Calibration curve
  for DPPH radicals, 286
  ED_{50} calculation, 325
  for RSA, 288
Canadian Diabetes Association (CDA), 260
Canadian oil, low acid, *see* Canola oil (Canadian oil, low acid)
Canadian Renewable Fuels Association (CRFA), 237
Canola, 2, 22, 59, 246, 252; *see also* Antioxidant; Canolol
  bioactive extraction, 147–155, 158, 160
  canolol content, 54
  clouding time at various sediment concentrations, 12
  crude oil in, 137
  development of, 3–4, 246
  essential amino acid content of, 61
  essential oil extraction, 155
  fathers of, 3
  fatty acids of, 139
  high-oleic, 205
  history, 2
  meal, 252
  minor components, 12–16
  phenolic compounds of, 281–282
  Polish type, 2
  production, 60
  protein content of oil-free, 59
  quality, 127
  room odour, 6
  saturated FAs, 107
  sedimentation phenomenon, 9–12
  sediment composition, 10
  sediment oil mixture DSC thermal curves, 11
  and soyabeans composition comparison, 60
  standard, 175

trace elements found in, 268
type oils, 104
Canola oil (Canadian oil, low acid), 2, 125, 183, 252, 317; *see also* Virgin canola oil processing
chlorophyll effect on, 126
components in, 9
consumers, 96–97
as cooking oil, 33
and CVD, 246
determination coefficients, 6
effect on lipid oxidation, 247–248
extractions, 125–126
fatty acids in extracted, 9, 151, 255
future research, 269
heating effects on chemical and sensory indices of oxidation of, 7
LNA into n-3 LC-PUFA, 248
low linolenic acid canola oil stability, 8–9
metabolic effects of, 261
minor components of, 268
obesity and insulin resistance, 252
oil, 2, 4–6
protein, 126
qualified health claim for, 95–96
regression equations for rancidity assessment methods, 6
response of serum lipids to, 246–247
shelf-life stability assessment, 16
storage effect, 8
titanium–hydroperoxide formation and absorption spectra, 5
tocopherols, 14–15
TPC over frying time for, 14
unique characteristic of, 246
Canola oil, cold-pressed; *see also* Virgin canola oil processing
influence of press parameters on quality, 179
influence of seed material on quality, 174
sensory assessment, 172–173
Canola oil fatty acids
as modulators of obesity and IR, 255
monounsaturated FA vs. saturated FA, 256–257
MUFA vs. carbohydrate, 260
polyunsaturated fatty acids, 257–260
synergistic effects of, 260–261
Canola oil metabolic effects, 261
adipose function and inflammatory markers, 266–267
fatty acid-independent mechanisms, 268–269
fatty acids and insulin signalling, 267–268
liver fatty acid metabolism, 265–266
PPAR and PUFAs, 262
relationship of MUFA to PPARs and SREBPs, 264
SREBP and PUFA, 263
tissue lipid accumulation and FA composition, 264–265
transcription factor regulation, 261
Canola protein, 62, 70
commercial canola processing, 66
dissolution of, 63
functional properties, 64, 65
isolation, 73, 75
Karr column, 69
meal, 65–68
membrane-based process, 74
membrane separation for, 71–73
protein concentrates, 68–70
protein isolates, 70
recovery, 71
Canola seed; *see also* Virgin canola oil processing
dehulling of, 180
deterioration by moisture, 178
Canolol, 24, 34; *see also* Canola; Vinylphenols
anti-alkylperoxyl radical activity of, 34
anticancerous effects, 32–33
antimutagenic activities, 32
antioxidant activity of, 28–29
bioactivities of, 32
content, 54
formation of, 24–25
generation from substituted cinnamic acid, 50–51
molecular structure of, 24
oxidative stability by, 323
production by thermal treatment, 54
protective effects on damages, 33–34
synthesis and estimation of, 25–27
Carboxylic acids, 39
decarboxylation, 40, 41–42, 44, 50
Cardiovascular disease (CVD), 245
hypertension and, 255
obesity and, 253
risk indicator, 248–249
Catalysts
alkoxides, 219
homogeneous acid, 219, 220
homogeneous base, 219
silver, 44
solid acid, 227
CDA, *see* Canadian Diabetes Association (CDA)
Cetane (Hexadecane), 226
Cetane number (CN), 226
of biodiesel, 223
of blended fuel, 225
CFPP, *see* Cold filter plugging point (CFPP)
Chemometric analyses, 131
Chemo-protective compounds, 162
Chlorophyll, 138, 179
in canola oil, 268
on canola seed quality, 126

Chlorophyll (*Continued*)
derivatives in canola seed, 138
measurement, 138–139
prediction by NIRS, 130, 133, 135, 136
reference method for, 139
Cinnamic acids, 49
decarboxylation of, 51
derivatives, 280
RSA and, 288
Clearfield®, 83
Cloud point (CP), 226
of biodiesel, 224
blended fuel, 225
CN, *see* Cetane number (CN)
Coefficient of variation (CV), 132
Cold filter plugging point (CFPP), 226
Conditional essential fatty acids, 301
Corn oil, 82
cholesterol reduction, 247
consumer preference, 96
tumour development, 332
COX-2, *see* Cyclooxygenase-2 (COX-2)
CP, *see* Cloud point (CP)
C-reactive protein (CRP), 255
CRFA, *see* Canadian Renewable Fuels Association (CRFA)
CRP, *see* C-reactive protein (CRP)
CV, *see* Coefficient of variation (CV)
CVD, *see* Cardiovascular disease (CVD)
Cyclooxygenase-2 (COX-2), 33

D

DAG, *see* Diacylglyceride (DAG); Diacylglycerol (DAG)
DAS, *see* Dow AgroSciences (DAS)
DBU, *see* 1,8-Diazabicyclo[5.4.0]undec-7-ene (DBU)
Decarboxylation, 40
β-ketocarboxylic acids, 40–41
canolol formation, 320, 321, 337
and canolol production, 54–55
of free carboxylic acids, 44
involving enzymes, 51–54
for vinylphenol generation, 49, 50
4-vinylphenols by, 26
Decarboxylation, transition metal-catalysed, 41
Barton decarboxylation, 46–47
copper-catalysed decarboxylation, 41
mercury-catalysed decarboxylation, 43
Pd-catalysed decarboxylation, 44–46
silver-catalysed decarboxylation, 43
substituted cinnamic acid transformation, 47–48
Deodorizer distillate fraction, 153
Deoiling process, 190, 192–193
Desolventizer toaster (DT), 66, 192
DF, *see* Diafiltration (DF)
DGAT, *see* Diacylglycerol acyltransferase (DGAT)
DGF, *see* German Society for Fat Science (DGF)
DGF Canola Oil Award, 182–183, 184
DHA, *see* Docosahexaenoic acid (DHA)
Diacylglyceride (DAG), 218
in biodiesel, 223
and rate-determining step, 232
transesterification, 218, 231–232
Diacylglycerol (DAG), 105, *see* Diacylglyceride
Diacylglycerol acyltransferase (DGAT), 105
Diafiltration (DF), 73
1,8-Diazabicyclo[5.4.0]undec-7-ene (DBU), 26, 50
Dietary antioxidants, 22; *see also* Antioxidants
Diet-induced obesity (DIO), 257
Differential scanning calorimetry (DSC), 11, 226, 230
Dimethylformamide (DMF), 44
Dimethyl sulfoxide (DMSO), 44
DIO, *see* Diet-induced obesity (DIO)
1,1-Diphenyl-2-picrylhydrazyl (DPPH), 285, 325
antioxidant activity of canolol, 324
for caffeic acid, 288
calibration curve for, 286
free radical scavenging, 285–286
measurement of the free radical, 326
scavenged by methanolic extract, 289–291, 324
DM2, *see* Type 2 diabetes mellitus (DM2)
DMF, *see* Dimethylformamide (DMF)
DMSO, *see* Dimethyl sulfoxide (DMSO)
Docosahexaenoic acid (DHA), 97–98, 263, 301
accumulation inhibition, 111
ALA into, 265
CVD reduction, 302
for human health, 109
oxidation, 304
Double low rapeseed, 4, 139, *see* Canola
Double zero rapeseed, 22
Dow AgroSciences (DAS), 83
analytical lab, 84
omega-9 canola oil in, 97–98
DPPH, *see* 1,1-Diphenyl-2-picrylhydrazyl (DPPH)
DSC, *see* Differential scanning calorimetry (DSC)
DT, *see* Desolventizer toaster (DT)
Dyslipidaemia, 254

E

EAR, *see* Estimated average requirement (EAR)
EHL, *see* Elastohydrodynamic lubrication (EHL)
Eicosapentaenoic acid (EPA), 109, 256
conditional essential fatty acids, 301
on serum cholesterol, 247
Elastohydrodynamic lubrication (EHL), 235

Elevated plus-maze (EPM), 31
EPA, *see* Eicosapentaenoic acid (EPA)
EPM, *see* Elevated plus-maze (EPM)
ERK, *see* Extracellular signal-regulated kinase (ERK)
Erucic acid, 80, 102, 220
in canola oil, 4
content, 139
control of, 3
and edibility, 278
elongation of, 112
to increase, 112, 114
industrial application, 111
inhibition, 104, 246
in mustard oil, 220
toxocity, 220
zero-erucic-acid, 111
Erwinia uredovora, 52
Essential fatty acids, 300
conditional, 301
Essential oil extraction, 155
SC-CO_2, 157–158
ultrasonication, 156
ultrasound, 155, 157
Estimated average requirement (EAR), 256
Ethanol polarity, 219
Ethanolysis, 219
Extracellular signal-regulated kinase (ERK), 33, 343

F

FA, *see* Fatty acid (FA); Ferulic acid (FA)
FAAE, *see* Fatty acid acyl ester (FAAE)
FACS, *see* Fatty acyl-CoA synthase (FACS)
FAE, *see* Fatty acid elongase (FAE)
FAMEs, *see* Fatty acid methyl esters (FAMEs)
FAO, *see* Food and Agriculture Organization (FAO)
FAS, *see* Fatty acid synthase (FAS)
Fathers of canola, 3
Fatty acid (FA), 102, 151, 158; *see also* Polyunsaturated fatty acid (PUFA); Saturated fatty acids (SFA); *Trans*-fatty acid; Triacylglyceride (TAG)
biosynthesis, 104
in canola oil, 9, 10
carbon–hydrogen bond positions in, 228
composition and tissue lipid accumulation, 264–265
dietary guidelines, 97
free fatty acids, 127
during frying, 209
frying stability, 13
furan, 309
hyperlipidaemia, 302
independent mechanisms, 268–269
and insulin signalling, 267–268
liver fatty acid metabolism, 265–266
medium chain saturated fatty acids, 108
of mustard oil, 220
oxidative stability of vegetable oils, 16
roasting effect, 324
in seed oil biosynthesis, 103
Fatty acid acyl ester (FAAE), 217
Fatty acid elongase (FAE), 104
Fatty acid methyl esters (FAMEs), 127
Fatty acid synthase (FAS), 104, 263
Fatty acyl-CoA synthase (FACS), 262
FDA, *see* U.S. Food and Drug Administration (FDA)
FDS, *see* Flash desolventizers (FDS)
Federation of Oils. Seeds and Fats Associations (FOSFA), 125
instrument calibration method, 128
oil extraction, 147
Ferulic acid (FA), 287
aroma compounds, 49
decarboxylase, 54
radical scavenging, 287
FFA, *see* Free fatty acid (FFA)
Filtration, 181
Flash desolventizers (FDS), 195
Flavour deterioration, 300
Flaxseed oil (FXCO), 95, 260
consumer preference, 96
Flow-mediated dialatation (FMD), 249
Fluidized bed, 196
Fluidized-bed desolventizer system, 196
batch, 200
continuous, 200
desolventized rapeseed meal, 199
economic data, 199
energy requirements, 198
operation modes, 197
small pilot-scale, 197
FMD, *see* Flow-mediated dialatation (FMD)
Food and Agriculture Organization (FAO), 188
FOSFA, *see* Federation of Oils. Seeds and Fats Associations (FOSFA)
Fourier-Transform (FT), 131
Fourier-Transform-NIR (FT-NIR), 131
Free fatty acid (FFA), 90, 150
analysis, 127
in canola oil, 208
in canola oil sediment, 9, 10
degradation, 179
during frying, 91, 209
insulin effect, 254
saponification prevention, 219
and sensory impression, 176
solubility, 147
storage condition and, 178
triglyceride solubility and, 150, 152

Free induction decay, 128
Free radicals, 22
Free radical scavenging, 286; *see also* Antioxidant
  DPPH radicals, 285–286, 289, 291
  rapeseed extracts, 288–291
  sinapic acid, 286–288
  sinapine, 286
  sinapoyl glucose, 286
Frying, 203–204
  doughnut, 93–94
  oil polymerization, 84–85
  oleic acid for high-stability frying, 102
  polar compounds formation, 90, 91, 207
  total tocopherols, 15
Frying medium, 203; *see also* High-oleic, low-linolenic oils (HOLL oils); Oil; Totox value
  alternatives to, 205
  chemical parameters, 206–208
  economical aspects, 203
  health aspects of, 204–205
  influence on fried product storage stability, 210–214
  linolenic acid, 205
  stability of, 203–204
Fry life, 85–86
FT, *see* Fourier-Transform (FT)
FT-NIR, *see* Fourier-Transform-NIR (FT-NIR)
FXCO, *see* Flaxseed oil (FXCO)

G

Gamma-linolenic acid (GLA), 110
γ-Oryzanols, 159
Gas chromatography (GC), 127
  static headspace, 292, 296
Gas chromatography-mass spectrometry (GC-MS), 306
Gas liquid chromatography (GLC), 3
GC, *see* Gas chromatography (GC)
GC-MS, *see* Gas chromatography-mass spectrometry (GC-MS)
GE, *see* Genetically engineered (GE)
Genetically engineered (GE), 102
German Society for Fat Science (DGF), 182
GL, *see* Glycerol (GL)
GLA, *see* Gamma-linolenic acid (GLA)
GLC, *see* Gas liquid chromatography (GLC)
Glucopyranosyl sinapate, 22, 23
Glycerol (GL), 218
  in transesterification, 233
sn-Glycerol-3-phosphate acyltransferase (GPAT), 105
GP, *see* Sinapoyl glucose (GP)
GPAT, *see sn*-Glycerol-3-phosphate acyltransferase (GPAT)
Grain Research Laboratory (GRL), 9
Green protocol, 47
GRL, *see* Grain Research Laboratory (GRL)

H

Half-seed method, 3
HDL, *see* High-density lipoprotein (HDL)
HDL-C, *see* High-density lipoprotein cholesterol (HDL-C)
HEAR, *see* High-erucic-acid rapeseed (HEAR)
Heterogeneous acid catalysts, 220
Heterogeneous base catalysts, 219
Hidden oxidation, 310
High-density lipoprotein (HDL), 204, 255, 302
High-density lipoprotein cholesterol (HDL-C), 246, 254
  T/HDL-C ratio, 248
High-erucic-acid rapeseed (HEAR), 111
High-oleic acid (Hi-OA), 247, 248
High oleic acid canola oil (HOCO), 13
  fatty acid profile, 252
  frying stability, 14
  oxidative stability, 278
  PUFAs for, 13
  response of serum lipids to, 247
High oleic and low linolenic acid canola oil (HOLLCO), 13
  PUFAs for, 13
  TPC formation, 14
High-oleic, low-linolenic oils (HOLL oils), 106, 209; *see also* Frying medium
  canola oil, 209
  during frying, 206
  frying media comparison, 208–210
  frying medium chemical parameters, 206–208
  frying performance, 206
  polar compounds in, 207
  product sensory quality, 206
  sensory evaluation, 207
High-oleic, low-*trans* (HOLT), 210
High-oleic rapeseed (canola) oil (HOCO), 95
High-oleic sunflower oils (HOSO), 205, 206
High-palmitic, low-*trans* (HPLT), 210
High pressure liquid chromatography (HPLC), 282
  crude soyabean oil, 306
  using Merck-Hitachi low-pressure-gradient system, 319
  methanolic extract estimation, 283, 284
  oxidized TAG molecule analysis, 304
  of virgin canola oil, 319
High-*trans* (HT), 210
Hi-OA, *see* High-oleic acid (Hi-OA)

HIPLEX®, 193
HOCO, *see* High oleic acid canola oil (HOCO); High-oleic rapeseed (canola) oil (HOCO)
HOLLCO, *see* High oleic and low linolenic acid canola oil (HOLLCO)
HOLL oils, *see* High-oleic, low-linolenic oils (HOLL oils)
HOLT, *see* High-oleic, low-*trans* (HOLT)
HOMA, *see* Homeostatic model assessment (HOMA)
Homeostatic model assessment (HOMA), 254, 259
Homogeneous acid catalysts, 219
Homogeneous base catalysts, 219
HOSO, *see* High-oleic sunflower oils (HOSO)
HPLC, *see* High pressure liquid chromatography (HPLC)
HPLT, *see* High-palmitic, low-*trans* (HPLT)
HT, *see* High-*trans* (HT)
HV, *see* Hydroperoxide value (HV)
HydCan, *see* Hydrogenated canola (HydCan)
Hydrogenated canola (HydCan), 87
Hydrogenated soyabean oil (HydSoy), 87
Hydroperoxide value (HV), 5, 8
Hydroxycinnamate decarboxylase, 54
Hydroxycinnamic acids, 49; *see also* Sinapic acid
    correlation between RSA of extracts and total, 288
    in food sources, 49
    4-vinyl derivatives of, 50
8-Hydroxy-20-deoxyguanosine (8-OHdG), 33
HydSoy, *see* Hydrogenated soyabean oil (HydSoy)
Hypertension, 255

I

Iatroscan, 16
IDL, *see* Intermediate density lipoprotein (IDL)
Ignition delay time, 222, 226
IL, *see* Interleukin (IL)
Inducible nitric oxide synthase (iNOS), 33, 344
Induction time, 229
Inflammatory mediators, 255
Infrared spectrum, 130
iNOS, *see* Inducible nitric oxide synthase (iNOS)
Insulin receptor substrate (IRS), 267
Insulin resistance (IR), 252, 253, 269
    assessment methods, 253–254
    canola oil fatty ac ids as modulators of, 255
    high SFA-diet, 256
    metabolic syndrome, 254–255
    effect of n-3 PUFAs, 264
Insulin signalling pathway, 267
Interferometers, 131
Interleukin (IL), 32, 255
Intermediate density lipoprotein (IDL), 255
International Organization for Standardization (ISO), 125
Iodine value (IV), 229
IP, *see* Isoelectric point (IP)
IR, *see* Insulin resistance (IR)
IRS, *see* Insulin receptor substrate (IRS)
ISO, *see* International Organization for Standardization (ISO)
Isoelectric point (IP), 190
Isolexx, 76; *see also* Canola protein
IV, *see* Iodine value (IV)

K

KA, *see* Kainic acid (KA)
Kainic acid (KA), 30
Karr column, 69
KAS, *see* β-Keto-acyl-ACP synthase (KAS)
KCS, *see* 3-keto-acyl-CoA synthase (KCS)
3-Keto-acyl-CoA synthase (KCS), 112

L

LA, *see* Linoleic acid (LA)
LDL, *see* Low-density lipoprotein (LDL)
LDL-C, *see* Low-density lipoprotein cholesterol (LDL-C)
Linoleic acid (LA), 104, 246, 252
    dietary, 257
    mono-hydroperoxide, 306, 308
    N-3, 258
    oils, 249
    oxidative stability, 304
Lipoprotein lipase (LPL), 254
LLCan, *see* Low linolenic canola (LLCan)
LLCO, *see* Low linolenic acid canola oil (LLCO)
LLSoy, *see* Low linolenic soyabean (LLSoy)
Long-chain omega-3 PUFA (n-3 LC-PUFA), 248
Low-density lipoprotein (LDL), 28, 152, 204
Low-density lipoprotein cholesterol (LDL-C), 245–246
LowLin, *see* Low α-linolenic acid canola (LowLin)
Low linolenic acid canola oil (LLCO), 13
    TPC formation, 13, 14
Low linolenic canola (LLCan), 86
Low linolenic soyabean (LLSoy), 87
Low α-linolenic acid canola (LowLin), 139
LPAAT, *see* Lysophosphatidic acid acyltransferase (LPAAT)
LPCAT, *see* Lysophosphatidylcholine acyltransferase (LPCAT)
LPL, *see* Lipoprotein lipase (LPL)
Lubricating property, fuel, 233

Lysophosphatidic acid acyltransferase (LPAAT), 105
Lysophosphatidylcholine acyltransferase (LPCAT), 104

M

MAG, *see* Mono-acyl-glyceride (MAG)
Magnetic nuclear resonance, 127
Malonyl-CoA, 263
Mass transfer, 146
- kinetics and seed moisture content, 150
- rates of fatty acids, 150
- resistance, 218
- of TAG, 219

MCFA, *see* Medium-chain saturated fatty acids (MCFA)
Meal desolventizing, 195
Medium-chain saturated fatty acids (MCFA), 108
- containing species, 109

MeLo, *see* Methyl linoleate (MeLo)
Membrane, 72
- based canola protein isolation, 73, 74
- processing, 72
- separation, 72
- technology, 71

Metabolic syndrome, 255
Methanolic extract fractionation, 282, 285
- DPPH radical scavenging activity, 291
- free radical scavenging activity, 288
- HPLC chromatograms of, 284
- phenolic content, 283

Methyl linoleate (MeLo), 27
MF, *see* Microfiltration (MF)
Microfiltration (MF), 72
Mid-infrared (MIR), 131
Mid oleic sunflower (MidSUN), 87
MidSUN, *see* Mid oleic sunflower (MidSUN)
MIR, *see* Mid-infrared (MIR)
Molecular weight cut-off (MWCO), 72
Mono-acyl-glyceride (MAG), 218, 219; *see also* Transesterification
Monounsaturated fatty acid (MUFA), 245, 252
- vs. carbohydrate, 260
- effects on adipose function, 266
- in preventing hepatic steatosis, 265
- relationship to PPARs and SREBP, 264
- role of dietary, 264
- vs. saturated fatty acids, 256

MUFA, *see* Monounsaturated fatty acid (MUFA)
Mustard oil, 229
- activation energy, 232, 235
- biodiesel production from, 229–230
- fatty acid compositions of, 221
- properties of, 230
- reaction step rate constants during transesterification of, 234

Mustards, 220; *see also* Biodiesel; *Brassica*
- Canadian production, 222
- fatty acid compositions, 220, 221

MWCO, *see* Molecular weight cut-off (MWCO)

N

NAFLD, *see* Non-alcoholic fatty liver disease (NAFLD)
Nanofiltration (NF), 72
Natural turbid oil, 181
Near-infrared (NIR), 130
- α-linolenic acid content analysis, 137
- chlorophyll content analysis, 136
- instruments, 131
- oil content analysis, 135
- protein content analysis, 135
- spectrophotometry, 127

Near-infrared analysis, 130; *see also* Oil content measurement
- α-linolenic acid analysis, 137, 139
- chlorophyll measurement, 138
- oil and protein measurements, 135, 136

Near-infrared spectroscopy (NIRS), 130; *see also* Oil content measurement
- advantages and disadvantages of, 133
- calibration model, 131
- diode array, 131
- of intact canola seeds, 132
- parameters affecting NIR results, 132
- verification result examples, 134

Nervonic acid, 112
NF, *see* Nanofiltration (NF)
n–9 Fatty acids, *see* Omega-9 fatty acids
NIR, *see* Near-infrared (NIR)
NIRS, *see* Near-infrared spectroscopy (NIRS)
n-3 LC-PUFA, *see* Long-chain omega-3 PUFA (n-3 LC-PUFA)
NMR, *see* Nuclear magnetic resonance (NMR)
Non-alcoholic fatty liver disease (NAFLD), 255
Nonvolatile degradation products, 177
n-Propyl gallate (PG), 228
Nuclear magnetic resonance (NMR), 92; *see also* Pulse NMR
- oil content analysis, 130
- pulse, 127

Nutraceutical-grade phospholipids, 162

O

OA, *see* Oleic acid (OA)
Obesity, 252
- assessment methods, 253–254
- canola oil fatty acids as modulators of, 255

high SFA-diet, 256
metabolic syndrome, 254–255
OCT, *see* Onset crystallization temperature (OCT)
Odour Intensity Value (OIV), 5
OGTT, *see* Oral glucose tolerance test (OGTT)
8-OHdG, *see* 8-Hydroxy-20-deoxyguanosine (8-OHdG)
Oil, 125, 128, 174; *see also* Canola oil; Essential oil extraction; Mustard oil; Oilseed; Omega-9 oils
polymerization, 84–85
Oil and bioactive component extraction, 147; *see also* Supercritical CO_2 (SC-CO_2)
conventional hexane extraction, 150
deodorizer distillate fraction, 153
explosions, 154
FOSFA method, 147
glucosinolates, 153
mechanical treatment, 154
SC-CO_2 operating parameter manipulation, 155
SFE, 147
Oil content measurement, 125; *see also* Near-infrared spectroscopy (NIRS); Near-infrared analysis; Pulse NMR
α-linolenic acid measurement, 139–140
chlorophyll measurement, 138–139
NIR analysis, 130–135, 136
oil and protein measurements, 136–138
pulse NMR, 127–129
Oil-in-water (O/W), 278, 296
Oilseed
bioactive extraction, 158
BOS, 101
components, 128, 337
inedible, 3
North American oilseeds complex, 81, 82
oil in, 128
production, 60
rape, 147
ultrasonic and SC-CO_2 applications in processing of, 145, 160
OIV, *see* Odour Intensity Value (OIV)
Oleic acid (OA), 80, 245, 252; *see also* High-oleic acid (Hi-OA); High oleic acid canola oil (HOCO); Omega-9 fatty acids
melting point, 220
position, 16
sources, 80, 81
Oleosins, 66
Omega-3 fatty acids, 332
in colon tissue, 333
tumour suppression, 333
Omega-9 fatty acids, 80; *see also* Oleic acid
Dow Agrosciences' Omega-9 Canola Programme, 83
list of, 80
North American oilseeds situation, 81–83
oilseeds complex, 82
shortening, 92–93, 94
U.S. food industry oil consumption, 82
ω–9 fatty acids, *see* Omega-9 fatty acids
Omega-9 oils, 79, 98
consumers, 96–97
and DHA blend, 97–98
doughnut frying, 93, 94
fatty acid profile and OSI, 83
frying, 85
fry life, 85
fry oil comparison, 86–91
health claim, 95–96
melting points of, 93
next generation of, 97
polymerization chart, 85
properties of, 84
spray oil application, 91–92
trans fat removal, 95
ultra low-saturated fat sunflower oil, 97
US dietary guidelines, 97
Onset crystallization temperature (OCT), 226
Oral glucose tolerance test (OGTT), 254
OSI, *see* Oxidative Stability Index (OSI)
O/W, *see* Oil-in-water (O/W)
Oxidative stability, 91, 106
antioxidants for, 279
by canolol, 323324
canolol effect on
fatty acid and, 300
and high oleic acid, 205, 308
HOLL canola oil, 209
for improved, 205
omega-9, 93
of PUFA, 304
as quality parameter, 173
of rapeseed and canola oils, 152, 278–279, 304–305
and unsaturation, 106
Oxidative Stability Index (OSI), 83
Oxidized LDL (ox-LDL), 247
ox-LDL, *see* Oxidized LDL (ox-LDL)

P

Palmitoyl thioesterase, 106
Palm olein (PO), 205, 206, 208
fatty acid profile and OSI of, 83
sensory evaluation with, 207, 214
Palmolein, *see* Palm olein (PO)
PAP, *see* Phosphatidic acid phosphatase (PAP)
Partial least squares regression (PLS), 131

Partially hydrogenated canola oil (PHCO), 206, 208
polar compounds, 207
sensory evaluation with, 207
Partially hydrogenated fats (PHF), 210
Partially hydrogenated vegetable oil (PHVO), 247
PC, *see* Phosphatidylcholine (PC)
p CA, see *p*-Coumaric acid (*p* CA)
p-Coumaric acid (*p* CA), 287
bacterial decarboxylation, 54
formation, 25
radical scavenging activity, 287
p-Coumaric acid decarboxylases (PDCs), 51
PDAT, *see* Phospholipid:diacylglycerol acyltransferase (PDAT)
PDCs, *see* *p*-Coumaric acid decarboxylases (PDCs)
PDCT, *see* Phosphatidyl choline:diacylglycerol choline phosphotransferase (PDCT)
PDHK, *see* Pyruvate dehydrogenase kinase (PDHK)
PDI, *see* Protein dispersibility index (PDI)
PDSC, *see* Pressurized differential scanning calorimeter (PDSC)
Pegylated zinc protoporphyrin (PEGZnPP), 32
PEGZnPP, *see* Pegylated zinc protoporphyrin (PEGZnPP)
Peptide bond, 137–138
Peroxide value (PV), 229, 278; *see also* Anisidine value
quality indicator, 158, 292
reversion, 308
totox value, 210–212
Peroxisome proliferator-activated receptors (PPARs), 261
EPA, 262
isoforms, 262
and PUFAs, 262–263
relationship of MUFA to, 264
Pesci reaction, 43
Petroleum diesel, 236
PG, see *n*-Propyl gallate (PG)
PHCO, *see* Partially hydrogenated canola oil (PHCO)
Phenolic acids
antioxidant activity of, 29
radical scavenging activity, 287
Phenolic antioxidants, 279
lipid oxidation inhibition, 279
from rapeseed, 22
Phenolic compound, 21; *see also* Antioxidants
in canola meal, 152
isolation of food-grade rapeseed, 152
as natural antioxidants, 281–282
naturally occurring, 22
properties, 281
quantification and characterization, 282–285
of rapeseed meal, 281–282
recovery, 152
SC-CO_2 extraction, 152
Phenolic compound antioxidative activity, 292
oxidation products, 294–296
effect of rapeseed meal extracts in purified rapeseed oil emulsion, 293–294
PHF, *see* Partially hydrogenated fats (PHF)
Phosphatidic acid phosphatase (PAP), 103, 105
Phosphatidyl choline (PC), 104
Phosphatidyl choline:diacylglycerol choline phosphotransferase (PDCT), 105
Phosphatidylinositol-3,4,5-triphosphate (PIP_3), 268
Phospholipid:diacylglycerol acyltransferase (PDAT), 105
Phospholipid recovery, 151
Phospholipids (PL), 179, 254
extraction, 151
nutraceutical-grade, 162
PHVO, *see* Partially hydrogenated vegetable oil (PHVO)
PIP_3, *see* Phosphatidylinositol-3,4,5-triphosphate (PIP_3)
PL, *see* Phospholipids (PL)
Plant proteins, 187
PLS, *see* Partial least squares regression (PLS)
PMM, *see* Protein micellar mass (PMM)
PO, *see* Palm olein (PO)
Polar compounds formation, 90, 91, 207
Polymorphic transition temperature, 226–227
Polyunsaturated fatty acid (PUFA), 13, 152, 245, 252; *see also* Omega-9 fatty acids; Very-long-chain polyunsaturated fatty acids (VLCPUFA)
ALA, 258
dietary n-6, 257
effect on IR, 264
formation of, 104
in inflammation and adipocyte function, 266
LA, 257, 258
and MUFA, 260
oxidation and off-flavour development, 205
PPAR and, 262–263
SREBP and, 263
triacylglycerols, 150
Polyvinylpyrrolidone (PVP), 74
Pour point (PP), 226
of omega-9 oils, 84
PP, *see* Pour point (PP)
PPARs, *see* Peroxisome proliferator-activated receptors (PPARs)
PPI, *see* Precipitated protein isolate (PPI)
Prairie Regional Laboratory (PRL), 3
Precipitated protein isolate (PPI), 63, 64
essential amino acid composition of, 73

Pressurized differential scanning calorimeter (PDSC), 229
PRL, *see* Prairie Regional Laboratory (PRL)
Pro-inflammatory cytokines, 266
Protein, 137
Protein dispersibility index (PDI), 192
Protein micellar mass (PMM), 75
Proteolytic enzymes, 67
Puccina graminis, 52
PUFA, *see* Polyunsaturated fatty acids (PUFA)
Pulse NMR, 127; *see also* Oil content measurement
    advantage, 128
    canola oil content analysis, 129
    free induction decay, 128
    oil content analysis, 135
PV, *see* Peroxide value (PV)
PVP, *see* Polyvinylpyrrolidone (PVP)
PY, *see* Pyrogallol (PY)
Pyrogallol (PY), 228
Pyruvate dehydrogenase kinase (PDHK), 113

Q

QTL, *see* Quantitative trait loci (QTL)
Quantitative insulin sensitivity check (QUICKI), 259
Quantitative trait loci (QTL), 112
QUICKI, *see* Quantitative insulin sensitivity check (QUICKI)

R

Rancimat test, 228–229, 323, 324
Rapeseed, 2, 22, 187, 278
    as antioxidant source, 278
    aqueous processing of, 67
    detoxified protein concentrate production, 69
    pH effect on nitrogen solubility of, 63, 64
    phenolics, 28, 152
    production, 60
    rancidity assessment, 6
    secondary plant substances, 190, 191
    storage proteins, 189–190
    4-vinylsyringol, 25
Rapeseed meal extract
    antioxidative activity of, 291–292
    fractionation, 282, 283
    free radical scavenging, 288–291
    HPLC chromatograms, 284
    phenolic constituents, 282, 283, 284, 285
    sinapic acid percent distribution, 284
Rapeseed oil
    factor affecting quality of virgin, 183
    phenolic compounds, 279, 281–282
    tocopherol levels in, 280
Rapeseed processing, value-added, 190, 202
    deoiling process, 190, 192–193
    protein fractionation process, 193–195
Rapeseed proteins, 188, 201
    commercially and fluidized-bed desolventized, 199
    extraction difficulty, 189
    meal desolventizing, 195
    ongoing projects, 199–201
    potential of, 188
    raw material for extraction, 195–199
    secondary plant substances, 190
    storage proteins, 189–190
    structure change and surface functionality, 189
    technical application possibilities, 188–189
    use of, 201
Rate-determining step (RDS), 232
    activation energy, 232, 235
    Arrhenius plot of, 235
RCO, *see* Regular canola (RCO)
RDA, *see* Recommended dietary allowance (RDA)
RDS, *see* Rate-determining step (RDS)
Reactive oxygen species (ROS), 32, 342
Recommended dietary allowance (RDA), 256
Regular canola (RCO), 13
Renewable fuel standard (RFS), 239
Renewable sources, 217
Response surface methodology (RSM), 158
Retinal pigment epithelial cells (RPE cells), 33
Reverse osmosis (RO), 72
Reversion, 308–309, *see* Peroxide value (PV)
RFM, *see* U.S. Renewable Fuel Mandate (RFM)
RFS, *see* Renewable fuel standard (RFS)
Rice bran oil, 159
RO, *see* Reverse osmosis (RO)
ROS, *see* Reactive oxygen species (ROS)
Roundup Ready®, 83
RPE cells, *see* Retinal pigment epithelial cells (RPE cells)
RSM, *see* Response surface methodology (RSM)

S

SA, *see* Sinapic acid (SA)
SAE, *see* Sinapic acid equivalent (SAE)
SAEs, *see* Sinapic acid esters (SAEs)
Saffron, 158
Saponification, 158–159, 219
Saturated fatty acids (SFA), 102
    in canola oil, 9, 139, 252
    CVD risk, 245
    dietary, 256
    in frying media, 204
    guidelines on, 97
    HOLL canola oil, 209
    MCFA, 108

SC-CO_2, *see* Supercritical CO_2 (SC-CO_2)
SDA, *see* Stearidonic acid (SDA)
SDS-PAGE, *see* Sodium dodecyl sulphate polyacrylamide gel electrophoresis (SDS-PAGE)
Secondary oxidation derivatives, 227
Secondary plant substances, 190
Sedimentation, 180
  purification by, 174
Seed oil
  composition modification, 106
  content modification, 112–115
  formation pathways, 102–106
Sensory attributes, 86
SFA, *see* Saturated fatty acids (SFA)
SFC, *see* Solid fat content (SFC)
SFI, *see* Solid fat index (SFI)
Shelf-life stability assessment, 16
SHMP, *see* Sodium hexa meta phosphate (SHMP)
Silver catalysts, 44
Sinapic acid (SA), 22, 23, 191, 281; *see also* Phenolic compound
  anticonvulsant effect of, 30
  as antioxidants, 22
  anxiolytic effect of, 30, 31–32
  canolol formation, 318
  comparison, 325
  DPPH radical scavenging, 290–291
  effect in purified rapeseed oil emulsion, 293–294
  on effect on broiler chickens, 30–31
  enzymatic reduction of, 26
  esterified forms of, 23
  fluidized-bed desolventizing, 198
  fractions of 70% methanolic extract, 283, 284
  free radical scavenging, 286–288
  heat effect on degradation of, 321
  to increase canolol, 54
  increase in, 55
  lignin and flavonoid production, 318
  neuroprotective effects of, 29
  as peroxyl radical scavenger, 27
  phenolic constituents of, 284
  precursor of canolol, 337
  propanal formation, 294, 295
  in rapeseed meal, 282
  SAE, 340, 341
  trans, 190
Sinapic acid equivalent (SAE), 283, 340
Sinapic acid esters (SAEs), 282
Sinapine, 22, 23, 34, 281; *see also* Phenolic compound
  analytical methods for, 26
  antioxidant activity of, 27–28
  as anti-radiation chemical, 30
  anxiolytic effects, 31–32
  on apoptotic rate, 30
  bioactivities of, 29
  on cell permeability, 29
  on digestibility and growth, 30–31
  distribution in Brassica, 23–24
  DPPH radical scavenging, 290
  fishy odours, 281
  on food intake in rats, 31
  as free radical scavenger, 30, 286
  inhibition of propanal, 293, 295
  neuroprotective effects, 29–30
  quantification and characterization of, 25
  sinapic acid equivalent, 283, 340
  source of, 24
Sinapoyl glucose (GP), 23, 284
  antioxidant activities, 286
  DPPH radicals scavenging, 290
  free radical scavenging, 286, 287
  heat effect on, 55
Sodium dodecyl sulphate polyacrylamide gel electrophoresis (SDS-PAGE), 194, 195
Sodium hexa meta phosphate (SHMP), 71
Solid fat content (SFC), 92
Solid fat index (SFI), 92
Soluble protein isolate (SPI), 63
  essential amino acid composition of, 73
  properties of, 64
Solvents, 44
Sonication, 145, 146, 158; *see also* Ultrasound
  extraction yield by, 158
  lipid extraction time, 156
  mechanical vibrations, 146
SOY, *see* Soyabean oil (SOY)
Soyabean oil (SOY), 87
  for biodiesel, 82
  Canadian, 87
  CLN content, 307, 308
  consumer preference, 96
  effect in French fries, 86
  HPLC analysis of, 305
  oxidative stability, 300
  resistance to oxidation, 304
  reversion, 308–309
  as shortenings, 92
Soyabeans
  composition, 60
  essential amino acid content of, 61
Soy protein products, 68
SPI, *see* Soluble protein isolate (SPI)
SREBPs, *see* Sterol regulatory element-binding proteins (SREBPs)
Stearidonic acid (SDA), 110
Sterol regulatory element-binding proteins (SREBPs), 261
  fatty acid regulator of, 263
  and PUFA, 263
  relationship of MUFA to, 264

Structural proteins, 62
Supercritical CO_2 (SC-CO_2), 146; *see also* Oil and bioactive component extraction
advantages of, 146, 149, 161
applications in oilseed processing, 160
biorefining model, 162
canola meal extraction, 151
chlorophyll concentration, 150
equipment design, 163
operating parameters, 148, 155, 158
phenolic compound recovery, 152
phospholipid recovery, 151
rice bran oil yield using, 159
solubility in, 147
tocopherol extraction, 159, 163
Supercritical state, 146

T

TAG, *see* Triacylglyceride (TAG); Triacylglycerol (TAG); Triglycerides (TAG)
TBHQ, *see* *Tert*-Butyl hydroquinone (TBHQ)
t-BuOOH, *see* *Tert*-Butyl hydroperoxide (*t*-BuOOH)
TC, *see* Total cholesterol (TC)
Tert-Butyl hydroperoxide (*t*-BuOOH), 32
Tert-Butyl hydroquinone (TBHQ), 228
TFs, *see* Transcription factors (TFs)
T/HDL-C ratio, *see* Total-to-HDL cholesterol ratio (T/HDL-C ratio)
TNF-α, *see* Tumour necrosis factor-α (TNF-α)
Tocopherol (Alpha-toco), 14, 211, 280, 287
canola fractionation, 155
degradation rates, 15
extraction, 159
in potato crisps, 212
quantification evaluation, 159
Total cholesterol (TC), 95, 245
Total polar compounds (TPC), 13, 14
Total polar material (TPM), 86
Total-to-HDL cholesterol ratio (T/HDL-C ratio), 248
Totox value, 210; *see also* Frying medium
in Berlin doughnuts, 212
in potato crisps, 211
TPC, *see* Total polar compounds (TPC)
TPM, *see* Total polar material (TPM)
Transcription factors (TFs), 113, 114, 261, 262, 268
Transesterification, 80, 217, 218
activation energy, 232, 235
alcohol used in, 218
biodiesel production, 229
catalysts used in, 219
ethanol polarity, 219
experimental and simulated FA concentrations, 233
intermediates, 227
kinetics of, 230
rate constants of, 234–235
stepwise, 218
Trans-fatty acid
and coronary heart diseases, 204
serum cholesterol, 247
source for, 204
Triacylglyceride (TAG), 217, 218; *see also* Fatty acid (FA)
Triacylglycerol (TAG), 102, 103, 254
Triglycerides (TAG), 125
in canola oil, 9
extraction, 152
Trolox, 280, 286
Tumour necrosis factor-α (TNF-α), 32, 255
Type 2 diabetes mellitus (DM2), 253

U

UF, *see* Ultrafiltration (UF)
Ultrafiltration (UF), 71, 72
batch, 72
Burcon's process, 75
canola protein isolation, 74
concentration of small molecules, 73
membrane, 72
Ultra Low Sat Omega-9 Sunflower Oil, 97
Ultrasonication, *see* Ultrasound
Ultrasound, 145–146, 155
applications in oilseed processing, 160
extraction, 157, 161
high-intensity, 160
United Nations Organization (UNO), 188
United States Department of Agriculture (USDA), 252
UNO, *see* United Nations Organization (UNO)
USDA, *see* United States Department of Agriculture (USDA)
U.S. Food and Drug Administration (FDA), 95, 204, 252
U.S. Renewable Fuel Mandate (RFM), 81

V

Vegetable oils, 147; *see also* Canola oil
anti-oxidant reagents, 228
biodiesel, 217
CLN in, 305, 306, 308
demand for, 59
fatty acid compositions of, 221, 306
omega-9 fatty acids, 80
oxidative deterioration, 296
oxidizability of, 304
phenolic compounds in, 318
waste, 239

Very long-chain marine n-3 PUFA (VLCMPUFA), 256
Very-long-chain polyunsaturated fatty acids (VLCPUFA), 102, 109
  pathways for, 110
  production of longer-chain, 111
Very-low-density lipoprotein (VLDL), 255
4-VG, *see* 4-Vinylguaiacol (4-VG)
Vinyl derivatives, 49
4-Vinylguaiacol (4-VG), 49, 50
Vinylphenols, 26; *see also* Canolol
  generation, 49, 50–51
4-Vinylsyringol (4-VS), 50; *see also* Canolol
Virgin canola oil processing, 171, 183–184; *see also* Canola oil, cold-pressed; Canola seed
  Canola standard, 175
  from dehulled seeds, 180
  DGF Canola Oil Award, 182–183
  filtration, 181
  influence of storage conditions, 176–178
  off-flavours, 172
  panel testing, 173
  pressing process, 171–172
  production difficulty, 174–175
  purification, 180–182
  sedimentation, 180
  seed material pre-treatment, 175–176
  sensory evaluation, 172–173
Virgin oil, 171
Vitalexx, 76; *see also* Canola protein
Vitamin E, 158
VLCMPUFA, *see* Very long-chain marine n-3 PUFA (VLCMPUFA)
VLCPUFA, *see* Very-long-chain polyunsaturated fatty acids (VLCPUFA)
VLDL, *see* Very-low-density lipoprotein (VLDL)
4-VS, *see* 4-Vinylsyringol (4-VS)

W

Waist circumference (WC), 253
Water-in-oil (W/O), 296
WC, *see* Waist circumference (WC)
WD, *see* Western diet (WD)
Western diet (WD), 95
WHO, *see* World Health Organization (WHO)
W/O, *see* Water-in-oil (W/O)
World Health Organization (WHO), 188

Z

ZDDP, *see* Zinc dialkyl-dithio phosphate (ZDDP)
Zinc dialkyl-dithio phosphate (ZDDP), 235